Palliative and Serious Illness Patient Management for Physician Assistants

Palliative and Serious Illness Patient Management for Physician Assistants

EDITED BY

Nadya Dimitrov, DPM, PA

Associate Clinical Professor and Assistant Director of PA

Post-Professional Masters Program

Department of Physician Assistant Education

Stony Brook University, NY, USA

AND

Kathy Kemle, MS, PA-C

Assistant Professor

Department of Family Medicine

Atrium Health Navicent, GA, USA

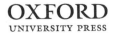

OXFORD
UNIVERSITY PRESS

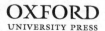

Oxford University Press is a department of the University of Oxford. It furthers
the University's objective of excellence in research, scholarship, and education
by publishing worldwide. Oxford is a registered trade mark of Oxford University
Press in the UK and certain other countries.

Published in the United States of America by Oxford University Press
198 Madison Avenue, New York, NY 10016, United States of America.

© Oxford University Press 2022

Library of Congress Cataloging-in-Publication Data
Names: Dimitrov, Nadya, editor. | Kemle, Kathy, editor.
Title: Palliative and serious illness patient management for physician assistants /
Nadya Dimitrov, Kathy Kemle.
Description: New York, NY : Oxford University Press, [2022] |
Includes bibliographical references and index.
Identifiers: LCCN 2021012196 (print) | LCCN 2021012197 (ebook) |
ISBN 9780190059996 (paperback) | ISBN 9780190060015 (epub) | ISBN 9780190060022
Subjects: MESH: Palliative Care | Physician Assistants
Classification: LCC R726.8 (print) | LCC R726.8 (ebook) |
NLM WB 310 | DDC 616.02/9—dc23
LC record available at https://lccn.loc.gov/2021012196
LC ebook record available at https://lccn.loc.gov/2021012197

DOI: 10.1093/med/9780190059996.001.0001

9 8 7 6 5 4 3 2 1

Printed by Marquis, Canada

This work is dedicated to all of our patients and their caregivers, our families who taught us the meaning of love and loss, as well as our mentors in palliative medicine and hospice care. We would also like to dedicate this book to all of our colleagues who found themselves treating the seriously ill patients in this country and abroad at a time when their fundamental training was suddenly challenged by events that taxed their communication skills and resilience. We sincerely hope that it will advance their compassionate care into this arena with new found confidence.

Contents

Section 5. Care Transitions Including End of Life

Section 6. Social, Cultural, and Legal Aspects of Care

Foreword

Palliative care is a relatively new and interdisciplinary medical and nursing specialty, achieving formal recognition in 2007. It is focused on relief of the pain, symptoms, and stresses of a serious illness in an effort to improve quality of life both for the patient and for those who care for the patient.[1] Eligibility for palliative care is based on need; hence, patients whose goal of care is cure (e.g., acute leukemia in a 20-year-old patient) or life prolongation (e.g., heart failure), or living as well as possible during a progressive disease (e.g., dementia) are all appropriate candidates for palliative care. The field grew in response to clinician observations of human suffering during treatment of a range of serious illnesses,[2] starting with cancer, but now inclusive of heart disease, neurodegenerative disorders, end-stage renal and liver failure, geriatric frailty, and multimorbidity and is applicable to patients of all ages and stages of illness.

Prior to the advent of the field of palliative care, the only model focused on relief of suffering in the United States was hospice. As a Medicare benefit, hospice eligibility is tightly constrained to include only patients with a prognosis of under 6 months (if the disease follows its usual course) who are willing to give up insurance coverage for "curative" or life-prolonging treatments in return for access to hospice. Because prognosis is highly variable and unpredictable, especially in noncancer diseases, hospice criteria privilege those patients who are very near death. The median length of stay in hospice in the United States is now about 18 days,[3] a time period so short that it misses most of the time a person is living with their serious illness. Because the majority of people living with a serious illness are chronically ill, and not predictably dying soon, and because most treatments that prolong life also improve its quality (e.g., diuretics for heart failure or dialysis for end-stage renal disease), the

1. https://getpalliativecare.org/whatis/
2. https://getpalliativecare.org/whatis/disease-types/
3. https://www.nhpco.org/hospice-facts-figures/

need for an open access model of palliative care was obvious. Hospice eligibility is based on prognosis. Palliative care eligibility is based on need.

In the last decade, palliative care teams have spread to more than 90% of large (>200-bed) US hospitals[4] and are also beginning to find a foothold in community-based settings,[5] including long-term care facilities, outpatient practices (e.g., cancer centers), and people's own homes. The main barrier to the spread and scale of palliative care to these settings, where the great majority of people with serious illness are living, is workforce.[6] Across the nation, palliative care programs are searching for clinical staff with training and expertise in the relief of suffering among people with serious illness. Physician assistants are essential to meet this challenge. This textbook is foundational to ensure the knowledge and skills necessary for physician assistants to deliver quality palliative care to the most medically complex and seriously ill people in our society.

Diane E. Meier, MD
Director Emerita and Strategic Advisor, Center to Advance Palliative Care
Professor, Department of Geriatrics and Palliative Medicine
Catherine Gaisman Professor of Medical Ethics
Icahn School of Medicine at Mount Sinai
New York, NY

May 4, 2021

---

4. https://reportcard.capc.org/

5. https://www.capc.org/mapping-community-palliative-care/

6. https://www.capc.org/blog/a-roadmap-for-workforce-training-to-meet-the-needs-of-patients-with-serious-illness/?clickthrough_doc_id=blog.blogpostpage.2235&clickthrough_req_id=rDAHulSVQbqfqliEzOwRWQ&clickthrough_query=workforce

Preface

This is the first edition of a comprehensive text for physician assistants/associates (PAs) in Palliative Care Medicine and Serious Illness Management. At its inception 50 years ago, the PA profession sought to define and establish its niche in health care. Both assistant and associate degree certificates were awarded during the first few years. But, over time PAs have proven their value to the public and other health care team members. At the 2021 AAPA House of Delegates meeting, the name was officially changed to physician associate. This was accomplished in order to better reflect the manner in which PAs collaborate with their physician colleagues in a patient centered approach to healthcare, and moreover to fully align with our peers in the international community. PAs are now well represented in all specialties, healthcare arenas and aspects of care, including that of the chronically and terminally ill. While there is a dramatic increase in frail patient populations, the current crisis in healthcare has accelerated and further focused attention on its global workforce shortage.

As compassionate listeners with an altruistic calling, PAs are trained in a medical model with fundamental patient-centered care that includes social and cultural competencies. There are many textbooks in Palliative Medicine. However, there has not yet been one written from the perspective of physician assistants. This textbook speaks to all PAs who treat patients with serious illness. It includes specific areas that have expanded in the PA profession as well as in the delivery of care. Specifically, it addresses integrative medical modalities for the management of pain and other symptoms, and a discussion of essential best practices in the telehealth/telemedicine arenas. It will serve as a resource for clinicians, educators, and researchers alike.

This textbook represents an essential step in fulfilling the need for all practitioners to understand how PAs function in this specialty and in the broader context of worldwide health care. Finally, it will empower all PAs to assume a leadership role in their management of serious illness patients on their respective palliative interdisciplinary teams.

Acknowledgments

We would like to thank all of our esteemed colleagues who have graciously contributed their time to serve as our chapter contributors. Their dedication in sharing their passion and expertise in palliative care of the seriously ill comes at a time when their own clinical expertise has been further exemplified in multiple healthcare arenas. We also would like to recognize our editorial team, Marta Moldvai and Tiffany Lu, who guided us through the editing and production of this text. Our family and friends who regard this initiative as not only a work of love but a demonstration of our own passion for the specialty are thanked for their patience and endless support.

Contributors

Richard Ackermann, MD
Hospice/Palliative Medicine Fellowship
    Director
The Medical Center, Navicent Health
Macon, GA, USA

Ebtesam Ahmed, PharmD
Clinical Professor
Clinical Health Professions
St. John's University College of Pharmacy
    and Health Sciences
Queens, NY, USA

Tonda Anderson, PA-C, MCHS, CCRN
Inpatient Palliative Care
Virginia Mason Hospital
Seattle, WA, USA

Ruth Ballweg, MPA, PA-C Emeritus
Department of Family Medicine
School of Medicine
University of Washington
MEDEX Northwest PA Program
Department of Family Medicine
School of Medicine
University of Washington
Seattle, WA, USA

Nicole Bates, MD
Acting Assistant Professor
Department of Psychiatry and Behavioral
    Sciences
University of Washington and Seattle Cancer
    Care Alliance
Seattle, WA, USA

Vanessa Battista, RN, MS, CPNP-PC
Pediatric Nurse Practitioner
Department of Neurology
Children's Hospital of Philadelphia
Philadelphia, Hazlet, USA

**Jamie Beachy, PhD MDiv, Certified ACPE
Educator**
Assistant Professor
Wisdom Traditions
Naropa University
Boulder, CO, USA

Joshua Briscoe, MD
Palliative Care Physician
Geriatric Research Education and Clinical
    Center (GRECC)
Durham VA Health Care System
Durham, NC, USA

Diane Bruessow, PA-C, MPAS, DFAAPA
Instructor
Physician Assistant Online Program
Yale School of Medicine
New Haven, CT
Healthy Transitions
Montclair, NJ, USA

Bonnie K. Cole-Gifford, JD, LMFT
Director, Behavioral Science
Department of Family Medicine
Navicent Health
Macon, GA, USA

Kimberly Angelia Curseen, MD, FAAHPM
Associate Professor
Department Family and Preventative
    Medicine
Emory School of Medicine
Atlanta, GA, USA

Lara Desanti-Siska, MD
Program Director
Hospice and Palliative Medicine Fellowship
Graduate Medical Education
Stony Brook Southampton Hospital
Southampton, NY, USA

Mark Deutchman, MD
Professor of Family Medicine and Dental
    Medicine and Public Health and Associate
    Dean for Rural Health
Department of Family Medicine
University of Colorado Health
    Sciences Center
Aurora, CO, USA

Nadya Dimitrov, DPM, PA
Associate Clinical Professor and Assistant
    Director of PA Post-Professional Masters
    Program
Department of Physician Assistant
    Education
Stony Brook University
Stony Brook, NY, USA

Shawn Fellows, PharmD
Associate Professor of Pharmacy Practice
Wegmans School of Pharmacy
St. John Fisher College
Rochester, NY, USA

**Betty Ferrell, RN, PhD, MA, FAAN,
FPCN, CHPN**
Professor and Director
Division of Nursing Research and Education
City of Hope National Medical Center
Duarte, CA, USA

Michael Fratkin, MD, FAAHPM, NAP
Founder and Medical Director
ResolutionCare Network
Eureka, CA, USA

Stefan J. Friedrichsdorf, MD
Professor in Pediatrics
Medical Director
Benioff Children's Hospitals Center of
    Pediatric Pain
Palliative and Integrative Medicine
University of California at San Francisco
San Francisco, CA, USA

**Myra Glajchen, DSW, MSW, BSW, ACSW,
APHSW-C**
Director of Education and Training
MJHS Institute for Innovation in
    Palliative Care
MJHS Hospice and Palliative Care
New York, NY, USA

Timothy Harrison, MArch
Associate Director for CBCT(r)
Center for Contemplative Science and
    Compassion-Based Ethics
Emory University
Atlanta, GA, USA

Jeremy Hirst, MD
Clinical Professor
Psychiatry
UC San Diego
San Diego, CA, USA

Scott A. Irwin, MD, PhD
Director Patient and Family Support
    Program and Professor of Psychiatry and
    Behavioral Neurosciences
Cedars-Sinai Cancer and the Department of
    Psychiatry and Behavioral Neurosciences
Cedars-Sinai Health System
Los Angeles, CA, USA

Catherine R. Judd, MS, PA-C, CAQ
Psychiatry
Clinical Assistant Professor
School of Health Professions
Department of PA Studies
University of Texas Southwestern
    Medical Center
Dallas, TX, USA

Kathy Kemle, MS, PA-C
Assistant Professor
Department of Family Medicine
Atrium Health Navicent
Macon, Georgia, USA

Farah Khalid, MPaed, MBBS
Consultant Pediatrician
Department of Pediatrics
University of Malaya
Kuala Lumpur, Malaysia

Min Ji Kim, MD
Physician
Supportive & Palliative Care
Baylor University Medical Center
Dallas, TX, USA

Calvin Krom, DO
Fellow in Hospice and Palliative Medicine
MJHS Hospice and Palliative Care
Brooklyn, NY, USA

Mary Ellen Lasala, PhD, RN
Chair
Undergraduate Program and Associate
    Professor
Nursing, Hofstra University
Hempstead, NY, USA

Britni Lookabaugh, MD
Physician
Hospice and Palliative Medicine
Ohio Health
Columbus, OH, USA

Jeffrey D. Myers, PA-C, MMSc, MIH
Assistant Professor
Palliative Care
Division of Hematology & Oncology
Knight Cancer Institute
Oregon Health & Science University
Portland, OR, USA

Noelle Noah, PA-C, MSHS
Trauma Services, Children's Minnesota
Masters of Physician Assistant studies
Physician Assistant—Pediatric Trauma
Minneapolis, MN, USA

Dipenkumar Patel, MD
Primary Care Physician
Family Medicine
Geriatrics
Macon, GA, USA

Holly Pilewski, MS, PA-C
Veterans Affairs
Asheville, NC, USA

Nicholas Polito, PharmD
Clinical Pharmacist
Department of Pharmacy
Highland Hospital of Rochester
Rochester, NY, USA

Marguerite R. Poreda, MD
Assistant Professor of Psychiatry and
    Behavioral Medicine
Department of Psychiatry and Behavioral
    Medicine
University of South Florida College of
    Medicine
Naples, FL, USA

Russell K. Portenoy, MD
Professor
Department of Neurology and Family and
    Social Medicine
Albert Einstein College of Medicine
New York, NY, USA

Michael L. Powe, BS
Vice President
Reimbursement & Professional Advocacy
American Academy of PAs
Adjunct Assistant Professor
Department of Physician Assistant Studies
George Washington University
Alexandria, VA, USA

**Christina M. Puchalski, MD, MS, OCDS,
FAAHPM, FACP**
Professor of Medicine and Health Sciences
Executive Director
The George Washington University's
    Institute for Spirituality and Health,
    Medicine
George Washington University
Washington, VA, USA

Denise Rizzolo, PhD, PA-C
Field Coordinator and Lecturer
Master of Public Health
Fairleigh Dickinson University
Florham Park, NJ, USA

Chase Samsel, MD
Attending Adult and Child Psychiatrist and
    Pediatrician
Department of Psychiatry and Behavioral
    Sciences
Boston Children's Hospital
Boston, MA, USA

Maureen J. Shelton, MDiv
Director of Education
Spiritual Health at Emory Healthcare
Emory University
Atlanta, GA, USA

Denis Snow, JD, RN
Clinical Associate Professor
School of Nursing
Stony Brook University
Stony Brook, NY, USA

Karl Steinberg, MD, HMDC, CMD
Chief Medical Officer
Mariner Health Care Central
Staten Island, NY, USA

**Harry S. Strothers III, MD, MMM,
CAQ-G, FAAFP**
Chairman and Professor
Department of Family Medicine
Mercer University School of Medicine
Macon, GA, USA

Jabeen Taj, MD
Site Director
Hospice and Palliative Medicine
Emory University Hospital
Medical Director
Cardiac Palliative Care
Assistant Professor, Medicine
Division of Palliative Medicine
Family and Preventive Medicine Emory
    School of Medicine
Atlanta, GA, USA

Kimberson Tanco, MD
Associate Professor
Palliative, Rehabilitation and Integrative
  Medicine
University of Texas MD Anderson
  Cancer Center
Houston, TX, USA

Manuel Trachsel, MD, PhD
Head of the Clinical Ethics Unit Basel; and
  Senior Research and Teaching Associate
Institute of Biomedical Ethics and History of
  Medicine
University of Zurich
Winterthurerstrasse, Switzerland

Charles von Gunten, MD, PhD
Vice President
Medical Affairs, Hospice & Palliative Care,
  OhioHealth
Columbus, OH, USA

Christine Wilkins, PhD, LCSW
Advance Care Planning Program Manager
Department of Nursing/Department of
  Social Work
NYU Langone Health
New York, NY, USA

Kathlyn F. Wohlrabe, LMFT
Behavioral Science
Department of Family Medicine
Navicent Health
Macon, GA, USA

Hunter Woodall, MD
Physician, Family Medicine Center
AnMed Health
Professor of Family Medicine
Medical University of South Carolina
Charleston, SC, USA

Essential Aspects of Serious Illness Patient Care

Structure and Processes

The Physician Assistant's Role in Palliative Care Medicine

Ruth Ballweg, Tonda Anderson, and Michael L. Powe

Introducing Palliative Care

From its beginning with Dr. Eugene Stead at Duke University in North Carolina, the mission of the physician assistant (PA) profession has been to create, increase, or expand health-care access in areas and populations with the greatest need.[1] Dr. Henry Silver's Child Health Associate Program at the University of Colorado is a good example, as is Dr. Hu Myer's Alderson Broaddus Program, which serves isolated rural communities in West Virginia.[2] Dr. Richard Smith's MEDEX (Medical Extender) Program at the University of Washington was also designed specifically to serve rural and medically underserved communities of the Pacific Northwest.[3]

Physician Assistants were among the first clinicians to staff public health and medical clinics serving HIV/AIDS patients and continue to be the permanent and ongoing providers in these clinical settings.[4] In 2016, PAs were part of the US Public Health Service response to Ebola in Liberia, providing care specifically for health professionals (including Liberian PAs) who were felled by the virus.[5,6] Volunteer PAs from the United States have been clinical first responders to major disasters, such as the hurricanes in Indonesia, Thailand, and Haiti.[7] In the current environment, the public health mission of the profession has been part of the redefinition in healthcare delivery for vulnerable and underserved populations. According to a PA workforce survey conducted early in the pandemic, between 40% and 52% of PAs have diagnosed and/or treated COVID-19 patients (AAPA [American Academy of Physician Assistants] PA Pulse Survey, May 19, 2020).

Fifteen years ago, healthcare leaders in the Netherlands recognized the need for the role of PAs and Nurse Practitioner in "keeping people healthy" when it became apparent that

Dutch citizens were living 10 years longer than had previously been estimated. There were insufficient numbers of doctors to provide care to this growing segment of the population. PA and NP programs were created in the country's five academic health centers as a strategy for the overall expansion of the healthcare system.[8]

In South Africa, the Ministry of Health recognized that physicians—already in short supply—could not meet the treatment and continuity needs of its regional rural hospitals.[9] The role of clinical associate was created in 2013, and three PA programs were established in Johannesburg, Pretoria, and the Eastern Cape. Additional programs are currently under development.

The provision of appropriate and cost-effective care to individuals with serious and chronic illness is today's emerging strategic priority in every country in the world. This philosophy of care is called palliative care/medicine; as such, it is yet another arena in which PAs and other non-physician healthcare providers are essential to address the yawning abyss in access to healthcare resources for which doctors are only part of the solution. In 2002 the World Health Organization (WHO) was one of the first proponents of palliative care, believing that systems of palliative care were appropriate in every country in the world. WHO saw palliative care as a public health strategy that could be integrated into existing healthcare systems and meet the needs of patients and their families.

The World Health Organization's Definition of Palliative Care, 2002

Palliative care is an approach that improves the quality of life of patients and their families facing the problems associated with life-threatening illness, through the prevention and relief of suffering by means of early identification and impeccable assessment and treatment of pain, and other problems, physical, psychosocial and spiritual.

Palliative Care

- Provides relief from pain and other distressing symptoms.
- Affirms life and regards dying as a normal process.
- Intends neither to hasten or postpone death.
- Integrates the psychological and spiritual aspects of patient care.
- Offers a support system to help the family cope during the patient's illness and in their own bereavement.
- Uses a team approach to address the needs of patients and their families including bereavement counseling if indicated.
- Will enhance quality of life, and may also positively influence the course of illness.
- Is applicable early in the course of illness in conjunction with other therapies that are intended to prolong life, such as chemotherapy or radiation therapy and include those investigations intended to better understand and manage distressing clinical complications.

Over time, the World Health Organization[10] has regularly modified its statement to align with the changes in healthcare systems and advancing technologies. The next section of this chapter applies the WHO guidelines to contemporary practice and describes US recommendations and projected policies.

Palliative care services have arisen not only because people are living longer but also because chronic illnesses and complex high-intensity illnesses such as cancer are now seen as "survivable"—rather than being quickly labels as "terminal." Healthcare systems intended to provide intensive and relatively short-term medical and surgical care for immediately terminal diseases are not designed to provide care specifically to assist patients in

adapting to their conditions. Palliative care changes the focus of healthcare to relieve symptoms and coordinate comprehensive care based on the patient's view of their prognosis and their life goals. This came about as part of the evolution in the treatment of HIV and survivable cancer care (survivorship medicine).[11]

Though somewhat less dramatic than HIV/AIDS, Ebola, and disaster care interventions, it is practical and realistic that PAs and NPs will provide the continuity and quality in relatively new palliative care infrastructures as they develop and grow throughout the United States.[12] While palliative and hospice care "services" have had somewhat parallel growth patterns in the United States, it important to note that palliative care and hospice care have different goals. Similarly, the Medicare reimbursement structure is different for the two types of care, with palliative care referring more to long-term care for chronic illnesses, while hospice care is directed at "end-of-life" care. Further in this chapter, Michael L. Powe, vice president of reimbursement and professional advocacy for the AAPA, provides a detailed discussion of reimbursement issues for palliative and hospice care.

Physician assistant programs have offered didactic content on palliative care and end-of-life care as part of their curriculum based on the accreditation and educational standards for the profession administered by accreditation review commission on education for the physician assistant (ARC-PA) beginning in 2010. Although the didactic component has been present, the challenge remained to find clinical sites and preceptors that are able to accommodate PA students. As of 2020, there are still few opportunities for PA program clinical rotations or postgraduate palliative care fellowships for PAs. As with physician providers, innovative ways to address workforce training are necessary to lead to optimal utilization in the full development of palliative care services.[13,14]

PAs as Palliative Medicine Champions

The demand for specialty trained palliative medicine practitioners continues to grow, with opportunities abounding for PAs to take on broad roles and responsibilities in palliative medicine. In addition to serving as independent providers and change agents on the interdisciplinary team, the PA may be the seasoned palliative care expert, educating medical residents, palliative medicine fellows, and team members alike, thus saliently demonstrating the keen skills of the PA.

At the same time, the palliative medicine PA must also take on the common burden of allaying misnomers about the role of palliative care in the healthcare continuum not only to patients and families, but also all healthcare providers, including specialists, residents, nurses, physicians, ancillary service teams, and administration. For example, palliative care is too often categorically and simplistically labeled as hospice care. WHO's definition of palliative care provides a springboard for the comprehensive nature of the palliative medicine clinician. Summarizing WHO's definition, the goal of palliative care excludes a preconceived agenda and provides the best possible care for patients, which reflects and empowers an individual's personal goals and values.[15]

The key for PA expansion into the realm of palliative care/medicine goes far beyond the clinic or bedside to include innovative fellowships in palliative care, as well as the development of medical educator roles to promote training and expertise in communication and complex symptom management. The teaching team ideally includes chaplains, social workers, PAs, NPs, and physicians. Palliative medicine fellowships for advanced practice providers are still scarce.[16]

Communication in palliative care debunks the fundamental power differential that often exists between learner and expert to that of collegiality, which ensures that each patient encounter encompasses high-quality communication. This is illustrated in teaching hospitals: PAs and other medical learners are in direct observation of each other, and this highlights the expertise of PAs in palliative medicine. The learners are in direct observation of the PA, and they receive real-time feedback in the post–patient experience that involves documentation of the encounter. This provides data regarding what the learner did well, what they might do differently, tips on nonverbal communication cues, as well as any feedback the learner might have for their preceptor. Furthermore, the customary group meetings that are an integral part of a palliative medicine team can serve as a venue for this interprofessional discussion.

A unique feature of palliative care involves eliciting a patient and family's values and concerns about the course of an illness (prognostication), which is a major component of palliative care training. Research on prognostication skills shows that medical providers who have developed close relationships with their patients and families often overestimate prognosis. Furthermore, many clinicians do not offer prognostics at all, even though literature shows patients desire this information. Serious illness conversations focused on prognostication may not be broached for a multitude of reasons: Generalists may have discomfort regarding initiating these conversations; they are often unaware of specific prognostication tools; and they may not know how to respond when the patient reacts emotionally. With expert communication skills, palliative care PAs fill the gap and navigate these conversations at a pace in tune with the patient's preferred communication style.

An essential role of the PA as a palliative medicine champion is to ensure that goal-concordant care is adhered to for the full course of the illness. Through their training in narrative medicine, PAs and NPs glean the patient's story; their priorities; what's important to them or gives life meaning, hopes, and worries; acceptable quality of life; previous experience with serious illness; and sources of strength, including the role of spirituality and/or religion. The patient is the "expert" on themselves, and the clinician is the liaison between their personhood and appropriate treatment recommendations. Palliative medicine PAs serve as role models not only in expert communication, but also perhaps most importantly by shifting the future of healthcare through aligning values-based care across the continuum.

Palliative medicine PAs should have knowledge and expertise in the eight domains of palliative care as outlined by the National Consensus Project (NCP) in their 2018 publication

Clinical Practice Guidelines for Quality Palliative Care (4th edition).[17] This description of palliative care is especially helpful:

> Palliative care is
> - Appropriate at any stage in a serious illness, and it is beneficial when provided along with treatments of curative or life-prolonging intent.
> - Provided over time to patients based on their needs and not their prognosis.
> - Offered in all care settings and by various organizations, such as physician practices, health systems, cancer centers, dialysis units, home health agencies, hospices, and long-term care providers.
> - Focused on what is most important to the patient, family and caregiver(s), assessing their goals and preferences and determining how best to achieve them.
> - Interdisciplinary to attend to the holistic care needs of the patient and their identified family and caregivers.

The eight domains that provide the structure for their report are as follows:

1. Structure and processes of care
2. Physical aspects of care
3. Psychological and psychiatric aspects of care
4. Social aspects of care
5. Spiritual, religious, and existential aspects of care
6. Cultural aspects of care
7. Care of the patient nearing the end of life
8. Ethical and legal aspects of care

The 165-page document is available online (free of charge) (https://www.nationalcoalitionhpc.org/ncp).[18] It is a valuable resource for anyone—and any agency—working with and supporting palliative care patients. For ongoing updates and skills in palliative care, PAs and PA students are encouraged to join Physician Assistants in Hospice and Palliative Medicine,[19] a nonprofit specialty organization affiliated with the American Academy of Physician Assistants. Members practice in clinical, research, and education settings.

Other resources include modules from the Center to Advance Palliative Care modules,[20] in which continuing medical education credits are also awarded, as well as joining the American Academy of Hospice and Palliative Medicine[21] as an affiliate, which gives equal access to clinicians for online tests and training modules.

Regulatory and Reimbursement Overview

From a clinical perspective, palliative care and hospice care are terms and care concepts often used interchangeably. In fact, both palliative and hospice care utilize many of the same medical and support services. However, from a Medicare regulatory and reimbursement standpoint, there are distinctions.[22] Palliative care is specialized medical care designed to help provide relief to both patients and the patient's family from the symptoms and side effects of serious disease or illnesses.[23] Those palliative services, which can include pain management, stress reduction, care coordination between members of the medical team, and mental/emotional support, are the types of services that may be covered by Medicare Part B and commercial insurers in a manner consistent with coverage for other medically necessary medical services delivered in hospitals, skilled nursing or rehabilitation facilities, the patient's home, or other settings. Generally, PAs are covered when delivering palliative care to Medicare beneficiaries.

Medicare's hospice benefit, in which the patient receives many of the same palliative care services, is a specialized Medicare program of care and support for people who are terminally ill with a life expectancy of 6 months or less.[24] Patients must qualify for Medicare Part A coverage in order to select the hospice benefit.

Patients receiving palliative care may or may not transition to hospice care. The more immediate focus of palliative care is on managing illness and creating an improved quality of life for patients and caregivers. As the need for palliative care increases, it is essential for the Medicare program and commercial insurers to become more attuned to the needs of this patient population from programmatic, benefit, and reimbursement perspectives. Presently, Medicare will pay on a fee-for-services (FFS) basis for services related to the provision of medically necessary palliative care services. However, generally there is no unique benefit coverage for comprehensive, interdisciplinary palliative care management under Medicare FFS. Medicare does reimburse for chronic care management services, which includes at least 20 minutes of non–face-to-face clinical staff time directed by a PA, physician, or other qualified healthcare professional for services such as answering patient's questions, refilling medications, reviewing laboratory results, coordinating referrals, and helping manage their care.

The Centers for Medicare and Medicaid Services (CMS), the agency with oversight responsibility for the Medicare and Medicaid programs, is best suited to lead the effort toward more comprehensive reimbursement and coverage policies for palliative care as a high percentage of Medicare patients need palliative care services. The Centers for Medicare and Medicaid Innovation, a government agency under the auspices of CMS, is testing, through a demonstration project, palliative care treatment and payment models that seek to reduce costs while maintaining or improving care quality and patient satisfaction in the delivery of palliative care services.[25] The data from these types of demonstration projects can then be shared with other stakeholders, health professionals, and organizations nationwide. As palliative services become more widely available and better understood, and coverage of these services increases, there will likely be a reduction in more expensive acute interventions and procedures resulting in cost savings to the health care system.

Palliative care can be provided in concert with curative treatment. However, curative care is generally not allowed when a patient has elected Medicare's hospice benefit. When patients elect the Medicare hospice benefit, they must agree to accept palliative versus curative care and waive all other Medicare benefits related to their terminal diagnosis. Under a new, very limited, pilot program, terminally ill patients will not have to give up curative treatment in order to receive Medicare-covered hospice care. The Medicare Care Choices Model, has been extended for further review through December 31, 2021, sought to determine if more patients would select hospice care and whether the quality of patient's lives would be improved by allowing the continuation of curative care after a patient elects the hospice benefit.[26]

Medicare FFS, also known as Original Medicare, will cover and pay for most of the services needed for care related to the terminal illness, but care must be provided by a Medicare-approved hospice provider. Patients may have to pay a copay for prescription drugs or a percentage of inpatient respite care, if needed. If a patient is covered by a Medicare Advantage (MA) plan and needs hospice care, they can elect Medicare's hospice benefit covered under Original Medicare and remain in the MA plan if you continue to pay your MA premiums. If you choose to leave hospice care, your Medicare Advantage Plan won't start again until the first of the following month.

Hospice care is usually provided in the patient's home, but it may also be covered in a hospice facility. Depending on the patient's terminal illness, the plan of care developed by the hospice team can include the following services:

- Medical services delivered by PAs, physicians and advanced practice registered nurses (APRNs)
- Nursing care
- Durable medical equipment (e.g., wheelchairs, walkers, oxygen)
- Medical supplies (i.e., bandages and catheters)
- Prescription drugs for symptom control and pain relief
- Physical and occupational therapy
- Speech-language services
- Social worker services
- Nutritional counseling
- Grief and loss counseling for the patient and family
- Short-term inpatient care (for pain and symptom management)
- Short-term respite care

Only the medical director of the hospice or the physician member of the hospice interdisciplinary group and the patient's physician (if the patient has one) can certify or recertify terminal illness. However, at the time a patient selects the hospice benefit, they are able to designate a health professional to serve as their "attending physician." PAs, physicians, and APRNs are the three types of health professionals authorized to serve in that attending physician role.

The hospice attending physician plays an essential role in the ongoing care of the patient and works closely with the hospice interdisciplinary team in developing and maintaining the patient's plan of care related to the terminal illness and routinely assessing the patient's status. The attending physician, who is not an employee of the hospice, can bill Medicare for their services.

Hospice organizations must have an Interdisciplinary Group (IDG) that is responsible for the overall well-being of the hospice beneficiary. The IDG works with the attending physician to develop and manage the plan of care and order medications as necessary. The IDG takes on a larger role when a hospice beneficiary has not designated an attending physician to manage their care. At a minimum, the IDG must include the following hospice employees who are qualified to practice in the following professional roles:

- Doctor of medicine or osteopathy
- Registered nurse
- Social worker
- Pastoral or other counselor

Although not required by regulation, PAs can be part of the IDG. While PAs have attained attending physician status for the Medicare hospice benefit, certain regulatory challenges remain that limit full PA utilization and reduce patient access to necessary hospice services. At the time of this printing, these restrictions prohibit PAs from

- Performing the required face-to-face patient visit prior to recertification after a patient has been under the hospice benefit for 180 days, and
- Initiating orders if they are employed by the hospice.

Hospice care is authorized in benefit periods. Hospice care is provided for two 90-day benefit periods, followed by an unlimited number of 60-day benefit periods, thereafter. Patients who live longer than 6 months can continue to receive hospice care if the hospice medical director or other hospice physician recertifies terminal illness. Presently, PAs and APRNs are not authorized to certify or recertify terminal illness.

Patients have the right to discontinue hospice care at any time. Improvements in their health status or illness progression can be reasons to stop hospice care. Discontinuing hospice will not prevent a patient from selecting hospice again at a later time if their health status worsens and they again meet the guidelines of having a terminal illness and an expected life span of 6 months or less.

The above regulatory and reimbursement information primarily reflects Medicare policy. Individual states may also have rules and regulations affecting the delivery of hospice care. In addition, commercial insurers may have coverage policies that differ from Medicare.

Looking Ahead

As compared to single national Medicare policies, there are a wide range of regulations covering palliative care across states. In some states, the regulation is through laws governing health facilities, civil rights, health professions, and hospice regulations. Many states' regulatory structures are silent on this topic. The best and most current information is to be found on the website for the National Academy for State Health Policy.[27]

As we move forward, health policy advisors see significant positive changes and additions to palliative care delivery. Some of these will be the result of technology (e.g., using telemedicine processes for diagnosis, care management, and data collection).

With insurance and healthcare delivery systems, there is increasing awareness that a major feature of a strong and effective palliative care system is a decrease in hospitalizations—and especially the decrease in emergency room visits and intensive care unit hospitalizations, where care is often the most costly in the entire health-care system.

Several US healthcare systems have already begun to expand their palliative care service beyond traditional hospital care to include coordination of care through system-based home health-care providers and "house calls" by PAs, NPs, and physical and occupational therapists.[28–32] While this coordinated palliative care approach may be utilized, it still features a patient's primary care provider as the key and consistent figure in their care.

References

1. Silver H, McAtee P. On the use of non-physician associate residents in overcrowded specialty-training programs. *New England Journal of Medicine*. 1984;*311*:326–328.
2. Myers H. The physician's assistant in the community hospital and in office practice. *Annals of the New York Academy of Sciences*. 1969;*166*(3):911–915.
3. American Academy of Physician Assistants (AAPA). MEDEX founder Richard A. Smith, MD on the PA concept's path. https:///www.aapa.org/about/history/medex-founder-richard-smith-and-pa-concepts-path/
4. Improving Patient Care. Quality of HIV care provided by nurse practitioners, physician assistants and physicians. *Annals of Internal Medicine* 2005, November 15. https://annals.org/aim/fullerarticle/718840/quality-hiv-care-provided-nurse-practitioners-physicanassistants--physicians
5. Wong K, Perdue C, Malia J, et al. Supportive care of the first 2 Ebola virus disease patients at the Monrovia Medical Unit. *Clinical Infections Diseases*. 2015;*16*(7):47–61.
6. Oliphant J. "Present": Ebola's impact on PAs in Liberia. *Clinician Reviews*. 2015;*25*(9):41–42.
7. PA Foundation. Donor profile: Don and Kathy Pedersen. 2020. https://pa-foundation.org/peedersen-profile/
8. Driesschen Q, Roo, F. Physician assistants in the Netherlands. *Journal of the American Academy of Physician Assistants*. 2014;*17*(9):10–11.
9. Couper, I. Physician assistants in South Africa. *Journal of the American Academy of Physician Assistants*. 2014;*27*(6).9–10.
10. Sepulveda C, Marlin A, Yoshida T, Ullrich, A. Palliative care: the World Health Organization's global perspective. *Journal of Pain and Symptom Management*. 2002;*24*(2):91–95.
11. Dzingina M. Public health and palliative care in 2015. *Clinics in Geriatric Medicine*. 2015;*31*:253–263.
12. Morton-Rias D. Certified PA-Cs integral to expansion of palliative medicine. *Provider Magazine*. 2019:*September*:1–3.
13. Accreditation Review Commission on Education for the Physician Assistant Inc. Accreditation standards for physician assistant education, fourth edition. First published March 2010, Effective September 1, 2010. http://www.arc-pa.org
14. Prazak K, Lester P, Fazzari M. Evaluation of physician assistant student knowledge and perception of competence in palliative symptom management. *Journal of Allied Health*. 2014;*43*(4):69–74.
15. World Health Organization. Palliative care, key facts. February 2018. https://www.euro.who.int/__data/assets/pdf_file/0003/98418/E82931.pdf
16. Mason V. Palliative care program. 2020. http://www.virginiamasonfoundation.org/palliative-care
17. Hallenbeck, J. Palliative care training for the generalist a luxury or a necessity? *Journal of General Internal Medicine*. 2006;*2*(9):1005–1006.
18. UW Professional and Continuing Education. Certificate in palliative care. January 2020. https://www.pce.uw.edu/certificates/palliative-care

19. Boucher NA, Nix H. The benefits of expanded physician assistant practice in hospice and palliative medicine. *Journal of the American Academy of Physician Assistants.* 2016;29(9):38–43.

20. National Consensus Project for Quality Palliative Care. *Clinical Practice Guidelines for Quality Palliative Care.* 4th ed. Richmond, VA: National Coalition for Hospice and Palliative Care; 2018. https://www.nationalcoalitionhpc.org/ncp

21. Physician Assistants in Hospice and Palliative Medicine (PAHPM). Home page. https://www.pahpm.org. Accessed January 15, 2020.

22. Center to Advance Palliative Care (CAPC). Welcome to the Center to Advance Palliative Care. https://www.capc.org. Accessed January 15, 2020.

23. American Academy of Hospice and Palliative Medicine (AAHPM). Expand your knowledge. Enhance your practice. http://aahpm.org/education/overview. Accessed January 15, 2020.

24. Centers for Medicare and Medicaid Services. Palliative care versus hospice care. https://www.cms.gov/Medicare-Medicaid-Coordination/Fraud-Prevention/Medicaid-Integrity-Education/Downloads/infograph-PalliativeCare-[June-2015].pdf

25. MedlinePlus. What is palliative care? https://medlineplus.gov/ency/patientinstructions/000536.htm

26. Centers for Medicare and Medicaid Services. Medicare hospice benefits. https://www.medicare.gov/Pubs/pdf/02154-medicare-hospice-benefits.pdf

27. Taylor DH Jr, Kaufman BG, Olson A, et al. Paying for palliative care in Medicare: Evidence from the Four Seasons/Duke CMMI Demonstration. *Journal of Pain and Symptom Management.* 2010;58(4):654–661. e2. https://www.sciencedirect.com/science/article/abs/pii/S088539241930363X

28. Centers for Medicare and Medicaid Services. Evaluation of the Medicare Care Choices Model. February 2020. https://downloads.cms.gov/files/mccm-secannrpt.pdf

29. National Academy of State Health Policy. Advancing palliative care for adults with serious illness: a national review of state health palliative care policies and programs. September 2018. https://www.nashp.org/wp-content/uploads/2018/12/NASHP_State-Palliative-Care-Scan_Appendix-B-New.pdf

30. Christakia N, Lamont E. Extent and determinants of error in physicians prognoses in terminally ill patients. *Western Journal of Medicine.* 2000;172(5):310–313.

31. Crossroads Hospice Blog. Trends in palliative care: looking ahead to 2019. December 2018. https://www.crossroadshospice.com/hospice-palliative-care-blog/2018/december/27/trends-in-palliative-care-looking-ahead-to-2019/. Accessed September 21, 2019.

32. Deerain P. What will emerging technologies mean for the future of palliative care? *Palliative Care Australia.* March 29, 2019. https://palliativecare.org.au/palliative-matters/what-will-emerging-technologies-mean-for-the-future-of-palliative-care. Accessed September 21, 2019.

2

Palliative Models of Care Delivery

Britni Lookabaugh and Charles von Gunten

Case

Mr. Smith is a 75-year-old man who initially presented to the emergency department (ED) due to worsening back pain leading to functional decline over the past several weeks. Imaging revealed diffuse metastatic disease to his bone with a large lung mass, and he was subsequently admitted to the hospital for further workup and treatment of his severe and debilitating pain. Biopsy revealed metastatic non–small cell lung cancer. The inpatient palliative care team was consulted to see Mr. Smith to address his uncontrolled pain. In addition to palliative physician and pharmacist evaluation for symptoms, the palliative social worker assisted with his completion of advance directives. He had one estranged son and chose his best friend as his power of attorney for healthcare. The team attempted to address his goals of care, but reeling from his new diagnosis, he was unwilling to discuss other alternatives despite cure of his cancer. After several days, the team was able to stabilize his pain with oral opioids and several adjuvants, and he was discharged home.

Because of the complexity of Mr. Smith's pain, which required active titration while he was undergoing palliative radiation, the outpatient palliative care team assisted with this during his appointments with his medical oncologist. With initiation of chemotherapy, he experienced severe fatigue, leading to functional decline and an additional hospitalization, where he was found to have malignant pleural effusions. He was discharged to a skilled nursing facility for rehabilitation. The palliative team in the skilled nursing facility over the course of time was able to discuss concerns about his declining functional status and discuss his hopes for his final weeks and months of life. When he had an acute episode of shortness of breath, he refused hospital transfer, and the palliative team facilitated a hospice referral at the nursing facility, where he had his symptoms managed during his last days of life.

This case demonstrates the ideal scenario for the longitudinal care for a palliative patient, with the provision of services spanning the care continuum from home, to community-based facility, to outpatient office, and to hospital setting. In addition, it emphasizes the need to coordinate this care across settings through the use of interdisciplinary teams as the patient transitions in an end-of-life scenario.

Inpatient Models

Inpatient models remain the most common location of delivery of palliative care.[1] Inpatient palliative care teams continue to grow throughout the United S. The number of hospitals with at least 50 beds with palliative care teams rose from 15% in 2001 to 67% in 2014. For larger hospitals with at least 300 beds, 90% had a palliative care team in 2014.[2] With recognition of the value of palliative care involvement earlier in the disease process, including at time of diagnosis of life-limiting illness, the demand for specialty palliative care has increased.

Inpatient palliative care teams are highly variable in structure. This includes interdisciplinary composition (as described in Chapter 3), consultative model versus primary service, and presence of an inpatient palliative care unit.[3] Recognizing the variability amid national growth, the National Quality Forum made consensus recommendations for hospital palliative care teams. The "must have" recommendations include integration with hospital management; consult service available at least Monday–Friday; staffing with board-certified palliative care physician, palliative care nurse, and/or advanced practice provider (APP) such as a nurse or physician assistant; and availability of social work and chaplain as part of the palliative team. In addition, the following are essential: tracked outcome metrics as well as quality improvement, marketing, education, bereavement, screening for palliative care for patients eligible for consultation, processes for transitions of care, and procedures promoting team wellness.[4]

Consultation Process

Hospitals with inpatient palliative care teams must first identify patients appropriate for palliative care. These include patients with chronic, complex, life-threatening illness with needs for symptom management; discussion regarding their goals and preferences for medical care; advance care planning; psychosocial and spiritual support; and end-of-life care. Identification of patients appropriate for palliative care consultation may follow attending physician identification, patient or family request, or a formalized consult trigger model.

There are many trigger tools presented in the literature for identifying palliative care patients; these tools may be general or disease specific. Several studies have advocated for a single-question approach, having clinicians evaluate, "Would you be surprised if the patient died within the next year?" to identify patients appropriate for palliative care.[5] Many studies have used this question as part of an assessment in identifying patients. In the intensive care unit (ICU) and ED settings, studies have reported on screening criteria such as metastatic cancer, age, length of ICU stay, length of mechanical ventilation, or family conflict.[6] In the ED, where patients may present with acute symptom management needs or where urgent discussion of goals of care may prevent undesired aggressive medical interventions and level of care, timely and streamlined identification of patients is key. Studies have evaluated screening by a nurse, an APP, or social worker. Many studies implementing screening tools emphasize patients with advanced cancer or dementia.[7]

Trigger tools have also been developed for different disease states. For heart failure patients, some consultation triggers may include candidacy for advanced therapies, such as an LVAD (left ventricular assist device) or transplant, recurrent hospitalizations, or dialysis.[8] For patients with chronic obstructive pulmonary disease patients, objective measures such as the forced expiratory volume in the first second of expiration, body mass index, or patient-specific subjective measures (e.g., shortness of breath) may be used.[9] One study found that for elderly trauma patients, the Palliative Performance Scale, may be a useful trigger and predictor of mortality and poor functional prognosis.[10]

Primary palliative care skills are essential for any provider regardless of medical specialty. These skills include communication with patients and families about serious illness, end-of-life decision-making, and straightforward pain and symptom management. Specialty palliative care provides an additional level of comprehensive interdisciplinary care for patients with complex, chronic, and life-limiting illness. Specialty palliative care teams navigate complex goals of care with expertise in communication regarding disease process, prognostication, advance care planning, and end-of-life education. Teams provide for complex psychosocial and spiritual contributors to disease as well.[11]

Many palliative care teams operate from a consultative model, with primary or specialty providers requesting inpatient consultation. Some palliative care teams operate from an embedded or mixed model. These teams are seen as arms of a primary service, such as within the ICU or oncology setting.

Patients in the ICU frequently have many palliative care needs, including psychosocial support, conversations regarding goals of care due to critical and life-threatening illness, symptom management, and end-of-life care as the ICU experiences a high volume of inpatient deaths. Mun and colleagues in 2018 implemented a process in their ICU to incorporate salient palliative care approaches into standard ICU practice, such as proactive goals of care and code status conversations, thereby allowing the ICU team to utilize primary palliative care skills and maintain specialty palliative care for complex cases.[12] Mosenthal and colleagues and the Center to Advance Palliative Care reported on surgical ICU interventions using an interdisciplinary team, including an APP, to provide psychosocial and bereavement support and to facilitate goals-of-care conversations with the surgical intensivist, among other interventions.[13]

Palliative Care Units

A dedicated acute palliative care unit (APCU) within the hospital serves multiple functions. The complex symptom management required for many palliative care patients necessitates a skilled interdisciplinary hospital team, especially nursing. For example, a patient with complex cancer pain may require high-level pain interventions such as ketamine or lidocaine infusions. A palliative care unit allows for specialty APP care in these situations. Staff on other units may not be as familiar or comfortable with these interventions. APCUs also allow for transfers from the ICU or ED when a patient's goals of care shift from aggressive medical interventions to comfort-focused care, thus facilitating for the hospital the availability for new patients needing the acuity of the ICU. When a patient's conditions necessitate ongoing end-of-life symptom management within the hospital setting, the trained staff of a palliative care unit provide this service. Some APCUs also care for hospice patients who require an inpatient level of care.[14] Many units employ physician assistants or advance practice nurses. For example, as described in a 2016 article, the palliative care unit at Dana-Farber Cancer Institute/Brigham and Women's Cancer Center (Boston, MA) is staffed with five physician assistants, who describe themselves as "first responders" for the patients on the unit.[15]

As described in 2011 by Elsayem and colleagues, the APCU at MD Anderson Cancer Center (Houston, TX) has a daily assessment of symptoms, utilizing the well-established Edmonton Symptom Assessment Scale and Memorial Delirium Assessment Scale.[16] Given the high symptom prevalence and severity within a palliative care population, an APCU allows for the identification, treatment, and monitoring that may not be present on another nursing unit in the hospital.

A 2011 study by Casarett and colleagues completed a nationwide telephone survey in order to compare the end-of-life care received between patients receiving a palliative care consult and patients receiving care on a dedicated palliative care unit. They found that for patients receiving care on a palliative care unit, families were more likely to report excellent care in the last month of life, patients were more likely to have do not resuscitate (DNR) orders, to have received a chaplain visit, and to have bereavement follow-up.[17]

Outcomes

An interdisciplinary approach to provide for palliation at the end of life has been well established, especially since the initiation of the Medicare Hospice Benefit. Intuitively, this comprehensive approach to the physical, psychosocial, spiritual, and practical needs for patients with complex and life-limiting illness allows for holistic care for patients, families and caregivers. Nevertheless, research has also shown the myriad benefits not only to patients and families but also hospitals. Despite this, barriers for access remain—such as disease category fitting within the hospice criteria and workforce shortages specifically with regard to employment of APPs by hospices.

Many studies have evaluated the financial aspects of inpatient palliative care programs. In contrast to procedural specialties, and given the vast amount of clinician time that is required to leverage the communication skills necessary to provide comprehensive palliative care, cost savings rather than direct fee-for-service calculations demonstrate the value of palliative care. Related to diagnosis related group (DRG) payment, cost avoidance associated with palliative care consultation and a transition to a lower level of care based on the patient's goals (e.g., from ICU to palliative care unit), tells the financial story. Additionally, the availability of an ICU bed when a palliative care patient transfers out based on their goals of care allows for another critically ill patient to take their place, allowing for further revenue to the hospital.[18]

In a 2008 multicenter study, Morrison and colleagues evaluated direct cost savings between patients with palliative care consultation and matched controls. They found that for patients who died, cost savings with palliative care consultation were $374 per day. Patients who were discharged alive had cost savings of $279 per day. The authors proposed several factors associated with cost savings, including fewer ICU days, as well as fewer diagnostic tests and procedures, when the patient's goals of care are appropriately addressed.[19]

A 2013 study assessing the cost avoidance associated with an APCU found that for their 12-bed unit at a 545-bed teaching hospital, in comparison to controls there was an annual cost avoidance of $848,556. Over half of this cost avoidance came from patients transferred from the ICU to the palliative care unit.[20]

Another 2008 study at one institution by Hanson and colleagues found cost savings as well. However, they also measured the clinical impact documenting new DNR/do not intubate orders and percentages of patients referred to hospice and also demonstrated statistically significant improvement in symptom scores for pain, dyspnea, and nausea.[21]

Similar results were also demonstrated through a prospective, randomized, multicenter study by Gade and colleagues in 2008, where patients with a life-limiting diagnosis and a physician answering in the affirmative to the question, "Would you be surprised if the patient died within 1 year?" were randomized to receive either usual care or inpatient palliative care consultation. This study also demonstrated lower costs for the palliative care group, but at the time frame of 6 months postdischarge related to decreased readmissions and decreased ICU days. There were also significant increases in hospice length of stay, completion of advance directives, and higher patient satisfaction in the palliative care consultation group.[22]

In the landmark 2010 trial by Temel and colleagues, patients with metastatic non–small cell lung cancer were randomized to receive either usual oncology care or palliative care early in diagnosis. Not only did the palliative care arm demonstrate higher quality-of-life scores, but also demonstrated a statistically significant longer median survival (11.6 months vs. 8.9 months) despite receiving less-aggressive interventions in comparison.[23] The outcomes of this study and others have led to oncology guideline recommendations for increased and earlier integration of palliative care for patients with advanced cancers.[24] A more recent review underlines the advantages of a palliative care approach to improve a patient's outcomes, including symptom burden and quality-of-life and end-of-life outcomes, all achieved with lower associated costs.[25]

Outpatient Models

A shift in payment models to one that penalizes hospitals and skilled nursing facilities in the United States for avoidable readmissions has led to more focus on the benefits of palliative care teams in providing care in the community, including outpatient clinics and home-based palliative care.[3] Patients with serious illness, as defined conceptually (and without regard to setting) in the *Journal of Palliative Medicine*, are those who have "a health condition that carries a high risk of mortality AND either negatively impacts a person's daily function or quality of life, OR excessively strains their caregivers."[26] For oncology patients whose care is primarily as an outpatient, access to palliative care teams in this setting is necessary to address the complex needs of patients with advanced cancer.[27] To maintain their credentialing level, the American Society of Clinical Oncology requires an outpatient supportive or palliative care clinic for cancer centers. The concept of the survivorship clinic has dynamically evolved from its cancer origins to a diversely accepted care model that encompasses all patients with serious illness. This is exemplified by the COVID survivorship care model now being developed in major health systems, and this interdisciplinary team also includes physician assistants.

Some teams have a stand-alone palliative care clinic, and others utilize an embedded clinic model within another specialty clinic. The embedded model allows for improved patient access with visibility for referrals, as well as ease for the patient who may have functional debility and may follow with multiple physician specialists. The embedded model also allows for improved collaboration between the specialist and palliative care. For example, at some institutions, outpatient goals of care conversations have been co-led by the patient's oncologist and their palliative care provider(s). This allows for real-time plans, including when there may be acute needs to address. Some teams also utilize an embedded approach within the heart failure clinic to similarly be able to collaborate successfully with the patient's cardiologist.

Depending on disease process, oncology-focused clinics may have more of an emphasis on symptom management, whereas a patient with end-stage organ disease may have more of a need for advance care planning and, especially as disease progresses, goals-of-care conversations.

One telephone survey of palliative care clinics highlighted the variability that exists in practice. Many were focused on oncology patients. Number of days of clinic per week varied, as did interdisciplinary support. Themes included challenges with funding and staffing, especially with experienced rapid growth when initiated.[28] In all cases, physician assistants have been used for the APP role in the outpatient palliative care team.

Community-Based Models

Many patients with palliative care needs require care that cannot be provided by either an inpatient palliative care team or outpatient palliative care and are not yet ready or eligible for hospice care. This gap may be filled by home-based palliative care teams or palliative care within nursing facilities. Another growing trend is the use of house calls to provide complex illness management within the home to patients with serious illness—regardless of the etiology or the age of the patient. This is especially true with trauma victims, rehabilitating patients from viral illness, and geriatric homebound patients. The potential exists for a paradigm of care delivery for pandemic survivors. Finally, this is an area where APPs have expanded the continuity of care and, as they are trained to be integral members of an interdisciplinary team, will be the essential link between the patient and the healthcare system.

Home-based palliative care programs also demonstrate significant variability. Home palliative care teams may be provided through home health or hospice agencies, with variation in components of interdisciplinary teams. One palliative care program utilizes nurses, social workers, and physicians as part of a Medicare Shared Savings Program Accountable

Care Organization and demonstrated significant cost savings, decreased hospitalizations at the end of life, and increased hospice enrollment.[29]

There have been other positive outcomes research on home teams. A 2013 Cochrane review concluded that home-based palliative care significantly increased the likelihood of death at home and improved symptom management.[30] A 2017 review evaluated studies to identify the components of care that led to patient and caregiver experience of home palliative care. The two major themes identified were presence and competence. Presence was inclusive of access of patients and caregivers to the teams, including at times 24/7 support. The theme of competence included the perception that the team was able to provide for effective symptom management and communication.[31]

Significant percentages of elderly patients die within skilled nursing or long-term care facilities and may have palliative care needs with significant functional debility and symptoms that cannot be fulfilled by hospice if the prognosis is longer than 6 months.[1] Many nursing homes report having palliative-focused interventions; however, little has been researched regarding specific nonhospice team models of care. Efforts in nursing homes have been focused on pain and symptom assessment, advance directive completion, interventions to reduce rehospitalizations at end of life, and increasing hospice enrollment.[32]

Carlson and colleagues mapped out three models of palliative care. The first model is an external palliative care consult service in which a program provides consultation to residents at the request of the patient's physician. A second model is a palliative care team employed by the nursing home. One example is Evercare Hospice and Palliative Care, which employs nurse practitioners to provide palliative care to contracted nursing homes. A third model emphasizes the positive downstream effects for all nursing home residents when there is a strong hospice presence within the facility.[33]

Physician assistants or advanced practice nurses have been employed in community-based models. In fact, cancer patients in the rural US South received substantially more care (56%) from APPs than physicians..[34]

International Models

Internationally, there are diverse palliative care models depending on country demographics, disease processes, and funding structures. Palliative care across the continuum of inpatient, outpatient and home-based services is highly variable by country. Additionally, palliative care provided by generalist and specialist models is highly variable. Hospice care also lacks a standard definition. Whereas in the United States, hospice is a model of care provided and patterned on the Medicare Hospice Benefit, in other countries hospice care may refer to a specific facility where end-of-life care is provided.[35]

A resolution at the World Health Assembly in 2014 named palliative care as a key component of health systems and advocated for improved international access to palliative care.[36] Advocates have further elevated this call by naming palliative care as a human right, as part of a comprehensive approach to disease, and its purpose to prevent and alleviate suffering.[37]

Within this response to the call for action, physician assistants are now part of the directory of global directory of educational programs in palliative and end-of-life training.[38]

The World Health Organization utilizes a public health strategy that advocates for "appropriate policies, adequate drug availability, education of health care workers and the public and implementation of palliative care services at all levels throughout the society."[39] Hannon and colleagues in 2007 linked these elements to experiences in several countries. Regarding appropriate policies, they noted an increase in palliative care services in Japan following the 2007 Cancer Control Act. Access to essential medications such as opioids remains very limited in many locations, such as sub-Saharan Africa. Yet, in sub-Saharan Africa, leveraging community volunteers has helped to provide home palliative care.[40]

Pediatric Models

Pediatric models of palliative care may be similar to adult models in the need for inpatient, outpatient, and home-based models of care; however, the population presents its own challenges for palliative care teams to address. Differences include, among others, a need for emphasis on developmental level (see Chapter 3 regarding the pediatric palliative interdisciplinary team); a greater level of medical technology, especially in the home setting with parent and nursing caregivers; a prolonged and unknown disease trajectory given the breadth and rarity of pediatric diagnoses[41]; and the intensity of psychosocial and bereavement concerns when a child dies.

One unique feature of pediatric palliative care is the ability for children to receive hospice services concurrently with disease-directed curative treatments. Recognizing that for children especially, forgoing life-sustaining treatment is rare earlier in a terminal illness trajectory; this allows for more patients to receive the benefits of hospice care. Through the Affordable Care Act, Medicaid and Children's Health Insurance Program, allow for coverage of both hospice services and curative treatments through the age of 21 for children with a terminal illness.[42]

Conclusion

Throughout the care continuum from inpatient to outpatient, to home and skilled nursing facilities, palliative care provides for enhanced quality of life and symptom management for patients with chronic, complex, and life-limiting illness. Physician assistants are rapidly expanding their role within the interdisciplinary palliative care team in all of these settings.

References

1. Kelley AS, Morrison RS. Palliative care for the seriously ill. *New England Journal of Medicine.* 2015;*373*(8):747–755.
2. Dumanovsky T, Augustin R, Rogers M, et al. The growth of palliative care in U.S. hospitals: a status report. *Journal of Palliative Medicine.* 2016;*19*(1):8–15.

3. Morrison RS. Models of palliative care delivery in the United States. *Current Opinion in Supportive and Palliative Care.* 2013;7(2):201–206.

4. Weissman DE, Meier DE. Operational features for hospital palliative care programs: consensus recommendations. *Journal of Palliative Medicine.* 2008;11(9):1189–1194.

5. Weissman DE, Meier DE. Identifying patients in need of a palliative care assessment in the hospital setting: a consensus report from the Center to Advance Palliative Care. *Journal of Palliative Medicine.* 2011;14(1):1–7.

6. Nelson JE, Curtis JR, Mulherin C, et al. Choosing and using screening criteria for palliative care consultation in the ICU: a report from the Improving Palliative Care in the ICU (IPAL-ICU) advisory board. *Critical Care Medicine.* 2013;41(10):2318–2327.

7. George N, Phillips E, Zaurova M, et al. Palliative care screening and assessment in the emergency department: a systematic review. *Journal of Pain and Symptom Management.* 2016;51(1):108–119.

8. Psotka MA, McKee KY, Liu AY. Palliative care in heart failure: what triggers specialist consultation? *Progress in Cardiovascular Diseases.* 2017;60(2):215 225.

9. Duenk RG, Verhagen C, Bronkhorst EM, et al. Development of the ProPal-COPD tool to identify patients with COPD for proactive palliative care. *International Journal of COPD.* 2017;12:2121–2128.

10. McGreavy CM, Bryczkowski S, Pentakota SR, et al. Unmet palliative care needs in elderly trauma patients: can the Palliative Performance Scale help close the gap? *American Journal of Surgery.* 2017;213:778–784.

11. Quill TE, Abernethy AP. Generalist plus specialist palliative care—creating a more sustainable model. *New England Journal of Medicine.* 2013;368(13):1173–1175.

12. Mun E, Umbarger L, Ceria-Ulep C, Nakatsuka C. Palliative care processes embedded in the ICU workflow may reserve palliative care teams for refractory cases. *American Journal of Hospice & Palliative Medicine.* 2018;35(1):60–65.

13. Mosenthal AC, Weissman DE, Curtis JR, et al. Integrating palliative care in the surgical and trauma intensive care unit (IPAL-ICU) project advisory board and the Center to Advance Palliative Care. *Critical Care Medicine.* 2012;40(4):1199–1206.

14. Lagman RL, Walsh D, LeGrand SB, Davis MP. The business of palliative medicine—part 6: clinical operations in a comprehensive integrate program. *American Journal of Hospice & Palliative Medicine.* 2011;28(2):75–81.

15. Drury L, Baccari K, Fang A, et al. Providing intensive palliative care on an inpatient unit: a full-time job. *Journal of the Advanced Practitioner in Oncology.* 2016;7:60–64.

16. Elsayem A, Calderon BB, Camarines EM, et al. A month in an acute palliative care unit: clinical interventions and financial outcomes. *American Journal of Hospice & Palliative Medicine.* 2011;28(8):550–555.

17. Casarett D, Johnson M, Smith D, Richardson D. The optimal delivery of palliative care: a national comparison of the outcomes of consultation teams vs inpatient units. *Archives of Internal Medicine.* 2011;171(7):649–655.

18. Smith TJ, Cassel JB. Cost and non-clinical outcomes of palliative care. *Journal of Pain and Symptom Management.* 2009;38(1):32–44.

19. Morrison RS, Penrod JD, Cassel B et al. Cost savings associated with US hospital palliative care consultation programs. *Archives of Internal Medicine.* 2008;168(16):1783–1790.

20. Albanese TH, Radwany SM, Mason H, et al. Assessing the financial impact of an inpatient acute palliative care unit in a tertiary care teaching hospital. *Journal of Palliative Medicine.* 2013;16(3):289–294.

21. Hanson LC, Usher B, Spragens L, Bernard S. Clinical and economic impact of palliative care consultation. *Journal of Pain and Symptom Management.* 2008;35(4):340–346.

22. Gade G, Venohr I, Conner D, et al. Impact of an inpatient palliative care team: a randomized control trial. *Journal of Palliative Medicine.* 2008;11(2):180–190.

23. Temel JS, Greer JA, Muzikansky A, et al. Early palliative care for patients with metastatic non-small cell lung cancer. *New England Journal of Medicine.* 2010;363(8):733–742.

24. Levy MH, Smith T, Alvarez-Perez A, et al. Palliative care, version 1.2014 featured updates to the NCCN guidelines. *Journal of the National Comprehensive Cancer Network.* 2014;12(10):1379–1388.

25. Dalal S, Bruera E. End-of-life care matters: palliative cancer care results in better care and lower costs. *Oncologist.* 2017;22:3613–3668.

26. Kelley AS, Bollens-Lund E. *Journal of Palliative Medicine*. Identifying the population with serious illness: the "denominator" challenge. 2018;*21*(S2):S7–S16. https://doi.org/10.1089/jpm.2017.0548

27. Hui D, Bruera E. Integrating palliative care into the trajectory of cancer care. *Nature Reviews. Clinical Oncology*. 2016;*13*(3):159–171.

28. Smith AK, Thai TN, Bakitas MA, et al. The diverse landscape of palliative care clinics. *Journal of Palliative Medicine*. 2013;*16*(6):661–668.

29. Lustbader D, Mudra M, Romano C, et al. The impact of a home-based palliative care program in an accountable care organization. *Journal of Palliative Medicine*. 2017;*20*(1):23–28.

30. Gomes B, Calanzani N, Curiale V, et al. Effectiveness and cost-effectiveness of home palliative care services for adults with advanced illness and their caregivers. *Cochrane Database of Systematic Reviews*. 2013;(6):CD007760. doi:10.1002/14651858.CD007760.pub2

31. Sarmento VP, Gysels M, Higginson IJ, Gomes B. Home palliative care works: but how? A meta-ethnography of the experiences of patients and family caregivers. *BMJ Supportive & Palliative Care*. 2017;*7*:390–403.

32. Ersek M, Carpenter JG. Geriatric palliative care in long-term care settings with a focus on nursing homes. *Journal of Palliative Medicine*. 2013;*16*(10):1180–1187.

33. Carlson MDA, Lim B, Meier DE. Strategies and innovative models for delivering palliative care in nursing homes. *Journal of the American Medical Directors Association*. 2011;*12*(2):91–98.

34. Coombs LA, Max W, Kolevska T, Tonner C, Stephens C. Nurse practitioners and physician assistants: an underestimated workforce for older adults with cancer. *Journal of the American Geriatric Society*. 2019;*67*:1489–1494. https://doi.org/10.1111/jgs.15931

35. Arias-Casias N, Garralda E, Rhee JY, et al. *EAPC Atlas of Palliative Care in Europe* 2019. Vilvoorde, Belgium: EAPC Press; 2019. http://hdl.handle.net/10171/56787. Accessed December 16, 2019.

36. World Health Organization. Noncommunicable disease and their risk factors: palliative care. https://www.who.int/ncds/management/palliative-care/en/. Accessed December 16, 2019.

37. Open Society Foundations. Public health fact sheet: palliative care as a human right. https://www.opensocietyfoundations.org/publications/palliative-care-human-right-fact-sheet. February 2016. Accessed December 16, 2019.

38. International Association for Hospice and Palliative Care (IAHPC). Global directory of educational programs in palliative care. https://hospicecare.com/global-directory-of-education-programs/programs/details/533/

39. Stjernsward J, Foley KM, Ferris FD. The public health strategy for palliative care. *Journal of Pain and Symptom Management*. 2007;*33*(5):486–493.

40. Hannon B, Librac SL, Zimmerman C. Palliative care program development: an international perspective. *Current Opinion in Supportive and Palliative Care*. 2013;*7*(2):192–194.

41. Feudtner C, Kang TI, Hexem KR, et al. Pediatric palliative care patients: a prospective multicenter cohort study. *Pediatrics*. 2011;*127*:1094–1101.

42. Keim-Malpass J, Hart TG, Miller JR. Coverage of palliative and hospice care for pediatric patients with a life-limiting illness: a policy brief. *Journal of Pediatric Health Care*. 2013;*27*(6):511–516.

3

Evolution of the Palliative Team

Britni Lookabaugh and Charles von Gunten

Palliative Team

As outlined in Chapter 2, the palliative care team has as many iterations as there are programs. However, at its core, the palliative team is inherently interdisciplinary to address all domains of palliative care. These include physical, psychologic, social, practical, and spiritual aspects of a patient's and family's (or those the patient identifies as family) care. A palliative care team will be able to comprehensively address the concerns commonly faced by patients and caregivers living with chronic, complex, life-limiting, or life-threatening illness with the expertise of the various disciplines at a specialty level of practice.[1,2]

Physicians

Most palliative care teams are physician led. As of 2012 in the United States, board certification in hospice and palliative medicine requires training via an accredited fellowship. Sponsoring primary specialty boards include the American boards of internal medicine, family medicine, pediatrics, obstetrics and gynecology, emergency medicine, anesthesia, surgery, psychiatry and neurology, radiology, physical medicine and rehabilitation, and emergency medicine.[3] Thus, hospice and palliative medicine physicians may have diverse primary specialty backgrounds prior to completion of palliative care fellowships and subsequent board certification.

As a member of the clinical team, the physician's role is one of medical consultant, primarily via communication with patients and families about serious illness and symptom management. Palliative medicine physicians are trained to address many of the inadequacies seen in end-of-life care in the landmark Study to understand prognoses and preferences for outcomes and risks of treatment (SUPPORT) study from 1995. For example, this study found that physicians knew of their patient's wishes to avoid cardiopulmonary resuscitation only 47% of the time.[4] Communication regarding diagnosis, prognosis, disease trajectory, and negotiation of the goals of a patient's medical care is a cornerstone of the palliative physician's role. The SUPPORT study also found that 50% of families felt their loved ones suffered from moderate-to-severe pain in their last days of life.[4] Symptom assessment and treatment, which can often be complex to manage, are also key components of the physician's role. This may involve the advanced practice provider (APP) in consultation and collaboration with the physician.

The physician's role may also include administrative functions, including program development and team development and education of fellows, residents, medical and APP students, and other staff. Depending on the program and interests, research may also be a component.

Advanced Practice Providers

Advanced practice providers, play a prominent role in most palliative care teams. They function in almost every setting, including in-patient and out-patient, community and home based and are embedded into other specialties such as pediatric and adult critical care. These roles are constantly evolving especially within the context of chronic disease management and a global pandemic. Some palliative care teams are led by an APP. Nurses may become a certified hospice and palliative nurse (CHPN) after qualifying based on practice and an examination.[5] Physician assistants (PAs) can also assume this role as their training and scope of practice is consistent with the medical model of the physician. Both professionals have similar enhanced clinical responsibilities which makes them a vital part of the team, and this is incorporated in their compassionate communication skills and complex symptom management.[2] They may also have a significant administrative component with program development and education, especially in programs led by an APP.[6]

Recognizing the need for more specific specialty training in palliative medicine, some institutional programs have developed formal post-graduate training curricula, including fellowships and master's degrees for APPs. An example is the interprofessional fellowship offered through Harvard Medical School, which is a 1-year fellowship with educational experiences aligned with palliative care physician, social work, and pharmacist fellows. Listed components of curriculum include bereavement, communication, ethics, hospice, medical education, psychosocial domain, sustainability and resilience, and spirituality.[7,8] A 2017 article characterized nurse practitioner residencies and fellowships and at that time identified four palliative care programs.[9] There are several programs that provide advanced training for PAs, clinical nurse specialists, and other members of the team in an interdisciplinary model; the University of Maryland and the University of Colorado are two examples. These and others represent a growing number of university-hospital–based settings in which PAs can earn either a graduate degree or certificate.

Nurses

The role of nurses on the palliative medicine team varies depending on the setting and what the patient and caregivers require. In the home setting, they may function similarly to a hospice case manager (described further under Hospice Team). In the inpatient setting, they may have a triage role for the consult team, as a bedside nurse in an acute palliative care unit, or assist the team with symptom assessment, patient and caregiver education, and communication. Specialty hospice and palliative care nursing may require unique and complex care based on the patient's disease process and symptom management, requiring significant care coordination, which is a primary role identified by palliative care nurses.[10] Symptom medications may involve administration routes and doses not ordinarily encountered in other settings. Examples include subcutaneous administration of opioids, initiation and titration of opioid and benzodiazepine infusions, or hypodermoclysis, which is the subcutaneous infusion of isotonic solutions.

Pharmacists

Depending on state laws and institutional policies, the pharmacist role on the palliative care team may range from consultant on medications, to provider status working in collaborative practice with the ability to initiate and titrate medications. The complexity of the patient population frequently requires creative and unique solutions to address symptoms. Pharmacists may use their expertise to guide off-label uses of medications, to strategize needs on route of administration, and to minimize risks from polypharmacy, as well as many other potential activities. In addition to making recommendations to the palliative care team, a key component of a palliative care pharmacist may be to act as a liaison with other pharmacists in the hospital or community setting who may not be familiar or comfortable with palliative care practice.[11] Pharmacist specialty training may include a residency training program in pain and palliative care.

Social Workers

Palliative care social workers assist with the psychologic and social challenges inherent in palliative care. In the psychological domain (as noted in the "National Consensus Project Guidelines, Domain 3: Psychological and Psychiatric Aspects of Care"), social workers provide emotional support and exploration of hopes and worries related to complex and life-limiting illness. Some social workers may assist with counseling. "Caregiver support is a key component as well, including practicalities of living arrangements, and the financial, legal and ethical components of a patient's care."[2] Social workers may assist with advance care planning including completion of advance directives. Stein et al. found that 96% of hospice and palliative social workers participated in advance care planning discussions.[12] They may also assist with bereavement interventions with grieving family members both before and after a patient's death.

A 2019 survey of hospice and palliative social workers identified the most important tasks of their role. These included, but were not limited to, facilitation of communication with the interdisciplinary team, patients, and families; assessment of support and coping skills; and provision of emotional support and education.[13]

Chaplains

Chaplains on the palliative care team help to address the spiritual aspect of the patient's care. In addition, they assist in meeting the spiritual needs of the interdisciplinary team—individuals with both the palliative and other related specialties that are caring for the patient. This role has been enhanced due to the moral distress and burnout that all healthcare providers are feeling as a result of the pandemic. While all palliative care clinicians should be able to perform a primary spiritual assessment and recognize the need for treatment of spiritual distress,[2] chaplains provide a comprehensive spiritual assessment. This often includes the psychosocial aspects of a comprehensive evaluation of the patient's pain and suffering. The chaplain is uniquely positioned to address these aspects of a patient's distress and can facilitate necessary consultations with other specialties and members of the team—such as social work, psychology, and other therapists. This suffering may require the facilitation of religious rituals such as prayer and connection to faith communities or the patient's own clergy. While religion may be a key component for some patients, the spiritual assessment for distress goes beyond religion. Hills et al. found that 87% of their palliative care patients identified as somewhat spiritual, while 77% identified as somewhat religious. They also found that negative religious coping was associated with increase in distress, depression, and reduced quality of life.[14] Spiritual distress may be associated with loss, not only of life, but also of role, dignity, and expectations. Chaplains may assist patients with existential suffering, such as the meaning of life and death, hopelessness, or guilt and regret.[2,15–17]

Other Disciplines

While no less important, these members from other disciplines are less commonly part of the core palliative care team, and they include psychologists; art therapists; music therapists; massage therapists; physical, occupational, and speech and language therapists; and volunteers.

In pediatrics, in particular, where the palliative care team may have a long-standing relationship with a patient and family dealing with chronic life-limiting illness, team members need to address issues on a developmental level. Developmentally appropriate communication and exploration of hopes and worries may be best facilitated by art therapists, music therapists, or child life specialists. Support for a patient's siblings and explanations of medical equipment are also facilitated by child life specialists. Achievement and maintenance of developmental milestones with the assistance of physical, occupational, and speech therapists are key components of quality of life for children with life-limiting illness.[18]

Hospice Team

The hospice interdisciplinary team is dictated by the Medicare Conditions of Participation and are not different from what is described here for palliative care teams. Hospices must also be able to contract with and provide for nutrition support if needed based on the patient's plan of care.[19] Some hospices provide other interdisciplinary support with massage, art or music therapy, or psychological or pharmacy support.

Nurse Case Manager

The hospice nurse case manager in many respects is the key component of the hospice team and the primary driver of the patient's hospice care plan. The nurse case manager provides education and support regarding disease process and caregiving as well as symptom and medication management. They coordinate the patient's interdisciplinary care plan and communicate with and receive orders from the hospice medical director and/or attending physician.

Volunteers

Medicare Conditions of Participation mandate that at least 5% of all care hours provided to hospice patients must be provided by volunteer support.[20] Volunteers may assist with providing respite for caregivers, sitting vigil with patients at the end of life, and assisting in life goal attainment for patients and their families. The means by which these are done may change depending on the local, national, and global health care circumstances, such as natural disasters and pandemics.

Unique Team Dynamics

The challenge for hospice and palliative care teams is to be able to move from multidisciplinary to interdisciplinary, rather than each discipline focusing on their area of expertise as it contributes to the patient's care, to a shared collaborative plan of care between the disciplines. For example, a cancer patient may have severe physical pain that is exacerbated by existential distress. Rather than the provider focusing on the medical treatment of physical symptoms and the chaplain addressing the spiritual pain associated with dying, the team when functioning at its best will be able to collaborate together about the underlying issues and develop a comprehensive plan together on how to best address the pain. This model in many respects can be a healthy departure from the hierarchical nature of the practice of medicine in the ways that the team can adapt to the needs of the patient and provide the different discipline support depending on the situation.[21] However, the inherent teamwork necessary to be able to utilize the skills of individual team members can impact team communication and role development and can even lead to burnout and conflict among the palliative care team.

Role Development

Development of a collaborative interdisciplinary team is key to the successful delivery of palliative care. As described by Periyakoil,[22] there are several factors associated with this type of team. The environment in which the team functions within the organization is important to consider and is described in more detail below. The team should have shared vision, purpose, and goals. This can be a foundation for team members to provide feedback to each other and navigate conflict, which are necessities and lead to team trust in one another.[22]

One qualitative study in 2011 looked at a palliative care interdisciplinary team and their perceived role for providing psychosocial care for patients, aptly named "Everybody thinks that everybody can do it and they can't." This study via interviews found an emerging theme of blurred role boundaries for which team members provide psychosocial support and the conflict that can arise within the team when the psychosocial support is provided by a non–psychosocial team member. The authors suggested that further support is necessary to help teams develop and function effectively.[23] Development of discipline roles and education between disciplines on the team can help build trust when there is overlap of the type of care provided between disciplines to allow for collaborative practice.

In an article citing the challenges in developing new teams[24] found the most important factors associated with successful team cooperation included team performance as indicated by smooth workflow, communication, and trust. These features, in addition to role clarity, help to balance the stressors for a team, which include conflict and the stress of the work of death and dying.

The exponential growth of palliative care as a specialty in the United States and globally has created opportunities for APPs to participate. For example, Dumanovsky et al. found that among US hospitals with 50 or more beds, the number of palliative programs increased from 15% of hospitals in 1998 to 67% of hospitals in.[25] Managing the growth of palliative care teams with high and increasing 2013.

demand can create unique and challenging situations for teams. Appropriate staffing is challenging for several reasons. First, given the large amount of time necessary to provide adequate palliative care for patients, it is difficult to measure productivity and patient volumes per team member on a given day. A high amount of care coordination is required between both primary and specialty teams and within the palliative care team to determine a plan of care and coordinate practical aspects of a patient's care. Much attention that is devoted to a patient's care is not at the bedside and therefore is difficult to quantify. A shortage of trained palliative care professionals has led to challenging recruitment and then staff onboarding and education. A 2010 study found that even to achieve appropriate physician staffing nationally there was a gap at that time of 2787 to 7510 hospice and palliative medicine physician full time equivalents (FTEs).[26]

Management of staff onboarding and team dynamics in the midst of a high volume of consults from primary care and other specialties can lead to burnout. Furthermore, based on the current projections of the increasing burden of serious chronic illness in the adult and pediatric populations, the gap in the supply of specialist palliative care providers will continue to increase. As calls for integration of palliative care increase, the worsening shortage of specialty physicians creates opportunities for APPs to play a role in meeting the needs for patient-centered, serious illness care.

Another important consideration is the incorporation of primary palliative medicine into all specialties—both medical and surgical. This presents another dynamic area for development, including consideration in the delivery of serious illness care in telemedicine/telehealth for all patients at risk or in recovery from illness in general.

Optimal Team Function

As described by Periyakoil,[22] the organizational environment is a key factor in the success of a palliative care team. There must be a leader who is respected within the organization to positively impact the system. Challenges also exist for making the financial case for palliative care for an organization in order to appropriately staff a palliative care team as demand grows. Strong relationships with consultant services are key to this success as well. At the present time, we author attributes our exponential growth in our palliative care service to our strong emphasis on consultant etiquette. We communicate extensively with consultant services on a daily basis, and because of this, consultants understand the lengths to which we go to coordinate care for their patients and explain the often complex goals of care. The appreciation of consultant services in turn leads to demand for more services from other teams to fund and further enhance growth.

Given the high emotional intensity of the patient care, burnout can be high for hospice and palliative professionals. A 2014 survey of members of the American Academy of Hospice and Palliative Medicine found 62% of members would meet criteria for burnout.[27] Therefore, developing team resilience is essential to a successful palliative care team.

In a seminal article that created a conceptual model and paradigm, the authors proposed building resilience in palliative care professionals through fostering balance of the "individual personal resources and work demands" to enhance clinician resilience skills in the workplace. Factors in the workplace they proposed include "enabling control, structuring rewards, building community, promoting fairness, recognizing values and calibrating workload."[28p287]

Conclusion

The effective comprehensive delivery of high-quality palliative care requires an optimally functioning interdisciplinary team. PAs, one of the disciplines included in the APP component, do play an important role. Teams provide the best care across all the domains of palliative care when they have clear and well-developed roles. Individual and team resilience and trust are keys to the successful development of the team.

References

1. Kelley AS, Morrison RS. Palliative care for the seriously ill. *New England Journal of Medicine.* 2015;*373*(8):747–755.
2. Ferrell BR, Twaddle ML, Melnick A, et al. National consensus project clinical practice guidelines for quality palliative care guidelines, 4th edition. *Journal of Palliative Medicine.* 2018;*21*(12):1684–1689. http://www.nationalcoalitionhpc.org/ncp. Accessed October 15, 2020.
3. American Board of Internal Medicine. Hospice & palliative medicine policies. https://www.abim.org/certification/policies/internal-medicine-subspecialty-policies/hospice-palliative-medicine.aspx. Accessed September 16, 2019.
4. SUPPORT Principal Investigators. A controlled trial to improve care for seriously ill hospitalized patients: The Study to Understand Prognoses and Preferences for Outcomes and Risks of Treatments (SUPPORT). *JAMA.* 1995;*274*(20):1591–1598.
5. Advancing Expert Care: Hospice & Palliative Nurses Association. Certified hospice and palliative nurse. https://www.advancingexpertcare.org/chpn. Accessed September 16, 2019.
6. Meier DE, Beresford L. Advanced practice nurses in palliative care: A pivotal role and perspective. *Journal of Palliative Medicine.* 2006;*9*(3):624–627.
7. Massachusetts General Hospital Division of Palliative Care and Geriatric Medicine. Palliative care nurse practitioner fellowship. https://www.massgeneral.org/palliativecare/education/NP_fellowship.aspx. Accessed September 13, 2019.
8. Harvard Medical School Center for Palliative Care. Harvard interprofessional palliative care fellowship program training. www.pallcare.hms.harvard.edu/training/curriculum. Accessed September 13, 2019.

9. Martsolf GR, Nguyen PG, Freund D, Poghosyan L. What we know about postgraduate nurse practitioner residency and fellowship programs. *Journal for Nurse Practitioners.* 2017;*13*(7):482–487.

10. Sekse RJT, Hunskar I, Ellingsen S. The nurse's role in palliative care: A qualitative meta-synthesis. *Journal of Clinical Nursing.* 2018;*27*:e21–e38.

11. Walker KA, Scarpaci L, McPherson ML. Fifty reasons to love your palliative care pharmacist. *American Journal of Hospice and Palliative Medicine.* 2010;*27*(8):511–513.

12. Stein GL, Cagle JG, Christ GH. Social work involvement in advance care planning: Findings from a large survey of social workers in hospice and palliative care settings. *Journal of Palliative Medicine.* 2017;*20*(3):253–259.

13. Head B, Peters B, Middleton A, et al. Results of a nationwide hospice and palliative care social work job analysis. *Journal of Social Work in End-of-Life & Palliative Care.* 2019;*15*(1):16–33.

14. Hills J, Paice JA, Cameron JR, Shott S. Spirituality and distress in palliative care consultation. *Journal of Palliative Medicine.* 2005;*8*(4):782–788.

15. Jeuland J, Fitchett G, Schulman-Green D, Kapo J. Chaplains working in palliative care: Who they are and what they do. *Journal of Palliative Medicine.* 2017;*20*(5):502–508.

16. Puchalski C, Ferrell B, Virani R, et al. Improving the quality of spiritual care as a dimension of palliative care: The report of the consensus conference. *Journal of Palliative Medicine.* 2009;*12*(10):885–904.

17. Boston P, Bruce A, Schreiber R. Existential suffering in the palliative care setting: An integrated literature review. *Journal of Pain and Symptom Management.* 2011;*41*(3):604–618.

18. Himelstein BP, Hilden JM, Boldt AM, Weissman D. Pediatric palliative care. *New England Journal of Medicine.* 2004;*350*(17):1752–1762.

19. Connor SR. Development of hospice and palliative care in the United States. *Omega.* 2007–2008;*56*(1):89–99.

20. Department of Health and Human Services, Centers for Medicare and Medicaid Services. *CMS Manual System.* Department of Health and Human Services, Centers for Medicare and Medicaid Services. October 1, 2010. https://www.cms.gov/Regulations-and-Guidance/Guidance/Transmittals/downloads/R65SOMA.pdf. Accessed September 16, 2019.

21. Corner J. The multidisciplinary team—fact or fiction? *European Journal of Palliative Care.* 2003;*10*(2):10–11.

22. Periyakoil VS. Growing pains: Health care enters "team"-age. *Journal of Palliative Medicine.* 2008;*11*(2):171–175.

23. O'Connor M, Fisher C. Exploring the dynamics of interdisciplinary palliative care teams in providing psychosocial care: "Everybody thinks that everybody can do it and they can't." *Journal of Palliative Medicine.* 2011;*14*(2):191–196.

24. Junger S, Pestinger M, Elsner F, et al. Criteria for successful multiprofessional cooperation in palliative care teams. *Palliative Medicine.* 2007;*21*:347–354.

25. Dumanovsky T, Augustin R, Rogers M, et al. The growth of palliative care in U.S. hospitals: A status report. *Journal of Palliative Medicine.* 2016;*19*(1):8–15.

26. Lupu D. Estimate of current hospice and palliative medicine physician workforce shortage. *Journal of Pain and Symptom Management.* 2010;*40*(6):899–911.

27. Kamal A, Bull J, Wolf S, et al. Burnout among palliative care clinicians in the United States: Results of a national survey. *Journal of Clinical Oncology.* 2017;*32*(15, suppl):e20530. doi:10.1200/jco.2014.32.15_suppl:e20530

28. Back AL, Steinhauser KE, Kamal AH, et al. Building resilience for palliative care clinicians: An approach to burnout prevention based on individual skills and workplace factors. *Journal of Pain and Symptom Management.* 2016;*52*(2):284–291.

4

Whole-Person Assessment of the Patient

Betty Ferrell and Vanessa Battista

Whole-Person Assessment

Comprehensive assessment of the patient with serious illness is the hallmark of palliative care. From the initial evaluation of the patient, whole-person assessment provides the foundation for meeting physical, psychological, social, and spiritual needs. An assessment, based on the fundamental goal of enhancing quality of life (QOL) for the duration of life and preparing for a peaceful death, will direct all care and serve to coordinate care across disciplines.[1-5]

Assessment of a patient with serious illness is in many ways similar to any excellent patient assessment. Identifying symptom concerns, assessing psychological issues, determining functional status, and conducting a complete physical examination form the basis of knowing the patient and identifying priority concerns. Palliative care assessment extends beyond basic patient evaluation. By recognizing the unique needs of patients who face serious illness and their family members, particularly if the illness is life limiting, a whole-person assessment can identify concerns early, create a trusting relationship between patient and clinicians, and prepare for future care needs.

A whole-person assessment in palliative care extends the basic evaluation to provide additional information regarding symptoms and other physical concerns; explores psychological concerns common in advanced disease; evaluates social factors such as family caregiver, parent/child, and sibling needs; and assesses spirituality, which is recognized as an important aspect of patient and family support in serious illness.[6-10] The following case study illustrates the role of the physician assistant (PA) in this assessment.

Case

Jane Green is a PA employed by an oncology medical practice in a community hospital setting. The medical oncologists have experienced intense workload increases in their growing practice, and given advances in cancer treatments, there is a need to focus their efforts primarily on new patient visits and treatment planning.

The oncology practice conducted an evaluation of their workflow and found that a large component of the oncologists' time was spent in symptom management and care coordination, resulting in a backlog in accepting new patients. This situation has created financial burden for the practice and impacted the quality of patient care. The oncology practice designated Jane as the clinic's lead to develop better practices and systems of care.

Over the past year, Jane has expanded her knowledge in palliative medicine through some online educational opportunities and by becoming involved in palliative care organizations. She has developed a collaborative relationship with the board-certified palliative care physician and palliative care advanced practice nurse in the hospital and spent 4 days observing their practice. She reports feeling much more confident in symptom management and addressing psychosocial and spiritual concerns.

Jane has led efforts to integrate palliative care within the oncology practice. This has included developing a symptom checklist, which is now integrated in the clinic's electronic medical record, and an initial assessment form, which expands the usual clinic assessment to gain more information regarding psychological, family, and spiritual needs. The oncology practice has designated a palliative care clinic 3 days per week run by Jane and the clinic's social worker; patients with palliative care needs are referred by the oncologists to the clinic. The oncology practice has developed new procedures, including triggers adopted by all clinic staff for referral to the palliative care clinic, which includes all stage IV patients and any patient with an urgent care visit for symptom concerns. Referrals can also be made by the clinic advanced practice registered nurses (APRNs). In addition, Jane has developed communication with the hospital palliative care service to refer patients requiring their care.

The first 6 months of this plan are evaluated by all clinic staff as a great improvement in patient care and clinic workflow. Jane and the oncologists have identified the next steps and longer-term goals, including the need for Jane to have greater access to the hospital pharmacist for symptom management issues and the need for better coordination with community hospices to ensure earlier and better care transitions.

Jane reports that she has recognized the critical need for comprehensive patient assessment to integrate palliative care within the oncology practice. Her initial experience has also identified the opportunities for interdisciplinary collaboration to best meet the patients' complex needs. She is working with the oncologists and APRNs to ensure that symptom management protocols are standardized across all providers in the clinic.

Elements of Whole-Person Assessment

Assessment of Physical Needs

Advanced diseases such as cancer; cardiac, pulmonary, gastrointestinal, and neurologic disease; and infection are recognized for their symptom burden and diminished QOL. In children, congenital syndromes and metabolic conditions also present distinct symptom subsets. Initial assessment of physical needs is essential to establish a baseline, determine symptoms associated with other comorbidities, and assess current medications being used to treat symptoms and the medications' effectiveness.[10-12] Physical examination and patient and caregiver interview are essential to establish the causes of symptoms and their frequency and severity. It is often helpful to include caregivers' perspectives in the assessment of the patient, regardless of the caregiver's age, if the patient is unable to communicate clearly details about their symptoms due to developmental stage or cognitive ability.

Physical assessment is also the time to anticipate future symptoms and develop a plan of care. For patients with advancing heart failure, for example, worsening dyspnea and diminished function should be anticipated and planned for in advance. Patient and caregiver fears and anxieties can be greatly reduced by having plans in place rather than having them experience acute symptom distress that create lasting fear without a plan in place. Having care plans can be especially helpful when patients are being cared for at home. Functional status assessment is also important and should be viewed from the perspective of palliative care and QOL goals rather than a traditional functional goal of rehabilitation or activity. For adults, the Palliative Performance Scale (PPS)[13] is often used as a guide to functional assessment in this population. For children, The PedsQL™ Measurement Model for the Pediatric Quality of Life Inventory™ is a useful tool to measure health-related QOL.[14]

There is growing recognition of the value of structured symptom assessment rather than relying only on what symptoms patients may report. Use of a structured tool such as the Edmonton Symptom Assessment Scale (ESAS) provides a list of common symptoms (e.g., pain, dyspnea, constipation, anxiety) that should be routinely assessed and quantified (e.g., 0–10), and inclusion of symptom assessments within the electronic medical record can provide for monitoring of symptom changes and treatment effectiveness.[15] Several pediatric-specific scales for symptom assessment are also available for use dependent on the patient's age, disease type, and functional ability.[16] Box 4.1 summarizes some key elements of physical assessment.

Management of symptoms at end of life is of special significance as symptoms may escalate at this time. Uncontrolled symptoms at the end of life significantly impact care at the time of death and create distress for both the dying patient and their family.[17-22] Table 4.1 presents a list of symptoms of special importance at the end of life.

Psychosocial Assessment

Psychological responses to serious illness are expected, and the challenge for clinicians is to assess normal responses versus those emotional responses warranting clinical interventions.[23-25] A commitment to whole-person, comprehensive care as the foundation of palliative care requires that psychosocial assessments be integrated into care. Asking patients

BOX 4.1 Physical Examination and PPS Score

General: Observe for patient disposition, acute distress, arousability; manner of dress, posture, body language, diaphoresis.

Vital Signs: Temperature, heart rate, respiratory rate, blood pressure, SpO_2 (oxygen saturation as measured by pulse oximetry), O_2 rate, O_2 delivery device, vent parameters.

HEENT (Head, Eyes, Ears, Nose/Neck, and Throat):

♦ Head. Observe for shape and evidence of trauma.
♦ Eyes. Observe pupils bilaterally for shape and reaction to light and accommodation, retinal fundi, sclera, icterus, discharge, tearing, glasses, contacts, reading glasses.
♦ Ears. Observe external ear, ear canal, tympanic membranes bilaterally, cerumen, discharge, hearing aids.
♦ Nose. Observe for inflammation, obstruction, discharge.
♦ Neck. Palpate cervical lymph nodes for palpable or fixed nodes and tenderness.
♦ Throat. Observe for jugular vein distention, thyroid location; palpate sublingual lymph nodes, thyroid; observe oropharynx, dentition, dental hygiene, dry or cracked lips. Auscultate carotid pulses bilaterally.

Respiratory: Observe chest excursion, use of accessory muscles, effort; palpate for tenderness; auscultate breath sounds in all lobes anterior/posterior, appreciate adventitious sounds, rales, rhonchi, wheezing; palpate fremitus, crepitus; percuss for dullness.

Cardiovascular: Observe posture, edema, cyanosis, cardiac assist devices; auscultate heart sounds; palpate peripheral pulses (radial, pedal) bilaterally.

Gastrointestinal: Observe for distention, abdominal ascites, ostomy, rectal tube, stool; auscultate bowel sounds in all four quadrants; palpate superficially and deep; observe for rebound tenderness; percuss for margins of abdominal organs.

Genitourinary: Observe for presence of urine, volume, color. Check external genitalia. Check for descended testes.

Musculoskeletal: Observe for spontaneous movements of extremities, muscle strength, spinal flexibility, temperature, deformities; left/right comparisons.

Neurological: Observe for level of consciousness, orientation, grossly intact cranial nerves II–XII, sensation in all extremities, full range of motion (ROM) in extremities, cerebellar reflexes, tremors, Romberg, gait.

Psychiatric: Observe for mood, affect, anxiety, disordered speech, language, delirium, hallucinations, capacity for decision-making, memory, attention span. An example tool for screening of cognition is the Saint Louis University Mental Status (SLUMS) examination.[32]

Integumentary: Observe for rashes, bruising, wounds, discoloration, mottling, lesions, nevi A asymmetry B border C color Dimension >6 mm (ABCD), venous access ports, complexion, makeup.

PPS: Determine the patient's current PPS score based on observations and collected data about the patient's ambulation, activity, and evidence of disease; self-care; intake; and level of consciousness.

Family: Assess and document the overall health of family members. Identification of the major health problems, physical limitations, and physical strengths of family members serves as a basis for care planning. The physical capabilities and constraints of the caregivers available to assist and support the patient may affect the plan of care, especially in relation to the most appropriate setting for care. This information also provides direction for the types of referrals that may be needed to provide care.

Adapted from Chovan John D. Principles of patient and family assessment. In: Ferrell BR, Paice J, eds. *Oxford Textbook of Palliative Nursing.* 5th ed. New York, NY: Oxford University Press; 2019:32–54.

TABLE 4.1 Common Physical Symptoms of Persons Who Are Actively Dying

Symptom	Definition
Agitation	Nonpurposeful movements associated with increased anxiety
Anorexia	No interest in eating or drinking
Confusion	Disorientation and lack of orderly thought
Delirium	An acute change in consciousness, cognition, and perceptual disturbances that can fluctuate throughout the day
Dyspnea	Shortness of breath
Fatigue	Overwhelming tiredness
Incontinence	Bladder, bowel
Insomnia	Difficulty sleeping
Mottling	Changes in skin color and temperature due to decreasing circulation that progresses from distal to proximal during the last 2–3 hours of life
Pain	PQRSTU (P is for pain and palliation, Q is for quality, R is for radiation, S is for severity, T is for timing, U is for understanding)
Restlessness	Uncontrollable increase in motor activity
Skin breakdown	Due to local ischemia secondary to immobility
Terminal secretions	Collection of saliva in the back of the throat that gurgles with each breath

Adapted from Chovan JD. Principles of patient and family assessment. In: Ferrell BR, Paice J, eds. *Oxford Textbook of Palliative Nursing.* 5th ed. New York, NY: Oxford University Press; 2019:32–54.

and caregivers about anxiety, depression, or fears is therapeutic in that it indicates that the clinician recognizes the stress of serious illness and considers these emotional responses to be important. When caring for pediatric patients, clinicians need to be mindful that children or adolescents may not identify with the words anxiety and depression, but it is still important to do a thorough psychological assessment using developmentally appropriate language (e.g., Do you feel sad? Do you worry about your parents? Do you enjoy spending time with your friends? Do you feel scared?).

Emotions often associated with serious illness include anxiety, depression, fear of the future, fear of being forgotten, death anxiety, and the stress of living with uncertainty. These emotions are intertwined with anticipatory grief, as patients and families face the many losses associated with serious illness and the ultimate future loss of life in terminal disease. When assessing psychological symptoms in pediatric and young adult patients, there may also be significant anxiety about a future life unfulfilled.[10,26,27]

It is also important to recognize that for caregivers, the experience of caring for a loved one with a life-threatening illness can cause increased psychological and emotional distress as well as feelings of guilt for not having enough time or energy to tend to other family members and tasks. Talking with patients and families and acknowledging the psychological and emotional stressors they may be experiencing offers an opportunity for relationship building and may be therapeutic in itself. Suggesting effective strategies to alleviate stress (e.g., self-care activities, community resources, relaxation techniques, meditation or prayer, yoga, memory making, journal writing, etc.) may help patients and families cope. Also, helping patients and families identify healthy coping strategies may enable them to effectively plan for the future when prognosis is unclear and life span may be limited.[28,29]

Patients and families should be assessed early in the illness for psychological concerns and emotional distress, especially given that the symptoms of anxiety and depression are common, treatable, and associated with distress and morbidity, yet are often unrecognized and undertreated, especially in children and adolescents.[30] As with physical symptoms, psychological symptoms can be assessed using structured instruments. Numerous detailed measures and screening tools exist. A common tool used in palliative care is the Distress Thermometer (National Comprehensive Cancer Network), which asks the patient to rate their overall distress on a scale of 0 to 10.[25] Simple rating scales are also often used for the most common symptoms of anxiety and depression. The Children's Depression Inventory[31] (CDI) and Beck Depression Inventory[32] are useful tools for assessing depression across the life span.

A key factor in psychosocial assessment is recognition of concerns that may have existed prior to the current serious illness as well as those symptoms associated with other comorbid disease. For example, chronic, well-managed depression or anxiety may be exacerbated once a new diagnosis is made or as the illness progresses. Assessing the presence of psychological symptoms early in the trajectory of care can facilitate early referral to support services such as social work, psychology, or psychiatry.

Spiritual Assessment

Spiritual care is one of the essential domains of quality palliative care.[2,8,9] Spirituality has been defined as "the aspect of humanity that refers to the way that individuals seek and express meaning and purpose and the way they experience their connectedness to the moment, to self, to others, to nature, and to the significant or sacred."[9]

Clinicians should include spiritual assessment as a component of their initial assessment for patients of all ages. One useful tool is the FICA (Faith, Import, Community, Address) instrument.[33]

The *FICA Spiritual History Tool* ©™ was developed by Dr. Christina Puchalski and a group of primary care physicians to help physicians and other healthcare professionals address spiritual issues with patients.[33] Spiritual histories are taken as part of the regular history during an annual examination or new patient visit, but can also be taken as part of follow-up visits, as appropriate. Patients and caregivers may feel challenged by or have doubts about their faith throughout the illness trajectory, and thus it is important to reassess spiritual aspects of care regularly. The FICA tool serves as a guide for conversations in the clinical setting.[34]

The acronym FICA can help structure questions in taking a spiritual history by healthcare professionals (Box 4.2).

BOX 4.2 FICA Acronym

F—Faith, Belief, Meaning

"Do you consider yourself spiritual or religious?" or "Is spirituality something important to you?" or "Do you have spiritual beliefs that help you cope with stress/difficult times?" (Contextualize to reason for visit if it is not the routine history.)

If the patient responds "No," the healthcare provider might ask, "What gives your life meaning?" Sometimes patients respond with answers such as family, career, or nature.

(The question of meaning should also be asked even if people answer yes to spirituality.)

I—Importance and Influence

"What importance does your spirituality have in your life?" "Has your spirituality influenced how you take care of yourself, your health?" "Does your spirituality influence you in your healthcare decision-making (e.g., advance directives, treatment, etc.)?"

C—Community

"Are you part of a spiritual community?" Communities such as churches, temples, and mosques, or a group of like-minded friends, family, or yoga groups can serve as strong support systems for some patients. Can explore further: "Is this of support to you and how?" "Is there a group of people you really love or who are important to you?"

A—Address in Care

"How would you like me, your healthcare provider, to address these issues in your healthcare?" (With the newer models including diagnosis of spiritual distress, the A in FICA also refers to the "Assessment and Plan" of patient spiritual distress or issues within a treatment or care plan.)

Understanding spiritual needs, spiritual distress, and the need for spiritual support assists clinicians in connecting patients to spiritual care providers in their communities or health settings. The growing diversity of the population means that clinicians care for patients from many different religions as well as for patients who have no identified religious preferences, yet may have important existential concerns when faced with serious illness. It is not possible for clinicians to be knowledgeable about all religions; therefore, an open approach to spiritual assessment is best. For example, a clinician might say, "I'm not really familiar with the Muslim faith, but I sense that this is important to you. How does your faith impact your present illness? How can we support you in your faith as we care for you?"

Recognizing spiritual beliefs early in the course of care can also be key to avoiding conflict later in the illness. For example, religious beliefs may be central to ethical dilemmas, such as a family decision regarding medically provided nutrition and hydration or discontinuing life support. Many cultural or ethical conflicts are deeply influenced by religious beliefs.

Many patients do not identify with a religious community, yet all people are considered spiritual, and a comprehensive assessment includes recognition of existential concerns. Assessing for spiritual and religious beliefs is an essential component of building trusting relationships with patients of all ages. It is helpful to ask even young children about their spiritual beliefs, using developmentally appropriate language, and to talk with other family members about their beliefs as well. This includes listening to concerns and using interdisciplinary colleagues such as chaplains and social workers to provide spiritual support. Table 4.2 includes common spiritual issues at end of life.

Adult Case Example

Jane Green, PA, described above, has been seeing Maria Gonzales in the palliative care clinic she coordinates. Maria is a 58-year-old patient with advanced breast cancer. Unfortunately, Maria has had numerous problems, including a recent aggressive metastasis of her disease involving her lungs and ribs. Her daughter reports that Maria has become very depressed, which has seemed to make her physical symptoms worse.

During the next clinic visit, Jane applies the principles described above of whole-person assessment. Jane uses the ESAS to measure Maria's symptoms and is able to initiate several treatments to manage her increasing dyspnea, constipation, and skin irritation associated with recent radiation for rib metastasis. She consults with the hospital palliative care team for input regarding Maria's pain, which has been difficult to control.

Jane also addresses Maria's depression and learns that her depression and distress are related to feeling that she has abandoned her elderly mother, who still resides in Mexico. She is unable to travel to visit her mother, as she can no longer tolerate the travel. Maria says she feels like such a "bad daughter" and "God will be so disappointed in me." Jane has included the clinic social worker in her plan of care as she knows these psychosocial and spiritual concerns will continue to be a predominant aspect of Maria's care and influence her physical and psychological symptoms.

Recognizing Maria's decline, Jane is also concerned about the future as Maria lives alone and has no advance directive, and Jane senses that Maria's daughter is extremely distressed. Jane recognizes that a plan is needed for care at the end of life, and she asks the social

TABLE 4.2 Spiritual Issues at the End of Life

Issues	Examples
Lack of meaning and purpose	"Why do I have to suffer on the way to death? Why couldn't I just go to my death in my sleep?" (meaninglessness of suffering) "I feel like I never really did anything important in life, and now it's too late." (purposelessness) "Why is my child suffering in this way? What is the point in a child suffering so much?"
Despair and hopelessness	"I just want to give up; it is not worth it anymore." (despair) Suicidal ideation (hopelessness)
Religious struggle	"Sometimes it is hard to believe there is a loving God upstairs that has my best interests in mind." "I used to believe . . . , but now how could I?" "How could God let this happen to our child?"
Not being remembered	"Death is just so final; I know my friends will eventually move on, and I'll have been like a blip on the monitor." "My parents will forget me. My friends will go on without me. Will anyone remember that I even existed?"
Guilt or shame	"I think my cancer is a punishment for something I did when I was young." (guilt) "I'm mortified that I'd get cancer in my private area." (shame) "I think we are being punished for not being better parents." "When I fought with my sibling I told him [her] I wish he [she] would die. This is my fault this is happening."
Loss of dignity	"Look and smell this body! It's so embarrassing. . . . It's not me anymore." "I'm such a burden now."
Lack of love, loneliness	"Everyone is so busy . . . too busy to take care of me." "Everyone is moving on with their lives, and I'm stuck here."
Anger at God/others	"Why would a loving God allow this to happen to me?" "Why did that corporation pollute the water where we lived for so long?" "How could God let this happen to my innocent child?"
Perceiving abandonment by God/others	"I feel like my prayers aren't being answered. . . . Where is God?" "The folks from church have stopped coming to visit; I guess I've been sick too long, and they are tired of me." "Having this disease makes me wonder if there even is a God."
Feeling out of control	"I'm ready to go . . . but it's not happening." "Why can't I do anything to stop this? I want to take care of my child. When will the suffering ever end?"
Need for reconciliation	Desire to be reunited with estranged family members "I haven't spoken to my father in a couple of years, but I want to see and talk with him before I die."
Grief from losses	Spiritual issues often accompany the various losses persons mourn when living with a terminal illness, such as the loss of independence; social roles and vocation; or body image and function. "I used to be the star of the team, and now I'm too sick and tired to even go to practice." "I always looked forward to attending the prom, but sadly I think I will have to miss it because I'm so sick."
Need for gratitude	"Now I have learned to appreciate the little things in life, and I'm just so happy for each new day that dawns." "I wish I didn't need to rely on others so much, but I am so thankful for how people do help me." "I love being surrounded by all the people who love me."

Adapted from Taylor EJ. Spiritual screening, history, and assessment, In: Ferrell BR, Paice J, eds. *Oxford Textbook of Palliative Nursing*. 5th ed. New York, NY: Oxford University Press; 2019:432–446.

worker if she can meet with Maria and her daughter to begin a conversation regarding end-of-life care and to discuss hospice referral. Jane will continue to follow Maria in the clinic until hospice is initiated.

Pediatric Case Example

Jane Green, PA, also has been following Emmanuel ("Manny") Chaning and his family, in the palliative care clinic. Manny is an 11-year-old boy with a progressive neurologic illness. He has a 7-year-old sister and a 2-year-old brother. His mother, Teresa, cares for Manny and his siblings full time and works part-time babysitting two other children in their home. She immigrated from Bolivia before Manny and his siblings were born. Manny's father, William, was born in the United States and works at a local factory. Both English and Spanish are spoken at home; although Manny has global developmental delays and says only a few words, he understands both English and Spanish. The family identifies as Catholic and says that their faith is very important to them. Manny is described by his mother as always being a very happy child. He gets physical, occupational, and speech therapy at home three times per week, as well as 12 hours of nursing assistance at home per week.

Unfortunately, Manny's condition, which is progressive in nature, has led to recent complications and subsequent overall worsening of his health status and quality of life. Manny has recently been having increasing difficulty breathing and now requires noninvasive respiratory support (i.e., bilevel positive airway pressure [BiPAP]) nearly 24 hours/day. He has had numerous health problems over the past year, including bilateral kidney stones, a pressure ulcer, and worsening scoliosis, and he was hospitalized three times for respiratory infections, including pneumonia.

Teresa (his mother) reports that Manny has not been acting "like himself" and hates wearing the BiPAP all the time; sometimes, he cries when it is being put on him. She and William (his father) are concerned that the pulmonologist brought up the option of a tracheostomy at Manny's last appointment. Maria reports that she has become very anxious while witnessing Manny's decline and is starting to feel like his care is getting to be more than she can handle at home. Additional nursing hours were denied by the insurance company, and Teresa would like to have her mother come from Bolivia to help with caring for the other kids at home, but her mother's visa has not yet been approved. William usually carries Manny up and down the stairs before and after work; he has been having back pain and is worried he will no longer be able to transport Manny, but they don't have room for a bed in the downstairs area of their apartment. Manny's parents tell Jane that they vowed that they would never "keep him alive on machines" if his quality of life couldn't be maintained and also promised Manny that they wouldn't let him suffer.

Jane is preparing for Manny's next clinic appointment and thinks about the physical, psychosocial, and spiritual aspects of care that are important to address at this time. She plans to have a Spanish interpreter present for the visit so that Teresa, who communicates fairly well in English, will have an opportunity to understand all of the details being discussed and to ask questions in her native language. Given the recent changes that Manny has experienced, Jane plans to do a very thorough assessment of Manny's physical status, focusing on the respiratory status changes. She prepares herself to talk with Manny's parents about the option of a tracheostomy if they seem ready to discuss it at this time. She consults with the hospital palliative care team to see if they will be available to participate in a goals-of-care discussion at the visit.

Jane also plans to assess Manny's mood. She knows that this may be difficult to do, given that he is nonverbal, but she plans to use the CDI with the assistance of Manny's parents to see if he is feeling anxious and/or sad. She will also ask Manny's parents if they or Manny's siblings have been feeling depressed or anxious and will refer them to appropriate community resources as needed. Jane remembers what Teresa and William told her at Manny's last appointment about how much they value Manny's quality of life and their promise to him not to let him suffer. Jane knows it will be important to keep those things in mind as she prepares to readdress Manny's goals of care with his family at his upcoming appointment. She also plans to ask the clinic social worker to be a part of this discussion.

Knowing that the family's Catholic faith is important to them, Jane also plans to use the FICA to do a thorough assessment of what spiritual resources may be most helpful at this time. Jane knows that there are a lot of things to discuss with Manny's parents at the upcoming appointment and is glad that she has built rapport with them over the past few visits and can use what they have shared about their values, goals, and wishes to guide their upcoming conversation. Jane recognizes that it will likely take more than one visit to address all of Manny's parents' concerns and plans to work with the clinic social worker and the hospital palliative care team to prioritize topics of conversation for Manny's upcoming appointment and subsequent visits.

Conclusion

Physician assistants and all clinicians caring for seriously ill patients and their families have a tremendous opportunity to improve the quality of care across the physical, psychosocial, and spiritual continuum. Comprehensive assessment of all domains is the foundation of this care, and documentation of patients' needs facilitates interdisciplinary collaboration. Designing palliative care initiatives for PAs builds on basic elements of patient assessment while recognizing unique patient, family, and caregiver needs.

References

1. Mazanec P, Reimer R, Bullington J, et al. Interdisciplinary palliative care teams. In: Ferrell BR, Paice J, eds. *Oxford Textbook of Palliative Nursing*. 5th ed. New York, NY: Oxford University Press; 2019:89–97.
2. Taylor E. Spiritual screening, history, and assessment. In: Ferrell BR, Paice J, eds. *Oxford Textbook of Palliative Nursing*. 5th ed. New York, NY: Oxford University Press; 2019:432–446.
3. Dahlin C, Coyne P, Ferrell B. *Textbook of Advanced Practice Palliative Nursing*. New York, NY: Oxford University Press; 2016.
4. Chovan J. Principles of patient and family assessment. In: Ferrell BR, Paice J, eds. *Oxford Textbook of Palliative Nursing*. 5th ed. New York, NY: Oxford University Press; 2019:32–54.
5. Maani-Fogelman P. Hospital-based palliative care. In: Ferrell BR, Paice J, eds. *Oxford Textbook of Palliative Nursing*. 5th ed. New York, NY: Oxford University Press; 2019:13–31.

6. Hui D, dos Santos R, Chisholm GB, Bruera E. Symptom expression in the last seven days of life among cancer patients admitted to acute palliative care units. *Journal of Pain and Symptom Management.* 2015;*50*(4):488–494.

7. Stajduhar K, Dionne-Odom N. Supporting families and family caregivers in palliative care. In: Ferrell BR, Paice J, eds. *Oxford Textbook of Palliative Nursing.* 5th ed. New York, NY: Oxford University Press; 2019:405–419.

8. Puchalski C, Ferrell B, Virani R, et al. Improving the quality of spiritual care as a dimension of palliative care: the report of the consensus conference. *Journal of Palliative Medicine.* 2009;*12*(10):885–904. doi:10.1089/jpm.2009.0142

9. Puchalski C, Ferrell BR. *Making Health Care Whole, Integrating Spirituality Into Patient Care.* West Conshohocken, PA: Templeton Press; May 2010.

10. Chrastek JJ, van Breemen C. Symptom management in pediatric palliative care. In: Ferrell BR, Paice J, eds. *Oxford Textbook of Palliative Nursing.* 5th ed. New York, NY: Oxford University Press; 2019:699–707.

11. McDaniel C, Desai JM. Pediatric goals of care. In: Ferrell BR, Paice J, eds. *Oxford Textbook of Palliative Nursing.* 5th ed. New York, NY: Oxford University Press; 2019:727–735.

12. O'Brien JH, Root MC. Pediatric pain. In: Ferrell BR, Paice J, eds. *Oxford Textbook of Palliative Nursing.* 5th ed. New York, NY: Oxford University Press; 2019:773–782.

13. Jang RW, Caraiscos VB, Swami N, et al. Simple prognostic model for patients with advanced cancer based on performance status. Palliative Performance Scale. *Journal of Oncology Practice.* 2014;*10*(5):e335–341. doi:10.1200/JOP.2014.001457. https://www.ncbi.nlm.nih.gov/pubmed/25118208/

14. Varni JW. PedsQLTM Measurement Model for the Pediatric Quality of Life InventoryTM. 2019. https://www.pedsql.org/about_pedsql.html

15. Bruera E, Kuehn N, Miller MJ, Selmser P, Macmillan K. The Edmonton Symptom Assessment System (ESAS): a simple method for the assessment of palliative care patients. *Journal of Palliative Care.* 1991;*7*(2):6–9. https://www.ncbi.nlm.nih.gov/pubmed/1714502

16. Dupuis LL, Ethier M-C, Tomlinson D, Hesser T, Sung L. A systematic review of symptom assessment scales in children with cancer. *BMC Cancer.* 2012;*12*:430. doi:10.1186/1471-2407-12-430

17. National Comprehensive Cancer Network. Adult cancer pain clinical practice guideline. 2016. https://www.nccn.org/. Accessed June 6, 2019.

18. Fink R, Gates R, Jeffers K. Pain assessment. In: Ferrell BR, Paice J, eds. *Oxford Textbook of Palliative Nursing.* 5th ed. New York, NY: Oxford University Press; 2019:98–115.

19. Collett D, Chow K. Nausea and vomiting. In: Ferrell BR, Paice J, eds. *Oxford Textbook of Palliative Nursing.* 5th ed. New York, NY: Oxford University Press; 2019:149–162.

20. Klinedinst R, Kurash-Cohen A, Dahlin C. Dysphagia, hiccups, and other oral symptoms. In: Ferrell BR, Paice J, eds. *Oxford Textbook of Palliative Nursing.* 5th ed. New York, NY: Oxford University Press; 2019:163–185.

21. Mooney S, Patel P, Buga S. Bowel management: constipation, obstruction, diarrhea, and ascites. In: Ferrell BR, Paice J, eds. *Oxford Textbook of Palliative Nursing.* 5th ed. New York, NY: Oxford University Press; 2019:186–205.

22. Lanz K, Gabriel M, Tschanz J. Medically administered nutrition and hydration. In: Ferrell BR, Paice J, eds. *Oxford Textbook of Palliative Nursing.* 5th ed. New York, NY: Oxford University Press; 2019:206–216.

23. Shwartz SK, Morris RD, Penna S. Psychometric properties of the Saint Louis University Mental Status (SLUMS) Examination. *Applied Neuropsychology. Adult.* 2019;*26*:101–110. doi:10.1080/23279095.2017.1362407

24. Salman J, Wolfe E, Patel S. Anxiety and depression. In: Ferrell BR, Paice J, eds. *Oxford Textbook of Palliative Nursing.* 5th ed. New York, NY: Oxford University Press; 2019:309–318.

25. National Comprehensive Cancer Network. *NCCN Clinical Practice Guidelines in Oncology (NCCN Guidelines) for Distress Management.* Version 1. 2017. https://www.nccn.org/about/news/ebulletin/ebulletindetail.aspx?ebulletinid=1120. Accessed July 1, 2019.

26. Wiener L, Kazak AE, Noll RB, Patenaude AF, Kupst MJ. Standards for the psychosocial care of children with cancer and their families: an introduction to the special issue. *Pediatric Blood and Cancer*. 2015;*62*:S419–S424.

27. Gatto M, Thomas P, Berger A. Anxiety. In: Dahlin C, Coyne PJ, Ferrell BR, eds. *Advanced Practice Palliative Nursing*. New York, NY: Oxford University Press; 2016:301–310.

28. Battista V, LaRagione G. Pediatric hospice and palliative care. In: Ferrell BR, Paice J, eds. *Oxford Textbook of Palliative Nursing*. 5th ed. New York, NY: Oxford University Press; 2019:708–726.

29. Battista V, Mosher PJ. Palliative care for the infant, child, or adolescent with spinal muscular atrophy (SMA). In: Ferguson V, ed. *Pediatric Life-Limiting Conditions*. Pittsburgh, PA: Hospice and Palliative Nurses Association; 2014:165–186.

30. Mullaney EK, Santucci G. Symptom management in pediatric palliative care. In: Santucci G, ed. *Core Curriculum for the Pediatric Hospice and Palliative Nurse*. 2nd ed. Pittsburgh, PA: Hospice and Palliative Nurses Association; 2017:73–107.

31. Helsel WJ, Matson JL. The assessment of depression in children: the internal structure of the Child Depression Inventory (CDI). *Behaviour Research and Therapy*. 1984;*22*(3):289–298. http://doi.org/10.1016/0005-7967(84)90009-3

32. Beck AT, Ward CM, Mendelson M, Mock JE, Erbaugh JK. An inventory for measuring depression. *Archives of General Psychiatry*. 1961;*4*:561–571.

33. FICA Spiritual History Tool. GW Institute for Spirituality and Health. 1996. https://smhs.gwu.edu/spiritually-health/program/transforming-practice-health-settings/clinical-fica-tool

34. Puchalski C, Romer AL. Taking a spiritual history allows clinicians to understand patients more fully. *Journal of Palliative Medicine*. 2000;*3*(1):129–137.

5

Enhanced Communication Skills

Myra Glajchen and Christine Wilkins

Introduction

Since its inception, palliative medicine has embraced good communication as the corner-stone of quality care and integrated communication techniques into best practices and clinical practice guidelines.[1] According to the National Consensus Project for Quality Palliative Care, communication is an essential requirement in palliative care and includes communication within the team, with patients and family caregivers, with other clinicians, and with community providers.[2] This chapter highlights definitions, evidence-based research, training, and best clinical practices in three areas of communication: narrative medicine, goals-of-care discussions, and the family meeting.

Narrative Medicine

Narrative medicine is an educational tool that integrates reading, writing, telling, and receiving stories. It invites healthcare professionals to be moved by the story of illness and promotes a healing relationship with patients, colleagues, and the self. For years, medical educators have attempted to train students in the more introspective and relational aspects of clinical practice to balance the impersonal, technological, and emotional demands of modern medicine.[3] Narrative medicine highlights listening, empathy, and reflection as key multidimensional concepts involving cognitive and affective domains. By promoting empathy, narrative medicine helps physicians build a trusting relationship with their patients and even enhance treatment outcomes. Narrative medicine was first introduced by Rita Charon in 2000 as a clinical practice defined by the ability to recognize, absorb, interpret, and act on the stories of others.[4]

Considerable overlap exists between narrative medicine and palliative care. Both emphasize patient-centered care, both help the patient derive meaning from their illness, both highlight humanistic practice, and both promote excellent listening skills. Palliative care trains team members in "life review," which presupposes that palliative care clinicians are willing and able to bear witness to the stories of dying patients as their final legacy. Ultimately, listening to patients' final stories enables palliative care professionals to develop a deeper understanding of the patient's priorities, validates patients' suffering, and acknowledges their common humanity.[5]

Research

Narrative medicine has been studied as a means of developing clinical skills of medical students, physicians, nurses, social workers, mental health professionals, chaplains, physician assistants, academics, and others. Training in narrative medicine develops and improves specific communication skills, enhances the capacity to collaborate, adopts a patient-centered approach, and helps physicians develop personally and professionally through reflection.[6] [8] But although research suggests that techniques like guided narrative writing can lead to reflective thinking and enhanced empathy, very few definitive studies have shown a causal relationship. In addition, studies have been modest in size, women have shown a greater increase in empathy scores compared to their male counterparts, the long-term effects of training can change over time, and increases in physician empathy have not been linked to better patient outcomes.[9]

In a review of 36 articles, the effectiveness of narrative medicine programs was assessed. Results showed a positive impact in changing medical students' attitudes, knowledge, and skills. But there was no definite evidence that narrative medicine training affected ongoing interaction with colleagues or that narrative medicine in the classroom positively impacted patient care.[10]

While narrative medicine holds great promise for enhancing communication in palliative care, further research is needed to identify and validate outcomes for practitioners and patients alike.

Training

Narrative medicine is taught through textbooks, undergraduate and graduate degree programs, workshops, and retreats. Nursing has shown promise by grounding training programs in narrative medicine theory.[11-13] Model narrative medicine programs for physicians are proliferating at medical schools across the United States (Columbia University, Harvard, University of California–Irvine, Baylor, Temple, others). At Columbia University in New York City, narrative medicine is offered through a full- or part-time master's program and through an online nondegree certificate program. A multidisciplinary curriculum is taught by clinicians and nonclinicians, with experts and specialists in creative writing, philosophy, film, anthropology, and history. In addition, to the coursework, students are provided with personalized career guidance to help them achieve their personal and professional goals. Courses are open to healthcare professionals, including physician assistants; trainees in clinical disciplines such as medicine, nursing, dentistry, social work, physical therapy, occupational therapy, psychoanalysis, and pastoral care; and students or alumni of graduate programs in other fields, such as literature, journalism, medical anthropology, and other social sciences.[14] The Accreditation Council for Graduate Medical Education has created a milestone evaluation to achieve competency in such areas as communication, collaboration, and professionalism, which has greatly spurred interest in narrative medicine training.[15] In addition, the Accreditation Review Commission on Education for the Physician Assistant (ARC-PA) standards mention education, self-care, reflection, and prevention of burnout.[16]

Best Practices

Best practices in narrative medicine help students improve their listening and observation skills and increase their capacity for empathy and reflection.[10] Narrative Medicine practices include reflective journaling, writing, essays, self-care, and self-reflection.[17] According to Charon, empathetic doctor-patient engagement, concerted training in self-reflective practices, and exposure to the arts—film, music, paintings, sculpture, or literature—lead to a better sense of self and more meaningful relationships with patients. Practicing narrative medicine techniques allows healthcare providers to reconnect to their passion for helping others and process the emotional stress of working with the sick and dying while also preventing burnout.

Narrative medicine has been used successfully in oncology practice settings. Through the use of narrative competence and empathy, several studies have shown improvements in clinical assessment of pain and other symptoms.[18] In addition, rather than adding time to clinical appointments, narrative medicine can save time through more targeted communication based on empathy and trust.

Serious Illness Communication and Goals-of-Care Discussions

Enhanced communication between providers, patients, and families is an essential component of caring for patients with serious illness. In the seminal report *Dying in America*, clinician-patient communication and advance care planning (ACP) form one of the five domains of quality patient care for individuals with serious illness.[19] Similarly, a review and synthesis of best practices in communication about serious illness care goals, conducted by the American College of Physicians High Value Task Care Force (2014), emphasized that, for patients facing serious illness, an understanding of their care goals allows clinicians to align care with what matters most to the patient.[20]

Definitions

Serious illnesses carry a high risk of death, adversely impact quality of life, and are burdensome in terms of patient symptoms, treatment, and caregiver stress.[21] Serious illness typically includes life-threatening conditions, advanced stages of chronic diseases, comorbidities, and frailty.[22] Serious illness communication addresses goals of care, ACP, and end-of-life care. Experts agree that a number of strategies are essential for serious illness communication, among them exploring goals, values, and preferences; discussing prognosis; responding to patient and family emotions; and recommending a plan aligned with the patient's values and priorities.[23]

Advance care planning supports adults in exploring, understanding, and sharing their personal goals, values, and preferences regarding future healthcare.[24-26] ACP is particularly important for individuals facing serious illness to clarify their preferences and promote goal-concordant care.[24] Quality ACP emphasizes person-centered conversations that result in meaningful advance directives (ADs) and actionable medical orders such as the Physician Orders for Life-Sustaining Treatment (POLST; www.polst.org). Ideally, person-centered conversations should begin early in the illness trajectory when patients can participate in a meaningful way and include healthcare agents, ensure that patients understand their medical condition and treatment options, and provide information about cardiopulmonary resuscitation (CPR) and other life-sustaining treatment. Such conversations are often documented on the POLST form, which provides medical orders to emergency personnel when the person is unable to communicate. POLST is appropriate for patients with serious illness or frailty.

Research

In a cross-sectional survey study of bereaved parents of children, adolescents, and young adults, parents reported that ACP was important.[27] The majority (70%) wanted ACP discussions earlier in the illness course. Parents who engaged in ACP were more likely to feel prepared for their children's final days of life and report their child's quality of life as good to excellent.

Despite the broad consensus among healthcare providers that quality conversations with patients are essential, research identifies gaps and barriers to care. Patients' emotions, especially anxiety and denial, combined with clinicians' own discomfort influence the quality and occurrence of serious illness conversations.[28]

The timing of ACP conversations is challenging. Most conversations occur during acute hospital admissions when patients and families have high distress and when patients' decision-making may be impaired due to illness, treatment side effects, or frailty. Findings from a prospective cohort study of 2155 patients with stage IV lung or colorectal cancer revealed that, although 87% of the patients who died had end-of-life discussions documented in the medical record, conversations took place only 1 month before death.[29] In addition, most of these conversations occurred in acute care and did not include the patients' oncologists or their primary care providers.

In another study, 118 healthcare professionals from community-based clinics participated in an online survey to evaluate policies, clinical routines, and workflow processes for ACP.[30] The results demonstrated that interprofessional team members played an important role in facilitating ACP, and despite most settings not knowing of or not having ACP policies, two-thirds of the respondents believed that addressing ACP was a high priority. The development of clinical routines to address ACP emerged as a priority for respondents.

Uncertainty about prognostic accuracy may pose a barrier to goals-of-care discussions.[28] Healthcare professionals commonly believe that sharing accurate prognostic information with patients will destroy hope. However, in a 2012 review, Mack and Smith[31] found that patients coped better when they were provided with honest prognostic information because this facilitated their ability to make informed healthcare decisions in keeping with their values, goals, and preferences.

Similarly, in a study conducted with 203 adolescents and young adults with cancer, 80% of newly diagnosed patients considered prognostic information extremely or very important.[32] Few found the prognosis details upsetting, and those who did wanted more information. Patients who received detailed prognostic information had higher odds of trust in the oncologist and hope with regard to physician communication.

Inadequate communication between healthcare professionals and patients leads to physical and psychological suffering.[19] When patients are not informed about their diagnosis, prognosis, and treatment options and they cannot meaningfully engage in discussions, they risk receiving care that is not concordant with their wishes.[33,34]

Patients suffer emotionally and physically from nonbeneficial treatments that prolong the dying process.[35] Family members experience distress as they are offered disease treatment while witnessing the patient's suffering. Healthcare providers experience moral distress as they accompany patients through life-sustaining interventions perceived as futile.[36] The term *moral distress* was first coined by Jameton, "who observed amongst nurses a tendency to feel distressed when they were forced to act, because of institutional constraints, in way that was contrary to their beliefs."[37] An Institute of Medicine report[19] emphasized the need for serious illness conversations to start earlier in the illness trajectory, facilitated by the primary care provider, who knows the patient best. Earlier conversations about goals of care are linked with better quality of life, reduced use of nonbeneficial medical care at end of life, goal-concordant care, positive patient and family outcomes, and reduced costs.[28]

Engaging patients and families in quality conversations to improve surgical decision-making is also important. In one study, a patient and family advisory council (PFAC) was created to identify decisions needed prior to surgery.[38] The PFAC included a panel with prior high-risk surgery experience as patients or family members. They developed a three-question prompt to assist future patients: "Should I have surgery?" "What should I expect if everything goes well?" and "What happens if things go wrong?" The importance of shared decision-making was emphasized in a second study designed to teach surgeons the best case/worst case framework to enhance person-centered communication during high-stakes surgical decisions.[39] Integrating discussion of the patient's overall quality-of-life goals and wishes into shared decision-making is essential.[40]

For children with serious illness, understanding the family's narrative about their child's illness and their definition of quality of life is essential for effective goals-of-care conversations.[41] Involving providers with a long-standing relationship with the child and family is essential. Particularly challenging for families of children with serious illness is prognostic uncertainty given that newer technologies and interventions allow children to live longer with increased medical complexities. This means that with pediatric patients, as with adult patients, goals-of-care conversations need to be ongoing and adapted over time.

Education and Training

All providers need training that prepares them for "basic" or "primary" palliative care. This training seeks to equip all providers with the skills for high-quality symptom management, as well as how to engage patients in quality conversations earlier in their illness trajectory and promote earlier referrals to palliative care or hospice when needed. Training for healthcare providers must focus on giving a direct, honest prognosis; recognizing and exploring emotions; and focusing on patients' quality of life, goals, fears, and concerns.[28]

Various programs provide quality training opportunities in palliative care. Among these are (1) the Center to Advance Palliative Care (CAPC) at the Icahn School of Medicine; (2) the Communication in Serious Illness Program, founded by Ariadne Labs, at Harvard Medical School and Dana-Farber Cancer Institute; and (3) Respecting Choices, founded by Gundersen Health System. Other programs include End-of-Life Nursing Education Consortium (ELNEC) training, a national education initiative whose mission is to improve palliative care in the United States and internationally; Education in Palliative and End-Of-Life Care (EPEC); and VitalTalk. See Table 5.1 for a summary of these programs

The essential aspects of these programs need to be incorporated into training for all healthcare providers as they prepare to become skilled in working with patients with serious illness.[12]

TABLE 5.1 Training Opportunities in Palliative Care

Program	Details
CAPC	■ Includes several online offerings as part of their Communication Skills Courses series, including ACP modules to train physicians and advanced practitioners. ■ Provides online training on how to facilitate family meetings, and deliver serious news. (https://www.capc.org/training/communication-skills/)
Communication in Serious Illness Program (Ariadne Labs)	■ Provides in-person "train-the-trainer" courses. This training includes the Serious Illness Conversation Guide, with review materials for patients and families. ■ The program focuses on sharing prognostic information, eliciting decision-making preferences, understanding fears and goals, exploring trade-offs and impaired function, and wishes for family involvement.[28] (https://www.ariadnelabs.org/areas-of-work/serious-illness-care/)
Respecting Choices	■ Provides facilitator certification training in staged approach to advance care planning called First Steps (FS), Next Steps (NS), and Advanced Steps (AS). Programs consist of daylong, in-person training sessions combined with online modules. Conversation guides, decision aids, and patient and family educational materials are included. ■ Offers the Shared Decision Making in Serious Illness (SDMSI) program, which is a newer program focused on physicians, residents, advanced nurse practitioners, and physician assistants. Whereas the Respecting Choices ACP programs focus on future healthcare decisions, the SDMSI program centers on decisions regarding current serious illness care. (https://respectingchoices.org/)
ELNEC	■ Offers in-person train-the-trainer courses and online training that helps equip nurses and other healthcare providers with skills for caring for individuals with serious illness. (https://www.aacnnursing.org/ELNEC)
EPEC	■ Focuses on educating healthcare professionals in the essential clinical competencies of palliative and end-of-life care to ensure that all patients receive the primary palliative care they need. (https://www.bioethics.northwestern.edu/programs/epec/)
VitalTalk	■ Provides evidence-based programs to train clinicians in communication that is culturally sensitive, interprofessional, and centered on patient values. (https://www.vitaltalk.org/)

Best Practices

System workflow redesign can improve serious illness communication.[43] Enhanced electronic medical record (EMR) systems make it possible to identify patients who would benefit from these valuable conversations and prompt clinicians to begin these conversations early in the illness trajectory. On the inpatient side, the mandatory surprise question that asks, "Would you be surprised if the patient died in the next year?" is a popular trigger for identifying patients appropriate for serious illness communication. Follow-up when the patient is discharged is also important. In a study that focused on ACP for patients with heart failure, a discharge order set that included a referral for ACP was created to ensure that patients received ACP follow-up.[44]

Better still, in primary care, creating a mechanism to promote interdisciplinary practice that helps identify patients expected to die in the next 1 to 2 years and an infrastructure that provides coordination among the varying care providers to facilitate serious illness communication are important.[45-48] Revisiting goals of care and preferences every year, when there is an acute event or change in functional or health status, when considering major procedures or interventions, and when there is a change in social support or living situation is important.[49] Other features include preparing both clinicians and patients for these conversations, receiving EMR reminders during routine care,[50] assigning a trained facilitator to conduct the discussions, and designating time for the conversation.[51]

In a study that focused on ACP conversations in primary care, interventions included staff training, physician coaching, and EMR enhancements.[52] In phase 1 of the study, ACP conversations were facilitated with 7200 unique patients. In phase 2, when ACP was initiated, and average of 29% of conversations led to an AD in the chart. There was a wide variety in the number of conversations that led to an AD being completed, from a low of 6% to a high of 70% for a 10-month period. In phase 3, 7589 new ACP conversations were conducted. Findings clearly demonstrated that this systematic approach resulted in an increase and sustained number of ACP conversations facilitated.

Further, a thorough discussion regarding the benefits and burdens of CPR and other life-sustaining treatment is essential in chronic and serious illness communication. Decision aids[53,54] and videos[55] demonstrating how CPR is conducted can be helpful in ensuring that patients make informed decisions.

The Family Meeting

The family meeting is an intervention frequently used in the context of advanced medical illness and end-of-life care. In specialist palliative care, the family meeting is usually initiated by the team to facilitate communication, discuss the illness experience, present treatment choices, and facilitate end-of-life decision-making. The family meeting, also called the family conference or the patient-family conference, is not rigidly defined in the literature. The term *family* is not strictly defined as blood relatives of the patient, but rather, whoever the patient considers family. Staff who attend the family meeting generally include members of several disciplines from the interdisciplinary team.[56]

Indications for the family meeting include transition points in care, ACP, surrogate decision-making, conflict resolution, and ethical dilemmas. The family meeting can also be used as a forum to communicate new information regarding prognosis, treatment options, and anticipated outcomes; determine the patient's goals of care; and provide emotional support.[57]

Research

Family meetings have been most widely used and studied in the intensive care unit (ICU) setting.[58,59] A growing body of evidence also points to the use of the family meeting in oncology and, more recently, in palliative care.[60-62]

Indications for the family meeting are generally setting specific. In the ICU setting, the family meeting is routinely arranged within 72 hours of admission for patients with a mortality risk greater than 25% and significant decline in functional status. Other indicators include a length of stay of 10 or more days in the hospital, older age (80+), and two or more life-threatening comorbidities. In the context of ICU family meetings, it is common to discuss procedures under consideration: tracheotomy, ventilator, or feeding tube.[63] In palliative care, the indications for the family meeting tend to include sharing new prognostic information, managing family conflict, addressing ethical issues, and seeking consensus for treatment decisions. The family meeting is also useful for surrogate decision-making, especially in the absence of a designated healthcare agent.[64-66] The family meeting is considered to be an ideal setting in which to introduce hospice and provide family support.

Research on family meetings in the ICU revealed a set of challenges obstructing high-quality communication, including missed opportunities for shared decision-making, domination of the discussion by physicians, lack of confidence by nurses and social workers about the extent of their participation, and a deemphasis on listening to families and acknowledging their emotions.

Although family meetings are prevalent in palliative care, little evidence currently exists to guide healthcare professionals in conducting the meeting. A systematic review of the literature analyzed 24 studies where the family meeting was the primary intervention. Patient and family outcomes included higher satisfaction, enhanced psychological well-being, and well-planned decisions regarding medical interventions. In further analyzing the relationship among variables, family satisfaction was increased by specific clinician communication behaviors, including a greater percentage of time for family speaking; clinician expressions of support, especially the assurances of nonabandonment, patient comfort and alleviation of suffering, and empathy for what family members were experiencing; shared decision-making; and support for family decisions. Direct participation in a family conference improved psychological well-being, as measured by pre- and postmeeting questionnaires. The authors concluded that the evidence is strong for improved family coping when their emotional and informational needs are effectively addressed during the family meeting.[67]

A systematic review of studies reporting empirical data from 1980 to 2015 reported low-level evidence to support family meetings. Only two quantitative pre- and poststudies used a validated palliative care family outcome measure, and only four other studies reported significant results using nonvalidated measures.[56] Because the family meeting is so labor intensive in terms of preparation and meeting and follow-up time and so emotionally charged for patients and families, more research and validated outcome measures are needed before this can be routinely integrated into palliative care practice. Similarly, a recent observational study reviewed 10 family meetings in the pediatric cardiac intensive care unit at the Children's Hospital of Philadelphia. In measuring and comparing the communication behaviors of interprofessional team members, physicians dominated the conversation; parents' understanding was infrequently checked; and parents expressed emotion an average of four times per meeting, and although the clinicians responded empathically to some statements, this was the least of their contribution. While the nurses and social workers complemented the skills of the physician, they only spoke when invited to do so by the physician. The authors concluded that role coordination and collaboration are essential for improving communication during the family meeting. In addition to responding to emotion and identifying parents' understanding and concerns, team members should clarify their role assignments by discipline and ensure that patients and families understand which team members are responsible for which follow-up activities.[68]

In spite of these limitations, existing studies showed promise in that the family meeting is associated with less time in ICU, earlier withdrawal of technology, and timely referral to palliative care and hospice[69-71]; model programs show the feasibility of changing practice patterns through upstreaming referrals[72]; tools to increase caregiver confidence can maximize the effectiveness of the family meeting; and the benefits of family meetings for bereaved caregivers cannot be overlooked. Bereaved family caregivers are at risk for prolonged grief disorder, depression, demoralization, and posttraumatic stress disorder following the loss of a loved one. The burden is especially high for surrogate decision-makers who make decisions during complex or urgent situations without clear guidance about the patient's preferences or goals of care. Family members may experience guilt or remorse over their decisions regarding tube feedings, resuscitation, and withdrawing or withholding life support, leaving them to manage additional emotional suffering during bereavement.[67,73] Shared decision-making during the family meeting can ameliorate these unfortunate outcomes.

Training

Most providers do not receive formal training in conducting family meetings and do not feel adequately prepared to lead them. The range of skills needed to lead productive meetings include skills on how to facilitate a group, empathic communication, family support, minimization of stress, and consensus-based decision-making.[74]

Healthcare tools can assist in standardizing family meetings and increase their effectiveness. Decision support aids, clinical templates, and checklists have been shown to improve screening/assessment, documentation, communication, and the family meeting, especially when they are incorporated into the electronic health record.[75,76]

Model training programs include the six-step SPIKES protocol used to train clinicians in giving bad news to patients and families; the Communication Skills Training Program at Memorial Sloan-Kettering; communication courses through the Center to Advance Palliative Care; communication skills training through California State University; and the webinar series called Palliative Care in the ICU: Critical Communication Skills through the

American Association of Critical Care Nurses. The Serious Illness Communication Program by Ariadne Labs and the Respecting Choices shared decision-Making program's SPIKES training includes templated guides for setting the stage, exploring what the patient knows, obtaining permission to share information, responding empathically to patient emotions, summarizing the discussion, and concluding with a plan.[77] The Com Skill curriculum provides training in breaking bad news, discussing unanticipated adverse events, discussing prognosis, reaching a shared treatment decision, responding to difficult emotions, coping with survivorship, running a family meeting, and transitioning to palliative care and end of life .[78–80]

Best Practices

Most family meetings are structured in the same way, with a preparation phase, a talk phase, and a follow-up phase. Prior to the meeting, team members are encouraged to preplan, review the medical chart, obtain a medical update from current and former providers, and get input from other disciplines, including the physician, nurse practitioner, physician assistant nurse, social worker, and chaplain. A quiet space should be arranged with dedicated uninterrupted time for all team members. Important a priori decisions include who will lead the meeting, who speaks for the family, whose agenda will be followed, who will take notes, who will summarize the meeting in the chart, and who will take responsibility for follow-up tasks.[61]

During the talk phase of the family meeting, a team member should introduce the purpose of meeting, explore what family caregivers wish to discuss, and make the agenda explicit. It is important to adopt a conversational tone and respond to difficult emotions.[73] During the course of the meeting, the team is likely to provide the patient and family with new information; it is important to tailor the information to the patient's and family's level and check their understanding along the way.

In the context of palliative care, the family meeting provides a forum through which both the primary and the palliative team validate the role of family caregivers and actively involve them in ACP. Making treatment decisions can be burdensome, especially during the terminal phase of illness. The family meeting provides opportunities to share the burden of decision-making with the family, review the benefits and burdens of different treatments, recommend against futile treatment, and reach consensus. If the patient is terminal, the family should be told what to expect during the dying process.

After the family meeting, the family should be offered support services (social work, patient advocacy, chaplaincy, ethics consultation, palliative care), and appropriate referrals based on their choices should be made. The team member who leads the family meeting should summarize the meeting content in person and in the medical record, summarize an action plan at the end, and check in with the patient and caregivers for any ongoing concerns. If possible, the team should debrief and clarify next steps.[61]

To the extent possible, it is advisable to identify the concerns of family caregivers ahead of time and allow staff and family to develop a joint meeting agenda. A Canadian study confirmed the value of planned multidisciplinary family meetings. The study utilized the Family Inventory of Needs to identify areas of greatest importance to family members before the meeting. In addition, a repeated self-report instrument showed reduction in concerns and increased confidence for family caregivers following their participation in the family meeting.[81]

Palliative care has been more readily available to adults than pediatric patients. Similarly, the family meeting is rarely used in pediatrics, and there is limited guidance about whether children should be included in the meeting. Certainly, such decisions should take the developmental needs of the child into account. Teenagers with HIV/AIDS and advanced cancer prefer to participate in their own ACP. Families who decided to speak with their children about death reported that they were pleased with that decision, while one-third of families who did not discuss death with their child regretted that decision later.[82] The literature suggests that missed opportunities exist for engaging in family conferences with parents of pediatric ICU patients who face life-altering decisions.[83] Promising lines of inquiry include the timing of the family meeting, the impact of meetings on length of stay and satisfaction with care, and evidence-based guidelines on decision-making and goals of care.[82]

Studies show the potential and the challenges in telehealth as a platform for family meetings in palliative care and hospice. One study compared web-based video and telephone meetings to include hospice caregivers in 200 hospice interdisciplinary team (IDT) meetings. The study showed the superiority of web-based video in image quality but less so in audio quality.[84] A second study showed the value of telemedicine in providing palliative care consultation for critically ill patients transferring from rural hospitals to tertiary care centers.[85] Because video and audio quality impact communication, preparation and technical expertise are essential for both staff and families. Future studies should focus on improvement of the technical quality of telehealth sessions in order to facilitate quality delivery of telemedicine.

Case Example

Mary was a 63-year-old Caucasian female diagnosed with a recurrence of breast cancer 8 months ago. Soon after she was given this news, and following a conversation with her oncologist about the diagnosis, treatment options, and prognosis, she was referred to the ACP program to discuss her goals of care and wishes regarding CPR and other life-sustaining treatments.

Mary was very clear that her goal was to get better and live well for as long as possible. Living well included spending quality time with her family, enjoying nature, visiting museums, and traveling. Her independence was very important to her. She emphasized that she would not want CPR should her heart or breathing suddenly stop. She was fine with a trial intubation if she experienced difficulty breathing; however, she would no longer want this if she was unable to recognize herself or her loved ones.

John, her partner and health-care agent, was encouraged to attend a follow-up session where he was able to ask questions and confirm that he could honor Mary's healthcare decisions. He was also encouraged to explore his own feelings and allow himself to begin the pregrieving process. An eMOLST (New York State electronic Medical Orders for Life-Sustaining Treatment) and healthcare proxy were completed and scanned in the Advance

Care Planning Navigator section of the EMR, and the corresponding code status order was entered in the EMR.

The names of the primary and secondary healthcare agents were entered in the ACP eNavigator, and an ACP note was completed. When the patient later presented to the emergency department, the care team was easily able to retrieve the eMOLST, code status, ACP note, and healthcare proxy. Building on previous serious illness communication efforts, the team, in collaboration with the healthcare agent, was able to honor the patient's wishes. Mary had sustained a massive stroke, and the medical team believed there was minimal chance that she would recover. Given this new diagnosis and poor prognosis, John agreed that Mary be allowed to die with dignity and not suffer. Mary was transitioned to inpatient hospice, where she died peacefully a few days later. John was sad but felt that he honored her wishes, and this allowed him to grieve more effectively.

Conclusion

Quality serious illness communication is essential as modern medicine contributes to increased survival of adults and children with serious illness. Quality healthcare mandates that all healthcare clinicians receive training in communication to ensure that treatment is patient and family centered. Enhanced communication in palliative care requires a systematic approach that incorporates (1) high-quality training for healthcare professionals across disciplines; (2) clearly defined indicators for serious illness conversations and family meetings; (3) documentation in the EMR; (4) metrics that document outcomes; (5) commitment from organizational leadership; and (6) recognition and reimbursement for these interventions by policymakers and insurers.

References

1. Wittenberg E, Ferrell BR, Goldsmith J, Smith T, Glajchen M, Handzo GF, eds. *Textbook of Palliative Care Communication*. Oxford University Press. 2015.
2. National Consensus Project for Quality Palliative Care. *Clinical Practice Guidelines for Quality Palliative Care*. 4th ed. Richmond, VA: National Coalition for Hospice and Palliative Care; 2018. https://www.nationalcoalitionhpc.org/ncp. Accessed September 6, 2019.
3. Miller E, Dorene D, Hermann N, Graham G, Charon R. Sounding narrative medicine: studying students' professional identity development at Columbia University College of Physicians and Surgeons. *Academic Medicine*. 2014;89(2):335–342.
4. Charon R. Narrative medicine: a model for empathy, reflection, profession, and trust. *JAMA*. 2001;286:1897–1902.
5. Stanley P, Hurst M. Narrative palliative care: a method for building empathy. *Journal of Social Work in End-of-Life & Palliative Care*. 2011;7:39–55.
6. Arntfield SL, Slesar K, Dickson J, Charon R. Narrative medicine as a means of training medical students toward residency competencies. *Patient Education and Counseling*. 2013;91:280–286.
7. DasGupta S, Charon R. Personal illness narratives: using reflective writing to teach empathy. *Academic Medicine*. 2004;79:351–356.
8. Charon R. Narrative medicine. Caring for the sick is a work of art. *JAAPA. Official Journal of the American Academy of Physician Assistants*. 2013;26(12):8.

9. Deen SR, Mangurian C, Cabaniss DL. Points of contact: using first-person narratives to help foster empathy in psychiatric residents. *Academic Psychiatry.* 2010;34:438–441.

10. Milota MM, van Thiel GJMW, van Delden JJM. Narrative medicine as a medical education tool: a systematic review. *Medical Teacher.* 2019;41(7):802–810.

11. End of Life Nursing Education Consortium. Home page. 2016. https://www.aacnnursing.org/ELNEC. Accessed September 3, 2019.

12. Ferrell B, Otis-Green S, Baird RP, Garcia A. Nurses' responses to requests for forgiveness at the end of life. *Journal of Pain and Symptom Management.* 2014;47:631e641.33.

13. Comfort Communication Project 2016. Home page. https://www.communicatecomfort.com. Accessed September 3, 2019.

14. Columbia University. Narrative medicine. https://sps.columbia.edu/academics/masters/narrative-medicine. Accessed September 8, 2019.

15. Arntfielda S, Slesar K, Dickson J, Charon R. Narrative medicine as a means of training medical students toward residency competencies. *Patient Education and Counseling.* 2013;91(3):280–286.

16. Accreditation Review Commission on Education for the Physician Assistant Inc. *Accreditation Standards for Physician Assistant Education©. 5th ed.* September 2019. http://www.arc-pa.org/wp-content/uploads/2021/03/Standards-5th-Ed-March-2021.pdf. Accessed November 22, 2019.

17. Braun UK, Gill AC, Teal CR, Morrison LJ. The utility of reflective writing after a palliative care experience: can we assess medical students' professionalism? *Journal of Palliative Medicine.* 2013;16(11):1342–1349.

18. Rosti G. Role of narrative-based medicine in proper patient assessment. *Supportive Care in Cancer.* 2017;25(Suppl 1):3–6.

19. Institute of Medicine (IOM). *Dying in America: Improving Quality and Honoring Individual Preferences Near the End of Life.* Washington, DC: National Academies Press; 2014.

20. Bernacki RE, Block SD, for the American College of Physicians High Value Care Task Force. Communication about serious illness care goals: a review and synthesis of best practices. *JAMA Internal Medicine.* 2014;174(12):1994–2003.

21. Kelly, 2014.

22. Austin CA, Mohottige DM, Sudore RL et al. Tools to promote shared decision making in serious illness: a systematic review. *JAMA Internal Medicine.* 2015;175(7):1213–1221.

23. Childers JW, Back AL, Tulsky JA, Arnold RM. REMAP: a framework for goals of care conversations. *Journal of Oncology Practice.* 2017;13(10):844–850.

24. Hammes BJ, Rooney BL. Death and end-of-life planning in one Midwestern community. *Archives of Internal Medicine.* 1998;383–390.

25. Houben CHM, Spruit MA, Groenen MTJ, Wouters EFM, Janssen DJA. Efficacy of advance care planning: a systematic review and meta-analysis. *Journal of the American Medical Directors Association.* 2014;154:477–489.

26. Sudore RL, Lum HD, You JJ, et al. Defining advance care planning for adults: a consensus definition from a multidisciplinary Delphi panel. *Journal of Pain Symptom Management.* 2017;53(5):821–832.

27. DeCourcey DD, Silverman M, Oladunjoye A Wolfe J. Advance care planning and parent-reported end-of-life outcomes in children, adolescents and young adults with complex chronic conditions. *Critical Care Medicine.* 2018;47(1):101–108.

28. Bernacki & Wolf, 2014.

29. Mack JW, Cronin MS, Taback N, et al. End-of-life discussions among patients with advanced cancer: a cohort study. *Annals of Internal Medicine.* 2012;156(3):204–210.

30. Arnett K, Sudore RL, Nowels D, Feng CX, Levy CR, Lum HD. Advance Care Planning: Understanding Clinical Routines and Experiences of Interprofessional Team Members in Diverse Health Care Settings. *American Journal of Hospice & Palliative Medicine.* 2017;34(10):946–953. doi:10.1177/1049909116666358

31. Mack JW, Smith TJ. Reasons why physicians do not have discussions about poor prognosis, why it matters, and what can be improved. *Journal of Clinical Oncology.* 2012;30(22):2715–2717.

32. Mack JM, Fasciano KM, Block SD. Communication about prognosis with adolescent and young adult patients with cancer: information needs, prognostic awareness, and outcomes of disclosure. *Journal of Clinical Oncology.* 2018;*36*(18):1861–1867.

33. Gawande A. Quantity and quality of life: duties of care in life-limiting illness. *JAMA.* 2016;*315*(3):267–269.

34. Tulsky, 2019.

35. Singer AE, Meeker D, Teno JM, et al. Symptom trends in the last year of life, 1998–2010: a cohort study. *Annals of Internal Medicine.* 2015;*162*(3);175–183.

36. Meltzer LS, Huckabay LM. Critical care nurses' perceptions of futile care and its effect on burnout. *American Journal of Critical Care.* 2004;*13*(3):202–208.

37. Morley G, Ives J, Bradbury-Jones C. Moral Distress and Austerity: An Avoidable Ethical Challenge in Healthcare. *Health Care Analysis.* 2019;*27*(3):185–201. doi:10.1007/s10728-019-00376-8

38. Steffens NM, Tucholka JL, Nabozny MJ. Engaging patients, health care professionals, and community members to improve preoperative decision making for older adults facing high-risk surgery. *JAMA Surgery.* 2016;*151*(10):938–945.

39. Taylor LJ, Brasel KJ, Kwekkeboom KL. A framework to improve surgeon communication in high-stakes surgical decisions: best case/worst case. *JAMA Surgery.* 2017;*152*(6):531–538.

40. Angelos P. 2017. The evolution of informed consent for surgery using the best case/worst case framework. *JAMA Surgery.* 2017;*152*(6):538–539.

41. Jordan M, Keefer PM, Lee YA. Top ten tips palliative care clinicians should know about caring for children. *Journal of Palliative Medicine.* 2018;*21*(12);1783–1789.

42. Back AL, Fromme EK, Meier DE. Training clinicians with communication skills needed to match medical treatments to patient values. *Journal of the American Geriatric Society.* 2019;*67*(52):435–441.

43. Auret K, Sinclair C, Wilkinson A, et al. Quality improvement report: project to improve storage, access and incorporation of advance care plans in a regional Australian hospital. *Australian Journal Rural Health.* 2019;*27*:104–110.

44. Schellinger S, Sidebottom, A, Briggs, L. Disease specific advance care planning for heart failure patients: implementation in a large health system. *Journal of Palliative Medicine.* 2011;*14*(11):1224–1230.

45. Curtis et al., 2018.

46. Lakin JR, Benotti E, Paladino J, Henrich N, Sanders J. Interprofessional work in serious illness communication in primary care: A qualitative study. *Journal of Palliative Medicine.* 2019;751–763. http://doi.org/10.1089/jpm.2018.0471

47. Lakin JR, Block SD, Billings JA, et al. Improving communication about serious illness in primary care: a review. *JAMA Internal Medicine.* 2016;*176*(9):1380–1387.

48. Paladino J, Bernacki R, Neville BA, et al. Evaluating an intervention to improve communication between oncology clinicians and patients with life-limiting cancer: a cluster randomized clinical trial of the serious illness care program. *JAMA Oncology.* 2019;*5*(6):801–809.

49. Dunlay SM, Strand JJ. How-to discuss goals of care with patients. *Trends in Cardiovascular Medicine.* 2017;*26*(1):36–43.

50. Paladino J, Bernacki R. Precision communication—a oath forward to improve goals-of-care communication. *JAMA Internal Medicine.* 2018;*178*(7):940–942.

51. Kirchhoff KT, Hammes BJ, Kehl KA, et al. Impact of a disease-specific advance care planning intervention on end-of-life care. *Journal of the American Geriatric Society.* 2012;*60*(5):946–950.

52. Rose BL, Leung S, Gustin J, Childers J. Initiating advance care planning in primary care: a model for success. *Journal of Palliative Medicine.* 2018;*20*(20):1–5.

53. Tulsky JA. Decision aids in serious illness: moving what works into practice. *JAMA Internal Medicine.* 2015;*175*(7):1221–1222.

54. Phillips G, Lifford K, Edwards A. Do published decision aids for end-of-life care address patients' decision-making needs? A systematic review and critical appraisal. *Palliative Medicine.* 2019;*33*(87):985–1002.

55. Volandes AE, Paasch-Orlow MK, Mitchell SL, et al. Randomized controlled trial of a video decision support tool for cardiopulmonary resuscitation decision making in advanced cancer. *Journal of Clinical Oncology.* 2012;*30*:1–8.

56. Cahill PJ, Lobb EA, Sanderson C, Phillips JL. What is the evidence for conducting palliative care family meetings? A systematic review. *Palliative Medicine.* 2017;*31*(3):197–2011.

57. Forbat L, Francois K, O'Callaghan L, Kulikowski J. Family meetings in inpatient specialist palliative care: a mechanism to convey empathy. *Journal of Pain and Symptom Management.* 2018;*55*(5):1253–1259.

58. Curtis JR, Patrick DL, Shannon SE, Treece PD, Engelberg, RA, Rubenfeld, GD. The family conference as a focus to improve communication about end-of-life care in the intensive care unit: Opportunities for improvement. *Critical Care Medicine.* 2001;*29*(2):N26–N33.

59. Curtis JR, Engelberg RA, Wenrich MD, et al. Studying communication about end-of-life care during the ICU family conference: development of a framework. *Journal of Critical Care.* 2002;*17*:147–160.

60. Hudson PL, Girgis A, Mitchell GK, Philip J, Parker-Oliver D et al. Benefits and resource implications of family meetings for hospitalized palliative care patients: research protocol. *BMC Palliative Care.* 2015;*14*:73. doi:10.1186/s12904-015-0071-6

61. Glajchen M, Goehring A. The family meeting in cancer care. *Seminars in Oncology Nursing.* 2017;*33*(5):489–497.

62. Sanderson CR, Cahill PJ, Phillips JL, Johnson A, Lobb EA. Patient-centered family meetings in palliative care: a quality improvement project to explore a new model of family meetings with patients and families at the end of life. *Annals of Palliative Medicine.* 2017;*6*(Suppl 2):S195–S205. doi:10.21037/apm.2017.08.11

63. Gay EB, Pronovost PJ, Bassett RD, Nelson JE. The intensive care unit family meeting: Making it happen, *Journal of Critical Care.* 2009;*24*(4):629.e1–629.e12, ISSN 0883-9441, https://doi.org/10.1016/j.jcrc.2008.10.003

64. Billings JA. The end-of-life family meeting in intensive care part I: Indications, outcomes, and family needs. *Journal of Palliative Medicine.* 2011 Sep;*14*(9):1042–1050. doi:10.1089/jpm.2011.0038. Epub 2011 Aug 10. PMID: 21830914.

65. Back A, Arnold R, Tulsky J. Conducting a family conference. In: *Mastering Communication With Seriously Ill Patients. Balancing Honesty With Empathy and Hope.* Cambridge University Press; 2009:79–91.

66. Hudson P, Quinn K, O'Hanlon B, et al. Family meetings in palliative care: Multidisciplinary clinical practice guidelines. *BMC Palliative Care.* 2008;*7*:12. https://doi.org/10.1186/1472-684X-7-12

67. Sullivan SS, da Rosa Silva CF, Meeker MA. Family meetings at end of life: a systematic review. *Journal of Hospice & Palliative Nursing.* 2015;*17*(3):196–205.

68. Walter JK, Schall TE, Dewitt AG, Miller VA, Arnold RM, Feudtner C. Interprofessional teamwork during family meetings in the pediatric cardiac intensive care. *Journal of Pain and Symptom Management.* 2019;*57*(6):1089–1098.

69. Black MD, Vigorito MC, Curtis JR, et al. A multifaceted intervention to improve compliance with process measures for ICU clinician communication with ICU patients and families. *Critical Care Medicine* 2013;*41*:2275.

70. Nelson JE, Puntillo KA, Pronovost PJ, et al. In their own words: patients and families define high-quality palliative care in the intensive care unit. *Critical Care Medicine.* 2010;*38*:808.

71. Shaw DJ, Davidson JE, Smilde RI, et al. Multidisciplinary team training to enhance family communication in the ICU. *Critical Care Medicine.* 2014;*42*:265.

72. Glajchen M, Lawson R, Homel P, DeSandre P, Todd KH. A rapid two-stage screening protocol for palliative care in the emergency department: a quality improvement initiative. *Journal of Pain and Symptom Management.* 2011;*42*(5):657–662.

73. Hannon B, O'Reilly V, Bennett K, Breen K, Lawlor PG. Meeting the family: measuring effectiveness of family meetings in a specialist inpatient palliative care unit. *Palliative & Supportive Care.* 2012;*10*(1):43–49.

74. Curtis JR, White DB. Practical guidance for evidence-based ICU family conferences. *Chest.* 2008;*134*(4):835–843.

75. Bryan C, Boren SA. The use and effectiveness of electronic clinical decision support tools in the ambulatory/primary care setting: a systematic review of the literature. *Informatics in Primary Care.* 2008;*16*(2):79–91.

76. Nelson JE, Walker AS, Luhrs CA, Cortez TB, Pronovost PJ. Family meetings made simpler: a toolkit for the intensive care unit. *Journal of Critical Care.* 2009;*24*(4):626.e7–e4.

77. Baile WF, Buckman R, Lenzi R, Glober G, Beale EA, Kudelka AP. SPIKES—a six-step protocol for delivering bad news: application to the patient with cancer. *Oncologist.* 2000;*5*(4):302–311.

78. Bylund CL, Brown R, Gueguen JA, Diamond C, Bianculli J, Kissane DW. The implementation and assessment of a comprehensive communication skills training curriculum for oncologists. *Psychooncology.* 2010;*19*:583–593.

79. Bylund et al., 2012.

80. Kissane DW, Bylund CL, Banerjee SC, et al. Communication skills training for oncology professionals. *Journal of Clinical Oncology.* 2012;*30*(11):1242–1247.

81. Kristijanson LJ, Atwood J, Degner LF. Validity and reliability of the family inventory of needs (FIN): measuring the care needs of families of advanced cancer patients. *Journal of Nursing Measurement.* 1995;*3*:109–129.

82. Miller EG, Levy C, Linebarger JS, Klick JC, Carter BS. Pediatric palliative care: current evidence and evidence gaps. *Journal of Pediatrics.* 2015;*166*(6):1536–1540.

83. Michelson KN, Clayman ML, Haber-Barker N, et al. The use of family conferences in the pediatric intensive care unit. *Journal of Palliative Medicine.* 2013;*16*(12):1595–1601.

84. Demiris G, Parker Oliver D, Kruse RL, Wittenberg-Lyles E. Telehealth group interactions in the hospice setting: assessing technical quality across platforms. Telemedicine and e-Health. *Journal of Nursing Measurement.* 2013;*19*(4):235–240.

85. Menon PR, Stapleton RD, McVeigh U, Rabinowitz T. Telemedicine as a tool to provide family conferences and palliative care consultations in critically ill patients at rural health care institutions: a pilot study. *American Journal of Hospice and Palliative Medicine.* 2015;*32*(4):448–453.

6

Decision-Making Toolkit

Jeffrey D. Myers

Introduction

One of the foundations of all physician assistant (PA) education is learning to perform and record a focused history along with a physical examination. Most PAs would agree that this was one of the skills that was driven home time and time again during training and recognized in their practice as a skill at which PAs should excel. Our collaborative and trusting relationship with our patients is a source of pride for many within our profession. This trust, this recognition that one needs to literally sit down and learn more about the whole story and whole patient is a skill that is critical to learning what is most important to our patients in terms of their health, their life, and their goals related to both. Advance care planning (ACP) is key in capturing these sentiments through thoughtful conversations, purposeful documentation, and meaningful relationships with the patients for which we care and the people closest to them.

In fact, waiting until one *is* at the end of life is often too late to begin these dialogues. These conversations and their documentation will enhance the care provided by PAs and their colleagues to better match the patients' and their loved ones' wishes. For example, during a conversation with a patient and their significant other or spouse about a worsening of a serious cardiac illness or a parent struggling with a new terminal diagnosis for their only child, there are some general approaches and tools that all of us should employ. However, one size does not fit all. One must find the right tool that is appropriate for the situation and health literacy level of the patient and those close to them. This takes time and experience. After reading this chapter, it is hoped the reader will be a bit closer to finding the right approach to a difficult conversation.

Advance Care Planning: Learning the Lingo, the Reasons Why, and the Tools Behind It

For several decades, there has been a growing awareness that healthcare providers in general have a poor grasp of patients' wishes when faced with important decisions in the setting of serious, life-threatening, and terminal illness. In 1990, the US Congress passed the Patient Self-Determination Act (PSDA) to affirm the right of patients to control their own medical care in situations when they lack decision-making capacity. Since that time, health providers and patients alike have attempted to define ACP. In 1995, the Study to Understand Prognoses and Preferences for Outcomes and Risks of Treatment indicated that the efforts to complete the process of advance directives was inadequate.[1] Subsequent research has sought to learn what patients and families are concerned about: (1) avoid prolongation of dying; (2) strengthen relationships with loved ones; (3) minimize burden; (4) manage pain and symptoms; (5) enhance patient-provider communication; (6) enhance completion of life and preparation for death; and finally (6) provide treatment as a "whole person."[2-4]

Perhaps the most meaningful way to define ACP is to think of it as a series of behaviors: conversations with family and medical providers; completion of advance directive; confirmation of a process by which patients and those close to them can continue goals-of-care discussions.[4-7] A recent consensus definition for ACP in adults provided an updated definition with a goal to ensure that the medical care patients receive is "consistent with their values, goals, and preferences during serious and chronic illness."[5] This group defined ACP as follows[5]:

1. A process that "supports adults at any age or stage of health in understanding and sharing their personal values, life goals, and preferences regarding future medical care."
2. "The goal of advance care planning is to help ensure that people receive medical care that is consistent with their values, goals and preferences during serious and chronic illness."
3. "This process may include choosing and preparing another trusted person or persons to make medical decisions in the event the person can no longer make his or her own decision."

Over the years, many have further explained the elements that belong in ACP that help determine the kind of treatment that a patient may want in a medical emergency, regardless of their age or health status. This includes informed consent about the benefits and burdens of medical treatments; clarification and understanding of the patient's values and preferences for treatment; and selection of a surrogate decision-maker when a patient cannot make complex medical decisions.[8-10]

For many providers, discussions about end-of-life decisions can be daunting, and we may worry that our patients feel the same way. However, research shows that patients want and really expect us to start these conversations.[4,11,12] They value a health system that makes time for this. The majority of providers do not know that their own patients have an existing advance directive—mostly because we are not asking. Unfortunately, in the United States, only about a third of adults have an advance directive, which is troubling when one realizes that more than 70% of adults may be unable to make their own decisions at the end of life.[13-15] Pediatric studies showed that while maybe a third of parents have discussed ACP with a medical provider, less than 3% have a written version.[16]

There is clearly a need to have these conversations and to elicit our patients' and families' wishes. Physician assistants are trained as compassionate listeners and are well poised to be involved in these conversations. As primary care providers, we have the opportunity to start the serious illness conversations early in the disease trajectory. Given our expanding role in healthcare and our unique training, we are able to transition into all medical and surgical specialties. This defines us as integral members of optimal team practice. Although we can feel "stuck in the middle" during difficult decision discussions with seriously and terminally ill patients,[17] specific tools exist to empower decision-making conversations, ensuring that our patient's values and preferences are honored.

Discussion Elements and Tools

For many PAs, especially those who work in the inpatient setting, conversations about "code status" and treatment preferences—Do you want us to resuscitate you? Do compressions, shock, intubate, and put you on life support?—are some of the more difficult and least rewarding. The default approach of "full-code" status avoids the fundamental issue of goals of care. The message becomes clear that the only option is to "do everything" or an implied "do nothing." The conversation then focuses on do not resuscitate (DNR) or do not intubate (DNI), which is important but complicated. It is essential to discuss with a patient and/or family and caregiver(s) what they *understand* about the serious illness or situation and their desired *outcomes* and *goals* for treatment. This assumes that a healthcare proxy or surrogate has been identified.[18] If the default setting of full care is understood by patients and families but they are not certain of limiting care in that situation, the topics will be revisited as more information is learned and the clinical situation evolves. The important thing to highlight is that aggressive management of symptoms will continue *regardless of code status*.

In the development of the goals of care, it is important to remember that a patient's life goals are an essential part of the conversation, as is the legacy they wish to leave. For example, they may want to complete a project, attend a wedding or graduation, witness a birth, arrange for the care of a pet, or other objectives. This will often clarify existential values and allow ideal alignment of values with treatment choices.

The SPIKES model was first introduced as an approach to breaking bad news to patients and families and has a series of six steps (Table 6.1): *setting up* the interview; assessing the patient's *perception*; obtaining the patient's *invitation*; giving *knowledge* and information; addressing and responding to the patient's *emotions*; and finally *strategy* and *summary* of the next steps.[19] Research has shown this to be an effective approach to breaking bad news, but it also can serve as a framework for any ACP discussions.[20]

There are other conversation tools and models for ACP discussions that are flexible and adaptable to a variety of settings. One of these is the "Serious Illness Conversation Guide."[21]

TABLE 6.1 SPIKES—A Protocol for Having Difficult Conversations

SPIKES	DOs	DON'TS
Setting	Set the scene, give yourself time, gather the right people	Interruptions
Perception	Find out what the patient/family understand, in their words	Assumptions
Invitation	OK to discuss? How do they want the information? All the details?	Blunt Disclosures
Knowledge	Use the patient's language to correct/clarify medical facts	Medical Jargon
Empathy	Be empathic: "This must be hard for you." They start crying—pause and let them; it's OK!	Destroying Hope
Strategy	Next steps, using their input. Summarize. Confirm when you will discuss this again.	Ignoring Patient-input

Adapted from Baile W F, et al. SPIKES—a six-step protocol for delivering bad news: application to the patient with cancer. *Oncologist* 2000; 5(4):302–311

This builds on a shared understanding of knowledge. It will involve incorporation of specific prognostic indicators and equalizing health literacy among the patient, caregivers, and other healthcare providers. The creators of the guide not only have worked to prove the model to be effective, but also have tested the language used in the discussion (Box 6.1).[22,23] Acknowledgment of the nuances of language and culture is important, and this can further facilitate difficult conversations.

Advance Directives and POLST/MOLST/ MOST Documentation

The main goal of the PSDA is to encourage the completion of documents known as advance directives. Advance directives include living wills and healthcare powers of attorney; these are legal instruments that allow patients to document their wishes (the living will part) and designate a proxy or healthcare surrogate in the event they are unable to make decisions for themselves or no longer have the capacity to do so.[14] Each state defines how it recognizes these documents; therefore, advance directives can vary in format from state to state and even within each state. Their intent is to capture what a patient would want in end-of-life situations and whom they would trust to make decisions for them. Some states include organ donation as part of their advance directives. PAs should be aware of the process of connection with the appropriate agencies in their facility.

Advance directives can be completed by anyone—regardless of their health. One doesn't need to be seriously ill, and preferably should not be, to complete an advance directive. Most states define an adult as anyone 18 years of age or older. Every adult should be encouraged to complete an advance directive. Studies have shown that even young adults are not only open to talking about but also often seek more information about ACP.[10,24] The activity of completing advance directives can be helpful to family. In one study, a "worst-case scenario" conversation between a son and his dad about his preferences revealed that there

BOX 6.1 Serious Illness Conversation Tips

The Conversation

Set up the conversation—Introduce purpose, ask permission

Assess understanding and preferences

Share prognosis—frame as "wish . . . worry," "Hope . . . worry" statements, allow for silence, explore emotion

Explore key topics—goals, fears and worries, sources of strength, critical abilities, trade-offs, family

Close the conversation—summarize, make a recommendation, check in with patient, affirm commitment

The Language

Setup up—"I'd like to talk about what is ahead with your illness and do some thinking in advance about what is important to you so that I can make sure we provide you with the care you want—is this OK?"

Assess—"What is your understanding now of where you are with your illness?" "How much information about what is likely to be ahead with your illness would you like from me?"

Share—"I want to share with you my understanding of where things are with your illness." "I hope you will continue to live well for a long time, but I'm worried." "I wish we were not in this situation, but I am worried that time may be short." "I hope that this is not the case, but I'm worried that this may be as strong as you will feel, and things are likely to get more difficult."

Explore—"What are your most important goals if your health situation worsens?" "What are your biggest fears and worries about the future with your health?" "If you become sicker, how much are you willing to go through for the possibility of gaining more time?"

Close—"I heard you say that ___ is really important to you. Keeping that in mind, and what we know about your illness, I recommend that we ___. This will helps us make sure that your treatment plans reflect what's important to you." "How does this plan seem to you?" "I will do everything I can to help you through this."

Adapted from Ariadne Labs. Serious illness conversation guide. 2019. https://www.ariadnelabs.org/wp-content/uploads/2018/04/Serious-Illness-Conversation-Guide.2017-04-18CC2pg.pdf. Accessed August 15, 2019.

was a discrepancy between wanting "everything" done and what was written: The dad actually did not want any life support in the worst-case scenarios they had discussed.[25]

Prior to completion of an advance directive, there are readily available tools in the community that can help start the conversation and document wishes around specific scenarios.[26] The Conversation Project was started in 2010 "to have every person's wishes for end-of-life care expressed and respected."[27] Other documents and booklets such as *Five Wishes* and *Voicing My Choices* can act as living wills and advance directives in many states. They approach the conversation with questions related to more person-specific situations (e.g., what kind of music, if any, would you want played while you were dying) and are designed for children and adults.[28]

In the early 1990s, the state of Oregon's healthcare leaders and patient advocates recognized a gap in having completed advance directives readily available for emergency personnel and medical providers. Thus, the birth of the POLST paradigm: Physician Orders for Life-Sustaining Treatment. Since then, other states have created forms and registries—some advanced enough to link up to emergency providers in the field and electronic medical record (EMR) systems—that capture a patient's wishes for life-sustaining treatments. The name may be different in some states—POLST, MOLST (Medical Orders for Life-Sustaining Treatments), and MOST (Medical Orders for Scope of Treatment). The goal is the same: a portable document that can be quickly accessed when needed and that provides a platform for decision-making for patients at risk for a life-threatening clinical event because they have a serious life-limiting medical condition, which may include advanced frailty.[29] While the POLST paradigm has not been without controversy, there have been numerous studies documenting their successful use in matching clinical care with patients' end-of-life wishes.[30-35]

An important difference between advance directives and POLST is the timing and appropriateness for the patient. While all capable adults (and children younger than 18 years of age with a parent or guardian who can legally execute the document) should be encouraged to complete an advance directive, which directs care preferences at the end of life, a POLST form is only for those with a serious illness or frailty for whom their healthcare providers would not be surprised if they died in the next year. Generally the default is "full care" and this means doing all the things, including cardiac resuscitation, intubation, and life-sustaining mechanical ventilation. When a serious or life-limiting illness is present, it is likely that the patient has faced the situation and has thought about limitations to care that match their life goals. Therefore, the POLST process is designed to create a portable document that could help any healthcare provider in any setting know what goals of care have been previously discussed and agreed on. It is not recognized with the same legal status in all states. However, it provides a way for medical providers to honor limits that are being set by patients. POLSTs should be reserved for not only those who healthcare providers might expect to die in the next year, but also those that may not be able to participate in their own care decisions in the next year—those with advancing dementia, risk of stroke, or neurodegenerative diseases like amyotrophic lateral sclerosis.

The key to a meaningful advance directive or POLST document is the conversations you have prior to completing them. Research shows that advance directives and POLSTs have the ability to make a difference in providing goal-concurrent care for patients. For example, it is much easier to complete a POLST when your patient has already told you they do not want to continue to return to the hospital, and if they do, they do not want to be hooked up to life-supporting machines and simply want to pass peacefully when their time comes. Knowing this up front allows you to start completing a POLST by saying, "After hearing what's important to you and knowing this, I don't think 'full care' fits your goals, and it makes sense to choose DNR and DNI on your POLST—would you agree?" There are times when it is more appropriate to be direct, such as "Do you want us to try to restart your heart if it were to stop?"

Legal and Ethical Issues: Surrogacy and Capacity

Decision-making in the context of serious illness requires a clinical ethics approach. Macauley summarized that there are two main principles: a determination of what a patient wants to do or would want done (autonomy) and what is best for the patient (beneficence).[36] Entire texts are written on ethics within palliative care, and for the purpose of our scope, this section focuses on two important topics that PAs encounter regularly, namely *surrogacy* and *capacity*.

In a recent review of statutes on surrogate or alternate decision-makers, it was noted that the definition and role of those who step in to speak for patients varies from state to state, particularly when it is not a legal family member.[37] There is broad ethical acceptance that others can make end-of-life decisions on behalf of patients who lack capacity. Research has demonstrated that ethics has shifted from a *paternalistic* approach to *patient-centered care* and *shared decision-making*. As already noted, advance directives give patients the opportunity to choose a designated surrogate decision-maker, sometimes referred to as an alternate healthcare representative; this is a trusted person or persons to make decisions for them if they are unable to speak for themselves.[5] This is different from a decision-maker who takes on this role without having been named legally in an advance directive or other legal document. Many states have a "surrogacy ladder" that names a hierarchical priority list of family and others who can serve as decision-makers.[37] For adults, the goal in choosing a surrogate or alternate decision-maker is to preserve patient autonomy.

Defining decision-making capacity should be our next step. It is important to note the difference between competency and capacity since they are related but *not* synonymous. Capacity is variable depending on the complexity of the situation. Patients can lack capacity in a variety of ways whether it is transient during episodes of delirium, uncontrolled symptoms, or other etiologies (e.g., sedated intubation) or more permanently in patients with dementia, in young children, or in those with cognitive disabilities.[38] Competency is a legal definition that determines an individual's mental capacity. Elements and definitions of capacity may vary by institution; however, as outlined by Grisso and Applebaum, patients with capacity should be able to

1. Communicate a choice
2. Understand relevant information

3. Appreciate the situation and its consequences
4. Explain the rationale behind their decision[39]

All medical providers should be able to determine decision-making capacity in most cases. Looking at the above elements more closely is important for PAs to be able to document these. The first, communication, is fundamental to the process. Every effort should be made to determine whether, through verbal or nonverbal means, patients can effectively communicate. Often, decisional patients are ignored or discounted. Patients should be able to understand their condition and, as the second element, explain the risks and benefits of the medical options that have been presented. Discussions should occur in their own language, not medical jargon. Third, patients should be able to understand the consequences of any choice they make and how it will impact them. Finally, the patient should be able to apply their own values and goals to their choice—why are they making that choice? It is, of course, helpful if their goals, values, and fears have already been documented in an earlier ACP discussion.

It is important to note the stark differences between the adult and pediatric world of decision-making, particularly when considering surrogacy and capacity. Most pediatric palliative care consultations are not for patients with cancer as they are in adults, but rather for congenital/genetic and neuromuscular disorders. Many of these patients survive for more than a year after palliative consultation—much longer than adults.[40,41] It is also important to note the greater variability within their prognoses: Some may die, some may have a premature death, and some may survive but with major impacts on quality of life. Given all this, there is a significant opportunity for providers to develop ongoing relationships with these families. Decisions about care and when to even talk about end-of-life topics will be more difficult to navigate. Consider the challenges of having a DNR/DNI plan in a school setting where school staff may be reluctant to honor wishes without feeling that they understand the full picture or feel comfortable enough to assess the situation.

In the pediatric world, the decision-maker is not ever the patient, and they do not get to choose their own surrogate. In 2003, the Institute of Medicine issued a report, *Improving Palliative and End-of-life Care for Children and their Families*, which sought to highlight this and the above-mentioned complexities.[42] One useful tool to frame end-of-life decision-making is offered by the Royal College of Paediatrics and Child Health to help determine when situations for not continuing treatment might be considered:

1. Limited quantity of life—when death is imminent and inevitable
2. Limited quality of life—who defines quality, and what is seen as a burden to some, may not be to others
3. The child has sufficient decision-making capacity and refuses further treatment[43]

There are limitations in this framework; however, it is a starting point. Two standards are often discussed and also used: the "best interest" standard and the "harm principle."[36] Parents are expected to act in the best interest of their child, the patient. This identifies a bias to parental values and belief systems. In reality, there are multiple options and rarely one best choice. However, when considered in the context of state statutes, the harm principle is identified as a social justice issue, which challenges parents to choose, but holds them to the standard that the choice cannot harm the child. Decision-making for children should include the child—according to his/her age and maturity level. While teens may not necessarily have decision-making capacity, they still have input. For example, children born with disability have a different definition of quality of life from others. This is often underappreciated. Ultimately, identification of some key components to the conversations have been found to help with decision-making[44]:

- Shared decision-making through open and honest communication
- Scheduled family meetings and follow-up
- Utilization of multidisciplinary teams, including music and art therapists to enhance health literacy with interactive, written, audio, and video formats
- Delineation of a care plan to encompass emergent (medical orders using POLST/MOLST) and future situations consistent with overall goals

Prognostication

One of the more challenging aspects of caring for those with serious illness is prognostication. It is important for the primary care or specialist PA to remain present and provide an honest answer when the patient and/or family and caregivers ask: "How much time do I have?" As Macauley noted, "The question is not only whether a patient qualifies for hospice but how to equip the patient to handle the realization that [they are] dying, as well as to empower [them] to live fully in whatever time [they have] left."[36p84] He writes that the three basic components to prognostication involve determining a prognosis with some accuracy, communicating this to the patient and their family, and using this information to make decisions. It is also important to utilize discussion tools such as SPIKES, which focus on "setting the stage" and ensuring that the patient wants to be a part of a prognosis discussion and who else should be present.

All patients have a unique illness narrative, and we know that certain disease states tend to follow a particular disease trajectory. Organ failure (e.g., cardiac, hepatic, pulmonary, renal) tends to follow a pattern of periodic acute events and exacerbations, including hospitalizations, and the patient may be stable but less functional than previously. This population is at risk for sudden death, in contrast to those with most cancers, which have a period of good function and then a sudden decline at the end. On the other hand, patients with debilitating illnesses (dementia, Parkinson disease, multiple sclerosis) tend to have a gradual decline and loss of function over time before death. These trajectories can provide us a map on which to place our patients' own stories to best predict where they are on these known paths.[45]

A number of tools have been created and found useful over the years to help document and track this, including the Eastern Cooperation Oncology Group Scale (0 = Normal, 5 = Dead); the Karnofsky Index (100 = Normal, 0 = Dead); and the updated Palliative Performance Scale version 2 (PPSv2) (0 = Dead, 100% = Normal).[46] All of these tools are commonly found online, and many are embedded into widely used EMR systems. These scales can help not only document a measurable change in performance over time but also serve as a communication tool among providers. They increasingly serve to illustrate the progression of disease for patients and families. Studies have shown the PPSv2 to be useful not only as a reliable tool in cancer but also in other disease states such as heart failure.[47,48]

There are also general guidelines for those developing complications from their cancer. Short median survival times in a number of these have been well documented.[49–59] There are a number of other disease-specific prognostication tools. For example, the Childs-Turcotte-Pugh and Model for End-Stage Liver Disease scores—both used in predicting prognosis for patients with decompensated chronic liver failure without liver transplantation. For example, the Advanced Dementia Prognostic Tool has been shown to more accurately predict 6-month survival in nursing home patients than hospice guidelines.[60] Pediatric tools also exist, such as the Pediatric Risk of Mortality Score, which is valuable in prognosis discussions.[61]

Another tool is the "surprise question," which is utilized primarily in adult patients in multiple settings. Clinicians are asked if they, "Would be surprised if the patient died in the next 12 months?"[62–64] This tool helps to prompt and guide conversations regarding goals of care and ACP because it requires clinicians to perform a comprehensive assessment of the patient.

Use of these tools will help patients and families reflect on the serious illness narrative. It is often what patients and families/caregivers can best understand since it relates directly to their own experience with the illness. They can interpret the disease trajectory in terms of what has changed in the care needs, for example, increasingly frequent admissions and escalating symptom burden as evidenced by increasing communication with service providers. They may not need but sometimes prefer to know further imaging or hear laboratory results to understand the decline in the patient's overall status. Near the end, an informed discussion about specific transitional symptoms with all involved in the care of the patient, including family members, can be a powerful tool that measures how quickly things are changing. It becomes important when there are unresolved emotions and allegiances among all involved in the patient's illness. Choice of the appropriate prognostication tool is important for the patient as well as the family and caregivers, who may all be in different stages of grieving. This may be the most meaningful part of the prognosis conversation.

Medical Documentation and Referral

Much emphasis has been placed on the conversations with patients and their families/caregivers. Reviews of tools such as POLST/MOLST have shown that even when there is goal concordance in care at the end of life, there are often many revisions that took place along the way, and this evolution should be documented.[35] Health systems are fragmented. Provision of care without a prior relationship with the patient is problematic and challenging. The opportunity to review documented discussions is invaluable for all healthcare providers—including therapists, discharge coordinators, nutritionists, and chaplains.

Although the EMR provides the opportunity and responsibility to review these conversations, they can also fail to highlight the ACP conversations.[65] Since 2016, Medicare has implemented a CPT (Current Procedural Terminology) code for ACP discussions that is utilized by all providers (Box 6.2).[66] Lack of reimbursement and time are no longer an excuse for failure to document these important conversations. Significant gaps in documentation regarding prognosis and goals exist between primary and palliative teams.[67] A number of studies and initiatives have shown that systemic changes in provider education, EMR templates and alerts, and embedding goals of care discussion into routine care can improve the concordance between patient outcomes and goals.[67,68]

BOX 6.2 Advance Care Planning: Billing for End-of-Life Discussions

The Centers for Medicare and Medicaid Services (CMS) pays for *voluntary* advance care planning (ACP). Medicare pays for ACP as either an element of an annual wellness visit or a separate Medicare Part B medically necessary service.[1] There are no limits to the number of times you can report ACP, just be sure to document the change in the patient's health status or wishes.

CPT Codes
99497 ACP including the discussion of advance directive forms by the healthcare professional; first 30 minutes, face to face with the patient, family, and/or surrogate

99498 ACP including the discussion of advance directive forms by the healthcare professional; each additional 30 minutes (list separately in addition to the code for the primary procedure)

Example
A primary care PA meets with their patient for a follow-up visit to a recent hospitalization for heart failure. The patient shares that given multiple hospitalizations this year, including time in the intensive care unit (ICU), he wants to know more about how to focus on his quality of life versus quantity. The PA talks about his treatment preferences, reviews an advance directive, and the two discuss limiting his care to not include ICU interventions, including cardiac resuscitation and life support when he returns to the hospital again in the future.

The PA documents the discussion, the patient's preferences, and the length (60 minutes). The PA then uses the standard code 99497 (for the first 30 minutes) as well as 99498 (for the second 30 minutes).

References
1. Jones CA, Acevedo J, Bull J, Kamal AH. Top 10 Tips for using advance care planning codes in palliative medicine and beyond. *Journal of Palliative Medicine.* 2016;19(12):1249-1253.
2. Centers for Medicare and Medicaid Services, Medicare Learning Network. Advance care planning. 2019. https://www.cms.gov/Outreach-and-Education/Medicare-Learning-Network-MLN/MLNProducts/Downloads/AdvanceCarePlanning.pdf. Accessed October 26, 2019.

Provision of quality healthcare is defined by specific goals and boundaries related to referral to other facilities, services, and resources. This is particularly the case with hospice. This may be as simple as understanding when to refer to hospice within your community or when symptoms and complex planning require a palliative medicine consultation. Given the complexity behind surrogate decision-makers and capacity, referral to a behavioral health specialist, the institutional ethics committee, or a local ombudsman may be not only helpful, but also part of your institution's policy.

Legacy Planning

An integral part of all of these discussions and decisions is an understanding of what patients are living for as well as how they want to be remembered. Patients and families with limited time often want to leave a legacy. Another way to consider a lasting legacy is to discuss organ donation. This is considered part of the ACP process. These decisions are based on the values of patients and families, and they may reveal themselves as legacies. This can be a "bucket list" for both children and adults through a foundation such as Make a Wish. More examples would be an ultrasound video of a fetus provided by a palliative team to allow a parent to share with another family member or the decision to harvest a kidney from a terminally ill patient. These all speak to legacy.[69]

We know that bereaved parents have noted that many children with cancer do things to be remembered. This can include writing letters, crafts, giving things away—legacy-making and planning has demonstrated to be a source of inspiration for both children with cancer or developmental illnesses and their loved ones.[70-72] Child life therapists, social workers, and others who help with legacy planning can help to provide activities such as digital diaries and dignity therapy to add meaning for children and adults alike. Studies have shown that many children living with advanced cancer were aware of their eventual death, and the opportunity to talk or act and share meaningful moments for family is important.[72]

The power of the ACP process cannot be underestimated. It provides meaning and reduces stress, anxiety, and depression for patients[12] and leaves a legacy of acceptance of one's death for families, caregivers, and loved ones.[73,74] ACP improves parent- and family-reported end-of-life outcomes and may be the first positive step in bereavement.[75] Pregrieving and bereavement are processes that are crucial to consider in order to aid in the management of caregiver distress and thus reduce potential liability.

Decisions, Decisions. Final Thoughts

Four Rules For Life:
Show up.
Pay attention.
Tell the truth.
Don't be attached to the results.
—Angeles Arrien, PhD

Summary

Patients and families/caregivers will make decisions that appear to them as a "best" or "least-harmful" option but will be contrary to professional medical advice. Parents will be faced with decisions that are aligned with their values of what is the best and least-harmful choice for their child, and the healthcare providers may be faced with stressful situations in which patients and families make what may seem to them as "bad" decisions. Additionally, the personal values and opinions of the healthcare providers who have intimate medical knowledge about their patients may differ substantially. It is essential to openly recognize this discrepancy as a potential source of stress for professional caregivers, who can become cynical and suffer from burnout as a result. Nonjudgmental listening can be difficult in these situations. Sometimes the act of "doing everything" or "waiting for a miracle" is the only way a family member or caregiver will know that they contributed to the care of their loved one. Healthcare providers may see these discrepancies as failures of care, whereas in fact the greatest tool is compassionate listening. PAs are trained to be attentive listeners and to provide care that aligns with their professional competencies.

References

1. A controlled trial to improve care for seriously ill hospitalized patients. The study to understand prognoses and preferences for outcomes and risks of treatments (SUPPORT). The SUPPORT Principal Investigators. *JAMA*. 1995;*274*(20):1591–1598.
2. Singer PA, Martin DK, Lavery JV, Thiel EC, Kelner M, Mendelssohn DC. Reconceptualizing advance care planning from the patient's perspective. *Archives of Internal Medicine*. 1998;*158*(8):879–884.
3. Steinhauser KE, Clipp EC, McNeilly M, Christakis NA, McIntyre LM, Tulsky JA. In search of a good death: observations of patients, families, and providers. *Annals of Internal Medicine*. 2000;*132*(10):825–832.
4. Kolarik RC, Arnold RM, Fischer GS, Tulsky JA. Objectives for advance care planning. *Journal of Palliative Medicine*. 2002;*5*(5):697–704.
5. Sudore RL, Lum HD, You JJ, et al. Defining advance care planning for adults: a consensus definition from a multidisciplinary Delphi panel. *Journal of Pain and Symptom Management*. 2017;*53*(5):821–832. e821.
6. Howard M, Bernard C, Tan A, Slaven M, Klein D, Heyland DK. Advance care planning: let's start sooner. *Canadian Family Physician*. 2015;*61*(8):663–665.
7. Institute of Medicine, Committee on Approaching Death: Addressing Key End of Life Issues. *Dying in America: Improving Quality and Honoring Individual Preferences Near the End of Life*. Washington, DC: National Academies Press; 2015. Copyright 2015 by the National Academy of Sciences. All rights reserved.
8. Hammes BJ. What does it take to help adults successfully plan for future medical decisions? *Journal of Palliative Medicine*. 2001;*4*(4):453–456.
9. Fried TR, Bradley EH, Towle VR, Allore H. Understanding the treatment preferences of seriously ill patients. *New England Journal of Medicine*. 2002;*346*(14):1061–1066.
10. Fried TR, Redding CA, Robbins ML, Paiva A, O'Leary JR, Iannone L. Stages of change for the component behaviors of advance care planning. *Journal of the American Geriatric Society*. 2010;*58*(12):2329–2336.
11. Horridge KA. Advance care planning: practicalities, legalities, complexities and controversies. *Archives of Disease in Childhood*. 2015;*100*(4):380–385.
12. Detering KM, Hancock AD, Reade MC, Silvester W. The impact of advance care planning on end of life care in elderly patients: randomised controlled trial. *BMJ (Clinical Research ed.)*. 2010;*340*:c1345.

13. Rao JK, Anderson LA, Lin FC, Laux JP. Completion of advance directives among U.S. consumers. *American Journal of Preventive Medicine.* 2014;*46*(1):65–70.

14. Yadav KN, Gabler NB, Cooney E, et al. Approximately one in three US adults completes any type of advance directive for end-of-life care. *Health Affairs (Millwood).* 2017;*36*(7):1244–1251.

15. Sudore RL, Fried TR. Redefining the "planning" in advance care planning: preparing for end-of-life decision making. *Annals of Internal Medicine.* 2010;*153*(4):256–261.

16. Liberman DB, Pham PK, Nager AL. Pediatric advance directives: parents' knowledge, experience, and preferences. *Pediatrics.* 2014;*134*(2):e436–e443.

17. Chuang E, Lamkin R, Hope AA, Kim G, Burg J, Gong MN. "I just felt like I was stuck in the middle": physician assistants' experiences communicating with terminally ill patients and their families in the acute care setting. *Journal of Pain and Symptom Management.* 2017;*54*(1):27–34.

18. White J, Fromme EK. "In the beginning . . .": tools for talking about resuscitation and goals of care early in the admission. *American Journal of Hospice and Palliative Care.* 2013;*30*(7):676–682.

19. Baile WF, Buckman R, Lenzi R, Glober G, Beale EA, Kudelka AP. SPIKES—a six-step protocol for delivering bad news: application to the patient with cancer. *Oncologist.* 2000;*5*(4):302–311.

20. Kaplan M. SPIKES: a framework for breaking bad news to patients with cancer. *Clinical Journal of Oncology Nursing.* 2010;*14*(4):514–516.

21. Ariadne Labs. Serious illness conversation guide. 2015. https://www.ariadnelabs.org/wp-content/uploads/2018/04/Serious-Illness-Conversation-Guide.2017-04-18CC2pg.pdf. Accessed June 17, 2021.

22. Lakin JR, Block SD, Billings JA, et al. Improving communication about serious illness in primary care: a review. *JAMA Internal Medicine.* 2016;*176*(9):1380–1387.

23. Lakin JR, Koritsanszky LA, Cunningham R, et al. A systematic intervention to improve serious illness communication in primary care. *Health Affairs (Millwood).* 2017;*36*(7):1258–1264.

24. Kavalieratos D, Ernecoff NC, Keim-Malpass J, Degenholtz HB. Knowledge, attitudes, and preferences of healthy young adults regarding advance care planning: a focus group study of university students in Pittsburgh, USA. *BMC Public Health.* 2015;*15*:197.

25. McMahan RD, Knight SJ, Fried TR, Sudore RL. Advance care planning beyond advance directives: perspectives from patients and surrogates. *Journal of Pain Symptom and Management.* 2013;*46*(3):355–365.

26. Abba K, Lloyd-Williams M, Horton S. Discussing end of life wishes—the impact of community interventions? *BMC Palliative Care.* 2019;*18*(1):26.

27. The Conversation Project. About us. https://theconversationproject.org/about/. Accessed July 1, 2019.

28. Wiener L, Ballard E, Brennan T, Battles H, Martinez P, Pao M. How I wish to be remembered: the use of an advance care planning document in adolescent and young adult populations. *Journal of Palliative Medicine.* 2008;*11*(10):1309–1313.

29. Zive DM, Jimenez VM, Fromme EK, Tolle SW. Changes over time in the Oregon Physician Orders for Life-Sustaining Treatment Registry: a study of two decedent cohorts. *Journal of Palliative Medicine.* 2019;*22*(5):500–507.

30. Brugger C, Breschi LC, Hart EM, et al. The POLST paradigm and form: facts and analysis. *Linacre Quarterly.* 2013;*80*(2):103–138.

31. Fromme EK, Guthrie AE, Grueber CM. Transitions in end-of-life care: the Oregon Trail. *Frontiers of Health Services Management.* 2011;*27*(3):3–16.

32. Nugent SM, Slatore CG, Ganzini L, et al. POLST registration and associated outcomes among veterans with advanced-stage lung cancer. *American Journal of Hospice Palliative Care Care.* 2019:1049909118824543.

33. Pedraza SL, Culp S, Knestrick M, Falkenstine E, Moss AH. Association of Physician Orders for Life-Sustaining Treatment form use with end-of-life care quality metrics in patients with cancer. *Journal of Oncology Practice.* 2017;*13*(10):e881–e888.

34. Collier J, Kelsberg G, Safranek S. Clinical inquiries: how well do POLST forms assure that patients get the end-of-life care they requested? *Journal of Family Practice.* 2018;*67*(4):249–251.

35. Hopping-Winn J, Mullin J, March L, Caughey M, Stern M, Jarvie J. The progression of end-of-life wishes and concordance with end-of-life care. *Journal of Palliative Medicine.* 2018;*21*(4):541–545.

36. Macauley RC. *Ethics in Palliative Care: A Complete Guide.* New York, NY: Oxford University Press; 2018.

37. DeMartino ES, Dudzinski DM, Doyle CK, et al. Who decides when a patient can't? Statutes on alternate decision makers. *New England Journal of Medicine.* 2017;*376*(15):1478–1482.

38. Epstein RM, Entwistle VA. Capacity and shared decision making in serious illness. In: Quill TE, Miller FG, eds. *Palliative Care and Ethics.* New York, NY: Oxford University Press; 2014:162–183.

39. Grisso T. *Assessing Competence to Consent to Treatment: A Guide for Physicians and Other Health Professionals.* New York, NY: Oxford University Press; 1998.

40. Kamal AH, Swetz KM, Carey EC, et al. Palliative care consultations in patients with cancer: a Mayo Clinic 5-year review. *Journal of Oncology Practice.* 2011;*7*(1):48–53.

41. Feudtner C, Kang TI, Hexem KR, et al. Pediatric palliative care patients: a prospective multicenter cohort study. *Pediatrics.* 2011;*127*(6):1094–1101.

42. Institute of Medicine Committee on Palliative and End-of-Life Care for Children and Their Families; Field MJ, Behrman RE, eds. *When Children Die: Improving Palliative and End-of-Life Care for Children and Their Families.* 2003. Washington, DC: National Academies Press. Copyright 2003 by the National Academy of Sciences. All rights reserved.

43. Larcher V, Craig F, Bhogal K, Wilkinson D, Brierley J. Making decisions to limit treatment in life-limiting and life-threatening conditions in children: a framework for practice. *Archives of Disease in Childhood.* 2015;*100*(Suppl 2):s3–s23.

44. Lotz JD, Daxer M, Jox RJ, Borasio GD, Fuhrer M. "Hope for the best, prepare for the worst": a qualitative interview study on parents' needs and fears in pediatric advance care planning. *Palliative Medicine.* 2017;*31*(8):764–771.

45. Amblàs-Novellas J, Murray SA, Espaulella J, et al. Identifying patients with advanced chronic conditions for a progressive palliative care approach: a cross-sectional study of prognostic indicators related to end-of-life trajectories. *BMJ Open.* 2016;*6*(9):e012340. doi:10.1136/bmjopen-2016-012340

46. Simmons CPL, McMillan DC, McWilliams K, et al. Prognostic tools in patients with advanced cancer: a systematic review. *Journal of Pain Symptom and Management.* 2017;*53*(5):962–970.e910.

47. Mei AH, Jin WL, Hwang MK, Meng YC, Seng LC, Yaw WH. Value of the Palliative Performance Scale in the prognostication of advanced cancer patients in a tertiary care setting. *Journal of Palliative Medicine.* 2013;*16*(8):887–893.

48. Masterson Creber R, Russell D, Dooley F, et al. Use of the Palliative Performance Scale to estimate survival among home hospice patients with heart failure. *ESC Heart Failure.* 2019;*6*(2):371–378.

49. Hodge C, Badgwell BD. Palliation of malignant ascites. *Journal of Surgical Oncology.* 2019;*120*(1):67–73.

50. Adam RA, Adam YG. Malignant ascites: past, present, and future. *Journal of the American College of Surgeons.* 2004;*198*(6):999–1011.

51. Sangisetty SL, Miner TJ. Malignant ascites: a review of prognostic factors, pathophysiology and therapeutic measures. *World Journal of Gastrointestinal Surgery.* 2012;*4*(4):87–95.

52. Belani CP, Pajeau TS, Bennett CL. Treating malignant pleural effusions cost consciously. *Chest.* 1998;*113*(1 Suppl):78s–85s.

53. Psallidas I, Kalomenidis I, Porcel JM, Robinson BW, Stathopoulos GT. Malignant pleural effusion: from bench to bedside. *European Respiratory Review.* 2016;*25*(140):189–198.

54. Chakraborty A, Selby D, Gardiner K, Myers J, Moravan V, Wright F. Malignant bowel obstruction: natural history of a heterogeneous patient population followed prospectively over two years. *Journal of Pain Symptom and Management.* 2011;*41*(2):412–420.

55. Weissman D. Fast facts and concepts #13: determining prognosis in advanced cancer. May 2015. https://www.mypcnow.org/fast-fact/determining-prognosis-in-advanced-cancer/

56. Lamont EB, Christakis NA. Complexities in prognostication in advanced cancer: "to help them live their lives the way they want to." *JAMA.* 2003;*290*(1):98–104.

57. Conroy S, O'Malley B. Hypercalcaemia in cancer. *BMJ (Clinical Research ed.).* 2005;*331*(7522):954.

58. Legrand SB. Modern management of malignant hypercalcemia. *American Journal of Hospice Palliative Care Care.* 2011;*28*(7):515–517.

59. Dosios T, Theakos N, Angouras D, Asimacopoulos P. Risk factors affecting the survival of patients with pericardial effusion submitted to subxiphoid pericardiostomy. *Chest.* 2003;*124*(1):242–246.

60. Mitchell SL, Miller SC, Teno JM, Davis RB, Shaffer ML. The Advanced Dementia Prognostic Tool: a risk score to estimate survival in nursing home residents with advanced dementia. *Journal of Pain Symptom and Management.* 2010;*40*(5):639–651.

61. Sayed HA, Ali AM, Elzembely MM. Can Pediatric Risk of Mortality Score (PRISM III) be used effectively in initial evaluation and follow-up of critically ill cancer patients admitted to pediatric oncology intensive care unit (POICU)? A prospective study, in a tertiary cancer center in Egypt. *Journal of Pediatric Hematology/Oncology.* 2018;*40*(5):382–386.

62. Gerlach C, Goebel S, Weber S, Weber M, Sleeman KE. Space for intuition—the "surprise"-question in haemato-oncology: qualitative analysis of experiences and perceptions of haemato-oncologists. *Palliative Medicine.* 2019;*33*(5): 536–540. doi:10.1177/0269216318824271

63. Javier AD, Figueroa R, Siew ED, et al. Reliability and utility of the surprise question in CKD stages 4 to 5. *American Journal of Kidney Diseases.* 2017;*70*(1):93–101.

64. Burke K, Coombes LH, Menezes A, Anderson AK. The "surprise" question in paediatric palliative care: a prospective cohort study. *Palliative Medicine.* 2018;*32*(2):535–542.

65. Wilson CJ, Newman J, Tapper S, et al. Multiple locations of advance care planning documentation in an electronic health record: are they easy to find? *Journal of Palliative Medicine.* 2013;*16*(9):1089–1094.

66. Jones CA, Acevedo J, Bull J, Kamal AH. Top 10 tips for using advance care planning codes in palliative medicine and beyond. *Journal of Palliative Medicine.* 2016;*19*(12):1249–1253.

67. Bear A, Thiel E. Documentation of crucial information relating to critically ill patients. *Journal of Palliative Care.* 2018;*33*(1):5–8.

68. Weissman D, Jessick T, McDonagh A, Feuling S. *Improving Generalist Palliative Care: For Hospitalized Seriously Ill Patients.* Palliative Care Network of Wisconsin; 2015 2015.

69. Kamrath HJ, Osterholm E, Stover-Haney R, George T, O'Connor-Von S, Needle J. Lasting legacy: maternal perspectives of perinatal palliative care. *Journal of Palliative Medicine.* 2019;*22*(3):310–315.

70. Akard TF, Dietrich MS, Friedman DL, et al. Digital storytelling: an innovative legacy-making intervention for children with cancer. *Pediatric Blood & Cancer.* 2015;*62*(4):658–665.

71. Foster TL. Personal reflections on legacy making. *Palliative and Supportive Care.* 2010;*8*(1):99–100.

72. Foster TL, Gilmer MJ, Davies B, et al. Bereaved parents' and siblings' reports of legacies created by children with cancer. *Journal of Pediatric Oncology Nursing.* 2009;*26*(6):369–376.

73. Wright AA, Zhang B, Ray A, et al. Associations between end-of-life discussions, patient mental health, medical care near death, and caregiver bereavement adjustment. *JAMA.* 2008;*300*(14):1665–1673.

74. Tilden VP, Tolle SW, Nelson CA, Fields J. Family decision-making to withdraw life-sustaining treatments from hospitalized patients. *Nursing Research.* 2001;*50*(2):105–115.

75. DeCourcey DD, Silverman M, Oladunjoye A, Wolfe J. Advance care planning and parent-reported end-of-life outcomes in children, adolescents, and young adults with complex chronic conditions. *Critical Care Medicine.* 2019;*47*(1):101–108.

Spiritual, Religious, and Existential Aspects of Care

7

Clinical Interprofessional Model of Spiritual Care

Assessing for and Treating Spiritual Distress

Christina M. Puchalski

Introduction

Spiritual care is based on the biopsychosocial spiritual model of care, first described by Dame Cicely Saunders, the founder of the hospice and palliative care model.[1] This model is also the basis of whole-person care,[2] a model required by many health systems that recognize the importance of attending to all factors that impact care and are interconnected—body, mind, spiritual, and community.[3] Saunders also cited the concept of total pain, including spiritual pain. Spiritual pain refers to the immensely intense suffering patients and families can experience. It includes existential pain, often summarized as "why me and why now"; hopelessness; grief; need for reconciliation; questions about meaning; faith-related questioning of beliefs; and isolation from God, a deity, and/or the transcendent or inability to engage in their usual spiritual practices.

The World Health Organization (WHO) passed a resolution for palliative care, referring to care for the seriously or chronically ill and those that are dying. The resolution further states that it is the "ethical obligation of all clinicians to attend to all the suffering of their patients as well as that of the families—psychosocial and spiritual as well as physical."[4] Attending to the suffering of a patient requires not only an assessment of that suffering within the whole-person model of care, but also the practice of compassionate presence and accompaniment of the patient in their suffering. Especially when experiencing deep suffering, no one wants to be alone in isolation with that intense pain. Sometimes the greatest intervention is for the clinician to be present, listen deeply, and commit to care until the person can find healing from the suffering within themselves.

Spiritual Care Model

While spiritual care has been important in models of hospice and palliative care, it was not fully integrated into care until more recently. In 2009, a national consensus conference, Improving the Spiritual Domain of Palliative Care, developed a model of interprofessional spiritual care. First a consensus-based definition for spirituality was developed to help achieve a broad definition that applies to all people—secular, religious, humanist, and others. Spirituality is defined broadly as a "dynamic and intrinsic aspect of humanity through which persons seek ultimate meaning, purpose, and transcendence, and experience relationships to self, family, others, community, society, nature, and the significant or sacred. Spirituality is expressed through beliefs, values, traditions, and practices."[5]

The model of interprofessional spiritual care integrates spiritually centered compassionate care into the biopsychosocial framework. The practice of spiritual care is based on a generalist-specialist model of care; healthcare providers address spiritual concerns and work with spiritual care specialists, such as trained chaplains, in treating spiritual distress. Thus, all clinicians should address patients' spirituality, identify and treat spiritual distress, and support spiritual resources of strength. In depth, spiritual counseling and exploration should be referred to the trained chaplain. All healthcare professionals should be trained in doing a spiritual screening or history as part of their routine history and evaluation.

The essential aspects of the interprofessional model of spiritual care are as follows:

- Spiritual screenings, histories, and assessments should be communicated and documented in patient records and shared with the interprofessional healthcare team. A spiritual history is taken by all clinicians who do clinical assessment and treatment plans—physicians, physician assistants, and advanced practice nurses. In some cases, social workers may also do a spiritual history.
- Follow-up spiritual histories or assessments should be conducted for all patients whose medical, psychosocial, or spiritual condition changes and as part of routine follow-up in a medical history.
- A spiritual issue becomes a diagnosis if the following criteria are met: (1) the spiritual issue leads to distress or suffering (e.g., lack of meaning, conflicted religious beliefs, inability to forgive); (2) the spiritual issue is the cause of a psychological or physical diagnosis, such as depression, anxiety, or acute or chronic pain (e.g., severe meaninglessness that leads to depression or suicidality, guilt that leads to chronic physical pain); and (3) the spiritual issue is a secondary cause or affects the presenting psychological or physical diagnosis (e.g., hypertension is difficult to control because the patient refuses to take medications because of his or her spiritual or cultural beliefs and values.
- Spiritual assessment is a more detailed assessment of spiritual issues and is done by a spiritual care professional such as a trained chaplain. Chaplains advise clinicians how to work with patients' spiritual issues and provide spiritual counseling as indicated. Chaplains also can coordinate the involvement of community spiritual care professionals, such as clergy, pastoral counselors, or spiritual directors. In addition, chaplains may interact with faith community nurses[6] if patients' religious communities have these providers.

- Treatment or care plans should include but not be limited to referral to chaplains, spiritual directors, pastoral counselors, and other spiritual care providers, including clergy or faith-community healers for spiritual counseling; development of spiritual goals, meaning-oriented therapy, mind-body interventions, rituals, spiritual practices, and contemplative interventions.

Symptom Management: Spiritual Distress

The WHO (2009) conference also defined spiritual distress as part of the overall distress diagnostic categories based on the National Comprehensive Cancer Network (NCCN) guidelines. NCCN defines distress as "A multifactorial unpleasant emotional experience of a psychological (cognitive, behavioral, emotional) social, and/or spiritual nature that may interfere with the ability to cope effectively with cancer/illness, its physical symptoms and its treatment."[7] In a systematic review study, the prevalence of spiritual distress within inpatient settings ranged from 16% to 63%, and 96% of patients had experienced spiritual pain at some point in their lives.[8] Table 7.1 lists the spiritual distress that includes the NCCN categories as well as those developed in the previously mentioned consensus conference.[9]

Studies have shown that spirituality can affect how a patient may cope with the illness, find meaning and peace, and define wellness in the midst of treatment of a serious illness such as cancer. Patients with cancer who had high levels of spiritual well-being reported more enjoyment in life and higher levels of meaning and peace, even in the midst of cancer-related symptoms such as fatigue or pain.[10] Spiritual distress is associated with poorer health outcomes, including greater physical pain, depression and anxiety,[11] poor emotional well-being,[12] diminished quality of life,[13] and lower satisfaction with life[14] and increased requests for euthanasia and physician-assisted suicide.[15] Untreated spiritual suffering may worsen the pain experience.[9] Since spiritual distress is a significant source of suffering, it is critical that clinicians address and attend to it in the course of their treatment of the whole patient.

Assessment of Spiritual Distress

Tools for assessing spiritual distress and spiritual concerns include the FICA (Faith, Import, Community, Address) tool, which was validated for cancer patients (Table 7.2).[16] During the visit, clinicians can ask about the spiritual history in the context of the personal or social history. Clinicians can also do a spiritual history in acute visits, such as breaking bad news. Spiritual distress and/or spiritual resources can be documented in the assessment and plan in the patient's chart. Clinicians can respond to the patient's sharing of spiritual distress by listening mindfully, offering presence, praying, or sharing a sacred moment with a patient. They should also consider referral to spiritual care professionals such as chaplains and also consider such referrals as meaning-oriented therapy,[17] multidignity therapy,[18] or other therapies such as mindfulness, art, narrative,[19,20] or music therapy as part of the treatment plan. Interprofessional Spiritual Care Education Curriculum (ISPEC) is a national

TABLE 7.1 Spiritual Distress

Diagnoses (Primary)	Key Feature From History
Existential	Lack of meaning/; questions meaning about one's own existence; /concern about afterlife/; questions the meaning of suffering/; seeks spiritual assistance
Abandonment by God or others	Lack of love, loneliness; not being remembered; no sense of relatedness
Anger at God or others	Displaces anger toward religious representatives/; inability to forgive
Concerns about relationship with deity	Closeness to God, deepening relationship
Conflicted or challenged belief systems	Verbalizes inner conflicts or questions about beliefs or faith; conflicts between religious beliefs and recommended treatments/questions moral or ethical implications of therapeutic regimen; express concern with life/death and/or belief system
Despair/hopelessness	Hopelessness about future health, life Despair as absolute hopelessness, no hope for value in life
Grief/loss	Grief is the feeling and process associated with a loss of person, health, etc.
Guilt/shame	Guilt is the feeling that the person has done something wrong or evil; shame is a feeling that the person is bad or evil
Reconciliation	Need for forgiveness and/or reconciliation of self or others
Isolation	From religious community or other
Religious specific	Ritual needs; unable to practice in usual religious practices
Religious/spiritual struggle	Loss of faith and/or meaning; religious or spiritual beliefs and/or community not helping with coping

and international online course and also a training program for clinicians and spiritual care professionals on interprofessional spiritual care based on the aforementioned generalist-specialist spiritual care model.[21]

Treatment of Spiritual Distress

Unlike physical pain, there are no "quick fixes" for spiritual pain or distress. As mentioned above, the most important intervention a clinician can provide is presence to the patient and a concept known as contemplative or compassionate listening. Contemplative listening is a discussion technique that facilitates a person's internal dialogue. Use of reflective inquiry can help patients focus more deeply on their own internal narrative.[22]

Within these moments of contemplative listening, the patient may come to an awareness about their suffering and maybe even a self-initiated way to address that suffering. Often patients note that "just being listened to" gives them strength to deal with the suffering and hope that it might at some point resolve or even "heal." Within this model of contemplative listening, often clinicians describe "sharing a sacred moment with a patient." In my own

TABLE 7.2 FICA Spiritual History Tool© Puchalski, 1996

F–Faith and Belief	• Do you consider yourself spiritual or religious? or • Do you have spiritual beliefs that help you cope with stress? • If the patient responds "No," the clinician might ask, "What gives your life meaning?" *Sometimes patients respond with answers such as family, career, or nature.*
I–Importance	• What importance does your faith or belief have in our life? • Have your beliefs influenced how you take care of yourself in this illness? • What role do your beliefs play in regaining your health
C–Community	• Are you part of a spiritual or religious community? • Is this of support to you and how? • Is there a group of people you really love or who are important to you? *Communities such as churches, temples, and mosques or a group of like-minded friends can serve as strong support systems for some patients.*
A–Address in Care/ Assessment	• How would you like me, your healthcare provider, to address these issues in your healthcare? • Use this category to assess for spiritual distress

experiences, the sense of something sacred or even holy occurs most often in these moments of deep silence and grace.

The process is first to still the mind and connect with our own spiritual values and our vocation to serve others. We focus on our intention to serve the other and be fully present. We raise our awareness to the patient as well as ourselves. We then practice contemplative listening by holding the space (silence, no fixing, no answer, no judgment). Then using our informed intuition or awareness, we transition back to the rest of the clinical visit.

One model that describes this approach to compassionate presence is GRACE, developed by Joan Halifax[23] (Box 7.1).

BOX 7.1 GRACE

G: Reminds us to pause and get grounded; focus our attention on the breath. On the inhale, we "gather attention"; on the exhale, we bring the attention to the body, getting stable and grounded.

R: Recalling our intention to serve others, to act with integrity and respect the integrity of others.

A: Attune to ourselves—our physical, emotional, cognitive experience and then, that of the patient. This is where boundaries enter in as the clinician needs to be aware when issues that are the clinician's get confused with the issues of the patient.

C: Considering which is a process of discerning using our intuition and insight about what is the appropriate response to the patient

E: Ethical engagement with the other in compassionate action, then when appropriate marking the end of the encounter.

The G.R.A.C.E. model has five elements:

1. **G**athering attention: focus, grounding, balance
2. **R**ecalling intention: the resource of motivation
3. **A**ttuning to self/other: affective resonance
4. **C**onsidering: what will serve
5. **E**ngaging: ethical enactment, then ending

Case Examples

Case 7.1

Jessica is a 27-year-old female who comes for a new-patient visit. She recently moved to Washington, D.C., to work with the government as a computer analyst. She is single and currently not in a relationship. Her chief concern is her anxiety, which she rates as 6–10/10. It is beginning to affect her sleep and work. She denies depression. She is beginning to make friends but has not yet established a good support system.

Her family history is significant for many members of family with anxiety disorders; her father was an alcoholic, and her sister had severe learning disabilities.

Her FICA spiritual history from the first visit is as follows:

- F: Not religious, does not relate to the word spiritual. Meaning: Has no meaning in life, no sense of purpose
- I: No values or beliefs that impact her health
- C: No spiritual community, very little support from family
- A: Not interested in talking with anyone

Jessica returns for a follow-up visit for anxiety. She raises the issue of meaning and purpose, saying, "I have been thinking about your questions about meaning in my life. It is sad I don't have any meaning." She wanted to discuss this further. From her narrative in this second visit, the following information was documented:

- **F**: Raised Catholic but not interested in going back to Catholicism or any faith. Her parents also left the church shortly after her brother was born. Meaning: Has no meaning in life, no sense of purpose, and since last visit has been exploring that and would like to find some meaning in her life and something that would guide her in her life.
- **I**: Sees a connection between lack of meaning and her anxiety.
- **C**: Interested in finding some spiritual ("in a broad sense") community.
- **A**: Would like some resources from her physician; not interested in therapy or chaplain visit.

TABLE 7.3 Jessica's Biopsychosocial-Spiritual Model Assessment and Plan

Jessica is a 27-year-old seen for a well visit and follow-up for anxiety. Interested in mind-body resources; searching for community; complicated issues with family.

Physical	Exercise, healthy eating, regular hours of sleep
Emotional	Suggested counselor; patient declined
Social	Encouraged building a support community of friends
Spiritual	Offer list of resources: mindfulness sessions; Adult Children of Alcoholics (ACOA) meeting given family history of alcoholism; Unitarian community as a potential community that is not specifically religious; consider meaning-oriented therapy

In this case, the clinician listened to Jessica's story without judgment. She elicited more about Jessica's understanding of the lack of meaning and how she sees that connected to her anxiety. The clinician also listened about the family issues at her home when she was young and how that might have affected her. Jessica mentioned that for reasons she did not know her parents left the church early in Jessica's life. Table 7.3 shows Jessica's whole-person assessment and plan based on the previous assessment.

Case 7.2

Frank is a 66-year-old male who presents for a new-patient visit with a physician assistant. Frank's wife of 35 years died suddenly from an aortic dissection 3 months prior to this visit. Frank moved from New York to Pennsylvania to be closer to his son, Jamison. Frank is a teacher in a junior college, where he has been mostly teaching online courses in creative writing. He took time off after his wife's death and his move. He noticed that he could not remember things as much and worried that maybe he was getting dementia as his mother had dementia when she was 76 years old. He also notes that 3 weeks after his wife died he had chest pain and shortness of breath. He has been treated for hypertension since age 45 and thought maybe he was having a heart attack. All the tests in the emergency room were negative. Subsequently, he had a cardiac stress test, which was negative. Frank was diagnosed with a panic attack. Frank has a history of mild anxiety, mostly exacerbated by stress, but says he never has felt as badly as he does now. Tearful, he notes that he feels like he cannot go on anymore, and that the "pain inside is too great." He denies suicidal ideation and affirms insomnia and decreased appetite since his wife died. He lost 10 pounds within 3 weeks of his wife's death. His FICA spiritual history is as follows:

- **F**: Raised Episcopalian, was very involved in his faith community but since his wife died, he cannot go back to church. He feels that maybe if he had not worked so hard he might have been able to notice something was wrong with his wife. His meaning is in his family and his work. He notes that "my son is grown up and settled now so I have not much more to help him with." When asked about his teaching, Frank notes that he is unsure.
- **I**: His faith is very important to him; he prayed and meditated all his life but less so since his wife's death. He talks about the intense emptiness he feels since his wife died. "Is there

TABLE 7.4 Frank's Biopsychosocial-Spiritual Model Assessment and Plan

Frank is a 66-year-old male with a history of hypertension and anxiety presenting for a new-patient visit. His wife died 3 months ago; he had one emergency department visit shortly after her death where he was diagnosed with a panic attack. He has depression and anxiety as well as spiritual distress.

Physical	Exercise, healthy eating, regular hours of sleep
Emotional	Referral to a therapist; begin antidepressant for his depression
Social	Encouraged building a support community of friends in his new area. Also suggested he begin reflecting on if and how he might continue teaching.
Spiritual	Grief, existential distress (why me?); conflicts about faith (God's presence, question of guilt). Referral to chaplain. Begin reflecting on this new phase in life on what would give meaning now.

really a God? Why would he do this to her and to me?" He also asks, "Am I still OK with God? I worked so hard; did I miss the fact that my wife was sick?"

- **C:** Would like to go back to church "eventually, just not now." Enjoys his son and son's family very much. Has friends back home and misses them.
- **A:** Would be interested in speaking with a chaplain or spiritual director.

During the visit, the PA was able to be present for Frank and created a sacred space where Frank was able to share his deep grief and his spiritual and existential distress. Not trying to fix him, the PA simply acknowledged his suffering by her presence and willingness to listen. After listening deeply, when it was clear that Frank fully expressed his needs and fears, the PA transitioned to the rest of the visit. First, the PA conveyed to Frank that she will be there with him in his difficult time. She also discussed resuming his meditation practice as studies have shown a benefit of meditation in the treatment of anxiety. Frank agreed that he has anxiety and maybe even depression. He was willing to start a low dose of an antidepressant. The PA also explored Frank's interest in reflecting on his meaning in his teaching and family and how that might look like now in his new phase of his life. The PA set up a follow-up appointment for 2 weeks and made referrals to a chaplain and a mental health counselor.

In this case, Frank's distress was both emotional (depression and anxiety) and spiritual distress. The latter was bereavement and loss, questioning about meaning in life, deep existential pain("why me"), and religion-specific distress in not being able to practice his prayer and meditation as well as wondering if he was being punished in some way (Table 7.4).

Conclusion

To standardize and institutionalize spirituality as a component of whole-patient care, the biopsychosocial-spiritual model must be integrated across the continuum of care for all patients. The biopsychosocial-spiritual model recognizes the distinct dimensions—biological, psychological, social, and spiritual—of a person and the fact that no dimension can be left out when caring for the whole person. For the same reason current practice includes psychosocial inquiries, spiritual inquiry also is needed in recognition that each person's history and illness are unique and will affect all dimensions of that person in unique ways. This chapter describes a consensus- and evidence-based model that enables clinicians to fully attend to the spiritual needs and the spiritual distress that patients and their families may experience.

References

1. Saunders C. The treatment of intractable pain in terminal cancer. *Proceedings of the Royal Society of Medicine.* 1963;56(3): 195–197.

2. Puchalski C, Ferrell B, Virani R, et al. Improving the quality of spiritual care as a dimension of palliative care: the report of the consensus conference. *Journal of Palliative Medicine.* 2009;12(10):885–904.

3. Allina Health. Whole person care. http://possible.allinahealth.org/whole-person-care. Accessed June 4, 2020.

4. World Health Assembly. Strengthening of palliative care as a component of comprehensive care throughout the life course. Report by the Secetariat. 2014. https://apps.who.int/iris/handle/10665/158962

5. Puchalski CM, Vitillo R, Hull SK, Reller N. Improving the spiritual dimension of whole person care: reaching national and international consensus. *Journal of Palliative Medicine.* 2014;17(6):642–656.

6. Center for Faith and Community Health Transformation. Faith community nursing (parish nursing): what is faith community nursing? 2020. https://www.faithhealthtransformation.org/resources-and-toolkits/faith-community-nursing/. Accessed June 10.

7. NCCN Guidelines for Patients: Distress®. https://www.nccn.org/patients/guidelines/content/PDF/distress patient.pdf. Accessed June 4, 2020.

8. Roze des Ordons AL, Sinuff T, Stelfox HT, Kondejewski J, Sinclair S. Spiritual distress within inpatient settings—a scoping review of patients' and families' experiences. *Journal of Pain and Symptom Management.* 2018;56(1):122–145.

9. Puchalski C, Ferrell B, Virani R, et al. Improving the quality of spiritual care as a dimension of palliative care: the report of the consensus conference. *Journal of Palliative Medicine.* 2009:12(10):885–904.

10. Norris L, Pratt-Chapman M, Noblick JA, Cowens-Alvarado R. Distress, demoralization, and depression in cancer survivorship. *Psychiatric Annals.* 2011;41(9):433–438.

11. Delgado-Guay MO, Chisholm G, Williams J, Frisbee-Hume S, Ferguson AO, Bruera E. Frequency, intensity, and correlates of spiritual pain in advanced cancer patients assessed in a supportive/palliative care clinic. *Palliative and Supportive Care.* 2016;14(4):341–348.

12. Salsman JM, Fitchett G, Merluzzi TV, Sherman AC, Park CL. Religion, spirituality, and health outcomes in cancer: a case for a meta-analytic investigation. *Cancer.* 2015;121(21):3754–3759.

13. Jafari N, Farakzadegan Z, Zamani I, Bahrami F, Emami H, Loghmani A. Spiritual well-being and quality of life in Iranian women with breast cancer undergoing radiation therapy. *Supportive Care in Cancer.* 2013;21(5):1219–1225.

14. Siddall P J, McIndoe L, Austin P, Wrigley PJ. The impact of pain on spiritual well-being in people with a spinal cord injury. *Spinal Cord.* 2017;55(1):105–111.

15. Radbruch L, Leget C, Bahr P, et al. Euthanasia and physician-assisted suicide: a white paper from the European Association for Palliative Care. *Palliative Medicine.* 2016;30(2):104–116.

16. Borneman T, Ferrell B, Puchalski CM. Evaluation of the FICA Tool for Spiritual Assessment. *Journal of Pain and Symptom Management.* 2010;40(2):163–173.

17. Lichtenthal WG, Catarozoli C, Masterson M, et al. An open trial of meaning-centered grief therapy: rationale and preliminary evaluation. *Palliative and Supportive Care.* 2019;17(1):2–12.

18. Chochinov HM, Hack T, Hassard T, Kristjanson LJ, McClement S, Harlos M. Dignity and psychotherapeutic considerations in end-of-life care. *Journal of Palliative Care.* 2004;*20*(3):134–142.
19. Rodriguez Vega B, Bayon Perez C, PalaoTarrero A, Fernandez Liria A. Mindfulness-based narrative therapy for depression in cancer patients. *Clinical Psychology and Psychotherapy.* 2014;*21*(5):411–419.
20. Rodriguez Vega B, Palao A, Torres G, et al. Combined therapy versus usual care for the treatment of depression in oncologic patients: a randomized controlled trial. *Psychooncology.* 2011;*20*(9):943–952.
21. Puchalski C, Jafari N, Buller H, Haythorn T, Jacobs C, Ferrell B. Interprofessional spiritual care education curriculum: a milestone toward the provision of spiritual care. *Journal of Palliative Medicine.* 2020;*23*(6):777–784.
22. Evers H. Contemplative listening: a rhetorical-critical approach to facilitate internal dialog. *Journal of Pastoral Care and Counseling.* 2017;*71*(2):114–121.
23. Halifax J. GRACE for nurses: cultivating compassion in nurse/patient interactions. *Journal of Nursing Education and Practice.* 2014;*4*(1):121.

8

Foundational Guidance in Grief and Bereavement

Jamie Beachy

Grief and Loss as a Normal Part of Life

In a 2016 interview on the public radio program *On Being*, B. J. Miller, a physician leader in the field of palliative medicine, shared insights about the human experience of grief and loss:

> We have these bookends of birth and death and in between feels like a guitar solo—in between, all sorts of crazy things can happen. But the song begins and the song ends, at least for this bodily life. And the fact that we share, that 100 percent of us across time and space, across cultures, that all of us share that version of fate is compelling to me. So finding a purchase, a toehold in what we share and all that we share opens me up in a way that I feel—that feels beautiful, that makes me love people more, not less, that makes me more open to people, not less, makes me more open to myself, not less.[1]

Miller's words serve to advocate for death awareness as a path toward greater connection with self and others—countering a tendency in North American culture to deny the reality of death. In many traditional cultures, the reality of death is honored in everyday life through ancestral family altars or observances such as *Día de los Muertos* ("Day of the Dead"). Modern cultures may approach death and loss as subjects to be avoided in everyday conversation. To speak of loss in dominant North American culture can be associated with weakness, fragility, or negativity. Yet, as Miller and many others who work in the field of palliative care have discovered, integrating an awareness of death and loss into everyday life can create greater connection with others and gratitude for life through the common and shared experience of vulnerability and impermanence. The living exist in the space between the bookends of birth and death—a space ripe with change, transition, loss and ultimately, death. Just as each person who has ever lived must face the reality of death for themselves and those they love, so, too, is the presence of loss woven into the fabric of each person's life, especially during times of illness.

The losses that come about as a result of an advanced illness can be destabilizing or even devastating, and the loss of a loved one can initiate a profound grief process. The loss will need to be integrated in order for a new sense of well-being to shape itself once again in the lives and hearts of those who grieve. Without adequate support and a capacity to adapt to the new reality, the experience of loss can lead to mental health problems, addictions, and ongoing existential suffering.

For those able to move through loss with a new sense of meaning and purpose, healthy coping strategies, and resilience, loss can become an opportunity for personal growth. The needs of those with advanced illness, the bereaved who must mourn their deaths, and the clinicians who care for them, are of central concern to this chapter. How clinicians can best navigate the inevitable losses and transitions that they will face in their own lives while caring for their grieving patients is an important consideration in light of the high rates of clinician burnout in the field of palliative care.[2]

For those with advanced illness, losses can range from seemingly small changes such as the loss of one's ability to eat certain foods or read a newspaper to more profound losses, such as a failed surgical treatment or missing the birth of a grandchild as a result of a terminal diagnosis. Although every life will necessarily include loss, the pace at which losses occur is accelerated with the onset of a chronic or serious illness. When a patient dies as a result of serious illness, the patient's bereaved loved ones will need support to navigate complex emotions, psychological challenges, and physical manifestations of grief. How palliative care clinicians can best support patients and their loved ones through the many losses that cascade from the onset of an advanced illness is the central consideration of this chapter. While the losses that result from advanced illness are disruptive and disorienting, grieving well with adequate support may hold opportunities for greater connection to sources of meaning and personal growth.

Grief, Bereavement, and Mourning

Before carefully considering the needs of palliative care patients and their loved ones who are experiencing grief and loss, it will be helpful to define key terms as they are utilized within the context of palliative care.

Grief is generally understood as a normal or expected response to loss and may include the presence of challenging emotions, such as sadness, anger, loneliness, regret, and numbness. A normal grieving process will include physical, emotional, cognitive, interpersonal, and spiritual responses to a significant loss or life change.[3] It is important to note that what constitutes a "normal" response to grief will vary depending on the particular cultural and religious context of the griever. Though more will be said about this further in the chapter, it is important from the outset to recognize that what is normative is located within a particular cultural context and social location. Loneliness as a response to the death of a loved one may be understood as normal in one culture and abnormal in another, for example. Here, the designation of *normal* is intended to differentiate normal grief from more complex forms of grief, such as traumatic, complicated, anticipatory, and disenfranchised grief. When assessing grief responses, clinicians should always be aware of cultural bias, which can lead to misinterpretation and cultural insensitivity, and approach patients and their loved ones from a position of cultural humility.

Mourning is the individual or communal expression of grief responses. One who has experienced the loss of a loved one may express a depth of sorrow through crying, rocking, or wailing. Mourning, as an individual or communal expression of grief, often includes culturally determined practices that invite the mourner to enact their grief in particular ways. Mourners may wear black clothing to a memorial service, send flowers to a loved one, create a home altar for remembrance, host relatives for a family meal, or compose a moving eulogy or song for the deceased. Healthy mourning allows those who are in an experience of grief to move through loss with social support and a path through the intensity of the grief experience. Yet, just as there is no clearly "normal" way of experiencing grief, what is considered normal mourning is also dependent on particular cultural norms and values. Within North American culture, for example, a quietly reflective, stoic, and individualistic expression of grief may be perceived by clinicians to be a normal mourning response while highly expressive and more communal expressions of grief, such as wailing and moaning, in large groups may be judged as unhealthy and outside of the preferred norm. It is generally understood that mourning with support from others is important for integrating a significant loss.

Bereavement refers to the condition of having lost a significant family member or loved one to death. Bereavement is not associated with any defined time period, and though most bereaved people will heal from the death of a loved one, some bereaved people will never be able to recover from such a loss.

Types of Grief and Clinical Interventions

Elizabeth Kubler-Ross, a Swiss American psychiatrist, was one of the first clinicians to address grief experienced by those with chronic illnesses. In her book *On Death and Dying* (1969),[4] Kubler-Ross first shared her research gathered from interviewing patients at the end of their lives. Her well-known five-stage model of grief describes patients' grief reactions as a linear sequence of denial, anger, bargaining, depression, and acceptance.[4] The Kubler-Ross model of grief has not been supported by bereavement research. In reality, grief does not follow a sequential and fixed process but is more often experienced in a dynamic and fluctuating way.[3(p21)]

Attending to the grief of palliative care patients and their loved ones is inherent to the whole-person model of palliative care that seeks to address and diminish physical, emotional, psychosocial, existential, and spiritual dimensions of suffering.

Skilled palliative care clinicians are attuned to assessing different types of grief, ensuring that the impact of loss in the lives of their patients is included in the overall care plan.

Each member of the team will bring particular insights and interventions to interdisciplinary planning. A palliative care chaplain, for example, might support a patient experiencing existential suffering after a major stroke by cocreating a ritual of transition, designed to provide a container for the patient's grief and a way for loved ones to express their support. Marking the end of the patient's prestroke identity and calling in a new way of living in the world will help the patient adapt to the difficulties of the loss in a more empowered way. In the case of a mother suffering from anticipatory grief after learning of her child's terminal diagnosis, the mother may benefit from meeting with a palliative care social worker trained in grief counseling.

For physician assistants (PA), listening to patients share their stories of grief provides important support for patients and loved ones. Each member of the palliative care team has the opportunity and responsibility to support those who are grieving as a way of contributing to the care of the patient and the overall well-being of their family unit.

In order to best support patients through the losses and changes that influence or come about as a result of serious illness, it will be helpful to consider different types of grief and the needs that are presented by each. The Clinical Practice Guidelines for Quality Palliative Care* affirm that grief assessments and services are fundamental components of the ongoing palliative plan of care.[5] All members of the palliative care team should have a foundational understanding of different types of grief and the ways that each may interact with the patient's and loved ones' experience of advanced illness.

Normal Grief

Patients with advanced illness will experience grief responses that are likely to manifest as physical, emotional, cognitive, psychosocial, and spiritual reactions to loss. Though grief can eventually bring about insight and personal growth, the experience of grief is initially one of disorientation and instability. Table 8.1 illustrates some of challenging grief responses that patients and their loved ones may experience.

Along with challenging responses to grief and loss, some individuals will experience positive grief responses and personal growth that comes about as a result of the experience of loss.[6] Patients may feel confused by the coexistence of challenging grief reactions and more positive manifestations of grief such as feelings of appreciation and connection. Patients approaching the end of life may experience a sense of being held by a benevolent presence or a deep appreciation for the preciousness of life. Though not all people will experience positive manifestations of their grieving, Table 8.2 illustrates potential growth responses that some grieving persons will experience in the course of an illness or bereavement process.

In their study of posttraumatic growth responses, researchers discovered that between 30% and 70% of individuals who experienced trauma also reported positive change and growth coming out of the traumatic experience.[6] Traumatic growth can be defined as the "the experience of positive change that occurs as a result of the struggle with highly challenging life crises. It is manifested in a variety of ways, including an increased appreciation

---

* The fourth edition of the guidelines was produced jointly by the National Coalition for Hospice and Palliative Care and the National Consensus Project for Quality Palliative Care.

TABLE 8.1 Common Grief Responses

Physical	Emotional	Cognitive	Psychosocial	Spiritual/Existential
Gastrointestinal disturbance	Helplessness	Disorientation	Isolation	Hopelessness
Heart palpitations	Hopelessness	Nightmares	Suicidal ideation	Crisis of meaning
Tightness in chest	Despair	Lack of concentration and focus	Increased substance use	Existential fear or despair
Breathlessness	Fear	Hallucinations	Risk-taking	Abandonment
Lack of energy	Numbness	Impaired memory	Avoidance	Feeling of being punished
Dry mouth	Anger	Rumination on the past	Worry about finances	Loss of faith
Loss of libido	Shock	Obsessive thoughts	Lost ability to work	Disconnection from community
Appetite changes	Shame	Feelings of victimization	Loss of social identity	Guilt
Dizziness	Guilt/regret	Disassociation	Change in family roles	
Weight changes	Sleepiness	Confusion	Identity crisis	
Sleep problems	Resentment	Insomnia		
Crying	Shock	Disbelief		
Shaking				
Chills/sweats				

Adapted from Strada EA. *Grief and Bereavement in the Adult Palliative Care Setting.* Oxford: Oxford University Press; 2013.

TABLE 8.2 Potential Growth Responses to Grief

Physical	Emotional	Cognitive	Psychosocial	Spiritual
Improved self-care habits	Redefined hope	Self-confidence	Gratitude	Hopefulness
Well-being that transcends physical limitations	Gratitude for life and loved ones	Spiritual dreams	Renewed purpose	Meaning-making
Greater attunement to physical health	Connection to common humanity	Visions	Self-acceptance	Connection with the transcendent or with nature
Appreciation for simple sensual experiences	A desire to leave a legacy	New insights	Forgiveness of self and others	Self-forgiveness
Gratitude for having lived an embodied human life	Peace in the midst of the storm	Increased self-awareness	Sense of completion	Shared common humanity
Feeling part of something larger than oneself	Courage	Increased agency	Greater connection to self and others	Stronger faith

for life in general, more meaningful interpersonal relationships, an increased sense of personal strength, changed priorities, and a richer existential and spiritual life."[7]

Growth is not an automatic or direct result of adversity, but is related to the conditions under which a person struggles as a result of the adversity.[7] Social support, genuine acceptance from others, the guidance of mentors and other supportive guides, and healthy coping strategies are factors that are more likely to lead to positive growth.

Calhounet et al. described how posttraumatic growth can be experienced in five areas following loss: (1) self-perception, where bereaved individuals may come to view themselves paradoxically as "more vulnerable, yet stronger"; (2) changed relationships in which bereaved persons may experience negative changes but often report positive changes; (3) new possibilities, whereby those who are grieving may develop new roles and new relationships; (4) appreciation of life, where bereaved individuals are able to live more fully in the present; and (5) existential elements, which can include religious and spiritual transformation and renewal. For Calhoun and colleagues, the five areas are not all inclusive but are often present in grieving persons who demonstrate posttraumatic growth following a loss.[7]

As Ira Byock, a physician leader in the field of hospice care, has articulated, terminal patients may experience tremendous growth as they near death. In their role, PAs can help facilitate this movement toward growth, contributing to healthy grieving for patients and their loved ones while enhancing the PA's own sense of purpose and well-being. Persons with a terminal diagnosis often develop a sense of completion with relationships; a new sense of meaning about life, love of self, love of others; an acceptance of finality; a new sense of self; and a surrender to the transcendent.[8] Competent palliative care clinicians address distress while recognizing that grief can also serve as a portal for personal and spiritual growth.[9]

Case

The following case illustrates one patient's experience of normal grief and the interventions that support his well-being, social and spiritual connection, and relief from unnecessary suffering.

Javier is a 58-year-old patient who entered a palliative care service on receiving a diagnosis of stage IV non–small cell lung cancer. For many years, Javier has worked as a woodworker and carpenter with a local company that designs and builds furniture. In the 2 weeks since his diagnosis was confirmed, Javier has retired from his company and moved into the ground level of his home—a home where he lives with his wife and two children, ages 15 and 12. Javier and his wife, Sarah, recently informed their children of Javier's diagnosis and the expected difficulties they expect to face as it progresses. As Javier's capacity for independent living decreases, he will be cared for at home by a caregiver hired with funds from their family savings. Javier has been told that he has a life expectancy of 1 year with the support of chemotherapy and radiation treatment.

In an initial family meeting with the palliative care team, the following dimensions of Javier's experience of grief and loss are explored:

> *Emotional Dimension*: "I have to say I am not doing well emotionally at all. I wake up
> in the morning with this feeling of a cold stone in the center of my heart. No matter

how much I cry or try to think positively, the feeling of heaviness does not go away. I am too young to die and too young to leave my family to live without me. When I am not overwhelmed with feelings of sadness, I am completely knocked over by fear. I am afraid of being in pain and having to rely on others. I am terrified of the future."

Physical Dimension: "Sometimes I can't tell the difference between the disease in my body and my grief about the disease. I have tremors, anxiety, shaking, a pain in my back, and this feeling like I can't breathe deeply. Every time something happens with my body, I think, oh no, the cancer is growing larger."

Psychosocial Dimension: "I don't know who I am anymore. I can't work like I used to. I can barely help around the house or mow the lawn. I feel like a constant burden to Sarah, and I feel more like her child than her husband. Sometimes I wish I had just been hit by a bus because it would be easier than this. Even though my friends come by to see me, none of them really understand what it's like. On the other hand, this illness has really brought my life into focus. All of the things I once thought were so important seem irrelevant now. I am so grateful for my family and for the beautiful life we have together. I am just angry that I can't see my children grow up or grow old with my wife. And I don't know how we are going to afford all of this care. How will my children go to college?"

Spiritual Dimension: "I have always been so connected with nature, and that's where my source of strength is coming from right now. If I can spend a few hours outside on our deck each day in the sunlight and near our stream, I feel like somehow I will make it through. I know that I am not alone. . . . It is just a feeling I have always had since I was a kid. I am not really religious, but I'm not afraid of death; I am just so sad and angry that my life will be cut short.

"My daughter has set up a little circle of rocks down by the stream where we can write down our hopes and our fears to leave there by the creek. She has such a deep spirit for a 15-year-old. I am so grateful for my family, and I know they will be OK even when I am gone."

Javier's experience of grief can be understood as a normal response to the myriad losses cascading through his life as a result of a serious, progressive, and terminal disease process. Assessing the various dimensions of grief—emotional, physical, psychosocial, and spiritual—will set the foundation for the team's ability to support a healthy grieving process for both Javier and his family. Addressing Javier's grief as part of an integrated care plan can prevent the onset of more complex mental health challenges, such as depression, suicidality, and existential anxiety from taking shape for Javier or his family members.

Brief Interventions for Normal Grief

The following interventions are examples of grief interventions that can be offered by any member of the palliative care team to facilitate a healthy grieving process for Javier and his family:

Emotional Dimension: In the initial palliative care team meeting, Javier reflects on how he is coping with his illness. After listening nonjudgmentally to Javier and Sarah without interruption or interpretation, the team registered nurse (RN) responds by validating and normalizing Javier's sadness and feelings of fear. The RN assures Javier that what he is feeling is normal and that the palliative care team will be there to help Javier and his family navigate this difficult time. The palliative care chaplain encourages Javier to take it one day at a time and to be gentle with himself.

Physical: In a follow-up appointment, the palliative care PA assesses Javier's ongoing physical symptoms associated with grief. After clarifying the treatment plan for his physical pain, she suggests a breathing practice to reduce anxiety before bedtime. She assures Javier that his symptoms will be addressed by the team.

Psychosocial Dimension: The psychosocial dimension of Javier's grief is yet another opportunity for the team to offer grief support. In one individual meeting with the PA, Javier expresses feeling burdensome to his family now that he is unable to work. The PA empathizes with Javier to reduce his feelings of isolation. He invites Javier to share more about his disappointment at no longer being able to work and listens for ways other than work that Javier finds purpose and meaning. The PA reflects on the importance of having a loving family and shares how he is moved by the ritual space set up by his daughter. The PA assures Javier that the team will be there as Javier and his family find their way through this difficult journey with his illness.

Spiritual Dimension: In a routine patient visit, the palliative care nurse affirms Javier's connection to nature as a resource for healthy coping. The nurse, an outdoor enthusiast, empathizes with Javier and validates his resources for spiritual meaning-making. The nurse lets Javier know that having time outside will be good for his grieving process as well as his physical health. In addition to each team member's attentiveness to Javier's spiritual needs and resources, the Palliative Care (PC) chaplain provides Javier and his family with the opportunity to explore their existential fears and their hopes for the future.

The team's support for Javier's grief process is woven into Javier's overall treatment plan. In addressing grief as a normal part of his journey with advanced illness, the team supports Javier's quality of life and overall health and well-being beyond just the physical manifestations of his disease process. Many patients and their families will experience normal manifestations of grief and loss. Many others will experience the following more nuanced and complex forms of grief.

Anticipatory Grief

When a patient or loved one knows or believes in advance that a significant loss will occur, they will often experience grief in anticipation of the loss. Anticipatory grief is very common in palliative care as patients look ahead to the natural outcome of serious or progressive illness. The loved ones of a patient will also experience anticipatory loss as they imagine life without the presence of their loved one.

Disenfranchised Grief

Grief is disenfranchised when the griever experiences a loss that cannot be openly acknowledged, socially sanctioned, or publicly mourned.[10] Grief can become disenfranchised for many reasons: (1) The loss isn't seen to be worthy of grief (e.g., a first-trimester miscarriage). (2) The relationship is stigmatized (e.g., the death of a same-sex partner). (3) The manner of death is stigmatized (e.g., complications from addictive behaviors). (4) The person grieving is not recognized as a griever (e.g., grief as a result of emigration). (5) The way someone is grieving is stigmatized (e.g., showing not enough or too much emotion). To convey sensitivity to grief among persons of different cultural and religious backgrounds or marginalized communities, it is important to ask the patient and their loved ones to describe their own experience of loss rather than assuming a common shared experience. Patients and loved ones can teach the palliative care team about their grief when they are listened to with calm and curious respect.

Complicated Grief

Sometimes grief is complicated by multiple losses, addiction, a history of trauma, or other complex coexisting influences. Complicated grief can impede decision-making and can make grieving more intense or difficult to navigate. Additionally, a current loss can trigger previous trauma experiences, and addictions or mental illnesses can add complexity to the grieving process.

Ambiguous Grief

Some losses bring up ambiguous feelings that can be confusing for the griever. Caregivers who have spent years caring for loved ones—sacrificing self-care, sleep, and personal interests, for example—may feel a mix of relief, sadness, and a loss of identity when the one they have cared for dies. Similarly, when a family member who has been abusive dies, surviving family members may feel a confusing mix of emotions. Though the family members of a patient are often referred to as the "loved ones," it is important to remember that the particular family member may have been resented, detested, and feared, but not necessarily loved.

Traumatic Grief

Traumatic grief can come about as a result of a sudden, unexpected, and traumatic loss such as an accident, a violent incident, a sexual assault, or a natural disaster. Though the majority of people with advanced illnesses experience a gradual illness progression, the suddenness of a terminal diagnosis can have a traumatic impact in the patient's life. Additionally, traumatic grief from the past or from a concurrent event can impact the patient or loved ones' grieving in important ways. Trauma is generally defined as a life-threatening event with lasting adverse effects.

The experience of receiving a serious or terminal diagnosis and the losses that follow can be a traumatic influence in the lives of patients and their loved ones. In addition to traumatic grief reactions that patients may experience as a result of the disease process, Edward Machtinger, a physician leader in trauma-informed medical care, articulated the following reasons for including a consideration of trauma into palliative care treatment and planning: (1) Childhood and adult trauma underlie and perpetuate many serious physical and psychosocial illnesses. (2) Data show that there is a striking association between trauma and illness. In 1994, the Centers for Disease Control and Prevention and Kaiser Permanente collaborated on a study of adverse childhood events (ACEs), assessing the relationship between adult health risk behaviors and childhood abuse and household dysfunction.[11] ACEs in childhood are strongly correlated with adult disease.[12] (3) Effective, evidence-based treatments exist that can be integrated into health-care settings and palliative care teams to help people heal from trauma and its consequence, posttraumatic stress disorder. Machtinger affirmed that the best way to support palliative care patients is to assume a history of trauma since half of all children have experienced one ACE, and 1 in 10 has experienced three or more. Offering statements of empathy and support while affirming the patient or loved one for having the courage to share their experience conveys respect and acceptance.[11]

Honoring the many forms of grief in the clinical context of palliative care allows for the possibility for patients and their loved ones to move through grief toward a new sense of meaning, purpose, and identity, contributing to positive health outcomes and a healthy journey with illness and death.

Bereavement

For many, the experience of losing a loved one to death is emotionally, physically, psychosocially, and spiritually destabilizing. Though a majority of people will recover from the death of a loved one through integrating the loss into a new sense of self, others will experience a more prolonged grief. As many who have lost a loved one well know, the death of someone dear is never truly healed, even when the intensity of the loss is integrated into a new sense of well-being.

Helping patients and loved ones integrate the loss of a loved one may take many months (and sometimes years). With support from friends, family, and professional bereavement counselors and support groups, most people will find a way to continue on in spite of the absence of the loved one in their lives.

Respecting the Mourner's Culture

Cultivating respect and humility in approaching the grieving or bereaved person's culture is a core dimension of quality care. Quality palliative care guidelines include a regard for the ways that culture shapes grief and bereavement, "Grief and bereavement support and interventions are in accordance with developmental, cultural, and spiritual needs and the expectations and preferences of the family."[5(p49)] For clinicians to gain competence in assessing the cultural needs of their patients, it is important that they first assess their own cultural beliefs about grieving and mourning to identify potential biases. A clinician who has learned to withdraw into privacy during times of significant loss may unintentionally judge or fail to support a grieving person who grieves communally and more emotively, for example.

When Children Grieve

Children are unique, and just like adults, they will grieve in their own way. Because children's grief responses are just as challenging as those of adults, their loved ones and the clinicians who care for them may be inclined to avoid asking about their grief. Like adults, children need to be invited to grieve in anticipation of their own deaths in order to diminish feelings of isolation and hold space for the possibility that the end of life may hold possibilities for their growth. The Hospice Foundation of America offers the guidelines that follow for supporting children who are grieving.[13]

Consider a child's age and ability to understand complex ideas. Very young children may not yet have a concrete understanding of death, so use language that is appropriate to the age of the child and let their questions guide the conversation. *It is okay to say you don't know the answer to a child's question.* It is best to be honest with children while affirming that they are safe and loved.

Use precise terms when talking about death. Children will become confused by vague terms like "passed away" or "we lost him to cancer." It is best to use language that is clear and age appropriate when speaking about death and dying. The same is true for speaking about illness and treatment plans. *Giving children information and choices when facing death and grief can be very helpful.* Children are curious and want to understand what is happening around them. *Remember that children cannot tolerate long periods of sadness.* Opportunities to create art and engage other types of play can give grieving children a break from talking directly about their sadness.

Bereavement groups may be an effective way for school-aged children to process their grief by participating with other children who have suffered losses.

Caring for children who are grieving requires sensitivity, close collaboration with the child's parents, respect for the family's beliefs and values, and a willingness to stay present to the child's questions and need for clear information about what is happening to them.

The Role of Physician Assistants in Assessing the Needs of Grieving Patients and Loved Ones

Assessing grief and bereavement is a necessary and important task for palliative care clinicians of all disciplines in order to monitor the severity of grief responses. Meaningful assessment allows the team to both recognize the extent of the grief reactions and the interaction with cultural, spiritual, and psychosocial dimensions of the care plan.[3]

Competent PAs attend to brief screenings as well as ongoing assessment of grief responses in order to identify patients and family caregivers who may be suffering from grief that they are not easily able to integrate. Box 8.1 highlights examples of screening questions that can be used to identify the potential for complex grief.

Once events or other influences are identified through screening, it is important for all members of the team to share information with each other. In a conversation with the palliative care PA, a patient with a progressive, terminal illness may share feelings of anxiety and guilt about abandoning an adult child who struggles with addiction and mental illness.

BOX 8.1 Sample Screening Questions for Complex Grief

Are other family members ill or currently experiencing distress in their lives?

Has anyone close to you died within the past 2 years?

Are there other stressors in your life that are difficult for you at this time?

Difficult life experiences, like growing up in a family where there was mental illness, drug/alcohol issues, or violence, can affect our health. Do you feel like any of your past experiences affect your experience of your illness?

Is there anything else that could be impacting your grieving?

Are other family members ill or currently experiencing distress in their lives?

It will then be important for the PA to share the patient's perspective with the team in order to contribute to a consistent narrative and care plan. Patients will become frustrated when approached by different members of the team asking the same questions, so identifying who will screen for complex grief responses can be helpful for the patient and the efficacy of the team's work together.

Assessing for Coping and Resilience

One simple way to determine how the patient or the bereaved loved one is integrating the experience of grief and loss is to invite the patient to share more about their resources for coping with an advanced illness. Spiritual assessment tools can help clinicians assess healthy and unhealthy coping with loss. One such scale, the Copiing Orientation to Problems Experienced (COPE) scale, includes 15 categories, including positive reinterpretation and growth, active coping, planning, seeking social support for emotional reasons, seeking social support for instrumental reasons, suppression of competing activities, religion, acceptance, mental disengagement, behavioral disengagement, focus on and venting of emotions, restraint coping, alcohol and drug use, and humor.[14] The FICA (Faith, Import, Community, Address) spiritual assessment tool addresses spirituality with simpler categories that include faith or beliefs; the importance and influence of faith and beliefs; connection to religious/spiritual community; and how faith and belief should best be addressed in the person's healthcare.[15] Such tools can support healthy spiritual and religious coping while identifying the potential for negative coping—as when a religious belief holds the potential to negatively influence a patient's well-being.

In Javier's case, as described above, Javier shares that his connection with the natural world and his family is helping him to cope with a difficult diagnosis and illness trajectory. Patients will share any number of resources for positive coping. Examples include choosing a positive mental outlook, focusing on gratitude and positive thoughts, setting aside time for prayer, connection with a pet, or relying on a particular friend during times of distress. Identifying coping strategies can lead to conversations about how often a patient is remembering to rely on their strategies and how well their strategies are working. Patients who feel helpless and unable to identify any positive coping strategies would likely benefit from the intentional support of a palliative care chaplain or social worker.

Additional Interventions

Nonjudgmental Listening and Nonverbal Communication

In screening and assessing grief, the ability to listen deeply with supportive, nonverbal body language can express genuine care and support to a grieving person who may be experiencing difficult grief responses. Sitting rather than standing, maintaining gentle and consistent eye contact, and offering an open body posture (without arms crossed or computers/notebooks/charts placed between the clinician and the patient) at a comfortable distance conveys warmth, attention, and care.[†] Listening attentively without introducing interpretations or additional questions ensures that a person who may be experiencing distress will feel heard and respected. Reflective listening—the practice of simply restating what was said so the speaker can feel heard and encouraged to continue—is the simplest and most effective method of responding to the needs of grieving and bereaved persons. Patients or loved ones who decline invitations to reflect on their grieving process can be referred to a social worker or chaplain for more specialized follow-up. In cases where the patient needs psychiatric support, outside consultation with a psychiatry service may be necessary.

Supporting Legacy Work

For many patients facing the end of life, support for shaping one's legacy can help bring an important sense of completion. Legacy-making assists in life review and gives loved ones a way to connect with the loved one after their death. Meaninglessness can lead to despair and hopelessness. Having the support to create a narrative record of one's values, beliefs, stories, advice, recipes, hopes, songs, and other unique contributions to future generations creates a sense of purpose and meaning that can relieve psychosocial suffering. One method for legacy-making is referred to as dignity therapy, a method developed by Harvey Chochinov to honor the dignity of dying patients.[16] One aspect of dignity therapy is the creation of an audio interview with patients aimed at discovering the values and beliefs that bring them meaning and purpose. Once the patients' answers are recorded, they are then transcribed and edited until a polished document is produced that is then passed on to their loved ones.

Some of the main considerations to take into account in determining the appropriateness of dignity therapy include the patient's cognitive capacity, energy level, expressed interest, ability to participate, beliefs about the afterlife, and beliefs about the role of legacy in the lives of their loved ones.

Grief and the Palliative Care Clinician

Living in the presence of death and dying can be challenging for palliative care clinicians, who may experience their own spiritual or existential crisis of meaning when caring for patients with difficult diagnoses or other challenging circumstances. Caring for pediatric patients or the children of dying patients can be particularly distressing for clinicians who may

---

† In certain culture contexts, direct eye contact may be seen as a sign of disrespect.

identify with the vulnerability of young patients. Empathic overload is a term that conveys the physical, emotional, and spiritual fatigue that can happen when clinicians empathize with the suffering of others without also cultivating an inner sense of resilience and well-being. Engaged compassion is one method for minimizing empathic fatigue through cultivating engaged open-heartedness. Engaged compassion affirms compassion toward self and others is a resource for remaining engaged without becoming burned out or overextended.

While empathy is the ability to emotionally resonate with the feelings of another, engaged compassion is a desire to alleviate suffering of another, as well as one's own, with a motivation to take action. Compassion research is clarifying how empathy in and of itself can place clinicians at greater risk for burnout, while compassion empowers clinicians through supporting connection and personal agency.[17]

In addition to the risks for burnout from empathic fatigue, clinicians will need to navigate their own grief responses when losses in their lives occur. Many clinicians have experiences of childhood trauma that may be triggered by difficult encounters with patients. Caring for patients with advanced illness while grieving losses in one's own life can be challenging. A nurse going through treatment for early stage breast cancer while working as a member of a palliative care team, for example, may find it challenging to navigate survivor's guilt and a tendency to overempathize with her patient's distress.

Healthy palliative care teams will have processes in place for supporting one another and debriefing after distressing cases. Through developing resilience practices that prevent burnout, clinicians can support each other through healthy grieving, while developing strategies for enhancing resilience and well-being.

Grief as a Lifelong Journey

To support the grieving of palliative care patients and their loved ones, clinicians must learn to embrace their own suffering with gentleness and a degree of acceptance for the journey through grief. Attending to grief supports a whole-person approach to care and allows for the opportunity to grow and make meaning in the midst of loss and change.

References

1. Miller B. Reframing our relationship to that we don't control. On Being. 2016. https://onbeing.org/programs/b-j-miller-reframing-our-relationship-to-that-we-dont-control/. Accessed July 1, 2019.
2. Kamal AH, Bull JH, Wolf SP, et al. Prevalence and predictors of burnout among hospice and palliative care clinicians in the U.S. *Journal of Pain and Symptom Management.* 2016;51(4):690–696.
3. Strada EA. *Grief and Bereavement in the Adult Palliative Care Setting.* Oxford: Oxford University Press; 2013.
4. Kubler-Ross stage theory.
5. National Consensus Project for Quality Palliative Care. *Clinical Practice Guidelines for Quality Palliative Care.* 4th ed. Richmond, VA: National Coalition for Hospice and Palliative Care; 2019. http://www.nationalcoalitionhpc.org/ncp. Accessed July 1, 2019.
6. Joseph S, Butler L. Positive changes following adversity. *PTSD Research Quarterly.* 2010;21(3).
7. Tedeschi R, Calhoun L. COMMENTARIES on "Posttraumatic Growth: Conceptual Foundations and Empirical Evidence". *Psychological Inquiry.* 2004;15(1):19–92. doi:10.1207/s15327965pli1501_02.

8. Byock, I. The nature of suffering and the nature of opportunity at the end of life. *Clinics in Geriatric Medicine.* 1996;*12*(2):237–251.

9. Weller F. *The Wild Edge of Sorrow: Rituals of Renewal and the Sacred Work of Grief.* Berkeley, CA: North Atlantic Books; 2015.

10. Cheung KC, Chan KY, Yap DY. Disenfranchised grief after the death of a palliative care colleague. *Journal of Palliative Medicine.* 2016;*19*(9):905.

11. Machtinger E. An interview with Dr. Edward Machtinger: lessons of trauma-informed care. In: Meier DE, CAPC National Seminar keynote speaker 2018.

12. Felitti VJ, Anda RF, Nordenberg D, et al. Relationship of childhood abuse and household dysfunction to many of the leading causes of death in adults: the Adverse Childhood Experiences (ACE) Study. *American Journal of Preventive Medicine.* 2019;*56*(6):774–786.

13. Hospice Foundation of America. Children and grief. 2019. https://hospicefoundation.org/Grief-(1)/Children-and-Grief. Accessed July 1, 2019.

14. Carver C, Scheier M, Weintraub K. Assessing coping strategies: a theoretically based approach. *Journal of Personality and Social Psychology.* 1989;*56*(2):267–283.

15. Puchalski C, Romer AL. Taking a spiritual history allows clinicians to understand patients more fully. *Journal of Palliative Medicine.* 2000;*3*(1) 129–137.

16. Montross-Thomas LP, Irwin SA, Meier EA, et al. Enhancing legacy in palliative care: study protocol for a randomized controlled trial of dignity therapy focused on positive outcomes. *BMC Palliative Care.* 2015;*14*:44.

17. Dodds SE, Pace TW, Bell ML, et al. Feasibility of cognitively-based compassion training (CBCT) for breast cancer survivors: a randomized, wait list controlled pilot study. *Supportive Care in Cancer.* 2015;*23*(12):3599–3608.

9

Caring for the Palliative Care Clinician

Fostering Resilience

Jamie Beachy, Maureen J. Shelton, and
Timothy Harrison

Case 9.1

Micah, a 28 year old physician assistant (PA), was drawn to the interdisciplinary focus of palliative care (PC) and the opportunity to support patients through meaningful decisions about quality of life, spirituality, and end-of-life decision-making.

Micah threw himself wholeheartedly into his work, learning as much as possible from the other members of his PC team. He felt a sense of closeness with his patients and worked diligently with the team to relieve their physical and emotional suffering.

At the end of each full day of family meetings and PC visits, Micah returned home feeling both energized and exhausted. He felt needed and appreciated and was committed to the work, even if it often left him feeling emotionally and physically fatigued.

As the years passed, Micah slowly began to feel less present with patients and their loved ones. Where he once had patience for difficult family members and profoundly sad patient cases, he now felt irritation and impatience. His patients' needs began to feel too great for the resources his small PC team had to offer.

Micah spoke with the PC team chaplain to discuss self-care strategies and to debrief his feelings of being overwhelmed, yet Micah's fatigue from difficult family conferences, a near-constant turnover of staff on the PC team, and a lack of safe and supportive discharge options for his patients slowly turned to apathy and feelings of disconnection. Micah no longer felt effective, and he began to imagine working in a different setting with a less-complex patient load and a better quality of life for himself and his significant other.

Case 9.2

Sonal, a 38-year-old PA, has been working for many years in the field of PC—a field that she loves. When Sonal began working for the busy PC service, she was concerned about the intensity of the position. She was encouraged to discover that the director of the PC team had developed a resiliency and burnout prevention program.

Over time, the intensity of the job has presented a challenge for Sonal. She sometimes finds herself overly involved with her patients, thinking of them after work hours and worrying about their well-being. Like Micah, Sonal feels frustrations with her position, including the increasing demands of an inefficient online documentation system and a lack of support for PC on the intensive care unit where she spends the majority of her time.

Though Sonal finds her work to be emotionally fatiguing and professionally frustrating at times, she finds her work to be incredibly rewarding even after many years. She is active on her hospital's ethics committee and her PC team's quality improvement committee. Like Micah, Sonal discusses self-care and healthy boundaries with the palliative team chaplain as well as the team social worker. Sonal experiences high levels of job satisfaction and is able to recover from difficult cases and work frustrations by approaching even the more challenging patients with a calm and warmhearted engagement.

Resilience and Well-Being in the Face of Suffering

The opportunity to help patients and their loved ones navigate complex palliative and end-of-life decisions can be rewarding, personally and professionally. Honoring patients' wishes, relieving their suffering, facilitating heartfelt conversations about what matters most in life, and working with caring colleagues on an interdisciplinary team can bring a sense of personal satisfaction, meaning, and purpose, leading to better patient outcomes and provider satisfaction. Yet, as revealed by a 2016 survey of American Academy of Hospice and Palliative Medicine (AAHPM) PAs, physicians, nurse practitioners, nurses, social workers, and chaplains, PC clinicians experience high rates of burnout, characterized by emotional fatigue, depersonalization, cynicism, and feelings of ineffectiveness.[1] In this study, 62% of the respondents met burnout criteria, with higher rates reported among nonphysician clinicians and an overall burnout rate higher than other subspecialties within medicine. PC clinicians' struggles with symptoms of burnout affect their patients by contributing to increased healthcare costs, medical errors, and poor patient outcomes. That one clinician (as demonstrated in the introductory case studies) will show signs of burnout while another leaves the hospital or clinic at the end of an equally rigorous workday with an inner sense of well-being is an important consideration when seeking to identify causes of and to prevent burnout.

Physician assistants are part of a relatively new discipline that lacks the extensive research on sources of and potential solutions for burnout available for nursing and physician cohorts.[1-3] Though data on the rates of burnout among PAs are limited, as the AAHPM study and the above anecdotal cases illustrate, burnout is a risk for PC clinicians in all professional disciplines. Cultivation of well-being to support resilience and prevent burnout is the central focus of this chapter.

As will become evident through considering the emerging science of compassion, *engaged compassion for self and others* is an effective resource for sustaining well-being and preventing burnout over time. Engaged compassion, which is understood as the embodied desire to alleviate distress or adversity, in contrast to empathy, which is understood as merely the awareness of or sensitivity to another's distress or adversity, can serve as a foundation for skillfully working with our own or others' stress and challenging situations while enhancing and supporting well-being and resilience. Before discussing the science of compassion in greater depth, it will be helpful to articulate the factors that contribute to burnout among PC clinicians and to clarify working definitions of well-being and resilience.

Being With Suffering and Loss

In order to offer interventions to relieve patient suffering, capable PC clinicians develop the skills to listen deeply and emotionally attune to difficult emotional responses to serious illness. Being present to emotions such as sadness, anger, despair, and fear can be emotionally challenging for clinicians who care for multiple distressed patients and loved ones in the course of a day. Despite the best efforts of the PC team, patients may not find immediate relief from distressing pain symptoms and discomfort. Clinician fears and sadness can surface as they treat patient suffering in relation to illness, loss, and death.

"Being present" to the suffering of another is a precious opportunity to connect with personal sources of meaning and comfort. Yet, connecting to difficult emotions can become destabilizing or emotionally fatiguing if the clinician has not learned to navigate their inner emotional landscape with skill and understanding. Skillful ways of engaging patients, loved ones, and colleagues who are suffering can be taught; this can prevent clinician burnout and contribute to professional and personal satisfaction over time.

Living Well in the Presence of Death and Dying

Caring for patients with a serious or terminal illness can stir difficult emotions and unresolved feelings about death and dying. Mainstream North American culture is largely a death-denying culture in which the end of life is not openly talked about and may be deeply feared. In order to engage in conversations about end-of-life care and terminal diagnoses, clinicians benefit by bringing awareness and a degree of acceptance of their own mortality. Helping patients to clarify goals and hopes in relationship to their dying process is one of the goals of PC and one that can be disruptive to clinicians who are not yet comfortable talking about death and dying with their own families and loved ones. Although the dying process is not a source of suffering for all patients—many will find relief at the end of life and a sense of closure and connection to the transcendent—living in the presence of death and dying can be challenging for PC clinicians, who may experience their own spiritual or existential crisis of meaning when caring for patients who approach dying from a place of fear or a lack of acceptance. Ira Byock, a physician pioneer in the field of hospice and palliative medicine, has coined the term *dying well* to refer to the ways that dying is a natural developmental stage in the life cycle of every person. When patients are given adequate support to address key developmental landmarks at the end of life, death can be a time of reconciliation and healthy closure.[4] To accept death as a natural part of life can allow for a greater sense of acceptance and well-being for PC clinicians and their patients. This can be particularly challenging when caring for pediatric patients and young adults, whose deaths may feel especially senseless or tragic. Compounding these difficulties, a caring PC clinician may develop a misleading mindset in which their sense of accomplishment depends on each of their patient's "dying well," when this outcome is neither predictable nor controllable even in the best of circumstances.

Well-Being and Resilience Defined

Although there is no consensus around a single definition, well-being is generally understood to include satisfaction with life, positive functioning, and the presence of positive emotions such as contentment and happiness.[5] Individual disciplines understand well-being through methodological lenses that emphasize the particular dimensions of well-being. Public health researchers, for example, generally focus on physical indications of well-being in interpreting data for particular populations, while social scientists research the social dimensions of well-being. Across all disciplines, the science of well-being has focused primarily on subjective well-being through relying on the self-reports of study participants to measure positive emotions such as happiness and fulfillment.

One of the earliest and most widely used well-being scales—the Ryff Scale of Psychological Well-Being (PWB), developed by Carol D. Ryff and colleagues at the Institute on Aging at the University of Wisconsin, Madison—is a method used to assess well-being in diverse disciplines within the healthcare professions.[6] Ryff's work, beginning with the psychological well-being scale in the late 1980s, recognized the need for an instrument to measure theoretically derived constructs of psychological well-being. Ryff developed a set of measurable constructs, including autonomy; environmental mastery; personal growth; positive relationships with others; purpose in life; realization of potential; and self-acceptance.[7] The 84-item Ryff PWB scale and the shortened 45-item version measure these constructs through the self-reporting of participants. Although the instrument does not measure all dimensions of well-being (distinctly physical measures are left out, e.g.), the knowledge of health practitioner's psychological well-being can aid healthcare teams and institutions in creating meaningful strategies to enhance these dimensions of well-being.

As the science of well-being has evolved, the focus has come to include not only how well-being is expressed, but also *what well-being is*, such as the ability to fulfill goals,[8] happiness,[9] and life satisfaction.[10] Consistent themes spanning definitions of well-being include positive emotions, a sense of connection to self and others, the perception of autonomy, and a positive outlook.[11]

We use well-being here to refer to *a state of positive psychosocial health*. This definition acknowledges physical, existential-spiritual, economic, and environmental dimensions of well-being that cannot truly be separated from psychosocial factors in the lived experience of clinicians and their patients. For the purposes of this chapter, defining well-being as a state of positive, psychosocial health will allow for an exploration of the ways that beliefs, practices, and attitudes can influence the experience of well-being for PC clinicians managing healthcare stressors.

In recent years, clinicians and researchers have come to a greater recognition of *resilience* as an influencer of psychosocial well-being. Unlike research on well-being, the study of resilience places the focus on the clinician's ability to recover from adverse experiences. Research and anecdotal wisdom aimed at supporting resilience approaches the problem of burnout with a recognition that while adverse experiences cannot be avoided, such experiences could be responded to in skillful ways that prevent lasting harm.

In a 2015 article on burnout among PC clinicians, a team of researchers identified risks as well as individual skills and workplace factors that contribute to resilience for clinicians in the field. In their article, Back et al. suggested it is important to view burnout among PC clinicians from both a personal lens that emphasizes skills and education and a systemic lens that accounts for systems-based stressors placed on PC clinicians.[2] Personal challenges include such factors as perfectionism and a failure to set healthy boundaries. Systemic challenges include factors such as failing to scale clinician workload to patient volume and acuity and restricting clinicians' input or influence into how their work is structured.[2]

Clinical leaders concerned with the personal and systemic influences on burnout and potential strategies to support resilience recognize that more research is needed to identify effective methods for recovering from the effects of stress and adversity in the rapidly expanding field of PC.

As explored in detail further in the chapter, a central element for supporting resilience is *compassion*. The provision of PC aligns naturally with the practice of sustained and extended compassion for others. The skills that support compassion also support a constructive response to a wide variety of stressors that are common to providing PC to patients and their loved ones and to collaborating with diverse colleagues in high-stress environments.

A working definition of resilience as *the ability to recover from stressful or adverse experiences without lasting harm* will serve to orient a consideration of clinician resilience and well-being. Although emotional and psychological stressors will never be eliminated in the personal and professional lives of clinicians working in the field of PC, learning to become resilient in managing stress and recovering from challenging events while remaining connected to deeper sources of meaning mediates fatigue and disconnection, creating benefit for clinicians and their patients.

Additional Factors That Contribute to Burnout

Personal and Interpersonal Factors

Individual personality and interpersonal habits may put clinicians at higher risk for burnout. In their work on the impacts of moral distress on burnout for nurses in situations of high intensity, Cynda Rushton and colleagues identified personal factors that contribute to burnout among nurses in high-intensity settings. For Rushton et al., moral distress as a crisis of meaning occurs when "one recognizes one's moral responsibility in a situation; evaluates the various courses of action; and identifies, in accordance with one's beliefs, the morally correct decision—but is then prevented from following through."[3] Clinical situations that can lead to a sense of moral distress might include being required to provide medical interventions and treatments that are perceived to be nonbeneficial to the patient; conflicts with institutional leaders in regard to the distribution of resources (as in the case of patients who are refused life-saving or life-enhancing treatments); and moral disagreements with other medical professionals that are resolved through hierarchical power structures. Personal factors that place nurses at higher risk of burnout from morally distressing work conditions include a perceived lack of autonomy (feelings of powerlessness), emotional exhaustion because of empathic "overload," a perceived lack of control in their professional lives, and poor physical self-care. Rushton suggests that protective factors may include the inverse of identified risks, including the ability to regulate emotions, higher levels of physical and spiritual well-being, and feelings of autonomy and a sense of control.[10] How protective factors can be cultivated by clinicians committed to developing resilience and healthy coping with stress are more thoroughly considered further in this chapter.

Systemic Factors

In the years following the AAPHM survey, there has been greater recognition of systemic factors that contribute to burnout among clinicians, including stressors such as work overload, loss of job autonomy, increased time spent in documentation, clinical inefficiencies, uneven training between clinicians and administrators, and a cultural shift from health values to corporate values.[11]

A recognition of systemic factors places much responsibility for the phenomenon of burnout on systemic failures that place clinicians at higher risk. A balanced approach to well-being and resilience recognizes both personal and systemic factors that lead to stress and burnout, while recognizing also that healthcare professions, especially PC, are inherently stressful and difficult to navigate even in the healthiest of systems.

Christine Maslach, a psychologist at the University of California, Berkeley, and one of the leading authorities on burnout, developed the Maslach burnout inventory—a burnout scale that takes systemic factors into consideration.[12] Maslach, who has written extensively on physician burnout, has identified six areas of work life that can put one at risk of meeting criteria for burnout:

> *Workload:* The demands of the job exceed the resources available to accomplish it.
> *Control:* Clinicians may have very little say over how they do their work—with a perception that no one is interested in their feedback.
> *Rewards:* Healthcare systems can lack clear rewards and recognition for a job well done. For Maslach, this extends beyond salary and benefits to include a lack of appreciation for the work that is expected of a clinician in the course of a day.
> *Community:* Unresolved conflicts and dysfunctional team dynamics can lead to a socially toxic environment that may include bullying and rudeness.
> *Fairness:* A perceived lack of equity in the workplace—that undervalues experience and expertise—can result in anger and hostility.

Values Conflicts: A disconnect between the values that give meaning to life and the day-to-day work realities can undermine a sense of well-being (often referred to as moral distress or moral injury).[12]

Additional stress factors for physicians, according to the National Academy of Medicine and the *Joint Commission Journal on Quality and Patient Safety* include staff ratios, incentive pay, requirements for documentation, and increasing productivity pressures.[13] How these factors relate to burnout for PAs is yet to be adequately studied. For all clinicians and for those working within the field of PC, the rapid growth of PC services in hospitals has resulted in small services that may be dependent on just one or two clinicians with high expectations for program growth,[9] while more established services face stressors, including increasingly acute cases and complex institutional politics.

A thorough consideration of systemic factors that place clinicians at risk for burnout is beyond the scope of this chapter. Because the field of PC is emotionally and spiritually intensive, it places pressures on clinicians to develop personal strategies for coping with unpredictable circumstances that are endemic to life-or-death situations. Such strategies—if effective and sustainable over the long term—are an invaluable consideration that determine whether clinicians will be able to approach challenges with the inner resources and wisdom needed to maintain well-being and resilience over the course of a clinical career.

Sustaining Well-Being and Resilience Through Compassion

The scientific study of compassion has drawn attention to the ways that engaged compassion holds potential to protect against burnout. In 2019, physician researchers Stephen Trzeciak and Anthony Mazzarelli reviewed the current literature on the science of compassion in an attempt to clarify whether or not compassion leads to tangible positive outcomes for clinicians and their patients.[14] Their findings were clear and surprising to some clinicians and researchers accustomed to conceiving of compassion as potentially fatiguing. Trzeciak and Mazzarelli found overwhelming evidence for the generative influence of compassion in the lives of healthcare clinicians and patients. They found that when clinicians are compassionate, they are happier and less burned out and their patients heal better and faster:

> After analyzing all of the evidence, we conclude with confidence: compassion matters—for patients, for patient care, and for those who care for patients. Compassion matters in not only meaningful ways, but also in measurable ways. Compassionate care is more effective than health care without compassion, by virtue of the fact that human connection confers distinct and measurable benefits. . . . Remember that these data are not what we *think,* nor are they what we *believe.* Rather, they are what we *found.* Compassionate care belongs in the domain of evidence-based medicine.[14(pp321,322)]

Reconsidering the anecdotal cases represented at the beginning of the chapter in the divergent experiences of Micah and Sonal highlights an important distinction in the research on compassion. What Trzeciak, Mazzarelli, and others have found is that the empathy experienced by Micah may actually place him at greater risk of burnout, while compassion, as expressed in Sonal's story of resilience, provides an antidote to burnout. Empathy is defined here as a response to the feeling state of another, either by seeing the other's perspective (cognitive empathy) or by mirroring the feelings that they are experiencing (affective empathy). Empathy plays a crucial role in providing the clinician information about the emotional state of the patient and thus is an invaluable part of the process of offering care. Maintaining affective empathy over time, however, and especially when the clinician is experiencing the same negative affect (whether fear, anxiety, sadness, frustration, etc.) as the patient, is not sustainable. Empathy on its own can promote empathic distress and may even lead to an experience of vicarious trauma and burnout over time, as in the case of Micah, who became burned out through his work as a PC PA.

While empathy can be understood as emotional resonance with the feelings of another or simply understanding their point of view, empathic concern (also known as compassion) is the desire to see their difficulties alleviated. It is this empathic concern, not the other forms of empathy, that fuels the motivation to act on their behalf. For compassion researchers, empathy in and of itself can place clinicians at greater risk for burnout while compassion empowers clinicians through supporting connection and personal agency as expressed in Sonal's experience.

Clinician training to develop emotional and psychological resilience is a crucial aspect in the prevention of empathic distress, which is a primary contributor to burnout. Empathic distress is a heightened level of empathy that is strong enough to contribute to unhealthy levels of stress. Unlike empathic distress, compassion is a state of empathic concern[15(p178)]—a state that sustains a human connection, remaining aware of their distress but not becoming overidentified, enmeshed, or disempowered by the distress. A common misunderstanding in clinicians is that increasing compassion leads to increased amounts of distress, but research on compassion is showing the opposite, that skills of compassion are actually an antidote to empathic distress and potential burnout.[14(p287)]

Conditions That Support Compassion

One of the central elements in developing the skills of compassion is the ability to feel compassion toward oneself. Self-compassion is the ability to sustain kindness and tenderness toward the self, especially when one faces difficulties, limitations, or vulnerabilities. Noticing when one may become overly harsh or judgmental in the interpretation of these limitations and difficulties is a fundamental skill in the development of self-compassion. Further, familiarizing oneself with the mental habits that can lead to feelings of helplessness can create a greater sense of agency about how to replace unhelpful mindsets with more accurate and less-debilitating mindsets. The broadening of perspective—in particular the ability to see and to easily recall that the ups and downs of life, such as loss, failure, death, and the like, are part of every human life—is the realistic mindset that allows for a sustained sense of self-kindness and self-acceptance.

In addition to developing more self-compassion, compassion for others is supported by an increased and more inclusive sense of closeness and tenderness toward them. Evolutionary psychology confirms that mammals in general, and primates in particular, are wired to react with compassion to those we feel close to when we see that they are struggling or in distress.[16] Thus, to enhance the compassionate response, clinicians can grow and sustain mindsets that enhance this sense of closeness. When one has an authentic sense of closeness with another and then develops empathic awareness of the suffering of this person, compassion cannot help but arise as a biological necessity that leads to engaged action. Such engaged compassion for others along with compassion that seeks the utmost well-being for the self has been demonstrated to sustain a clinician's capacity to respond effectively to their patients over time. In further articulating the importance of compassion for self and other, it will be helpful to address myths about compassion toward the self.

Myths About Self-Compassion

Most clinicians enter the field of healthcare with the motivation to provide care and compassion to people in need of support. An admirable virtue highly esteemed by the world's religious and spiritual traditions, compassion is associated with mercy, sympathy, tenderheartedness, and selfless love for others. Many healthcare providers strive to embody the virtue of compassion in their work with vulnerable people. As Kristen Neff, a PhD psychologist, has demonstrated through her research on compassion, both compassion toward other and *self-compassion* are strongly related to mental health, healthy behaviors, resilience, and an increased satisfaction with one's caregiving role.[17]

While compassion is a noble virtue involving a degree of sacrifice, healthcare practitioners may feel that to be compassionate toward themselves is indulgent and selfish. Yet Neff argued that self-compassion is better for healthcare workers and the patients they serve by preventing and addressing burnout—a condition that undermines the well-being of both healthcare clinicians and their patients.

Neff named several myths about self-compassion that can prevent clinicians from including themselves in a practice of compassion; these include the following[18]:

Myth: Self-compassion is a form of pity. Compassion is often confused with pity, and similarly, self-compassion is confused with self-pity. Self-pity suggests an attitude of victimhood that sustains negative emotional responses to setbacks and shortcomings, while self-compassion includes an attitude of kindness that makes it easier to release negativity and find agency in the face of (or even because of) distressing or limiting experiences.

Myth: Self-compassion is an expression of weakness. For clinicians who are accustomed to prioritizing the care of others, taking time to extend tenderness and kind support toward oneself may seem like a form of weakness or indulgence. In reality, repressing emotions and putting on a façade of strength can create greater vulnerability to burnout, while self-compassion, which allows the acknowledgment and acceptance of weakness as inherent to the human condition, increases resilience and healthy coping, supporting resilience and preventing burnout over time.

Myth: Self-compassion makes people complacent and lazy. Rather than creating complacency, self-compassion helps clinicians find the energy they need to be present to others. Tenderly attending to challenging emotions and reactions in oneself creates greater energy and feelings of well-being that carry forward in relationships with others.

Myth: Self-compassion is self-centered and narcissistic. This final myth about self-compassion claims that self-compassion is indulgent through prioritizing the needs of the self over the other, who may have a greater need for support. As Neff's research and the research on compassion demonstrates, caring for the self is important to sustaining an inner sense of well-being[17] that allows clinicians to remain genuinely oriented toward others in their work. Without self-compassion, clinicians are at risk of becoming cynical, emotionally exhausted, and emotionally unavailable—qualities that do not benefit patients and their loved ones or clinical colleagues and may even cause harm. Self-compassion is fundamental to the well-being of the self *and* the other and is central to resilience, well-being, and the ability to respond to the needs of the other with caring wisdom and insight.

Cultivating Compassion

In the same way that a person seeks a vaccination to boost immunity to a disease in advance of encountering that disease in the wild, a healthcare practitioner may seek to strengthen the capacity to sustain compassion prior to encountering challenging circumstances in the hospital or examination rooms. Such a "vaccination" could confer psychosocial immunity, which is the goal of several programs that have been developed to train or cultivate compassion in recent decades. One of the most researched and established methods is CBCT®, Cognitively-Based Compassion Training,[19] which has similarities to other programs of this type, including mindful self-compassion (mentioned above) and compassion cultivation training (CCT). As practitioners and teachers of CBCT, we share theoretical and practical aspects of CBCT in order to provide insight into supporting greater self-care, particularly for the PC clinician.

In 2004, Lobsang Tenzin Negi, PhD, a professor at Emory University in Atlanta, Georgia, developed CBCT as one of the first contemplative protocols to enact a systematic and rigorous study of the effects of compassion training on physiological, psychological, and behavioral outcomes. Dr. Negi brought to this development his 27 years as a monk studying Indo-Tibetan Buddhist psychological practices along with his study of emotion science through his academic research and doctoral work at Emory. In the development of CBCT (as with the aforementioned CCT protocol), psychological insights are distilled from the *lojong* tradition—a 1200-year-old series of practices focused on the goal of becoming the most compassionate human being that one can be. In the translation, CBCT was also designed to be useful for people of any or no faith tradition.[19] A brief overview of CBCT follows in order to illustrate the potential benefits of a targeted skills training program for PC clinicians to prevent and address clinician burnout.

The understanding of compassion utilized in most compassion training protocols and in the emerging field of compassion science centers on the motivation to be of benefit to others in their distress. We here define compassion as *the desire to alleviate the distress or adversity of others, arising from a sensitivity to their challenges and rooted in warmheartedness.* A foundational insight, drawn from the field of evolutionary psychology, is that people have an inherent, biologically based capacity for compassion for those in a person's "in-group" or close family and friends.[16] This inherent capacity can be expanded through training aimed at expanding the "in-group" to ever-widening circles of individuals. Taking an approach that utilizes human intelligence and the ability to shift perspectives, CBCT targets two specific mindsets for the purpose of enhancing a sense of belonging or closeness with others, including strangers: (1) identifying with them through the recognition of shared humanity and (2) recalling how much one depends on them for well-being and livelihood. These shifting mindsets constitute a cognitive reframing process that gives CBCT its moniker, "cognitively based," even though the program squarely aims for change at emotional and behavioral domains as well. By cultivating a consistently tenderhearted relationship with a wider and more inclusive circle of others, one becomes naturally moved to action by their struggles. This inner state is what CBCT refers to as *engaged compassion.*

Learning Model: Three Levels of Understanding

Cognitively-Based Compassion Training relies on a pedagogical model that begins with intellectual learning but then moves toward embodiment of skills through practice. The three levels of learning are referred to as *content knowledge, personal insight,* and *embodied understanding.*

Content knowledge is the aspect of learning that takes place as knowledge and information received from external sources such as lectures and readings. *Personal insight* occurs when the participant applies these insights to their own experience and has what are sometimes called "ah-hah" moments, or a felt sense of the truth of the insight. One primary approach to achieving such insight is through a contemplative practice called analytical meditation, which uses meditation and critical thinking to create the conditions for personal insights to arise. The third stage, *embodied understanding,* unfolds as the participant sustains the insight over time and thus is more able to recall it—that is, to sustain mindfulness of the insight—in the midst of daily experience.

Although the desired long-term outcome is a more spontaneous and inclusive compassion, the learning model acknowledges that it takes time to embody such skills, much as it would to learn expertise with a musical instrument or a complex medical procedure. The amount of time will be shorter if the clinician has motivation to practice the self-cultivation practices and if the insights are being reinforced by the day-to-day culture or community in which they are embedded. Palliative clinicians who belong to clinical care teams with an overt commitment to the cultivation of resiliency and compassion will much more easily develop and sustain the benefits of the practices over time.

Contemplative Practice for Training Compassion

Contemplative practices can support the cultivation of compassion, and CBCT depends on two types of practice: present moment practice and analytical practice. The present moment practices, comprising Modules I and II (see Table 9.1), help to stabilize the participant's focus as well as help to provide greater availability to the moment-to-moment arising of mental experience. Growing out of this heightened availability, analytical practice serves as the basis for Modules III to VI and relies on critical thinking to consider unhelpful mindsets and encourage mindsets that support kindness toward oneself and an ability to relate more inclusively to a broader circle of individuals. This sequential process leads to more spontaneous access to the concepts and application of the skills, especially in postmeditation moments of distress or crisis when they are arguably most needed.

Skills and Insights of Compassion Training for PC Clinicians

While the practices of CBCT are taught formally in multiday courses (with a minimum 15 contact hours), the protocol is described here to introduce PAs who are members of PC teams to the components of a systematic approach to sustaining compassion. Table 9.1 summarizes the exercises that comprise the foundational practice and six sequential modules of CBCT. Engaging the practices of the early CBCT modules (Foundational Practice, I, II, and III) cultivates a sense of security, reduces emotional disturbances, sets realistic expectations of self, and thereby enhances resilience. The engagement with the later modules (IV, V, and VI) enhances closeness and connection with others through both identification and gratitude and leads naturally to a more sustainable and inclusive compassion. These two primary outcomes, resilience and compassion, buffer against burnout and contribute to the practitioner's flourishing and development of well-being over time.

Importantly, compassion training does not predict or instruct what a compassionate action should be in response to suffering. Rather it helps to prepare the clinician to be able to stay focused and resilient in the midst of suffering and to sustain their connection to the person who is in distress. This warmhearted connection is in fact the essential catalyst for a compassionate response. The resulting action or behavior will necessarily depend on the existing skills of each individual as well as the given context, even though the underlying compassionate motivation is the same. Thus, the cultivation of a sense of connectedness with or affection toward others, which results in the motivation to help, is a central focus of compassion training.

Clinical Applications of Compassion Training

Skills developed through contemplative practices can be used by PAs to address the identified factors leading to burnout and distress named throughout this chapter and lead to relief and a sense of increased agency when confronted with these sources of distress. For examples of such skills, refer to Table 9.2. The sequential repeated engagement with compassion practices

TABLE 9.1 Summary of Compassion Training Practices (Based on CBCT)

Foundational practice: resting in a moment of nurturance	Each CBCT practice period begins with recalling a time of feeling safe and secure—a moment of nurturance—from past experience and sustaining this in the mind's eye in order to allow feelings of soothing and comfort to arise. First, this practice connects the practitioner with a feeling of warmth and support, sometimes called grounding, as they prepare for later practices and gives a place to return to if later practices are destabilizing. Second, this practice motivates the cultivation of compassion as the practitioner focuses on the value of feeling nurtured and supported in their own life and reflects on how it feels positive to help others to have the experience of being supported and cared for.
Module I: attentional stability and clarity	Here the practitioner does an exercise to stabilize attentional focus and promote clarity of perception of internal experiences. This skill is developed through focusing on sensations (typically of the breath as it follows its natural rhythm) as a way to train in the skill of noticing when distractions arise, disengaging from the distraction, and refocusing the attention on the intended object of focus. This is a present moment practice, as physical sensations are experienced in the here and now.
Module II: insight into the nature of mental experience	The focus here remains in the present moment but broadens the focus of attention to include awareness of any sensations, images, feelings, or thoughts that arise in the mind. Increasing the ability to observe mental activity gives insight into mental habits and provides greater flexibility and choice to respond constructively to mental events, appraisals, and internal triggers.
Module III: self-compassion and self-acceptance	Here analytical methods are employed to examine how mental habits or patterns may be increasing distress via overly harsh self-judgment or exaggerated expectations of perfection or control. Then, to shift these mental habits for greater well-being over time, the practice offers techniques for replacing unhelpful and unrealistic mindsets with more helpful and realistic ones. By relating to difficult experiences in the context of shared human vulnerability, the participant gains confidence that they can sustain an attitude of kindness and informed acceptance toward self in the face of their imperfections, adversities, and vulnerabilities.
Module IV: impartiality and inclusivity	Turning toward their relationships with others, the practitioner examines the harm that occurs from excessive liking and disliking of certain groups or individuals. By becoming aware of the habit of categorizing others as friends, strangers, and difficult people and then recalling fundamental similarities between self and all others—in particular the shared desire for well-being and freedom from harm and distress—the practitioner naturally widens the circle of those with whom the practitioner identifies and thus will experience a sense of connection and greater empathic understanding.
Module V: gratitude and affection	Here the practitioner recalls and sustains awareness of dependence on others for sources of well-being and freedom from harm. Through analysis and critical thinking, the practitioner attunes to the reality of interdependence, thereby cultivating stronger feelings of gratitude and affection for others. The strengthening of such feelings naturally leads to a greater appreciation of and sense of closeness with others, even strangers and sometimes even those who are difficult. The practitioner also reflects on the drawbacks of narrow self-focus, both personally and societally. By embracing these more realistic mindsets, a more stable and inclusive sense of closeness and tenderness toward others is cultivated and sustained.
Module VI: empathetic concern and engaged compassion	Having cultivated a stronger and more inclusive sense of affection for others, the practitioner now calls to mind their difficulties and vulnerabilities. The instruction is to allow compassion naturally to arise and to sustain it. This requires also noticing and applying antidotes to competing internal experiences that are impediments to compassion (i.e., empathic distress, pity, blame, fear, frustration, self-criticism, etc.). The practitoner uses the many CBCT insights and skills to keep navigating back to a simple wish, focused on the other person, that they could be free from their distress or suffering. In this way, the practitioner learns to sustain a compassionate motivation without negative impacts of empathetic distress, such as exhaustion or secondary trauma. Finally the practitioner begins to sustain the insight that compassion is energizing, not fatiguing, and that feeling connected to the other with the motivation to alleviate their suffering—even when it seems that nothing more can be done at that moment—is a replenishing experience for the care provider and often for the care seeker as well.

TABLE 9.2 CBCT Components to Counteract PC Clinician Burnout

Maslach's Burnout Inventory Category[12]	Common contributors to burnout for PC clinicians[2]	Relevant skill or insight cultivated via compassion training (relevant CBCT modules are indicated in parentheses)
Workload	Continual transitions	Able to recall feeling safe and secure and sustain that awareness over time (Foundational Practice); increased ability to notice distractions, disengage, and return to intended focal point without judgment or criticism (Module I); embracing the reality that things are constantly changing and that the events of my life are not 100% in my control (Module III)
Workload	Emotional exhaustion	Acknowledging thought and emotions without becoming overly entangled (Module II); accepting my limitations and vulnerabilities with kindness and understanding (Module III)
Community	Depersonalization	Approaching others as "just like me" on a fundamental level, despite differences, and seeing that others have the same basic desire to flourish and avoid distress that I do (Module IV); attuning to the reality of interdependence and interconnectedness (Module V); deepening and extending gratitude and appreciation for others (Module V)
Workload	Overidentification with the sadness of patients	Understanding empathy as necessary for compassion, but not the same as compassion (Module VI); acknowledging thoughts and emotions without becoming overly entangled (Module II)
Control, Value Conflicts	Lack of safe and supportive discharge options	Accepting my limitations with kindness and understanding (Module III); sustaining a compassionate motivation even when I cannot see an immediate solution to alleviate someone's troubles or difficulties (Module VI)
Rewards	No longer feeling effective	Resolving to change from within and to cultivate inner sources of well-being, replacing misleading and harmful thought patterns with more realistic and constructive attitudes (Module III); sustaining a compassionate motivation even when I cannot see an immediate solution to alleviate someone's troubles or difficulties (Module VI)

can help to build the familiarization with skills that clinicians can draw from in the midst of challenging circumstances.

To reflect on the potential benefit of these inner skills for a PC clinician, it is helpful to return to the story of Micah from the beginning of the chapter. For a moment, we can imagine that Micah is given the opportunity to learn and practice compassion cultivation skills early in his career. Perhaps he is now able to avoid the depersonalization and perceived inefficacy that led to his experience of burnout. Micah is now more able to notice when his thoughts wander repetitively to the more difficult and unsolvable cases or situations as he now redirects his attention to many parts of the job that are going well, including his growing skill set as a clinician. This mental flexibility now serves as a primary resource to support his emotional resilience, especially on tough days. Now more resilient in the face of frustrations, Micah is more open to connecting to patients and colleagues as fellow humans who share with him the imperfections and vulnerabilities that are part of every life. In the end, it is this felt and real sense of connection, closeness, and support that sustains the warmheartedness to motivate and energize his daily engagement with the valuable and rewarding work of caring for others in their times of need, whether or not things turn out well in every case.

Through the daily reflection on and practice of self-compassion, Micah's sense of well-being is now freed from a need to control outcomes or to be the "perfect" care provider as he comes to an acceptance of inevitable flaws and vulnerabilities. While these supportive skills and insights can certainly be learned or developed simply by living life and reflecting on its lessons over time, compassion training provides Micah the structured support needed to bring compassion more efficiently and directly into his everyday work context.

For Sonal, who did not experience burnout even after years of practice, training in compassion may allow her to find an even stronger sense of meaning and purpose in her work. This could strengthen her ability to support these skills in her colleagues and to build a community of like-minded others who share a commitment to the kind of self-care practices that make it possible to face the challenges inherent to PC with less discouragement and empathic fatigue. For both Micah and Sonal, a variety of benefits may arise through training in compassion. Table 9.3 highlights statements from healthcare staff who were interviewed after taking a CBCT course, demonstrating the potentially beneficial effects of CBCT training for clinicians from varied disciplines.

The Implementation of CBCT in Healthcare and in Other Settings

Compassion training has proven meaningful in a variety of contexts within healthcare. For example, since 2014 CBCT courses have been offered at the Emory School of Medicine to faculty and staff twice annually and even more frequently to students. A tailored course for nurses is offered regularly through Emory's Professional Development Center, and courses have been brought to healthcare professionals in contexts such as the pediatric intensive care unit, neonatal intensive care unit, and a center for autism, as well as in medical centers in Ohio, Massachusetts, California, and Brazil. In 2015, the University of Illinois College of Medicine (UICOM) of Peoria sent six faculty to Emory to become certified CBCT instructors so that they could teach regularly to medical students, faculty, and staff, and this program will expand in 2020 to all four UICOM campuses. Continuing education credits are available for nurses (CNE, continuing nursing education), and physicians (CME, continuing medical education), and others.[20]

Since 2016 CBCT has been adopted as central to the chaplain-training programs of Spiritual Health at Emory Healthcare, one of the largest such programs in the nation. The venture has grown into a program, Compassion-Centered Spiritual Health, and is being researched to determine impact on chaplain well-being, burnout, and efficacy. A bedside spiritual health intervention, based on CBCT, has been developed and is under study.

To support the research programs that require faithful offering of the protocol, a rigorous CBCT Instructor certification program certifies dozens of teachers annually through Emory's Center for Contemplative Science and Compassion-Based Ethics.

Addressing Distress on the PC Team

Though PC clinicians work one-on-one with patients, PC services are organized into interdisciplinary or transdisciplinary clinical teams. Because of the team-oriented nature of the

TABLE 9.3 Case Studies Paired With Compassion Training Skills and Insights

This table highlights the ways that clinicians from varied disciplines felt supported by compassion training and more able to support their patients in return. The module numbers refer to the CBCT modules explained in Table 9.1: Summary of Compassion Training Practices.

Comments From CBCT Participants	Paired CBCT Skills or Insights
Nurse: "After 30 years of nursing I now have more of a sense of inner strength to care for others without becoming caught up in all of the emotions of those around me. As a result, I can compassionately communicate to my patients and colleagues while maintaining my care of self. I have more energy now for my work and a sense that I can do my work with more compassion both for others and for myself."	Resolving to change from within and to cultivate inner sources of well-being, replacing misleading and harmful thought patterns with more realistic and constructive attitudes (Module III) Sustaining a compassionate motivation even when I cannot see an immediate solution to alleviate someone's troubles or difficulties (Module VI)
Chaplain: "Taking this course in CBCT has given me access to skills which have been life changing for me as I have looked at my sources of distress from broader perspectives. Taking this course for just a few weeks has been equivalent to many years of therapy!"	Able to recall feeling safe and secure and sustain that awareness over time (Foundational Practice) Increased ability to notice distractions, disengage, and return to intended focal point without judgment or criticism (Module I) Embracing the reality that things are constantly changing and that the events of my life are not 100% in my control (Module III)
Physician: "After taking CBCT, I realized that I had a misperception of my role as a physician. Prior to CBCT, I perceived that my success as a care provider was only tied to whether or not the patient fully recovered. Now, I have more of an insight that my presence and my ability to be with the suffering of my patients (not turning away automatically) is a crucial part of my role. This insight has allowed me to have more self-compassion as well as an increased sense of meaning and purpose in my day-to-day work."	Resolving to change from within and to cultivate inner sources of well-being, replacing misleading and harmful thought patterns with more realistic and constructive attitudes (Module III) Sustaining a compassionate motivation even when I cannot see an immediate solution to alleviate someone's troubles or difficulties (Module VI)
Healthcare clinician: "I had a traumatic event in my work involving a patient and this course has helped me listen to the advice that I am able to give to support others and apply it to myself. The insight that there are so many things that I can't control but that I can have a sense of agency to choose what to focus on, or what I can do, has brought me relief."	Accepting my limitations and vulnerabilities with kindness and understanding (Module III) Understanding empathy as necessary for compassion, but not the same as compassion (Module VI)

work, that broader well-being of the PC team as a whole has an important influence on the way clinicians will engage patients and their loved ones. The following initiatives represent resources in addition to compassion training that provide support for interdisciplinary teams and the larger healthcare communities where they practice.

The Role of the Chaplain on the PC Team

Well-developed PC services include a professionally certified chaplain. As members of the clinical PC team, chaplains attend to the spiritual dimension of the patient's care plan. In addition to providing direct spiritual care to patients and their loved ones, chaplains also attend to the spiritual health and well-being of the PC team as a whole. Chaplains receive in-depth training to respond to clinicians' experiences of grief, loss, and transition with a nonjudgmental, supportive presence. Chaplains are available to debrief difficult cases and support clinicians who may face challenging group dynamics and other stressors that can develop when teams are under pressure. Chaplains support clinicians through losses and other upheavals that may occur in their personal lives and are skilled at listening to the spiritual distress or moral questions that may arise for clinicians when caring for patients with difficult diagnoses, challenging symptoms, or a lack of support. They may recommend or teach supportive spiritual practices that connect to the clinicians' own spiritual or religious belief systems and can help refer clinicians to services available through the healthcare system including professional counseling or other crisis benefits that may be provided by the healthcare system's human resources department.

Schwartz Rounds

The Schwartz Rounds' program, sponsored by the Schwartz Center for Compassionate Care, is offered in more than 470 healthcare organizations in the United States, Canada, Australia, New Zealand, the United Kingdom and Ireland. Trained Schwartz Rounds leaders offer regularly scheduled times for healthcare clinicians to come together to openly discuss social and emotional issues they face in their clinical work; this is done in a confidential, supportive, and compassionate environment where clinicians share and gain insight into challenging patient cases with the help of skilled facilitation.[21]

Critical Incident Stress Debriefing

Critical Incident Stress Debriefing (CISD) is a specific, 7-phase, small group, supportive crisis intervention process included under the umbrella of a Critical Incident Stress Management program. CISD offers a supportive opportunity to process and move beyond a traumatic event (frequently called a critical incident). CISD was developed exclusively for small groups that have encountered a critical incident, such as a particularly difficult patient case or violent event. CISD aims at reduction of distress and a restoration of group cohesion and unit performance.[22]

Ethics Consultation as a Strategy for Preventing Moral Distress

Palliative care teams are part of larger healthcare systems that may offer on-site ethics consultation services to help clinicians reflect on the ethical implications of clinical situations, including those that produce moral and ethical distress for clinicians. Reaching out to ethics consult services can help to create a greater sense of empowerment and clarity when there are competing values and complex ethical dilemmas.

Well-Being Beyond the Walls of the Institution

Ultimately, any consideration of resilience and well-being will account for the well-being of communities beyond the walls of healthcare institution. As PC services continue to expand into community and outpatient contexts, the health of the larger communities in which they function is of increasing importance. Clinicians empowered to develop their compassion, while simultaneously strengthening their well-being and resilience, are better able to address the challenges of the broader communities in which they serve, ultimately benefiting patients and the larger society.

References

1. Kamal AH, Bull JH, Wolf SP, et al. Prevalence and predictors of burnout among hospice and palliative care clinicians in the U.S. *Journal of Pain and Symptom Management*. 2016;*51*(4):690–696.
2. Back AL, Steinhauser KE, Kamal AH, Jackson VA. Building resilience for palliative care clinicians: an approach to burnout prevention based on individual skills and workplace factors. *Journal of Pain and Symptom Management*. 2016;*52*(2):284–291.
3. Rushton CH, Batcheller J, Schroeder K, Donohue P. Burnout and resilience among nurses practicing in high-intensity settings. *American Journal of Critical Care*. 2015;*24*(5):412–420.
4. Byock I. *Dying Well: The Prospect for Growth at the End of Life*. New York, NY: Riverhead Books; 1997.
5. National Center for Chronic Disease Prevention and Health Promotion DoPH. Well-being concepts. 2018. http://www.cdc.gov/hrqol/wellbeing.htm#three. Accessed July 1, 2019.
6. Ryff CD. Psychological wellbeing revisited: advances in the science and practice of eudaimonia. *Psychotherapy and Psychosomatics*. 2014;*83*(1):10–28.
7. Ryff CD. Happiness is everything, or is it? Explorations on the meaning of psychological wellbeing. *Journal of Personality and Social Psychology*. 1989;*57*(6):1069–1081.
8. Kirkwood TBL, Bond J, May C, McKeith I, Teh M-M. Foresight mental capital and wellbeing project. In Wellbeing CL, Cooper (Ed.). 2014. https://doi.org/10.1002/9781118539415.wbwell092
9. Pollard EL, Lee PD. Child wellbeing: a systematic review of the literature. *Social Indicators Research*. 2003;*61*(1):59–78.
10. Diener E, Suh E. Measuring quality of life: economic, social, and subjective indicators. *Social Indicators Research*. 1997;*40*(1/2):189–216.
11. Rotenstein LS, Torre M, Ramos MA, et al. Prevalence of burnout among physicians: a systematic review. *JAMA*. 2018;*320*(11):1131–1150.
12. Maslach C, Leiter MP. New insights into burnout and health care: strategies for improving civility and alleviating burnout. *Medical Teacher*. 2017;*39*(2):160–163.
13. Additional stress factors for physicians, according to the National Academy of Medicine and the Joint Commission Journal on Quality and Patient Safety.
14. Mazzarelli A, Trzeciak S, Booker C. *Compassionomics: The Revolutionary Scientific Evidence That Caring Makes a Difference*. Fire Starter; 2019.
15. Zaki, J. *The War for Kindness: Building Empathy in a Fractured World*. New York, NY: Crown; 2019
16. De Waal F. *The Age of Empathy: Nature's Lessons for a Kinder Society*. New York, NY: Three Rivers Press; 2009.
17. Neff K. The Five Myths of Self Compassion. *Greater Good Magazine*. September 30, 2015. https://greatergood.berkeley.edu/article/item/the_five_myths_of_self_compassion. Accessed August 1, 2019.
18. Neff KD. The role of self-compassion in development: a healthier way to relate to oneself. *Human Development*. 2009;*52*(4):211–214.
19. More than a dozen randomized controlled trials have been published from research on CBCT. The initial study with Emory undergraduates indicated that participants experienced a healthier response to stress after engaging the CBCT course in those participants who spent the most time doing the contemplative practices. A study with children in the Atlanta foster care system further demonstrated a reduction in inflammatory biomarkers and increased hopefulness after the practice of CBCT. Subsequent randomized controlled trials have shown promising outcomes with CBCT as an intervention for specific populations, including medical students, veterans with posttraumatic stress disorder, and breast cancer survivors in Arizona and Spain. Additional feasibility trials suggest promising outcomes with suicide survivors, as do several pilot trials with NICU nurses, HIV-positive individuals, public school

teachers, parents of children with autism, and transgender youth. Overall, research measures suggest that the practice of CBCT may decrease loneliness and depressive symptoms, improve hopefulness, increase empathic accuracy, moderate the effects of trauma, help with sleep, and improve resiliency for professionals in stressful workplace contexts or other difficult environments. From Negi LT. CBCT' Compassion Training. Center for Contemplative Science and Compassion-Based Ethics website. 2020. https://compassion.emory.edu/cbct-compassion-training/index.html. Accessed May 15, 2020.

20. Pace TWW, Negi LT, Adame DD, et al. Effect of compassion meditation on neuroendocrine, innate immune and behavioral responses to psychosocial stress. *Psychoneuroendocrinology.* 2009;*34*(1):87–98.

21. Hughes J, Duff AJ, Puntis JWL. Using Schwartz Center Rounds to promote compassionate care in a children's hospital. *Archives of Disease in Childhood.* 2018;*103*(1):11–12.

22. International Critical Incident Stress Foundation. What is critical incident stress management (CISM)? 2019. https://icisf.org/about-us/. Accessed August 1, 2019.

Illness Burden and
Its Management

Physical Aspects of Care

10

Constitutional Symptoms

Lara Desanti-Siska, Shawn Fellows,
and Nicholas Polito

Fatigue

Definition and Etiology

Fatigue is defined as a "subjective state characterized by feelings of tiredness and a perception of decreased capacity for physical or mental work."[1] The National Comprehensive Cancer Network defines cancer-related fatigue as a "distressing, persistent, subjective sense of physical, emotional, and/or cognitive tiredness or exhaustion related to cancer or cancer treatment and is not proportional to activity and interferes with usual functioning."[2] It is one of the most common symptoms seen in palliative care patients who have advanced illness[3] and is also one of the most underreported and undertreated symptoms in this population of patients.[4] In advanced illness, fatigue is typically not relieved by rest; therefore, it negatively impacts quality of life and activities of daily living.[5] This debilitating symptom is prevalent in patients with cancer, ranging from 60% to 90% of patients,[6] but it can also be seen in other diagnoses, such as chronic heart, pulmonary, and renal disease. In a meta-analysis of 84 studies, which involved a total of 144,813 patients, the pooled prevalence of cancer-related fatigue was found to be 52% and was more common in the patients older than 65 years of age.[7] This study also documented several physical symptoms (poor performance status), chemoradiotherapy, insomnia, pain, and psychological distress (depression) as risk factors for the development of cancer-related fatigue.[7]

The pathophysiology of fatigue is multifactorial and is not fully understood. Saligan et al. in 2015 illustrated the complexity of cancer-related fatigue and possible pathways involved in its etiology, including the immune response, inflammatory response, metabolic and neuroendocrine functions, hypothalamic-pituitary-adrenal (HPA) axis, and genetics.[8] Cancer and its treatments can lead to immune activation with a release of pro-inflammatory cytokines contributing to inflammation, alterations in endocrine functions,

HPA axis dysfunction, as well as mitochondrial impairment in the peripheral and central nervous systems.[8] Noncancer conditions that are characterized by fatigue also produce pro-inflammatory cytokines.[9] Physical and cognitive function mutually affect and are affected by deconditioning, depression, sleep disturbance, and cognitive impairment. All are also associated with worsening symptoms of cancer-related fatigue.

Assessment

Fatigue is subjective, and therefore its intensity can vary from one person to another. One of the scales that is used frequently by palliative care clinicians is the Edmonton Symptom Assessment Scale, which rates symptoms on a numerical scale from 0 to 10. Scores of 4 or greater should trigger further investigation. It is important to distinguish fatigue from other common conditions, including depression and delirium; however, this can be difficult at times. A comprehensive history and physical examination are essential to understanding the impact of the fatigue on the patient's quality of life and to investigate contributing factors. Screening will identify reversible conditions such as anemia, polypharmacy, hypotension, low testosterone, deconditioning, and malnutrition. If an underlying condition is identified and treated, fatigue may successfully be reversed. However, if the fatigue is chronic, as seen in patients with advanced cancer, the causes are usually multifactorial and less likely to be reversed. Some diagnostic workup may be necessary to confirm clinical suspicion. Medication review is critical, and this includes prescribed drugs, supplements, and over-the-counter medications. Fatigue may be a known side effect of a medication, or a drug-drug interaction may contribute to the fatigue. By dose reduction, discontinuation, or even medication rotation, fatigue may be significantly improved. An interdisciplinary approach to diagnosis will also enhance the treatment plan.

Management

Nonpharmacological Interventions

Education, energy-conserving strategies, and exercise are paramount in the approach to treatment of fatigue. Patient and caregiver education on fatigue in the context of progressive serious illness will help them develop realistic goals, establish boundaries, and prioritize activities. Short periods of rest can encourage patients to conserve their energy, and they will be more empowered to participate in the activities they truly enjoy. This also enhances patient autonomy at a critical time of serious illness. Patients also need to understand that excessive rest may contribute to fatigue. The benefits of engaging in a structured exercise program has been shown to reduce fatigue and also to help to improve function, strength, and overall well-being.[10] Stress, anxiety, and depression have also been associated with increased intensity of fatigue, and psychological interventions in the form of cognitive behavioral therapy have shown benefits in this population of patients.[11] Increased physical activity and reduced psychological stress help to increase resiliency by emphasizing the impact of fatigue on the overall longevity and quality of life of the patient.

Pharmacological Interventions

There are a limited number of medications that have demonstrated efficacy in the treatment of fatigue. A Cochrane review concluded that no specific drug could be recommended for the treatment of fatigue in palliative care patients due to the limited evidence.[12] However, psychostimulants and corticosteroids show promising results in the treatment of fatigue.

Psychostimulants that have shown the most benefit in treating fatigue in the palliative care patient population are methylphenidate (Ritalin), modafinil (Provigil), and armodafinil (Nuvigil). These medications tend to be tolerated well and are more beneficial in patients with severe fatigue than in those with mild-to-moderate fatigue. Off-label use of methylphenidate is usually started at an oral dose of 5 mg twice daily with breakfast and lunch in order to minimize nighttime insomnia. If no improvement is achieved within 1 week, the dose may be increased to 10 mg. After 2 weeks, if there is no improvement in fatigue symptoms, the medication should be discontinued. Methylphenidate has shown the most benefit in treating fatigue related to opioid-induced sedation and cognitive failure in patients for whom dose reduction or dose rotation is impractical or inappropriate.[13] Methylphenidate is well tolerated and quick acting, and patients may get some relief of their fatigue within 24 hours. The most common adverse side effects were agitation, restlessness, tachycardia, palpitations, delirium, confusion, and insomnia. One serious but uncommon adverse effects is arrhythmia, which is reversible with discontinuation.[13]

Modafinil, better known as Provigil, is a Schedule IV nonamphetamine psychostimulant approved for excessive daytime somnolence associated with obstructive sleep apnea, narcolepsy, and shift work sleep disorder. Off-label use of modafinil for the treatment of fatigue is usually started as a single oral 250-mg dose in the morning. Armodafinil, which is an enantiomer of modafinil, is also used off label for treatment of fatigue, and the daily dose is 150 mg orally. Side effects of both modafinil and armodafinil include headache, nausea, dry mouth, reduced appetite, dizziness, anxiety, and insomnia. Care needs to be taken when prescribing these medications to avoid unintended side effects, and if they should arise, the medications should be discontinued.

Glucocorticoids may also help to relieve fatigue in patients who are in the terminal phases of advanced cancer or other serious life-limiting illnesses. These medications have been shown to have only modest effects in improving fatigue and are used for only a short period of time, typically 2–4 weeks. Dexamethasone appears to be the most widely studied, with a starting daily dose of 1–2 mg orally. Megestrol acetate, which is used for the treatment of anorexia-cachexia, has been shown to improve fatigue and can be considered for short-term usage[14]; a usual starting dose is 400 mg daily by mouth. Prednisone has also shown some modest benefit in improving fatigue; a starting dose of 7.5–10 mg per day can be titrated to an effective dose if needed. Common side effects from all glucocorticoids include elevations in blood pressure and glucose, upper gastrointestinal (GI) upset, agitation, insomnia, and delirium.[12] Therefore, in clinical practice, the use of glucocorticoids should only be considered as a short-term therapeutic option in the treatment of fatigue.

Other treatments have been studied in advanced illness and lack the convincing evidence to support their use in the treatment of fatigue. The provider is cautioned in these instances where fatigue symptoms are recalcitrant, and they should only be considered following consultation with a pharmacology specialist. The potential for life-threatening adverse events is great. These agents include amantadine (an antiviral agent commonly used for influenza treatment); pemoline (a stimulant used for attention deficit hyperactivity disorder and narcolepsy); donepezil (an acetylcholinesterase inhibitor used to treat Alzheimer dementia); as well as supplements such as L-carnitine.[12]

Conclusion

Fatigue is one of the most common symptoms that is seen in palliative care, but because of its subjectivity, it is a symptom that tends to be underreported and therefore undertreated. The etiology of fatigue is complex and multifaceted and therefore requires an interdisciplinary approach to treatment. Optimizing contributing conditions will help to improve symptoms, but if no specific cause can be identified, symptomatic treatment with a multimodal approach is recommended along with educational strategies, physical and psychological interventions, and careful use of pharmacological therapies.

Fever and Sweating
Definition and Etiology

Fever is defined as a temperature of 383°C on three occasions at least an hour apart or in excess of 38.5°C once is considered clinically significant and requires further investigation.[15] The pathophysiology of fever is a fine balance between heat production, heat conservation, and heat loss in an effort to control core body temperature. A fever develops when a pyrogen elevates the thermoregulatory set point for the core body temperature above normal. In older adults, an elevation of 2°C above their baseline is considered an indication for further investigation. The associated cutaneous vasoconstriction causes heat retention, and shivering generates additional heat to achieve the new set point.[1]

The prevalence of fever in advanced illness varies greatly. However, the causes of fever can be infectious in nature, tumor related, or medication induced. Infectious causes also need to be ruled out since it is not uncommon for a patient to develop a wound infection, pneumonia, or urinary tract infection at the end of life. Many terminally ill patients receive antimicrobial therapy in the days to weeks before their death in an effort to provide symptom relief and improve quality of life.[16] The pathophysiology of tumor-related fever is thought to be the result of hypersensitivity reactions, pyrogen production, primary cytokine production, and tumor necrosis.[1] Lymphoma, both Hodgkin and non-Hodgkin; leukemia; and renal cell carcinomas are among the more common malignancies to present with fever; however, it is seen in other cancers.[17] Drug-induced fever is most commonly the result of a hypersensitivity reaction, and its characteristics resemble an allergic reaction. The fever usually occurs 7–10 days after initiation of the medication and will dissipate within 72 hours once the medication is discontinued. There are a number of medications that can cause a drug-induced fever, but the agents most commonly associated with fever include sulfa-containing medications (trimethoprim-sulfamethoxazole, sulfasalazine), diuretics (furosemide), antiepileptics (phenytoin), H_2 blockers, opioids, β-lactams (penicillins), and carbapenems.[18]

Sweating is a normal bodily function used to help regulate temperature and prevent hyperthermia. Sweating can be either localized or generalized, and it can occur only during the day or predominantly at night and is not always associated with fever (pyrexia). The prevalence of sweating in patients with advanced illness is not well delineated, however, in those with advanced cancer, receiving palliative care, the prevalence ranges from 14% to 28%, is frequently nocturnal and is moderate to severe in intensity.[1] Along with cancer, there are many other conditions that can cause hyperhidrosis, including infections; endocrine disorders (hypoglycemia, thyrotoxicosis, pheochromocytoma, diabetes mellitus, and hypopituitarism); hormone suppression treatments (antiestrogen and antiandrogen therapy); or medications (opioids, naproxen, acyclovir) or may be a paraneoplastic phenomenon. The causes of sweating in the cancer patient may be the tumor, treatment of the neoplasm, or unrelated disorders. Episodes of sweating that occur independently of fever are often hormonally mediated or related to pharmacotherapy.[1] Causes of localized hyperhidrosis include spinal cord disease, cerebrovascular disease, or peripheral neuropathy.

Assessment

A thorough history and physical examination will provide a differential diagnosis to inform targeted laboratory and imaging modalities. Identification and treatment of the reversible causes of hyperhidrosis are essential. If there are no identifiable causes, then symptomatic treatment is indicated.

Management

The management of fever consists of nonspecific therapies to lower temperature, including acetaminophen and/or nonsteroidal anti-inflammatory drugs (NSAIDs) and cooling treatments; tepid water can also help to lower temperature as well as use of cooling blankets. Oral hydration is also important to reduce risks of dehydration. However, directed treatment aimed at the underlying cause is the primary goal.

In the absence of fever, treatment options for sweating alone consist of histamine receptor antagonists, such as cimetidine 400–800 mg twice daily; antimuscarinics (thought to act directly on the sweat glands); NSAIDs (ibuprofen 400 mg every 6 hours or 600 mg every 8 hours or diclofenac 50 mg orally two or three times per day); and selective serotonin reuptake inhibitors, such as paroxetine 20 mg orally per day, sertraline 50 mg orally per day).[19] All have been shown to reduce sweating in the palliative care population with serious and advanced illness.

Conclusion

Fever and sweating can be very distressing symptoms to patients and their families. Effective management of these symptoms includes identification of the underlying and contributing factors; discussion of potential treatments with the patient and their caregivers; and tailoring treatment according to the patient's stated treatment goals of care. Therapeutic management of these symptoms can reduce them and their concomitant distress and suffering, and this will improve the patient's overall comfort level and reduce their symptom burden.

TABLE 10.1 International Forum for the Study of Itch (IFSI) Clinical Classification of Itch

Category 1	Dermatological disease	<ul><li>Psoriasis</li><li>Atopic dermatitis</li><li>Xerosis (dry skin)</li><li>Scabies</li><li>Urticaria</li></ul>
Category 2	Systemic disease	<ul><li>Drug-induced pruritus</li><li>Pruritus arising from disease of the internal organs - Liver (cholestasis) - Kidney (uremia) - Blood (leukemia, lymphoma, polycythemia) - Metabolic diseases (hypothyroidism, hyperthyroidism, diabetes mellitus)</li></ul>
Category 3	Neurological disease	<ul><li>Systemic (multiple sclerosis)</li><li>Peripheral (nerve damage, nerve compression or irritation)</li></ul>
Category 4	Psychiatric or psychosomatic disease	<ul><li>Tactile hallucinations</li><li>Delusional parasitosis</li><li>Somatoform pruritus</li><li>Anxiety</li></ul>
Category 5	Mixed disease	<ul><li>Overlap of several diseases</li></ul>
Category 6	Other pruritus of undetermined origin (acute or chronic)	

Pruritus

Definition and Etiology

Pruritus (itching) is defined as a sensation that leads to the desire to scratch and is the predominant symptom of many diseases. It can lead to significant distress for the patient, resulting in insomnia, agitation, depression, and skin infections and scarring. When the cause of the pruritus is known, management is straightforward as long as there is an effective treatment available for the condition. However, in the 8%–15% of affected patients, the cause of the pruritus is unknown, making effective relief of the symptom difficult to achieve. According to the International Forum for the Study of Itch (IFSI), pruritus is defined as being acute with symptoms less than 6 weeks to chronic at greater than 6 weeks.[20] The data regarding the prevalence of pruritus in the general population are limited. However, it is more common in the elderly, estimated to affect up to 60% of those 65 years and older.[21] Pruritus is a common symptom in the palliative care population due to their older age, comorbid conditions, and/or resultant polypharmacy.

A classification system for categorizing diseases that are known to cause pruritus has been proposed by IFSI (see Table 10.1).[1]

> Category 1: dermatological disease, including psoriasis, atopic dermatitis, xerosis (dry skin), scabies, and urticaria

Category 2: systemic disease, including drug-induced pruritus and pruritus arising from disease of the internal organs, such as liver (cholestasis), kidney (uremia), blood (leukemia, lymphoma, polycythemia), and from metabolic diseases (hypothyroidism, hyperthyroidism, diabetes mellitus)

Category 3: neurological disease, including pruritus arising from diseases or disorders of the central or peripheral nervous system, such as multiple sclerosis, nerve damage, nerve compression, or nerve root irritation

Category 4: psychiatric or psychosomatic disease, including tactile hallucinations, delusional parasitosis, somatoform pruritus, anxiety

Category 5: mixed disease, involving overlap of several disorders

Category 6: other pruritus of undetermined origin or chronic pruritus of unknown origin

Pathophysiology

The complex pathophysiology of pruritus is only partially understood and involves the interplay between numerous mediated pathways. The thick myelinated type II sensory receptors transmit tactile sensations, whereas the thin myelinated A-delta and unmyelinated C-polymodel fibers are mainly involved in conducting thermal pain and itch sensation. The C fibers are located more superficially near the dermoepidermal junction and are therefore more sensitive to pruritogenic substrates than pain receptors. Neurotransmitters for these nerves—many of which are activated by inflammation—include histamine, calcitonin gene–related peptide, neuropeptide substrate P, serotonin, bradykinin, proteases (mast cell tryptase), neurokinin (KN1), and endothelin (which stimulates the release of nitric oxide). Nerve impulses are then transmitted from the dorsal root ganglion to the spinothalamic tract and eventually to the thalamus.[22] Neurogenic and systemic itch caused by the toxic effects of diseased organs does not show any neuronal pathology but may cause pruritus through the central nervous system and is thought to be the result of endospinal endogenous opioid release. Neuropathic itch is caused by damage to either peripheral or central sensory nerve fibers themselves, without any cutaneous stimuli. The pathophysiology of psychogenic itch continues to remain elusive.[2] As more is known about the pathways involved in the pruritic response, more novel therapies can be developed. Therapies currently used to treat pruritus target many of these known pathways.

Management

As part of the initial management, a thorough clinical history and physical examination is required to identify possible etiologies of the pruritus. There may be clues that are uncovered in the patient's history that may lead toward the source or cause(s). Ask simple questions, such as the duration of symptoms (acute vs. chronic), location (localized vs. systemic), timing (intermittent vs. constant) and any known triggers. Be sure to take a detailed medication history, and identify any treatments that have been tried in the past and were or were not effective. Obtain a full medical and family history to help define a differential diagnosis. Basic laboratory testing is necessary, including complete blood count with differential, erythrocyte sedimentation rate, C-reactive protein (CRP), complete metabolic panel, and thyroid-stimulating hormone, to rule out metabolic or end organ failure. If a cause is identified, then specific treatment for that cause should be initiated. However, in up to 20% of patients the cause of the pruritus is unknown,[23] making the treatment of the condition more complicated.

Patients should be educated on the nonpharmacological interventions that can be initiated for general pruritus relief. These include ensuring that the living environment is cool and humid. Apply moisturizers, particularly after bathing, to improve the skin barrier. Emollients or moisturizers with active ingredients such as urea (5%–10%) and glycerol (20%) that have been best studied, but those with propylene glycol (20%) and lactic acid (1.5%–5%) may also be helpful and can be applied multiple times per day. Reduce bathing frequency and use lukewarm water; mild, slightly acidic pH cleansers; and oatmeal baths, which help to soothe irritated skin. Herbal remedies, including aloe, have also been shown to soothe the skin and reduce pruritus. Clothing should be lightweight, washed in unscented detergent, and made of breathable fabrics. Trim the nails or wear cotton gloves to help reduce risk of infection due to scratching and avoid vasodilators, such as caffeine, alcohol, spices, and hot water. If pruritus persists despite conservative measures, topical pharmacological intervention offers additional treatment efficacy.

Topical pharmacological interventions are useful and should be tried first to provide some initial relief. There are many agents that are available over the counter and via prescription. Table 10.2 summarizes some of the possible topical interventions that may be appropriate for use.

Systemic pharmacological intervention may be required if topical agents fail to relieve the patient's symptoms. Again, there are many options available over the counter and by prescription. Care must be taken in the older adult population to try to avoid polypharmacy interactions as well as heavily anticholinergic preparations as they are additive or superlative as in 1 + 1 = 4. Table 10.3 lists a summary of some of the agents used, mediating pathways, common uses, and common side effects.

Opioid-Induced Pruritus

Opioid-induced pruritus is caused by a complex pathogenesis, involving the histamine, 5-hydroxytryptamine-3 (5-HT$_3$), prostaglandin E$_1$ (PGE1), PGE2, and C fibers. This pruritus is most commonly seen in the initiation of opioid therapy, but can also be seen in long-term use. The incidence is high in intrathecal or epidural administration and is less frequently seen with fentanyl use. The data are inconclusive on the most effective way to treat this condition. During the initiation of therapy, symptoms can be managed conservatively with systemic antihistamines, ondansetron, or gabapentin and are likely to resolve within a few days to weeks. However, if pruritus develops in the setting of long-term opioid use, dose reduction and opioid rotation can be considered and seem to be effective. Use of opioid receptor antagonists, such as naltrexone, naloxone, butorphanol, and methylnaltrexone, has been studied and showed mixed results with the potential of precipitating a withdrawal syndrome.

TABLE 10.2 Topical Pharmacological Interventions

Anti-inflammatory	Steroid-based creams; avoid long-term use due to risk of skin atrophy Salicylic acid 2%–6%; for lichen simplex chronicus; avoid in acute inflammatory dermatoses
Cooling sensation	Menthol 1%–2% cream/lotion Sarna Original or Men-Phor Lotion (active ingredients: 0.5% menthol + 0.5% camphor) Calamine lotion (zinc oxide compound); also a mild antiseptic
Antihistamine	Diphenhydramine 2% cream; apply 4 times daily Doxepin 5% cream, apply 4 times daily; avoid use in children and older adults, may cause sedation
Anesthetic	Lidocaine products: (especially beneficial for neuropathic pruritus) - Lidocaine patch 5% - Lidocaine cream 4% (Lidocaine Plus with aloe vera) - EMLA cream (eutectic mixture of 2.5% lidocaine and 2.5% pilocaine) Pramoxine products: (especially beneficial for uremic pruritus) - Pramoxine 1%–2.5% twice daily, available in gel, spray, cream, foam, solution, and pads; do not use on open wounds Example Sarna Sensitive Lotion(1% pramoxine) Sarna Ultra Cream(1% pramoxine + 0.5% menthol + 20% white petroleum)
Antidepressants	Doxepin (tricyclic antidepressant) 5% apply 4 times daily for up to 8 days; can cause sedation and allergic dermatitis
Nerve block	Capsaicin 0.025%–0.1% cream, apply 3 times daily (beneficial for neuropathic and uremic pruritus); can cause a transient burning sensation, but usually resolves within a few weeks; do not use on open wounds
Calcineurin inhibitors	Tacrolimus 0.1% ointment apply 2 times per day Pimecrolimus 1% cream apply 2 times per day
Phototherapy	Ultraviolet B irradiation; initial daily dose of 200–400 mJ/cm²; increase by 100 mJ/cm² at each session to a maximum daily dose of 1500

Coping Strategies

Chronic pruritic conditions are associated with high levels of stress and definitely impacts a patient's quality of life. Stress has also been proven to exacerbate itch, leading to what is known as the itch-scratch-itch cycle. This vicious cycle results in continuous scratching, worsening disease prognosis, and decreased quality of life.[24] Adjunctive psychosocial programs, in the forms of relaxation techniques, stress management/mindfulness, music therapy, cognitive behavioral therapy, and healing touch, may help to break the cycle by changing stress-related behaviors and thought patterns. Acupuncture, an integrative medicine modality, has proven to be successful in helping to treat pruritus.[25] The association between stress and pruritus has been well established, despite our incomplete understanding of the mechanism of action. Therefore, adjunctive strategies that can be used to reduce stress and anxiety will ultimately help to break this cycle and bring relief to patients with pruritus.

Conclusion

Pruritus is a distressing symptom that can be seen in many palliative care patients. Often the etiology is unknown and multifactorial, therefore making an effective treatment plan more challenging. It is essential to educate patients on effective strategies that can help to reduce

TABLE 10.3 Systemic Pharmacological Interventions

Medication	Medications	Uses	Side Effects
Antihistamines 1st generation 2nd generation	Diphenhydramine 12.5–50 mg by mouth/SC every 6–12 h Hydroxyzine 10–50 mg by mouth/SC every 4–12 h Cetirizine 10 mg every day Loratadine 10 mg every day Cimetidine 300 mg by mouth at bedtime Cyproheptadine 4-mg tablet; 2 mg/5 mL syrup; 4 mg by mouth three or four times a day	Urticaria, mastocytosis, and opioid pruritus	Sedation, confusion/delirium, headache, dry mouth, and nausea
Steroids	Dexamethasone 2–8 mg by mouth/SC every day Prednisone 10–30 mg every day	Inflammatory skin disease, systemic inflammatory disease	Gastrointestinal upset, insomnia
Antidepressants	Mirtazapine 15–45 mg by mouth at bedtime Paroxetine 10–40 mg by mouth every day Sertraline 75–100 mg by mouth every day Doxepin 25–75 mg by mouth at bedtime[a]	Psychogenic, paraneoplastic pruritus, urticaria	Drowsiness, fatigue, headache
Anticonvulsants	Gabapentin 100–300 mg by mouth every day to three times a day Pregabalin 50–100 mg by mouth twice or three times daily	Neuropathic itch, pruritis associated with chronic kidney disease	Altered mental status, unsteady gait
Antipsychotics	Seroquel 12.5–50 mg by mouth every day to three times daily Haloperidol 2.5–5 mg by mouth three times daily	Tactile hallucinations	Sedation,
Other mechanisms of action	Ondansetron 4–8 mg by mouth every 8 h Cholestyramine 4 g by mouth three times daily	Cholestatic pruritus, opioid-induced pruritus, pruritus induced by chronic kidney disease	

[a]Doxepin is very anticholinergic and should be avoided in older adults.

their symptoms regardless of the cause. A multiprong approach should be utilized and has been shown to relieve symptoms and improve the quality of life in this fragile population.

Anorexia-Cachexia

Definition and Etiology

Anorexia-cachexia syndrome (ACS) is a phenomenon that is commonly seen in patients with advanced or terminal illness and can be considered a natural part of the end-of-life process. ACS is a multifactorial syndrome, mediated by a cascade of inflammatory responses creating a negative energy balance that leads to loss of body mass and loss of appetite for food.[26] This syndrome is largely misunderstood by patients and their families and can lead to a great deal of emotional distress for those caring for the patient. It is the role of the palliative care clinician to recognize the condition, assess for any reversible causes, and if none are identified, educate the patient and their caregivers on the dying process to alleviate further emotional distress.

Anorexia is defined as the loss of appetite, while cachexia is a hypermetabolic state defined as accelerated loss of skeletal muscle in the context of a chronic inflammatory response. This is commonly seen in cancer diagnoses, but can also be seen in chronic infections, AIDS, heart failure, and chronic obstructive pulmonary disease (COPD).[27] The prevalence of cachexia is high, ranging from 5% to 15% in congestive heart failure and COPD to 60% to 80% in advanced cancer.[28] The diagnostic criterion for cachexia is weight loss greater than 5% within 1 year or weight loss greater than 2% in individuals already showing depletion (body mass index < 20 kg/m^2). Additionally, reduced skeletal muscle mass (sarcopenia) plus three of the following criteria is diagnostic of ACS[29]:

1. Decreased muscle strength.
2. Low fat-free mass index. The low fat-free mass index is a measure much like body mass index, but instead it measures the amount of muscle related to the patient's height, which helps to distinguish muscle and fat.[30]
3. Fatigue.
4. Anorexia.
5. Abnormal biochemistry (increased inflammatory markers (CRP > 5.0 mg/L and interleukin [IL] 6 > 4.0 pg/mL); anemia (<12 g/dL); and low serum albumin (<3.2 g/dL). The inflammatory markers, which tend to rise with age and are associated with age-related diseases (cardiovascular disease, diabetes, and cancers), increase over time and are associated with greater mortality risk,[31] as well as psychological stressors.[32] CRP and IL-6 levels within individuals vary over time, and increases in CRP are associated with greater mortality risk. Three-year changes in inflammatory markers are better predictors of mortality than baseline measures.

Anorexia cachexia syndrome is incorporated into numerous prognostication scales, and it is considered a common manifestation on the terminal illness pathway and is associated with a prognosis of less than 3 months.[33] Clinicians therefore should utilize the presence of anorexia-cachexia to help improve prognostication skills and help to guide clinical recommendations.

Dietary intake patterns in the terminally ill naturally decrease in frequency of eating, reduction in the variety of foods, and unusually high proportions of liquids.[34] While the loss of appetite and weight loss are common in most patients with serious illness, the profound weight loss suffered by patients with cachexia cannot be entirely attributed to poor caloric intake alone. This is why cachexia in advanced illness is typically not responsive to nutritional supplementation, which can be surprising to families and to some practitioners. Patients and families should be reassured that eating extra calories does not reverse the underlying process in patients with advanced disease, and that loss of interest in food is a natural occurrence as the illness progresses. In these cases, the social aspects of eating and the pleasure of food should be emphasized over the nutritional benefits.

Assessment

The palliative care provider should focus on trying to identify reversible conditions that are contributing to ACS. A careful history and physical exam should always be performed, focusing on weight loss history, calorie count or food diary, management of treatable physical conditions (oral ulcers or thrush, poor dentition), associated psychosocial issues and spiritual concerns. The role of the palliative care provider is often to educate the patient and their caregivers on aspects of the patient's condition that are amenable to treatment and those that are not. Understanding that ACS is part of the disease process and is a natural part of the dying process, can help with acceptance.

Management

While ACS can be considered completely normal in advanced illness, impaired oral intake can be impeded by other potentially reversible causes, such as dry mouth, taste or smell alterations, stomatitis, odynophagia, dysphagia, severe constipation, nausea or vomiting, and uncontrolled symptoms, such as pain, depression, dyspnea, or delirium. Other catabolic states, such as hyperthyroidism, B_{12} deficiency, adrenal insufficiency, and hypogonadism, are also potentially reversible conditions that could contribute to the ACS.[35] It is also the case that side effects from various medications and treatments—including chemotherapy and radiation therapy—can affect a person's appetite and ability to eat. It is vitally important for palliative care providers to identify and control these reversible causes of ACS as other interventions are considered. Early in the disease process, consultations with supportive therapists, including nutrition specialists, speech and language therapists, occupational therapists, and physical therapists, help to provide additional management options for the patient and their caregivers.

Some general recommendations that palliative care clinicians can offer families and caregivers include allowing patients to guide their intake by eating what they want, how much they want, and when they want. Offer their favorite foods that are easy to swallow, such as soups, puddings, smoothies, and liberalize dietary restrictions as appropriate for the individual. Some initial strategies could be offering smaller, more frequent meals; adding additional proteins (i.e., natural peanut butter, hummus) and fats (i.e., avocado, cooking with olive oil) to usual meals to enhance caloric content; and changing the environment where they are provided. Since socialization, in many families and cultures, is centered in food, providers can also encourage alternative ways to enjoy this activity and time together with other people—such as listening to music, telling stories, or reading together. This is an area of expertise that is addressed by activities directors in long-term care facilities.

Role of Appetite Stimulants

Appetite stimulants may be considered when no identifiable reversible causes of anorexia have been identified or once those causes have been addressed. Unfortunately, the literature demonstrates limited efficacy for a variety of medications used for this purpose. However, the use of appetite stimulants in the setting of cancer-related anorexia-cachexia has been well demonstrated, while there is still less-strong evidence to support use in other types of advanced illness. If there is no demonstrated benefit at the end of the agreed-on trial period, the medication should be discontinued. The primary benefits associated with these drugs are increased appetite and modest weight gain, not improved survival or quality of life. When initiating appetite stimulants, clinicians must make it clear to the patient and family that medications will be initiated as a trial following a discussion regarding realistic treatment goals and a time frame.

Nevertheless, the treatments listed in Table 10.4 may be beneficial.

Glucocorticoids can be administered orally or parenterally and are capable of improving appetite, nausea, and energy for brief periods of time. Dexamethasone (Medrol) (4 mg) or prednisone (20 mg) are often recommended when short-term treatment is being considered, up to 4–8 weeks. Dexamethasone seems to be the steroid most often used due to its minimal mineralocorticoid effects and ease of dosing (usually 2 to 8 mg orally daily). Equivalent prednisone dosing is 20 to 40 mg orally daily. The side-effect profile includes hyperglycemia, insomnia, fluids retention, gastritis, and delirium.

Megestrol acetate (Megace) improves appetite and body weight by increasing fat and water retention, not lean muscle mass. However, there is no strong evidence to suggest that

TABLE 10.4 Pharmacologic Appetite Stimulants

	Dosing	Common Side Effects
GLUCOCORTICOIDS		
Dexamethasone (Medrol)	2 to 8 mg by mouth/ IV daily	Hyperglycemia, insomnia, fluid retention, GI upset (gastritis), delirium
Prednisone	20 to 40 mg by mouth/ IV daily	Hyperglycemia, insomnia, fluid retention, GI upset (gastritis), delirium
PROGESTIN		
Megestrol acetate (Megace)	400 mg by mouth daily	Venous thrombosis, adrenal insufficiency, and possible severe androgen deficiency
CANNABINOIDS		
Dronabinol (Marinol)	2.5 to 10 mg by mouth twice daily	Hypotension, ataxia, somnolence, dry mouth, gastroparesis, euphoria, poor concentration, and hallucinations
GHRELIN RECEPTOR AGONIST		
Anamorelin HCL	50 to 100 mg by mouth daily	Elevated LFTs, headache, GI upset
NORADRENERGIC/SELECTIVE SEROTINERGIC REUPTAKE INHIBITOR (NaSSRI)		
Mirtazepine (Remeron)	7.5 to 15 mg by mouth daily	Dry mouth, constipation, sedation
ANTIPSYCHOTICS		
Olanzapine (Zyprexa)	2.5 to 10 mg by mouth daily	Delirium, sedation, agranulocytosis, tardive dyskinesia

megestrol improves nutritional status or quality of life.[37] When prescribing megestrol acetate, consider a starting oral dose of 400 mg daily. If there is no improvement in appetite within 2 weeks, increase to 600 or 800 mg orally daily. Oral suspension (40 mg/mL) is less expensive and has greater bioavailability; therefore, it is the preferred formulation when prescribing. Megestrol acetate maintains its clinical effectiveness longer and is better tolerated than glucocorticoids, but there are significant side effects to use, including a significant risk of developing venous thrombosis,[38] adrenal insufficiency, and possible severe androgen deficiency in male patients.

Cannabinoids, such as dronabinol (Marinol), significantly improve appetite in AIDS patients with anorexia-cachexia but have limited efficacy in cancer-associated anorexia-cachexia.[39] If a trial is warranted, start with oral dronabinol 2.5 mg twice a day, before lunch and dinner. Dosing can be titrated as high as 10 mg orally twice a day but is usually limited by adverse side effects, which include hypotension, ataxia, somnolence, dry mouth, gastroparesis, euphoria, poor concentration, and hallucinations.

Ghrelin is a growth hormone–releasing peptide that is secreted in the stomach; it stimulates appetite through the activation of the hypothalamus, promoting GI motility and therefore decreasing nausea and vomiting, and increasing insulin-like growth factor to maintain muscle mass. It has a central role in regulation of energy balance by reducing thermogenesis in brown adipose tissue, resulting in a positive energy balance and weight gain.[40] Multiple clinical trials showed promising results for the effectiveness of anamorelin HCl, a potent and selective ghrelin receptor agonist that mimics the effects of ghrelin. However, long-term efficacy and safety outcomes of this novel class of medication need to be further understood.[9]

A number of other pharmacological interventions have been studied. L-Carnitine supplementation used intravenously or in high oral doses has been studied in the context of serious cardiomyopathies, severe weight loss, and wasting syndromes, but there are no definitive regimens and multiple side effects (see guideline from the National Institutes of Health at https://ods.od.nih.gov/factsheets/Carnitine-HealthProfessional/#ref). Both mirtazapine (Remeron) and olanzapine (Zyprexa) treat mood disorders that can affect patients with advanced illness, which may contribute to ACS, and they are also known to cause weight gain.

Role of Artificial Nutrition

The great majority of patients in the terminal phases of an advanced, serious, or life-limiting illness will experience reduced oral intake. Family members and caregivers often experience high levels of emotional distress when a terminally ill patient becomes unable or unwilling to take fluids and nourishment orally, fearing that dehydration and malnutrition will contribute to suffering and hasten death. While artificial nutrition supplementation may appear ideal to control or reverse malnutrition, for the vast majority of patients, there is no evidence to support that artificial nutrition prolongs life or improves functional status; therefore, it is not indicated.[41] For a subset of patients who might otherwise have a prognosis that is measured in months—such as those with head and neck cancer undergoing chemo-/radiation therapy, acute cerebral vascular accident, or neurological disorders (i.e., amyotrophic lateral sclerosis)—home parenteral nutrition support may be considered.[42]

There are two forms of artificial nutrition/hydration that could be considered. Parenteral nutrition is provided via an intravenous route (total parenteral nutrition), and enteral nutrition is provided via nasogastric tube (NG), percutaneous endoscopic gastrostomy (PEG) tube, or postpyloric or jejunostomy tube. Once installed, risks and benefits need to be considered along with periodic reevaluations. Risks associated with artificial nutrition and hydration include increased risk of aspiration; GI upset, including nausea, vomiting, and diarrhea; skin breakdown due to increased urinary and bowel output; infection of the intravenous site; and the presence of a tube, limited mobility, and tolerance by the patient. If the benefits are outweighed by the risks, it should be discontinued. Maintaining or improving a patient's quality of life, even in the short term; reducing pain and suffering; and providing access for hydration or medication delivery may be reasonable goals of PEG tube placement, even in patients with a terminal illness, as long as it aligns with the patient's stated wishes and goals of care. There have been some studies to support the role of artificial nutrition and hydration for improvement in healing rates of decubitus ulcers.[43] In such cases, the role of artificial nutrition must be carefully considered. Specifically in the population of those with dementia, and according to the American Geriatric Society recommendations, Choosing Wisely (https://www.choosingwisely.org/societies/american-geriatrics-society/) recommends against feeding tubes in advanced dementia.

Conclusion

Anorexia-cachexia syndrome is a multifactorial syndrome that requires a multimodal approach to treatment. In the early stages of the syndrome, improving intake with the help of nutritional consultation, speech and language therapy, appetite stimulants, and incorporation of supportive care in the form of physical and occupational therapy can all help to improve quality of life for patients with serious illness. However, in advanced illness, these modalities will not reverse the process. Patients and caregivers need to be educated on the limitations and risks of treatment considerations, and decisions should be made based on the patient's goals-of-care discussions and stated wishes.

Hiccoughs

Singultus, more commonly referred to as hiccups or hiccoughs, comes from the Latin term *singulf*, meaning, "to catch one's breath while sobbing."[44] An involuntary contraction of the diaphragm in consequence with sudden glottis closure results in its characteristic "hic" sound. In concert with these actions is activation of inspiratory intercostal muscles. Several theories exist to explain the physiologic existence of hiccups. Most commonly, hiccups are cited to be advantageous perinatally, acting as respiratory training in utero or a reflex mechanism meant to avoid aspiration of meconium at birth.[45] Postnatal hiccups have no known physiological purpose and may only be the result of an underlying syndrome rather than a diagnosis in isolation.[46]

Epidemiology and Etiology

Despite being ubiquitous among humans, no internationally agreed-on definitions exist to describe hiccups. Most literature classifies hiccups by duration and whether acute, persistent, or intractable. "Persistent" hiccups are typically those lasting longer than 48 hours, while "intractable" describes hiccups lasting for greater than 1 month.[47] "Acute" hiccups are generally considered those lasting less than 2 days. When evaluating literature on therapy to terminate hiccups, it is important to denote the definitions used in order to determine if the therapy is applicable to patients with variable or unknown durations.

Hiccups may be further broken down by suspected origin and whether peripheral or central.[47,48] Determining the source of the hiccup in combination with duration has been suggested as a useful modality to provide treatment options for patients. The causes of hiccups can be organic, psychogenic, and idiopathic. Psychogenic and idiopathic hiccups should be diagnosed only once organic reasons have been excluded.[49]

Pathophysiology

The pathophysiologic mechanism by which hiccups occur is known as the "hiccup reflex arc." Included in this pathway are the phrenic, vagus, and sympathetic nerves.[47] Both afferent and efferent nerves are involved in the nerve conduction pathway. Centrally, the brainstem processes and relays information through the efferent pathway of the phrenic nerve, which is the sole motor nerve responsible for diaphragmatic muscle contraction. The phrenic nerve originates from cranial nerves III–V.[50] Injury or insult to any of the areas known to be in the reflex arc can contribute to the development of hiccups. Almost all of the body's neurotransmitters can be found in these pathways, with γ-aminobutyric acid-ergic and dopaminergic pathways the most frequent targets for hiccup pharmacotherapy. Gastroesophageal reflux disease also contributes to the development of hiccups.[51]

Implications

Physical harm as a result of prolonged hiccupping episodes is rare. Hiccups typically occur during inspiration and cause abrupt cessation of the inspiratory phase. A small case series of patients with active hiccups measured lung volume as well as effects on arterial blood gases.[52] The impact of hiccups on all values was determined to be insignificant by the study authors. Preoperatively, hiccups may make surgery challenging or even dangerous due to increased motion. Ventilation may also potentially be more challenging due to intermittent glottic closure.[53] However, hiccups tend to be most consequential on palliative care patients' quality of life as the hiccups can negatively impact their ability to perform activities of daily living. If prolonged and severe enough, especially in deconditioned patients, hiccups can lead to fatigue, impaired sleep, dehydration, weight loss, malnutrition, and aspiration syndromes.[54] If left untreated, intractable hiccups can cause severe discomfort, depression, and reduced physical strength.[55] The risk of death as a direct result from hiccups is remote. However, hiccups may be a symptom of a more significant underlying pathology that could result in significant patient harm if not diagnosed and treated.[56]

Diagnosis

Hiccups may be due to an isolated cause or multifactorial. Over 100 causes have been cited in the literature, including singularly or in combination with medication, psychogenic, or organic reasons.[54,57] A review of 220 cases in patients with persistent hiccups found that 61% of cases were due to a combination of etiologies.[58] Authors suggested in patients with persistent or recalcitrant hiccups that greater than one underlying cause should be considered. Oncology patients may be uniquely challenging as both individual cancers and their treatments are known to induce hiccups. Furthermore, corticosteroids, used to ameliorate chemotherapy-induced nausea and vomiting, are also associated with hiccup development.[59] The diagnostic approach for hiccups is best described by Georg Petroianu, "hiccup is not a disease but a symptom."[46] Evaluation of hiccups should emphasize identification of the underlying cause while providing symptom relief. A detailed approach to identify hiccup etiology is found in Figure 10.1.

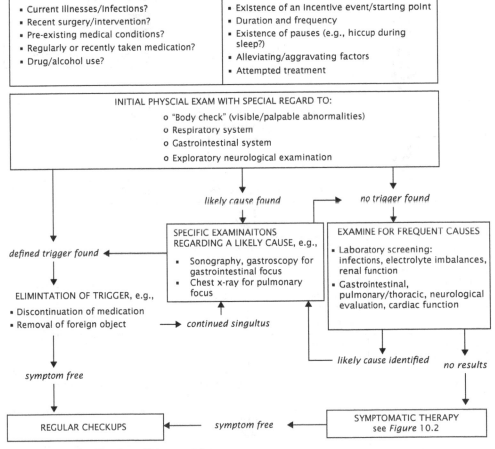

FIGURE 10.1 Identification of hiccup etiology.

Treatment

General

A number of treatments and techniques are available to manage hiccups. Unfortunately, many treatments are not supported by high-quality randomized controlled trials.[60] A 2013 Cochrane review found insufficient evidence to support either pharmacological or nonpharmacological interventions.[61] From the available evidence, direct oropharyngeal stimulation and pharmacological manipulation of the GI tract to reduce acidity or modulate the hiccup reflex arc may be the most effective treatment modalities.[47,62,63] While no guideline endorsed treatment algorithms dedicated solely to hiccup management are available, most literature agrees choice of treatment should be directed by etiology.[48,63] Figure 10.2 is a treatment algorithm proposed by Jeon and colleagues for patients with intractable hiccups in the palliative care setting. A more in-depth explanation of treatment options can be found next.

Palliative patients with recurrent episodes of hiccups causing distress and unresponsive to physical maneuvers (e.g., vagal maneuvers, supra-supramaximal inspiration)

If patient is in last days of life, consider midazolam

Explore underlying causes and treat as appropriate. See Figure 10.1 for diagnostic approach

During workup or if no cause found, Consider PPI

	First line	Second line	Alternatives
Peripheral (gastric)	Metoclopramide or proton pump inhibitor (when suspecting reflux)	Baclofen or Gabapentin	Chlorpromazine, lidocaine, midazolam, or methylphenidate or nimodipine,
Peripheral (nongastric)	Metoclopramide		
Central	Baclofen	Gabapentin	Haloperidol or nimodipine

If no response, consider procedural intervention

FIGURE 10.2 Treatment algorithm. (Adapted with permission from Reference 48.)

Nonpharmacological Methods

Evidence supporting most nonpharmacological methods is anecdotal. Options range from folk remedies such as attempting to startle the individual with hiccups to the bizarre, which includes forced traction of the tongue, the Heimlich maneuver, applying pressure to the eyes, and drinking water while upside down.[64,65] Interventions such as these should be avoided due to limited evidence and the potential for patient harm. A more systematic and less-aggressive nonpharmacological approach has been proposed: supra-supramaximal inspiration. This technique involves hypercapnia, diaphragm immobilization, and positive airway pressure. This is accomplished by inspiring maximally and holding one's breath for 10 seconds. After 10 seconds, additional small supramaximal inspiration is added, followed by another 5 seconds of breath holding. The third step is to take one additional supra-supramaximal breath and hold for 5 seconds.[66] Vagal maneuvers, including the Valsalva maneuver, carotid massage, and initiation of the diving reflex with cold water or ice are thought to help mitigate hiccups by directly activating the vagus nerve, which is believed to be integral to the hiccup reflex arc.[46] *In patients with underlying cardiovascular or other diseases that increase susceptibility to the negative consequences of temporary reduction in blood oxygen levels, interventions involving alteration of a patient's respirations or cerebral blood flow should be used with caution.* Acupuncture has been shown to be successful in a number of small trials and provides a more favorable risk-benefit profile, particularly in patients with hiccups associated with cancer or stroke.[67,68] Conflicting reports of phrenic and vagus nerve stimulation, in either isolation or combination, have also shown variable success.[69-71]

Interventional Methods

More aggressive interventional treatments have been described, although evidence for their use is limited to case reports and series. Their utility may be limited by publication bias. The use of ultrasound-guided phrenic nerve blocks in the operative and nonoperative setting have been shown to be successful.[72-74] This may be used as a method for refractory cases as many of the reports have shown successful hiccup cessation in patients who failed aggressive pharmacological therapy. In anesthetized patients, direct pharyngeal stimulation is considered an alternative option for refractory cases. This use of this modality was first described in a large case series published 1967 and successfully terminated nearly 100% of cases.[53,62] Several newer reports have shown similar results.[75-77] Careful consideration of the potential risks versus uncertain benefits must be weighed on a case-by-case basis after failure of more reasonable treatment modalities prior to initiating invasive interventional treatment. Stronger consideration should be given for interventional therapy in palliative care patients with longer life expectancy as there is a high risk for medication-related adverse effects with pharmacological therapy.

Pharmacological Methods

Over two dozen medications with unique mechanisms of action have been identified as being useful for the treatment of hiccups.[60] Medications directly targeting the GI tract or the neurotransmitters involved in the hiccup reflex arc, dopamine and GABA, have the strongest data to support their use for intractable hiccups. Patients with recurrent hiccups due to a known illness should receive therapy directed at resolving the underlying cause. To control hiccup symptoms while an underlying cause is being investigated, pharmacotherapy can be selected based on suspected hiccup etiology: peripheral (gastric), peripheral (nongastric), or central (Figure 10.2).[48] When a suspected cause is unknown, acid suppression therapy with a proton pump inhibitor (PPI) is recommended as initial treatment.

Despite the impressive list of reported treatments, few medications used to treat intractable hiccups are supported by prospective or randomized controlled evidence. In fact, only chlorpromazine, which has not been studied in a randomized controlled manner, is approved by the Food and Drug Administration for the indication of treating hiccups. A small case series published in 1955 is the basis for the approved indication.[60,78] Although chlorpromazine works on the hiccup reflex arc to antagonize dopamine activity, it also has significant anticholinergic and alpha 1 antagonist properties.[79] Even with acute dosing, this has led to considerable side effects, including orthostatic hypotension, QTc prolongation, and movement disorders. *Due to its significant side-effect profile and limited data supporting its efficacy, chlorpromazine is not recommended as a first-line therapy by some authors* (Figure 10.2).[63] However, due to familiarity and clinical experience, many providers continue to advocate for its indiscriminate use. Metoclopramide and baclofen are reasonable options for patients with hiccups due to an unknown etiology. They are the only drug therapies to have been studied prospectively in randomized controlled trials, and both have been shown to be more effective than placebo.[80,81] Baclofen should be considered as a first-line treatment option for hiccups suspected to be caused by a centrally occurring pathology and may be particularly useful in poststroke patients.[81] Gabapentin has also been studied prospectively in a large cohort of patients and should be considered as an alternative therapy to metoclopramide and baclofen.[82]

Patients with a peripheral GI etiology should receive agents that directly target this underlying cause. If hiccups are thought to be related to gastroesophageal reflux or gastric distention, PPIs may provide relief. These agents are generally well tolerated and are associated with a relatively benign side-effect profile. To date, no study has explored the effect of acid suppression monotherapy to relieve hiccup symptoms. Providers should have a low threshold to add or change therapy in patients initially receiving PPIs.[60] Metoclopramide is a reasonable choice after a sufficient trial of a PPI has failed for patients with hiccups related to a peripheral GI etiology.[48] For patients with hiccups due to a suspected peripheral etiology in which reflux or distension is not suspected, the likely cause is irritation of the vagus or phrenic nerve. In such cases, metoclopramide should be considered the first-line pharmacological treatment option. Metoclopramide is a prokinetic agent with central dopamine antagonism and serotonin agonism. Metoclopramide is generally well tolerated, although development of extrapyramidal symptoms can occur.[83] Dystonia and akathisia can occur even after a single dose of metoclopramide. Oral therapy, lower doses, and slower intravenous infusion rates may mitigate some of the risks. Diphenhydramine can also be administered prior to metoclopramide to mitigate extrapyramidal side effects. Tardive dyskinesia and parkinsonism are usually only associated with long-term use.[84] Metoclopramide is eliminated primarily through the urine, and dose adjustment may be warranted in patients with poor renal function.

For patients with a peripheral, non-gastric-related source of hiccups, the most likely culprit is irritation of the vagus or phrenic nerve. In such cases, metoclopramide should be considered the first-line pharmacological treatment option, followed by baclofen as a second-line agent. As mentioned previously, patients with hiccups believed to be caused by a central mechanism should receive baclofen as a first-line treatment. Baclofen is a centrally acting muscle relaxant and GABA analog that acts to hyperpolarize neurons, inducing a blockade of neural transmission.[85] As a result, baclofen can cause somnolence, weakness, and respiratory depression, especially with higher doses. Conservative starting doses and escalation of baclofen dosing should be used for patients with impaired renal function as the drug can accumulate, leading to toxicity. According to one case report, a patient on peritoneal dialysis receiving several days of baclofen for hiccup treatment required mechanical ventilation due to substantial respiratory depression.[86] Baclofen can be used as a second-line therapy for hiccups related to peripheral causes.[48]

Gabapentin can be considered a second-line option for patients with either peripherally or centrally mediated hiccups. The exact mechanism by which gabapentin alleviates hiccups is unclear, but it is likely through its action on the GABA pathway. Gabapentin is generally well tolerated but can cause sedation and is renally cleared.[87] Like baclofen and metoclopramide, dose adjustment of gabapentin should be considered in patients with impaired kidney function due to renal elimination.

Several alternative pharmacological options are reasonable to try if first-line and second-line options fail (Figure 10.2). However, patient-specific factors may require a more tailored approach, and alternative therapies may be indicated early in the treatment course. Midazolam, a short-acting benzodiazepine, may be reasonable as monotherapy for patients receiving end-of-life care. Midazolam is associated with dose-dependent adverse effects and may require additional monitoring due to its potency.[88] Metoclopramide, gabapentin, and baclofen have alleviated hiccups within 1 day of initiation but may take longer.

The exact time frame to expect a response to therapy is unknown. Providers should not expect all patients to have hiccup termination after the initial dose. In fact, some patients have required prolonged maintenance therapy, depending on hiccup etiology. It is reasonable to assume a positive effect within the first several doses of treatment start or with dose escalations. When this does not occur, alternative or combination therapy should be explored. If combination therapy is chosen, patients should be monitored for drug-drug interactions and synergistic side effects. A dosing chart is provided in Table 10.5 for first- and second-line pharmacotherapies. Insufficient evidence is available to make empiric dosing recommendations for alternative therapies. It is reasonable to begin a selected therapy at low-to-moderate doses, titrating up every 1–2 days as tolerated. Interventional therapy should be considered in patients refractory or unable to tolerate pharmacotherapy and those at high risk due to ongoing complications of hiccups.

TABLE 10.5 Medication Dosing and Clinical Trial Success

Pharmacological Intervention	Improvement of Hiccups	Complete Relief of Hiccups	Failures	Starting Doses (consult drug reference for renal dose adjustments)
Baclofen (n = 84)[1-14]	78	66	6	Oral: 5–10 mg three times daily (maximum of 75 mg/d)
Gabapentin (n = 60)[1-3]	58	52	2	Oral: 100–400 mg three to four times daily (maximum of 1200 mg/d)
Metoclopramide (n = 31)[1,2]	25	2	6	Oral: 5–10 mg three times per day (maximum 40 mg/d) Intravenous: 5–10 mg three times per day (maximum 30 mg/d)

Polito NB, Fellows SE. Pharmacologic Interventions for Intractable and Persistent Hiccups: A Systematic Review. J Emerg Med. 2017 Oct;53(4):540–9.

References
Baclofen
1. D'Alessandro DJ, Dever LL. Baclofen for treatment of persistent hiccups in HIV-infected patients. AIDS 1997;11:1063–4.
2. Mirjello A, Addolorato G, D'Angelo C, et al. Baclofen in the treatment of persistent hiccup: a case series. Int J Clin Pract 2013;67:918–21.
3. Petroianu G, Hein G, Petroianu A, et al. Idiopathic chronic hiccup: combination therapy with cisapride, omeprazole, and baclofen. Clin Ther 1997;19:1031–8.
4. Zhang C, Zhang R, Zhang S, et al. Baclofen for stroke patients with persistent hiccups: a randomized, double-blind, placebo-controlled trial. Trials 2014;15:295.
5. Guelaud C, Similowski T, Bizec JL, et al. Baclofen therapy for chronic hiccup. Eur Respir J 1995;8:235–7.
6. Boz C, Velioglu S, Bulbul I, et al. Baclofen is effective in intractable hiccups induced by brainstem lesions. Neurol Sci 2001;22:409.
7. Neuhaus T, Ko YD, Stier S. Successful treatment of intractable hiccups by oral application of lidocaine. Support Care Cancer 2012;20:3009–11.
8. Hadjiyannacos D, Vlassopoulos D. Hadjiconstantinou. Treatment of intractable hiccup in haemodialysis patients with baclofen. AmJ Nephrol 2001;21:427–8.
9. Burke AM, White AB. Baclofen for intractable hiccups. N Engl J Med 1988;319:1354.Walker P, Watanabe S, Bruera E. Baclofen, a treatment for chronic hiccup. J Pain Symptom Manage 1998;16:125–32.
10. Krahn A, Penner B. Use of baclofen for intractable hiccups in uremia. Am J Med 1994;96:391.
11. Yaqoob M, Prabhu P, Ahmad R. Baclofen for intractable hiccups. Lancet 1989;2:562–3.
12. Seker MM, Aksoy S, Nuriye Y, et al. Successful treatment of chronic hiccup with baclofen in cancer patients. Med Oncol 2012;29:1369–70.
13. Choo YM, Kim GB, Choi JY, et al. Severe respiratory depression by low dose-baclofen in the treatment of chronic hiccups in a patient undergoing CAPD. Nephron 2000;84:546–7.
14. Peces R, Navascues RA, Baltar J, et al. Baclofen neurotoxicity in chronic haemodialysis patients with hiccups. Nephrol Dial Transplant1998;7:1896–7.

Gabapentin
1. Moretti R, Torre P, Antonello M, et al. Gabapentin as a drug therapy of intractable hiccup because of vascular lesion: a three-year follow-up. Neurologist 2004;10:101–6.
2. Porzio G, Aielli F, Verna L, et al. Gabapentin in the treatment of hiccups in patients with advanced cancer: a 5-year experience. Clin Neuropharmacol 2010;33:179–80.
3. Liang CY, Tsai KW, Hsu MC. Gabapentin therapy for persistent hiccups and central post-stroke pain in a lateral medullary infarction-two case reports and literature review. Tzu Chi Med J 2005;5:365–8.

Metoclopramide
1. Wang T, Wang D. Metoclopramide for patients with intractable hiccups: a multicentre, randomised, controlled pilot study. Intern Med J 2014;44:1205–9.
2. Madanagopolan N. Metoclopramide in hiccup. Curr Med Res Opin 1975;3:371–4.

Nausea and Vomiting

Definition and Etiology

Nausea and vomiting are common symptoms that patients experience, with a variety of causes in the seriously ill population. These symptoms are very unpleasant and can cause a great deal of psychological distress for the patient and their family and can significantly impact quality of life. Nausea is defined as a feeling of sickness with an inclination to vomit,[89] which can occur alone or in conjunction with vomiting, dyspepsia, or GI symptoms. Vomiting is the forcible voluntary or involuntary emptying of the stomach contents through the mouth.[89] There are multiple causes of nausea and vomiting in the palliative care population; therefore, treatments need to be multifactorial. In cancer patients, nausea and vomiting may be related to the treatment of the cancers, as in chemotherapy, radiation therapy, represent a complication of the cancer. The prevalence of nausea and vomiting in the palliative care population has been mostly studied in cancer, with approximately 20%–30% of patients with advanced cancer reporting nausea, and up to 70% of patients in the last week of life reporting nausea[90.] Approximately 50%–80% of patients having undergone radiation therapy experience nausea and/or vomiting in the absence of appropriate antiemetic prophylaxis.[91] However, the prevalence of nausea has also been documented in noncancer diagnoses, such as AIDS (43%–49%), heart failure (17%–48%), and chronic renal disease (30%–43%).[92] This is a very common and distressing symptom that can be seen in patients with advanced illness and may often be caused by more than one issue.

Vomiting is mediated centrally through the vomiting center (VC), an anatomically indistinct area that includes the nucleus of the tractus solitaris and the reticular formation of the medulla oblongata. Neural inputs from the following pathways send impulses to the VC and trigger nausea and vomiting. The chemoreceptor trigger zone, in the postrema in the floor of the fourth ventricle and center of the brain, senses changes in the level of chemical stimuli in the blood and cerebrospinal fluid, vestibular system. This reacts to changes in positions, and peripheral signals from receptors in the GI tract, which respond to mechanical stretch and chemical stimuli, and all stimulate the VC, leading to emesis. There are many etiologies that can cause nausea and vomiting, including medications such as opioids; delayed gastric emptying; mechanical bowel obstruction; increased intracranial pressure; vestibular dysfunction; metabolic issues; and/or cortical effects such as anxiety and/or depression (see Table 10.6).[93] These signals are mediated by neurotransmitters, such as serotonin, dopamine, acetylcholine, and histamine. Therefore, therapies used to treat nausea and vomiting are multifactorial and focus on mitigating the activation of the VC.

Assessment

Clinical assessment starts with a careful medical history and physical examination. Be sure to ask about alternative therapies that have been attempted, and a detailed medication history may also be helpful to understand which medications have been tried in the past and those that may be potential triggers of the nausea. Psychological and spiritual assessment is also important to assess for anxiety that contributes to the patient's symptoms. Investigation with routine laboratory work, including an electrolyte panel, serum urea nitrogen (BUN)/creatinine, liver function tests (LFTs), and calcium, may help to uncover the underlying cause of the symptom. Also, plain abdominal radiography may help to identify constipation, ileus, or GI obstruction. A computed tomographic (CT) scan of the abdomen with oral and intravenous contrast is more specific and sensitive for identifying an obstruction. CT scan or magnetic resonance imaging of the brain may also be needed if a patient is exhibiting signs and symptoms of intracranial pathology in the presence of nausea and vomiting.

TABLE 10.6 Causes, Symptoms, and Treatment of Nausea and Vomiting[a]

Etiology	Symptoms	Treatment
Cortical		
Tumor in central nervous system and meninges	Focal neurological signs or mental status changes	• Dexamethasone • Radiation therapy
Increased intracranial pressure	Headache and vomiting	• Dexamethasone • Prednisone
Anxiety	Anticipatory nausea/vomiting	• Counseling • Benzodiazepines
Uncontrolled pain	Pain and nausea	• Opioids, other pain medications
Vestibular		
Vestibular disease	Vertigo, vomiting with head movement	• Meclizine • Epley maneuvers • Ear, nose, throat referral
Middle ear infections	Ear pain/bulging tympanic membrane	• Antibiotics as appropriate
Motion sickness	Nausea with traveling	• Scopolamine • Diphenhydramine
Chemoreceptor Trigger Zone		
Medications (i.e., opioids, chemotherapeutic agents, antibiotics)	Nausea worse after medication is taken or exacerbated by an increase in dose	• Decrease medication or discontinue medication
Metabolic (renal/liver failure)	Increased BUN, creatinine, LFTs, bilirubin	• Haloperidol
Gastrointestinal Tract		
Gastritis	Use of NSAIDs, iron, alcohol, and antibiotics	• Discontinue medication • Add proton pump inhibitor
Constipation	Bloating, abdominal distension, nausea	• Laxative • Enema
Obstruction—tumor/reduced motility	Increased secretions, no bowel movements, nausea	• Metoclopramide • Scopolamine • Octreotide
Tube feeding	Abdominal distention, diarrhea	• Reduce feeding volume
Thick secretions	Cough-induced vomiting	• Nebulized saline expectorant • Anticholinergics
Gastroesophageal reflux	Cough and nausea	• Proton pump inhibitors • H_2 blockers

[a]From Reference 5.

Management

Due to the multifactorial etiologies of nausea and vomiting, there are many modalities that can be used to treat the symptoms, including nonpharmacological and pharmacological interventions.

Nonpharmacological Interventions

Since nausea and vomiting are distressing not only to the patient, but also to their caregivers, it is important to educate the patient and caregivers on the potential triggers that have been identified by the history and ways in which to provide emotional support. Eating can be very difficult for patients who are suffering with nausea. Offer small, frequent meals that the patient desires and encourage fluids, which can help reduce the risk of dehydration. Present foods in settings where the patient can avoid the triggering medication and those that can trigger anticipatory nausea, thus allowing for reduction in overall intake. The interdisciplinary team can be helpful in identifying psychological, social, and spiritual concerns that can exacerbate the symptom. Therefore, modalities such as relaxation techniques, which are useful as adjunctive therapy, especially when anxiety is a contributor; and manipulative techniques, including massage, acupuncture, and acupressure, can also be effective adjunctive therapies to aid in reducing symptoms. However, the evidence to support their use is lacking in the setting of advanced illness.[94]

Pharmacological Interventions

Pharmacological therapies can be very effective at reducing symptoms and improving quality of life. Below is a list of the common medications, based on their mechanism of action, used to help treat nausea and vomiting. Many of the medications affect multiple receptors in the body, and, depending on the potential cause of the symptoms, an empiric approach to treatment can be enacted (see Table 10.7).

Specific Conditions

Chemotherapy- and Radiation Therapy–Induced Nausea and Vomiting

Among patients with cancer, chemotherapy and radiation therapy are common causes of nausea and vomiting. For patients receiving moderately emetogenic chemotherapy, neurokinin 1(NK-1) receptor antagonist, a $5\text{-}HT_3$ receptor antagonist, and dexamethasone have been successful in preventing vomiting; however, this regimen has not been effective in preventing nausea.[95] A recent study demonstrated that the addition of olanzapine to an NK-1 receptor antagonist, $5\text{-}HT_3$ receptor antagonist, and dexamethasone for patients receiving highly emetogenic chemotherapy was effective in preventing both emesis and nausea, and this is now recommended by various international guidelines for chemotherapy-induced nausea and vomiting.[96] While there are limited clinical trials available that studied the prevention of nausea and vomiting in radiation therapy, the American Society of Clinical Oncology antiemetic guidelines suggest the use of dexamethasone plus a $5\text{-}HT_3$ receptor antagonist for total body radiation and a $5\text{-}HT_3$ receptor antagonist alone for radiotherapy to the upper abdomen.[97]

Anticipatory Nausea and Vomiting

Anticipatory nausea and vomiting occur when patients have a poor experience with the initial cycle of therapy, which resulted in nausea and vomiting. This is considered a conditioned, learned response and is more difficult to control with subsequent cycles of the same chemotherapy. Use of antiemetic medications along with antianxiety medications, such as lorazepam or another benzodiazepine, may be considered prior to the first course of chemotherapy in order to prevent anticipatory nausea and vomiting.

TABLE 10.7 Classes of Medications Used to Treat Nausea and Vomiting

Class of Medications	Initial Dose		Comments
	Oral	Parental	
PROKINETICS			
Metoclopramide (Reglan)	5–20 mg by mouth every 4–6 h; maximum 60 mg/d	SC/IV available; same dosing	Improves gastric motility Blocks dopaminergic and 5-HT$_3$ receptors Antiemetic dose is slightly higher than prokinetic dose
ANTIHISTAMINES (H$_1$)			
Diphenhydramine (Benadryl)	25–50 mg by mouth every 4–6 h	SC/IV available; same dosing	Also has anticholinergic properties
Hydroxyzine (Atarax)	50–100 mg by mouth every 6–8 h; maximum 600 mg/d	IM available; same dosing	
Meclizine (Antivert)	12.5–50 mg by mouth every 6–8 h		Used for vertigo
Promethazine (Phenergan)	12.5–50 mg by mouth every 6–8 h	IM/PO/per rectum (PR) available	Best used for vertigo and gastroenteritis
DOPAMINERGIC (D$_2$) ANTAGONISTS			
Haloperidol (Haldol)	0.25–1.0 mg by mouth twice daily; maximum 5 mg/d	0.5–1.5 mg SC/IV available; maximum 10 mg/d	Typical antipsychotics Tardive dyskinesia, sedation side effects
Chlorpromazine (Thorazine)	10–25mg by mouth every 8 h; maximum 50 mg/dose	IM 12.5 mg IV 2 mg every 2 min; maximum dose 25 mg	
Prochlorperazine	5–10mg by mouth every 6–8h ; maximum 40 mg/dose	IM 5–10 mg IV 2.5–10 mg slow rate PR 25 mg every 12 h	Helpful for opioid-induced nausea
Olanzapine (Zyrexa)	2.5–10mg by mouth daily	Oral preparation tablet and ODT	Atypical antipsychotic
SEROTINERGIC 5-HT$_3$ RECEPTOR ANTAGONISTS			
Ondansetron (Zofran)	4–8 mg by mouth/oral disintegrating tablet (ODT) every 8 h; maximum dose 8 mg	SC/IV available; maximum dose 8 mg	
Granisetron (Kytril)	1 mg by mouth every 12 h	IV infusion 10 µg/kg over 5 min or 10 µg; IV push over 30 s SC 10 mg extended release every 7 days Transdermal patch 34.3 mg every 7 days	Ideal for chemo- and radiation-induced nausea; to be given by mouth 1 h prior; IV/SC to be given 30 min prior; transdermal patch to be initiated 24 h prior to therapy
NK-1 RECEPTOR ANTAGONIST			
Aprepitant (Cinvanti)	125 mg by mouth day 1; then 80 mg by mouth days 2 and 3	IV infusion 130 mg over 30 min or IV push over 2 min	Helpful for chemo- and radiation-induced nausea; to be given 30 min prior Very costly

TABLE 10.7 Continued

Class of Medications	Initial Dose		Comments
	Oral	Parental	
BENZODIAZEPINES			
Diazepam	2–5 mg by mouth every 6 h; maximum dose 10 mg	IV and PR preparations	Useful for anticipatory nausea; long half-life
Lorazepam	0.5–1 mg by mouth every 8 h; maximum 4 mg/dose	IV and SL preparations	Useful for anticipatory nausea; shorter half-life
CORTICOSTEROIDS			
Dexamethasone	10-mg loading dose by mouth/IV; then 2–4mg by mouth every 8–12 h	IM and IV preparations available	Useful in reducing cerebral edema; response usually takes 12–24 h Side effects include GI upset, mood swings, weight gain
Prednisone	5–60 mg by mouth		
CANNIBINOIDS			
Dronabinol	2.5 mg by mouth twice daily up to 20 mg/d		Can cause dysphoria, drowsiness, or hallucinations
ANTICHOLINERGICS			
Scopolamine	Transdermal preparation: 1.5-mg patch every 72 h	0.006 mg/kg/dose every 6 h IV/SC	Helpful for motion-related nausea; well tolerated; often causes dry mouth, blurred vision, confusion/sedation
ANTISECRETORY			
Octreotide	100–400 mg SC every 8 h		Reduces GI secretions in the presence of inoperable GI obstruction

Conclusion

Nausea and vomiting are common symptoms seen at the end of life and can cause substantial physical and psychological distress for both patient and caregivers, thereby impacting their quality of life. Despite the potential causes, efforts should be made to identify and correct any reversible causes and then to tailor therapy to the patient's stated goals. Nonpharmacological therapies can help reduce symptoms but are best used with targeted pharmacological therapies. Depending on the potential cause, medications can be used to modulate the inputs to the VC and thus control the symptoms.

Ascites

Definition and Etiology

Ascites is considered an ominous sign of end-organ failure and is defined as an abnormal collection of fluid in the abdomen, greater than 25 mL. Ascites can be seen in many conditions, including liver failure (75%–80%), heart failure (10%–15%), and malignancies (10%).

Ascites is seen most commonly in ovarian, pancreatic, uterine, gastric, and colorectal cancers. Associated symptoms include increased abdominal size, increased weight, abdominal discomfort, and shortness of breath. Complications of ascites can encompass spontaneous bacterial peritonitis, abdominal cellulitis, and umbilical hernia. The pathophysiology of ascites from liver failure causes fibrosis of the liver parenchyma, and this leads to portal hypertension. The increased portal pressure increases the release of nitrous oxide and other vasodilators, which in turn leads to splanchnic arterial vasodilation and low arterial blood volume and triggers the kidneys to conserve sodium, thereby increasing the amount of fluid retained in the body, which worsens the ascites.[98] It is this physiologic pathway that further leads to acute renal injury that is sometimes seen with severe hepatic disease, known as hepatorenal syndrome (HRS).

In cancer-related ascites, the presence of peritoneal carcinomatosis can lead to blockage of draining lymphatic channels, increased vascular permeability, and tumor cell production of fluid. Additionally, liver metastases can cause obstruction and external compression of the portal veins. The degree or severity of ascites is graded based on detectability:

Grade 1 ascites: mild and only detectable by ultrasound examination
Grade 2: moderate and manifested by moderate symmetrical distension of the abdomen
Grade 3: large or gross ascites with marked abdominal distension, also known as being "tense"

Severe ascites is associated with poorer health-related quality of life scores and increased risk of mortality.[99] Ascites can also be referred to as refractory, which indicates that the fluid does not recede or reaccumulates quickly with standard treatments, discussed further in this section. Because of the severity of the condition, HRS is a definite indication for intensive palliative care and referral to hospice. Patients can receive dialysis while awaiting liver transplant. For further reference regarding the management of the symptoms of end-stage liver disease.[100]

Assessment of Ascites

Performing a complete history and physical examination is an essential first step in the assessment of a patient with ascites. Information should be gathered to identify the etiology of the ascites as well any associated symptoms that impact the patient's quality of life. The presence of as little as 100 mL of ascites can be detected on abdominal ultrasound or CT scan; however, ascites is not usually detectable with traditional physical examination techniques, such as shifting dullness to percussion, until there is more than 500 mL of fluid collected. The fluid analysis is useful in determining the cause of the ascites. Ascitic fluid with a high serum albumin gradient is usually caused by cirrhosis. However, ascitic fluid with malignant cells on cytology and high fluid protein levels is more likely a result of cancer. The presence of ascites, whether it occurs acutely or chronically, usually indicates poor prognosis; therefore, it is important to have a goals-of-care discussion to review the patient's desire for more conservative versus invasive treatment options.

Management

Several options for treatment are available for the treatment of ascites and have consistently been shown to improve symptoms and quality of life. When symptoms are well controlled, patients feel better and enjoy increased mobility, have reduced shortness of breath, and feel less abdominal discomfort, which increases oral intake.[2] It is important to review the patient's stated goals of care when considering conservative, interventional, and pharmacological treatments that are available and includes a discussion of the risks and benefits, which informs the choice of therapeutic options.

Conservative Approaches

Conservative measures, such as diet modification, with reduced sodium intake to less than 2000 mg per day, helps to reduce fluid retention. Fluid restriction, however, is generally not recommended since patients are usually volume depleted, which requires the intravascular fluid to maintain adequate blood pressure. If liver disease is related to alcohol, it is important to discuss abstinence and may require further involvement with substance use disorder consultants or counselors. Alcohol cessation can reverse the changes in the liver architecture, normalize portal pressures, and improve diuretic treatment response. Whenever possible, a nutritionist is a critical member to include on the interdisciplinary team. Patient education regarding these conservative measures that emphasize lifestyle modifications is the first-line approach to symptom management.

Pharmacological Approaches

Diuretics effectively reduce symptoms in about 40% of cases; however, these medications are more effective in cirrhosis-related ascites versus malignant ascites.[100] This difference may be related to the correlation between the efficacy of the diuretics versus levels of plasma renin-aldosterone, which are elevated in portal hypertension and normal in malignant ascites.[3] Spironolactone (Aldactone) and furosemide (Lasix) are used most frequently together and are effective in reducing fluid accumulation. Adverse effects of diuretics include nausea and vomiting, which can cause or exacerbate electrolyte imbalance; hypotension; and renal insufficiency. Serial laboratory monitoring is necessary to assess for ongoing electrolyte imbalances and renal insufficiency. Starting oral of spironolactone 50 mg and Lasix 20 mg are usually effective, but they can be titrated up to spironolactone 100 mg and Lasix 40 mg if needed. The combination of the two medications works to reduce risk of potassium imbalance.

Interventional Approaches

Intermittent paracentesis is also a viable first-line therapy if diuretics are ill advised. Paracentesis is widely used by providers and found to be very effective in reducing the volume and symptoms of ascites. Unfortunately, it provides only temporary relief of symptoms, requiring repeated treatments, since symptoms tend to return in as little as 72 hours as the ascites reaccumulates. Complications of paracentesis include pain at the site, perforation of viscera, hypotension secondary to large-volume fluid shifts, drainage of protein and electrolytes, secondary peritonitis, and bleeding.[101] Therefore, it is important for patients to understand the risks and benefits of the procedure. There are no specific guidelines regarding how much fluid to remove and how often to perform paracentesis. In general, it is recommended that removal of more than 5 L of fluids at a single session should be avoided; wait until the patient develops tense symptomatic ascites before performing the procedure. This allows for reduced visits to the hospital, safe drainage of the ascites, and maximum benefit from each drainage session.[102] If frequent procedures are needed over time, the placement of intraperitoneal drainage catheters ease intermittent drainage. The frequency of this procedure and the timeline should both be considered in determining the type of intervention to follow, in conjunction with a thorough discussion of goals of care with the patient and caregivers.

There are numerous types of catheters available that can be placed to help with intermittent drainage of ascites. Tunneled catheters are usually preferred due to their significantly reduced risk of infections and peritonitis versus nontunneled catheters. When ascites is tense or refractory and requires frequent drainage, use of catheters needs to be determined by the team and related specialists involved in ascites management. If the patient has a prognosis of more than 1 month, then the use of a more permanent peritoneal catheter for home drainage should be considered. However, it is important to discuss this in depth with the patient's caregivers to ensure that they are willing and capable to assume the care and management of the catheter. The catheter is placed under fluoroscopic, ultrasound, or CT guidance as an outpatient and allows patients to control their ascites at home without frequent facility visits—both inpatient and outpatient. This is also dependent on their geographic location and social determinants of health. Indwelling catheters also allow for more frequent fluid drainage (up to daily) and removal of less fluid (1–2 L) at a time, and this achieves better symptom control.[103] Quality-of-life scores improve significantly with the placement of a tunneled intraperitoneal catheter, which relates directly to the benefits listed above.[104] Contraindications to placement of an indwelling catheter include coagulopathy, loculated ascites, and current intraperitoneal infection.[105] Common complications seen with the placement of an indwelling catheter are abdominal pain; catheter-related infection (cellulitis, bacterial peritonitis); leakage at the catheter site; and catheter dislodgement or obstruction. Patients and their caregivers may have varying availability of hospice services. This can help with the decision-making process regarding the use of indwelling catheters for long-term management of ascites. These services should be able to educate and support the patients and caregivers in the home regarding catheter management. These decisions are also part of the POLST/MOLST (Physician Orders for Life-Sustaining Treatment/Medical Orders for Life-Sustaining Treatments) process and are considered in the management of the seriously ill patient.

More advanced techniques are available but are utilized less in palliative care. These include intraperitoneal port placement and peritoneovenous shunt placement. The intraperitoneal port is a subcutaneous implantable reservoir and attached intraperitoneal catheter that allows for the effective, intermittent drainage of ascites. Surgical implantation is required for the placement of the port, but once placed it is an easily accessible, durable option for patients, and it remains in place for an average of 53 days.[106] Infection rates are quite low, ranging between 0% and 4%.[107] Access to the port requires an inpatient or outpatient visit to a specialist provider; therefore, it is not considered a realistic or cost-effective method for the home-based setting. Another option specifically for noncardiogenic ascites is the placement of a peritoneovenous shunt. This procedure allows the peritoneal fluid to be returned to the superior vena cava via a one-way, pressure-sensitive valve. These shunts can be placed percutaneously with local anesthetic under ultrasound, fluoroscopic guidance, or surgical laparoscopy. The most recent guidelines from the American Association for the Study of Liver Diseases recommends peritoneovenous shunting should only be considered if the patient is resistant to diuretics, is not a transplant candidate, and is not a good candidate for serial therapeutic paracentesis.[108] These shunts also provide symptom improvement in many patients; however, they have the highest rate of serious adverse effects, including infection, leakage of ascites fluid, occlusion, and deregulation of the blood-clotting mechanism (e.g., disseminated intravascular coagulopathy).[109] There are several options for control of the chronic ascites in palliative care patients.

Conclusion

Ascites is present in many different palliative care conditions, including liver disease, congestive heart failure, and malignancies; it is often a poor prognostic indicator and represents end-organ failure. There are many options available for treatment of ascites, with the goal of symptom burden reduction and improved quality of life. These treatments include the use of diuretics, intermittent paracentesis, indwelling catheters, and more advanced interventions. It is always important to review all of these options, including significant risks and benefits, with the patient and family. Ultimately, a comprehensive treatment plan is necessary that both supports the patient's wishes and is reasonable given the resources available to them along their palliative care journey.

References

1. Stone P, Richards M, Hardy J. Fatigue in patients with cancer. *European Journal of Cancer*. 1998;*34*:1670.
2. National Comprehensive Cancer Network. Cancer related fatigue version 2.20. http://www.ncc.org/professionals/physicians_gls/PDF/Fatigue.pdf. Accessed 9.1.2020.
3. Cella D, et al. Cancer-related fatigue: prevalence of proposed criteria in the United States sample of cancer survivors. *Journal of Clinical Oncology*. 2001;*19*:3385.
4. Aapro M, et al. A practical approach to fatigue management in colorectal cancer. *Clinical Colorectal Cancer*. 2016;*16*(4):275.
5. Cella D, et al. Progress toward guidelines for the management of fatigue. *Oncology*. 1998;*12*(11A):369.
6. Gleeson A. Management of less common symptoms in palliative care. *Medicine*. 2019;*48*(1):43.
7. Ma Y, et al. Prevalence and risk factor of cancer related fatigue: a systematic review and meta-analysis. *International Journal of Nursing Studies*. 2020;*111*:1.
8. Saligan LN, et al. The biology of cancer related fatigue: a review of the literature. 2015;*23*:2461.
9. Moss RB, et al. TNF-alpha and chronic fatigue syndrome. *Journal of Clinical Immunology*. 1999;*19*:314.
10. Pyszora A, et al. Physiotherapy programme reduces fatigue in patients with advanced cancer receiving palliative care: randomized controlled trial. *Support Care Cancer*. 2017;*25*:2899.
11. Poort M, et al. Study protocol of TIRED study: a randomized controlled trial comparing either graded exercise therapy for severe fatigue or cognitive behavioural therapy with usual care in patient with curable cancer. *BMC Cancer*. 2017;*17*:81.

12. Mucke M, et al. Pharmacological treatments for fatigue associated with palliative care. *Cochrane Database of Systematic Reviews*. 2015;2015(5):CD006788.

13. Onishi E, Baigioli F. Methylphenidate for management of fatigue in the palliative care setting. *American Family Physician*. 2014;89(2):126.

14. Ruiz Garcia V, et al. Megestrol acetate for treatment of anorexia-cachexia syndrome. *Cochrane Database of Systematic Reviews*. 2013;CD004310.

15. Zhukovsky DS. Fever and sweats in the patient with advanced cancer. *Hematology/Oncology Clinics of North America*. 2002;16:579.

16. Morioka S, et al. Determinants of physicians' attitudes toward the management of infectious diseases in terminally ill patients with cancer. *Journal of Pain and Symptom Management*. 2020;60(6):1109–1116.e2.

17. Cunha CB, Cunha BA. Fever of unknown origin (FUO). In: *Infectious diseases*. 4th ed; 2017:611.

18. Vodovar D, et al. Drug-induced fever: a diagnosis to remember. *La Revue de Médecine Interne*. 2014;35(3):183–188.

19. Pittelow MR, et al. Puritis and sweating in palliative medicine. In: Cherney N, Fallown M, Kassa S, Portenoy R, Currow D, eds. *Oxford textbook of palliative medicine*. Oxford:Oxford University Press, 2015;chap 11.2.

20. Stander S, et al. Clinical classification of itch: a position paper of the International Forum for the Study of Itch. *Acta Dermato-Venereologica*. 2007;87(4):291.

21. Weisshaar E, et al. European S2k guideline on chronic pruritus: in cooperation with the European Dermatology Forum(EDF) and the European Academy of Dermatology and Venereology(EADV). *Acta Dermato-Venereologica*. 2019;99:469.

22. Andrafe A, et al. Intervention for chronic pruritus of unknown origin (review). *Cochrane Database of Systemic Reviews*. 2020;1(1):CD013128.

23. Weisshaar E, et al. Epidemiology of itch: add to the burden of skin morbidity. *Acta Dermato-Venereologica*. 2009;89(4):339.

24. Golpanian RS. Effects of stress on itch. *Clinical Therapeutics*. 2020;42(5):745.

25. Pfab F, et al. Complementary integrative approach for treating pruritus. *Dermatologic Therapy*. 2013;26:149.

26. Tisdale MJ. Mechanisms of cancer cachexia. *Physiological Reviews*. 2009;89:381.

27. Arguiles JM, et al. The cachexia score(CASCO): a new tool for staging cachectic cancer patients. *Journal of Cachexia, Sarcopenia, and Muscle*. 2011;2(2):87–93.

28. Von Haehling S, Anker SD. Cachexia as a major underestimated and unmet medical need: facts and numbers. *Journal of Cachexia, Sarcopenia, and Muscle*. 2010;1(1):1–5.

29. Evans WJ, et al. Cachexia: a new definition. *Clinical Nutrition*. 2008;27:793.

30. Arenas CB. Fat free mass index: importance and maintaining the right levels. 2019.

31. Alley DE, Crimmins E, Bandeen-Roche K, Guralnik J, Ferrucci L. Three-year change in inflammatory markers in elderly people and mortality: the Invecchiare in Chianti study. *Journal of the American Geriatrics Society*. 2007;55(11):1801–1807.

32. Donoho CJ, Crommins E, Seeman TE. Marital quality, gender, and markers of inflammation in the MIDUS cohort. *Journal of Marriage and Family*. 2013;75(1):127–141.

33. Maltoni M, et al. Prognostic factors in advanced cancer patients: evidence-based clinical recommendations—a study by the Steering Committee of the European Association for Palliative Care. *American Society of Clinical Oncology*. 2005;23:6240.

34. Hutton JL, et al. Dietary patterns in patients with advanced cancer: implications for anorexia-cachexia therapy. *American Journal of Clinical Nutrition*. 2006;84:1163.

35. Del Fabbro E, et al. Clinical outcomes and contributors to weight loss in a cancer cachexia clinic. *Journal of Palliative Medicine*. 2011;14(9):1004–1008.

36. Prommer E. Oncology update: anamorelin. *Palliative Care: Research and Treatment*. 2017;10:1–6.

37. Lopez AP, et al. Systemic review of megestrol acetate in the treatment of anorexia-cachexia syndrome. *Journal of Pain and Symptom Management*. 2004;27(4):360–369.

38. Kropsky B, Shi Y, Cherniack EP. Incidence of deep-venous thrombosis in nursing home residents using megestrol acetate. *Journal of the American Medical Directors Association*. 2003;4(5):255–256.

39. Badowski ME, Yanful PK. Dronabinol oral solution in the management of anorexia and weight loss in AIDs and Cancer. *Therapeutics and Clinical Risk Management*. 2018;*14*:643–651.

40. Esposito A, et al. Mechanisms of anorexia-cachexia syndrome and rationale for treatment with selective ghrelin receptor agonist. *Cancer Treatment Reviews*. 2015;*41*:793.

41. Good P, Cavenagh J, Mather M, Ravenscroft P. Medically assisted nutrition for palliative care adult patients. *Cochrane Database of Systematic Reviews*. 2008;(4):CD006274.

42. Dev R, Dalal S, Bruera E. Is there a role of parenteral nutrition or hydration at the end of life? *Journal of Supportive and Palliative Care*. 2012;*6*(3):365–370.

43. Saghaleini SH, et al. Pressure ulcer and nutrition. *Indian Journal of Critical Care Medicine*. 2018;*22*(4):283–289.

44. Cole JA, Plewa MC. Singultus(hiccups). In: StatPearls. Treasure Island, FL: StatPearls;2019.

45. Howes D. Hiccups: a new explanation for the mysterious reflex. *Bioessays*. 2012;*34*(6):451–453.

46. Petroianu GA. Treatment of hiccup by vagal maneuvers. *Journal of the History of the Neurosciences*. 2015;*24*(2):123–136.

47. Steger M, Schneemann M, Fox M. Systemic review: the pathogenesis and pharmacological treatment of hiccups. *Alimentary Pharmacology and Therapeutics*. 2015;*42*(9):1037–1050.

48. Jeon YS, Kearney AM, Baker PG. Management of hiccups in palliative care patients. *BMJ Supportive and Palliative Care*. 2018;*8*(1):1–6.

49. Friedman NL. Hiccups: a treatment review. *Pharmacotherapy*. 1996;*16*(6):986–995.

50. Marieb EN, Wilhelm PB, Mallatt JB. *Human anatomy*. Pearson Higher Education;2016.

51. Marshall JB, Landreneau RJ, Beyer KL. Hiccups: esophageal manometric features and relationship to gastroesophageal reflux. *Amercan Journal of Gastroenterology*. 1990;*85*(9):1172–1175.

52. Davis JN. An experimental study of hiccup. *Brain*. 1970;*93*(4):851–872.

53. Salem MR. Hiccups and pharyngeal stimulation. *JAMA*. 1968;*204*(6):551.

54. Marinella MA. Diagnosis and management of hiccups in the patient with advanced cancer. *Journal of Supportive Oncology*. 2009;*7*(4):122–127, 130.

55. Nausheen F, Mohsin H, Lakhan SE. Neurotransmitters in hiccups. *Springerplus*. 2016;*5*(1):1357.

56. Goldin M, Hahn Z. A hiccup in holiday plans. *BMJ Case Reports [Internet]*. 2016;*2016*:bcr2015213288. doi:10.1136/bcr-2015-213288

57. Kohse EK, Hollmann MW, Bardenheuer HJ, Kessler J. Chronic hiccups: an underestimated problem. *Anesthesia and Analgesia*. 2017;*125*(4):1169–1183.

58. Souadjian JV, Cain JC. Intractable hiccup. Etiologic factors in 220 cases. *Postgrad Medicine*. 1968;*43*(2):72–77.

59. Ross J, Eledrisi M, Casner P. Persistent hiccups induced by dexamethasone. *Western Journal of Medicine*. 1999;*170*(1):51–52.

60. Polito NB, Fellows SE. Pharmacologic interventions for intractable and persistent hiccups: a systematic review. *Journal of Emergency Medicine*. 2017;*53*(4):540–549.

61. Moretto EN, Wee B, Wiffen PJ, Murchison AG. Interventions for treating persistent and intractable hiccups in adults. *Cochrane Database of Systematic Reviews*. 2013;(1):CD008768.

62. Ramez Salem M, Baraka A, Rattenborg CC, Holaday DA. Treatment of hiccups by pharyngeal stimulation in anesthetized and conscious subjects. *JAMA*. 1967;*202*(1):32–36.

63. Woelk CJ. Managing hiccups. *Canadian Family Physician*. 2011;*57*(6):672–675, e198–e201.

64. Chang F-Y, Lu C-L. Hiccup: mystery, nature and treatment. *Journal of Neurogastroenterology and Motility*. 2012;*18*(2):123–130.

65. Heymann WR. The Heimlich maneuver for hiccups. *Journal of Emergency Medicine*. 2003;*25*(1):107–108.

66. Morris LG, Marti JL, Ziff DJ. Termination of idiopathic persistent singultus(hiccup) with supra-supramaximal inspiration. *Journal of Emergency Medicine*. 2004;*27*(4):416–417.

67. Yue J, Liu M, Li J, et al. Acupuncture for the treatment of hiccups following stroke: a systematic review and meta-analysis. *Acupuncture in Medicine*. 2017;*35*(1):2–8.

68. Choi T-Y, Lee MS, Ernst E. Acupuncture for cancer patients suffering from hiccups: a systematic review and meta-analysis. *Complementary Therapies in Medicine*. 2012;*20*(6):447–455.

69. Schulz-Stübner S, Kehl F. Treatment of persistent hiccups with transcutaneous phrenic and vagal nerve stimulation. *Intensive Care Medicine*. 2011;*37*(6):1048–1049.

70. Okuda Y, Kitajima T, Asai T. Use of a nerve stimulator for phrenic nerve block in treatment of hiccups. *Anesthesiology.* 1998;*88*(2):525–527.

71. Grewal SS, Adams AC, Van Gompel JJ. Vagal nerve stimulation for intractable hiccups is not a panacea: a case report and review of the literature. *International Journal of Neuroscience.* 2018;*128*(12):1114–1117.

72. Kuusniemi K, Pyylampi V. Phrenic nerve block with ultrasound-guidance for treatment of hiccups: a case report. *Journal of Medical Case Reports.* 2011;*5*:493.

73. Arsanious D, Khoury S, Martinez E, et al. Ultrasound-guided phrenic nerve block for intractable hiccups following placement of esophageal stent for esophageal squamous cell carcinoma. *Pain Physician.* 2016;*19*(4):E653–E656.

74. Zhang Y, Duan F, Ma W. Ultrasound-guided phrenic nerve block for intraoperative persistent hiccups: a case report. *BMC Anesthesiology.* 2018;*18*(1):123.

75. Mangar D, Patil VU. Elimination of hiccups with a nasopharyngeal airway. *Journal of Clinical Anesthesiology.* 1992;*4*(1):86.

76. Orlovich DS, Brodsky JB, Brock-Utne JG. Nonpharmacologic management of acute singultus (hiccups). *Anesthesia and Analgesia.* 2018;*126*(3):1091.

77. Kranke P, Eberhart LH, Morin AM, Cracknell J, Greim CA, Roewer N. Treatment of hiccup during general anaesthesia or sedation: a qualitative systematic review. *European Journal of Anaesthesiology.* 2003;*20*(3):239–244.

78. Friedgood CE, Ripstein CB. Chlorpromazine(thorazine) in the treatment of intractable hiccups. *JAMA.* 1955;*157*(4):309–310.

79. Muench J, Hamer AM. Adverse effects of antipsychotic medications. *American Family Physician.* 2010;*81*(5):617–622.

80. Wang T, Wang D. Metoclopramide for patients with intractable hiccups: a multicentre, randomised, controlled pilot study. *Internal Medicine Journal.* 2014;*44*(12a):1205–1209.

81. Zhang C, Zhang R, Zhang S, Xu M, Zhang S. Baclofen for stroke patients with persistent hiccups: a randomized, double-blind, placebo-controlled trial. *Trials.* 2014;*15*:295.

82. Moretti R, Torre P, Antonello RM, Ukmar M, Cazzato G, Bava A. Gabapentin as a drug therapy of intractable hiccup because of vascular lesion: a three-year follow up. *Neurologist.* 2004;*10*(2):102–106.

83. Wijemanne S, Jankovic J, Evans RW. Movement disorders from the use of metoclopramide and other antiemetics in the treatment of migraine. *Headache.* 2016;*56*(1):153–161.

84. DiPalma JR. Metoclopramide: a dopamine receptor antagonist. *American Family Physician.* 1990;*41*(3):919–924.

85. Ertzgaard P, Campo C, Calabrese A. Efficacy and safety of oral baclofen in the management of spasticity: a rationale for intrathecal baclofen. *Journal of Rehabilitation Medicine.* 2017;*49*(3):193–203.

86. Choo YM, Kim GB, Choi JY, et al. Severe respiratory depression by low-dose baclofen in the treatment of chronic hiccups in a patient undergoing CAPD. *Nephron.* 2000;*86*(4):546–547.

87. Bockbrader HN, Wesche D, Miller R, Chapel S, Janiczek N, Burger P. A comparison of the pharmacokinetics and pharmacodynamics of pregabalin and gabapentin. *Clinical Pharmacokinetics.* 2010;*49*(10):661–669.

88. Reves JG, Fragen RJ, Vinik HR, Greenblatt DJ. Midazolam: pharmacology and uses. *Anesthesiology.* 1985;*62*(3):310–324.

89. *Oxford English Dictionary.* s.vv. "nausea" and "vomiting" Oxford University Press; 2019.

90. Walsh D, et al. 2016 updated MASCC/ESMO consensus recommendations: management of nausea and vomiting in advanced cancer. *Supportive Care in Cancer.* 2017;*25*(1):333.

91. Feyer P, et al. Radiation induced nausea and vomiting. *European Journal of Pharmacology.* 2014;*722*:165.

92. Solano JP, et al. A comparison of symptoms prevalence in far advanced cancer, AIDs, heart disease, chronic obstructive pulmonary disease and renal disease. *Journal of Pain and Symptom Management.* 2006;*31*:58.

93. Navari RM. Nausea and vomiting in advanced cancer. *Current Treatment Options in Oncology.* 2020;*21*:14.

94. Walsh D, et al. Updated MASCC/ESMO consensus recommendations management of nausea and vomiting in advanced cancer patients. *Supportive Care in Cancer.* 2017;*25*(1):333–340.

95. Navari RM. Nausea and vomiting in advanced cancer. *Current Treatment Options in Oncology.* 2020;*21*:14.

96. Zhong Z, et al. Effects of low-dose olanzapine on duloxetine-related nausea and vomiting for the treatment of major depressive disorder. *Journal Clinical Psychopharmacology.* 2014;*34*:495–498.

97. Hesketh PJ, et al. ASCO antiemetic guidelines. *Journal of Clinical Oncology.* 2017;*35*:3240–3261.

98. Hodge C, Badgwell BD. Palliation of malignant ascites. *Journal of Surgical Oncology.* 2019;*120*:67–73.

99. MacDonald S, et al. Quality of life measures predict mortality in patients with cirrhosis and severe ascites. *Alimentary Pharmacology and Therapeutics.* 2019;*49*:321–330.

100. Hodge C, Badgwell BD. Palliation of malignant ascites. *Journal of Surg Oncology.* 2019;*120*:67–73. https://doi.org/10.1002/jso.25453

101. Fleming ND, et al. Indwelling catheters for the management of refractory malignant ascites: a systemic literature overview and retrospective chart review. *Journal of Pain and Symptom Management.* 2009;*38*(3):341–349.

102. Stephenson J, Gilbert J. The development of clinical guidelines for ascites related to malignancy. *Palliative Medicine.* 2002:*16*(3):213–218.

103. Courtney A, et al. Prospective evaluation of the PleurX catheter when used to treat recurrent ascites associated with malignancy. *Journal of Vascular and Interventional Radiology.* 2008;*19*(12):1723–1731.

104. Cote Robson P, et al. Quality of life improves after palliative placement of percutaneous tunneled drainage catheter for refractory ascites in prospective study of patients with end-stage cancer. *Palliative and Supportive Care.* 2019;677–685.

105. Narayanan G, et al. Safety and efficacy of PleurX catheter for the treatment of malignant ascites. *Journal of Palliative Medicine.* 2014;*17*(8):906–912.

106. Coupe NA, et al. Outcomes of permanent peritoneal ports for the management of recurrent malignant ascites. *Journal of Palliative Medicine.* 2013;*16*(8):938–940.

107. Stukan M. Drainage of malignant ascites: patient selection and perspectives. *Cancer Management and Research.* 2017;9:115–130.

108. American Gastroenterological Association. Home page. https://gastro.org. Accessed November 12, 2020.

109. *Encyclopedia of Surgery.* s.v. "Peritoneous venous shunt." https://www.surgeryencyclopedia.com/Pa-St/Peritoneovenous-Shunt.html. Accessed November 12, 2020.

11

Gastrointestinal Symptoms

Kimberly Angelia Curseen, Denise Rizzolo, and Mark Deutchman

Introduction

Management of gastrointestinal symptoms in palliative care can be challenging. The pathophysiology of the symptoms can be complicated, and many of the medical interventions have difficult side effect profiles. However, the majority of patients with advanced illness will experience several of these symptoms as they approach the end of life. Poorly controlled gastrointestinal symptoms may not only interfere with a patient's quality of life but also have the potential to shorten the length of life if not evaluated and managed properly.[1,2]

Oral Health
Taste Disturbances

Taste disturbances occur with chronic illness but are commonly seen in cancer patients. Loss of taste can be seen with direct radiation to the tongue or adjacent structures or as a result of chemotherapy. Direct radiation to the oral cavity can alter taste due to damage to the innervation to the tongue. It is unclear the exact cause of taste alternation with chemotherapy, but some research suggests it may be due to zinc deficiency. Lack of salivary flow contributes to changes in taste as well. Patients may completely lose their taste or have changes in taste to sweet, sour, and salty food. Once taste is altered, patients may eat less, leading to malnutrition.

Treatment is limited, and there is a chance taste will not return to normal after radiation. Typically, it will return after chemotherapy. Some nonpharmacological treatment strategies include eating smaller and more frequent meals, adding sauces and/or condiments to food, and adding sweets to meats to improve overall taste.[3] Research has suggested that zinc supplementation before undergoing cancer treatment may help with alterations in taste.[3]

TABLE 11.1 Medications That Alter Taste or Cause Dry Mouth[4]

Medication	Alter Taste	Dry Mouth
Bronchodilators: albuterol		x
Antibiotics, including ampicillin, azithromycin, ciprofloxacin, clarithromycin, griseofulvin, metronidazole, tetracycline	x	
Anticonvulsants: carbamazepine and phenytoin	x	
Antidepressants: tricyclics	x	x
Antihistamines and decongestants	x	x
Antihypertensives and cardiac medications, including captopril, diltiazem, enalapril, hydrochlorothiazide, nifedipine, nitroglycerin, propranolol, spironolactone	x	
Diuretics	x	x
Lithium	x	
Antineoplastics	x	
Antiparkinsonians	x	
Antipsychotics	x	
Lipid-lowering agents: statins	x	
Muscle relaxants: baclofen and dantroline	x	
Antithyroid agents: methimazole and propylthiouracil	x	
Pain medication: oxycodone and acetaminophen		x

Patients should be counseled that they may have taste alterations and begin to try different foods that may help stimulate their appetite before undergoing cancer therapy.[4]

Nonrelated cancer taste disturbances can occur in patients on long-term medications, specifically medications that can cause dry mouth. Medications that can cause taste disturbances are listed in Table 11.1. Treatment for taste disturbance when caused by medications is first to try to discontinue the agent if possible. Additional treatment is similar to the above.

Denture-Related Problems

Denture-related problems are common during end-of-life treatment. For example, many immunocompromised patients can develop mucositis. This can often cause the hard palate to become friable and irritated; as well this can cause ulceration of the tongue, buccal surfaces, and lips. Mucositis is not a contraindication to denture use, but a patient may find it uncomfortable to wear them.

Patients who are severely immunocompromised may also develop dry mouth and oral ulcers. When severe dry mouth occurs, dentures may become ill-fitting as they will not adhere to the mouth well. Treatment is similar to that for patients with xerostomia and consists of keeping the mouth moist and increasing salivary flow. Additionally, dentures should be kept in a water solution overnight. Dentures should be cleaned periodically. Avoid using abrasive materials such as brushes with stiff bristles, whitening toothpastes or products containing bleach as this may cause damage to the dentures. It is also not recommended to boil dentures as they may become warped and then fit incorrectly. Literature is mixed on what denture solution should be used.[5] Some general guidelines to follow when cleaning dentures are as follows: Dentures should be cleaned daily by soaking and brushing with an effective, nonabrasive denture cleanser. Denture cleansers should ONLY be used to clean dentures outside of the mouth. Dentures should always be thoroughly rinsed after soaking and brushing with denture-cleansing solutions prior to reinsertion into the oral cavity. Always follow the product usage instructions.[6]

The treatment of mucositis should begin as soon as the patient becomes symptomatic. The first step of treatment is good oral care, obtained by keeping the mouth moist, brushing twice a day, and flossing. If the patient is experiencing localized pain, a topical anesthetic can be used. Other therapies have included rinsing with diphenhydramine elixirs, sucralfate solutions, and topical anesthetics. One topical solution that can be used is called "magic mouthwash." Magic mouthwash is a combination that can be made with different medications but what is commonly prescribed is equal parts of diphenhydramine suspension, Maalox, and viscous lidocaine. It can be swished in the mouth, and then the patient should spit it out. This combination may vary by institution. If the topical anesthetic fails, the patient can be given nonsteroidal anti-inflammatories at the recommended dose.[6]

Oral Fungal Infections

Many factors can promote fungal infections in patients receiving palliative care. First, xerostomia from lack of salivary flow or salivary dysfunction can increase the risk of developing fungal infections, particularly candidiasis. Once the lining of the mouth becomes inflamed, the tissues can weaken, increasing the risk of candidiasis and other viral or bacterial infections. Depending on the patient's immune status, fungal infections can become invasive, and the patient can develop esophageal candidiasis. In many seriously ill patients, nutritional status may decrease, and this contributes to more extensive and/or systemic fungal infections.

The cornerstone of treatment is prevention with good oral hygiene. If a patient develops an oral candida infection, treat with topical antifungal agents such as nystatin rinse/pastilles and clotrimazole troches. Patients should avoid drinking or eating 30 minutes after the use of the troches.[5] If the fungal infection is resistant to topical treatment or is beyond the oral cavity, treatment with a systemic antifungal agent such as fluconazole is indicated. Fluconazole dosage should be adjusted for age, but in adults it can be given as follows: 200 mg by mouth daily on day 1 and then 100 mg daily for 2–3 weeks.[7]

Nausea and Vomiting

Nausea and vomiting are common symptoms in cancer patients as well as patients with advanced serious illness, and the etiology is often multifactorial.[8] Up to 70% of patients with cancer experience these symptoms secondary to cancer therapies, obstruction, medications, and psychological factors.[9,10] Congestive heart failure, organ failure, acquired immunodeficiency virus, and gastroparesis can all increase nausea, particularly as patients progress toward end of life and during disease flares.[11]

There is a lack of strong evidence to manage nausea and vomiting based on mechanism. However, understanding the etiology of the symptoms can help guide treatment, especially when it is secondary to reversible conditions such as uncontrolled constipation, medication side effects, gastric reflux disease, gastrointestinal dysmotility or obstruction, and anticipatory nausea caused by psychological distress.[2] In these cases, tailoring the treatment plan to the mechanism may be the most appropriate way to start.[12]

The vomiting center is located in the medulla. This center can receive direct and indirect input from several areas of the brain, which explains the wide variety of medications that are used to target this area. The vomiting center can receive direct input from medications, signals from the gastrointestinal tract, metabolic disturbances, and toxins in the blood through the chemoreceptor trigger zone (CTZ) or by direct stimulation from the cerebral cortex, vestibular apparatus, and sensory organs. The CTZ is located on the floor of the fourth ventricle, which is outside of the blood-brain barrier. Through neurotransmitters serotonin, dopamine, histamine, and acetylcholine, CTZ mediates the nausea and vomiting response to the vomiting center (Figure 11.1).[13,14]

Starting with an appropriate assessment is important before initiating therapy. Careful history and physical examination can often lead to a symptom's etiology. History should include evaluation of nausea and vomiting patterns. Frequency, onset duration, exacerbating factors, consistency of vomitus (including presence of blood), pain, and nausea-relieving factors should be evaluated. Each of these factors may provide clues to the etiology of nausea and vomiting. Comorbid factors should be noted as well.[15] Patients with gastroparesis, constipation, functional ileus, peptic ulcer disease, gastric reflux, poorly controlled heart failure, diabetes, migraine headache, acute visual changes, or end-stage renal and liver disease have an increased risk of intermittent/chronic nausea and vomiting.[16] Anticipatory nausea is defined as being triggered by the thought of an event (i.e., chemotherapy, smells, and sights associated with anxiety).[17]

Physical examination should focus on the gastrointestinal examination. Oral examination should be performed to evaluate for thrush and dental health. Distention and reduced bowel sounds on the abdominal examination could be signs of obstruction or ascites. Pain and fever could denote bowel perforation, infection, sequela of cancer progression, and possible need for surgical consultation. Patients should always be evaluated for constipation and fecal impaction. Ophthalmic examination should be performed to rule out papilledema, which could be a sign of increased intracranial pressure. Neurological examination, including vestibular examination, to evaluate for neurological deficits that may reveal the etiology or lead to cerebral imaging to evaluate for a brain mass or other abnormalities.[13,14,16] Laboratory evaluation should include a comprehensive metabolic panel, which assesses liver/renal function, calcium levels, and drug levels if applicable. Imaging, if appropriate, should include an upright abdominal x-ray to evaluate for obstruction (air-fluid level), and fecal impaction/obstipation. An abdominal ultrasound can determine the presence of ascites and hepatomegaly. Abdominal computed tomographic (CT) scan can evaluate for obstruction, perforation, megacolon, infection, and organomegaly.[10,14,16]

Completing a careful medication review is also key to assessing patients who are experiencing nausea and vomiting. It is important to evaluate for emetogenic medications and therapies (Box 11.1). Opioid therapy commonly used in palliative care for pain or dyspnea management can be very emetogenic. The symptoms usually resolve in 3–5 days, but for some patients it can be intolerable. Opioids also cause constipation, which can contribute to nausea.

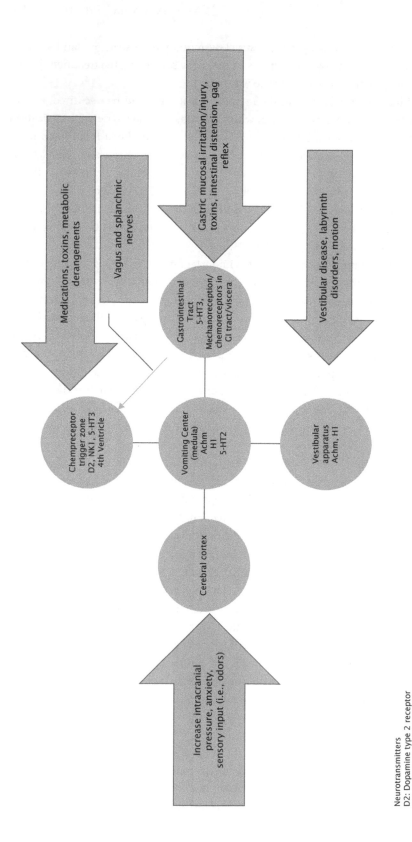

FIGURE 11.1 Pathophysiology of nausea and vomiting. GI, gastrointestinal. (From References 13 and 14.)

Neurotransmitters
D2: Dopamine type 2 receptor
H1: Histamine type 1 receptor
NK: Neurokinin type 1 receptor
5-HT2: 5-hydroxytryptamine type 2 receptor; 5-HT3: 5-hydroxytryptamine type 3 receptor
Achm: Muscarinic acetylcholine receptor

BOX 11.1 Emetogenic Medications[9,18]

Chemotherapy
- Cisplatin
- Carmustine
- Cyclophosphamide
- Dacarbazine
- Mechloretamine
- ABVD (adriamycin, bleomycin, vinblastine, dacarbazine)
- AC (adriamycin, cyclophosphamide)
- BEP (bleomycin, etoposide, platinum)

Medications
- Opioids
- Antidepressants
- Cholinesterase inhibitors
- Metformin
- Vitamins/iron
- Antibiotics
- Calcium channel blockers
- Nonsteroidal anti-inflammatories

A useful acronym is *A VOMIT*, which can be used to guide a comprehensive nausea/vomiting evaluation[19]:

A Anxiety or anticipatory
V Vestibular
O Obstructive
M Medication/metabolic
I Infection/inflammation
T Toxins

There are two approaches to treating nausea and vomiting: empiric treatment and cause-based treatment. Empiric treatment is choosing an antiemetic regardless of etiology, and cause-based treatment is choosing an antiemetic that best fits the possible etiology. There is limited evidence for non-chemotherapy-induced nausea and vomiting for either approach. However, all treatment plans start with identification and removal of reversible causes and offending agents.[16,20]

There are several classes of drugs available to manage nausea and vomiting in patients with advanced illness (Table 11.2). Dopamine (D_2) antagonists have potent effects that minimize dopamine on the CTZ. This results in reduced stimulation of the vomiting center.

TABLE 11.2 Cause and Management Strategies for Nausea and Vomiting[10,16,17,21-24]

Anatomy	Clinical Presentation	Treatment	Medications	Receptors
Vestibular - Labyrinthitis - Vertigo	Symptoms with motion, ear pain	Antihistamine and anticholinergics	Diphenhydramine 25–50 mg IV/oral Hyoscyamine 0.135–0.25 mg IV/oral, SL Scopolamine 1.5-mg transdermal every 72 h	H1 Achm Achm
Chemoreceptor trigger zone - Medications - Toxins (infection, ischemia - Metabolic: renal/liver failure, hypercalcemia, hyponatremia	Constant nausea, intermittent vomiting. drug toxicity, organ failure	D$_2$ receptor antagonist Serotonin receptor antagonist Neurokinin 1 receptor antagonist	Haldoperidol oral/SC/IV 0.5–5 mg every 4–8 h Promethazine oral/IV/Supp 12.5–25 mg every 6 h Prochloroperazine oral/IV/Supp 5–10 mg every 4–6 h; 25 mg Supp every 6 h Ondansetron oral/ODT/IV 4 mg every 6 h; 8 mg every 8 h Palonosetron IV/oral 0.25 mg IV 1 h prior to chemotherapy; 0.5–1 mg oral 1 h prior to chemotherapy	D2 D2, Achm, H1 D2 5-HT3 5-HT3
Cortical	Anticipatory nausea Meningeal irritation	Thienobenzodiazepine Benzamine analogues/prokinetic		5-HT3
Gastrointestinal tract - Constipation - Peritoneal carcinomatosis - Bowel obstruction - Ascites - Gastroparesis	Headache, falls, projectile vomiting, mental status changes, pain Constipation Projectile vomit Early satiety Gag reflex Epigastric irritation Large-volume emesis: high obstruction Low-volume emesis/fecal matter: colonic obstruction	Cannabinoids Benzodiazepines Corticosteroids Radiation Pain management Cognitive behavioral therapy Laxatives Prokinetic Agent Proton pump inhibitors, H$_2$ blockers Hydration	Granisetron IV/oral/SC/transdermal 2 mg before chemo orally; 1 mg twice daily orally 10 mg SC 30 min prior to chemo with steroid Transdermal patch; apply 24–48 h before chemo, duration 7 days Aprepitant oral 125 mg first day, 80 mg oral for 3 days Fosaprepitant IV 130 mg prior to chemo Olanzapine oral/ODT/IM 2.5–10 mg oral/ODT; IM 5 mg Metoclopramide oral/IV: 5–10 mg every 6 h or AC at bedtime Dronabinol oral 2.5–10 mg every 4 h Nabilone oral 1 mg every 12 h to maximum 2 mg every 8 h; start 3 h prior to chemo	NK-1 D2, 5-HT3, H1, Achm D1, 5-HT3 5-HT$_{1A}$ GABA Reduction in inflammation and prostaglandin production D1, 5-HT3
- Tumor infiltration - Organomegaly - Autonomic dysfunction			Lorazepam 0.025–2 mg IV prior to chemotherapy; 0.5–1 mg oral every 8 h as needed for nausea (caution: respiratory depression with opioid; risk for dependence) Dexamethasone: 12 mg day 1 chemo or prechemo, 8 mg days 2–4; 6–4 mg oral every 6 h brain metastases with taper Treatment for brain metastasis Opioid and nonopioid analgesia Osmotic, stimulants, opioid receptor antagonist, surfactants, bulking agents Metoclopramide oral/IV: 5–10 mg every 6 h or AC at bedtime Omeprazole, esomeprazole, famotidine IV fluid hydration with normal saline or lactated Ringer's	

A common antipsychotic medication used in palliative care is haloperidol which uses this pathway. Other dopamine receptor agonists are promethazine, prochlorperazine, and chlorpromazine. Although these medications are effective, the side-effect profile can include sedation, extrapyramidal side effects, neuroleptic malignant syndrome, delirium, orthostasis, altered cardiac conduction, and delirium. They can also potentiate the sedating effects of opioids.[9,16] Metaclopramide is a prokinetic agent that acts on D_2 receptors and at higher doses on serotonin and muscarinic receptors. It can be a good choice if dysmotility is the primary cause of nausea. However, obstruction must be ruled out. It also has a similar side-effect profile to antipsychotics and can cause drug-induced parkinsonism.

The atypical antipsychotic olanzapine (thienobenzodiazepine) has a growing evidence base for chemotherapy-induced and cancer nausea. Olanzapine blocks multiple neurotransmitter receptors involved in the pathophysiology of nausea and vomiting, which include the dopaminergic D_1 and D_2 brain receptors; serotonergic at 5-$HT_{2a,c}$, 5-$HT_{3,6}$; catecholamines at alpha$_1$ adrenergic receptors; acetylcholine at muscarinic receptors; and histamine at H_1 receptors. It also is not a cytochrome p450 inhibitor, which limits drug interactions. It is supplied as an oral disintegrating tablet and an intramuscular preparation. The side-effect profile includes weight gain, anticholinergic side effects, hyperglycemia, sedation, increased appetite, orthostasis, extrapyramidal symptoms (EPS), altered cardiac conduction, and reduction in seizure threshold.[21] Typical and atypical antipsychotics carry a black box warning for increased risk for stroke and death for patients with dementia.[25,26]

There are several agents that target the vestibular systems. Two categories are anticholinergics (scopolamine, hysoscyamine) and antihistamines (meclizine, diphenhydramine, hydroxyzine). These medications block histamine (H_1) and acetylcholine (Achm, muscarinic acetylcholine) receptors located on the vestibulocochlear nerve. The side-effect profile can be difficult to tolerate, especially for elderly patients, secondary to anticholinergic side effects, which include delirium, urinary retention, falls, dry mouth, sedation, depressed mood, and blurred vision.[27] These medications are also used for secretion management.

A serotonin antagonist (5-hydroxytryptamine-3 [5-HT_3]), such as palonosetron and ondansetron, in combination with dexamethasone has shown evidence for prevention of chemotherapy-induced nausea.[22] The combination has a more favorable side-effect profile than other antiemetics and is well tolerated. Common side effects are constipation and fatigue. They do have risk for prolongation QTc and should be used cautiously with other QTc-prolonging agents.[28,29] 5-HT_3 medications can also potentiate headaches, which can make them difficult to use in patients prone to migraines. 5-HT_3 also can come in intravenous, oral (disintegrating), and transdermal preparations.[9,16,22]

Steroids can be effective for patients with intractable nausea and vomiting. The etiology is thought to be a reduction in prostaglandin and inflammation around tumors. They are often seen in combination with 5-HT_3 or other antiemetics. Steroids have the potential to increase appetite and improve fatigue in patients with serious illness. They are not appropriate for long-term treatment for patients who are not at end of life; this is secondary to a poor side-effect profile with prolonged use, which includes suppression of the hypothalamic-pituitary axis, cortisol suppression, easy bruising, Cushing symptoms, and osteoporosis. Immediate side effects are hyperglycemia, steroid psychosis, insomnia, and epigastric burning.[14,16,30]

A neurokinin (NK) type 1 receptor antagonist such as aprepitant has been shown to prevent delayed emesis after treatment with cisplatin and improve acute nausea if used with steroid and 5-HT$_3$. It works on receptors in the gastrointestinal tract and the vomiting center by blocking binding of substance P. It comes in intravenous and oral preparations and is expensive. Common side effects are hiccups, constipation, anorexia, fatigue, and headaches. Usually, NK-1 antagonists are used in oncology infusion centers with chemotherapy.[16,31]

Synthetic cannabinoids such as dronabinol and nabilone have been shown to have some efficacy for nausea patients with AIDs and cancer, although evidence for efficacy for AIDS is stronger. The studies using traditional cannabis for nausea has been mixed, and further research is required despite the animal models being promising. It is thought to work through indirect activation of somatodendritic 5-HT$_{1A}$ receptors in the dorsal raphe nucleus.[23,32] Use can be limited by side effects and legality. Marijuana remains federally illegal despite being legalized by several states. Marijuana is not currently regulated by the Food and Drug Administration, and preparations have the risk of lacking quality and safety controls. Also, there is a significant amount of product variability. They have been used successfully as adjuvants for nausea treatment for patients intolerant to traditional antiemetics.[24]

For patients experiencing intractable nausea and vomiting, a closely supervised intravenous fluid hydration trial can help break the nausea cycle, especially if dehydration has led to a reduction in creatinine clearance. This can be particularly true when patients are on opioids or other medication with emetogenic metabolites.

Constipation and Diarrhea

There are several factors that contribute to constipation in patients with advanced illness (Table 11.3). Poorly managed constipation is associated with nausea, anorexia, abdominal pain, early satiety, fatigue, and abdominal bloating and can be a causative factor for delirium in the elderly. Opioid-induced constipation has high prevalence in palliative care and hospice patients. The prevalence of constipation for all patients with terminal illness ranges from 32% to 87%.[33] In a study evaluating constipation in hospitalized cancer patients, the prevalence ranged from 10% to 70%. Half of patients admitted to hospice noted constipation on admission.[34] Patients with reduced or no oral intake should still have bowel movements. Fifty percent of stool is intestinal slough and water as the colon draws in approximately 7 L of fluid daily. Gut transit is normally 24 to 48 hours in healthy individuals but can be about 12 days in palliative care patients with serious illness, secondary to that illness and medications for symptom management.[35]

Undertreatment of constipation may lead to lower gastrointestinal complications, such as urinary retention, gastrointestinal obstruction, bowel ischemia and/or perforations, hemorrhoids, fecal overflow, anal tears/fissure, rectal bleeding, and rectal prolapses.[36] Constipation is also associated with psychological distress, social isolation, and possible catastrophic thinking.[37,38]

Constipation has been defined as having less than three bowel movements per week, although there is no consensus definition. Symptoms of straining, hard stool, and feelings of incomplete evacuation are signs just as significant as decrease in stool frequency. There are several assessment tools for constipation, but two tools, the Rome Criteria for Constipation

TABLE 11.3 Constipation Etiology in Palliative Care[16,33,34]

Cause	Medical Condition or Population
Preexisting constipation	Common in older adults
Neurologic disorders	Spinal cord injuries Multiple sclerosis Parkinson disease Peripheral neuropathy Amyotrophic lateral sclerosis
Gastrointestinal structural disorders	Tumors Radiation fibrosis Adhesions Stricture Hemorrhoids Rectal prolapse Anal fissures Obstruction
Gastrointestinal functional disorders/ metabolic	Gastroparesis - Diabetes - Mitochondrial disorders - Hypoparathyroidism - Hypothyroidism
Medications	Opioids/opiates Chemotherapy - Alkylating agents Iron supplements Calcium channel blocker Diuretics Anticholinergic medications Psychostimulants Ipratropium bromide Anticonvulsants Calcium supplements Antiarrhythmic Antacids 5-HT_3 antiemetic Dopaminergic medications
Electrolyte abnormalities	Hypercalcemia Hypokalemia Uremia
Patient factors/behaviors	Poor fluid intake Immobility Emotional distress Diet

and the Bowel Function Index, appear to be helpful for the advanced illness population (Table 11.4).[39,40]

In addition to the assessment tools for constipation, the history and physical will be important to determining an etiology. In addition to identifying the stool pattern, a careful history and medication review should be performed to develop the differential diagnosis. Often, the etiology is multifactorial for constipation in palliative care patients. Patients are often on multiple constipating medications for symptom management, including but not limited to opioid analgesics and antiemetics. Chronic illness often accompanies gastrointestinal

TABLE 11.4 Constipation Assessment Tools[39,40]

Rome Criteria	At least two of the following *symptoms* over the preceding 3 months: - Fewer than three spontaneous bowel movements per week - Straining for more than 25% of defecation attempts - Lumpy or hard stools for at least 25% of defecation attempts
Bowel Function Index	Validated specifically for opioid-induced constipation (OIC). It is a physician-administered, easy-to-use scale made up of three items (ease of defecation, feeling of incomplete *bowel* evacuation, and personal judgment of constipation)

dysmotility, decreased function, and decreased oral intake, especially as a patient approaches end of life.[33,41]

Patients should undergo a thorough physical examination focused on identifying abdominal abnormalities, including distention, diminished bowel sounds, organomegaly, and ascites. It is important to evaluate for signs of obstruction. A rectal examination may be warranted to evaluate for fecal impaction, anal fissures, rectal tone, and fecal seepage. Fecal seepage can happen when loose stool flows around an impaction. Some patients with fecal incontinence may actually have constipation. Constipation can also be a warning sign for spinal cord compression, and patients with risk factors should undergo a neurologic evaluation.

Radiological imaging may be helpful to confirm fecal impaction or obstipation. A plain upright radiograph and/or CT scan can evaluate for obstruction prior to initiating an aggressive bowel regimen for a patient at risk of colonic obstruction.[16,34,42]

Management strategies for constipation should include an effort focused on correcting any reversible causes.[1,43] Treatment plans should be tailored to the patient's clinical condition, goals, and etiology of constipation. Nonpharmacological strategies should be implemented with patients when appropriate (Box 11.2).[37]

Opioid-induced constipation is common in patients receiving palliative care services. This symptom can usually be managed with a proactive bowel regimen that consists of a stimulant and osmotic laxative. Opioids bind to mu receptor in the colon. This causes an inhibition of acetylcholine from the myenteric plexus, which interrupts and slows colonic peristalsis. The stool spends a protracted time in the colon, and water/electrolytes are absorbed from the stool, causing hardening. Opioids decrease gastric, pancreatic, intestinal, and biliary secretions in addition to decreasing the defecation reflex. Opioids also interfere with rectal sensation sensitivity, which makes evacuation harder and decreases tone at the ileocecal valve.[16,43]

It is universally accepted that patients who are started on opioid therapy should be started on laxatives, preferably a stimulant and osmotic laxative combination to prevent and manage opioid-induced constipation, although there is limited evidence to support this currently.[37,45] There is strong evidence for peripherally acting mu-opioid receptor antagonists for opioid-induced constipation.[37] As opioids are increased, often there is a need for an accompanying laxative increase. However, it is not clear that the relationship between opioid and laxative dosing is completely linear. Escalation of laxatives every 2 days is a reasonable strategy to implement with close monitoring.[16,37,38] Opioid rotation should be considered; there is evidence that transdermal fentanyl and tapentadol may be associated with less

---

BOX 11.2 Nonpharmacological Constipation Strategies[44]

- Increase fluid intake 2–3 L/d: oral hydration
- Avoid caffeinated beverages (secondary to diuretic properties)
- Exercise: increase physical activity
- Avoid use of bedpan
- Bowel routines; timed toileting
- ± Increase in fiber intake
- Prunes (rich insoluble fiber and sorbitol)
- Manual disimpaction (often used with a lubricant [i.e., spinal cord injuries, weakness, end-stage dementia])[3]

---

constipation.[46–48] Other studies did not find improvement in constipation with transdermal fentanyl over other opioid therapy.[49]

The choice of pharmacological intervention should take the etiology of constipation into consideration. There are several classes of medication available to treat constipation (Table 11.5).[16,34,36,37,50,51]

The Palliative Care Study Group of the *Multinational Association for Supportive Care in Cancer* (MASCC) collaborated to produce 15 evidence-based recommendations published in 2020 for the management of constipation in patients with advanced cancer.[37] There were only two recommendations that had evidence stronger than a suggestion. Peripherally acting mu-opioid receptor antagonists should always be considered in patients with opioid-induced constipation, and conventional laxatives should be considered as first-line treatment in patients with functional constipation (Table 11.6).[37,51–53]

Diarrhea

Diarrhea is not an uncommon symptom encountered in seriously ill patients. Diarrhea is defined as loose, watery bowel movements that occur three or more times in 1 day. Often it is managed in the setting of cytotoxic and targeted chemotherapy agents and after radiation (Table 11.7). However, palliative care providers may also manage patients with diarrhea for other etiologies, such as short-gut syndrome, dumping syndrome, bacterial overgrowth, lactose deficiency, AIDS, diarrhea-predominant irritable bowel syndrome, infections, medications, endocrinopathies, and autoimmune diseases. Untreated diarrhea can lead to electrolyte abnormalities and dehydration, which can worsen a patient's already fragile condition. It can also limit a patient's ability to tolerate life-prolonging therapies they wish to pursue and lead to unwanted hospitalizations.

Volume loss and electrolyte abnormalities, including hypokalemia and metabolic alkalosis that result from diarrhea, place patients at risk for cardiac arrhythmias, renal failure, orthostatic hypotension, fatigue, and falls. Poorly controlled diarrhea can also cause patients to become isolated for fear of fecal incontinence, which leads to or potentiates anxiety and

TABLE 11.5 Laxative Medications[16,34,36,37,50,51]

Drug Classification	Agent	Mechanism of Action	
Bulk-forming agents	Psyllium, methylcellulose	Increase bulk, draw water	Avoid in dehydrated, OIC, and terminally ill patients can worsen constipation. May cause bloating, flatulence, pain.
Stimulants	Senna Bisacodyl	Increases colonic peristalsis by stimulating the myenteric plexus	Senna can cause abdominal cramping, colic, melanosis coli; may develop tachyphylaxis; may use 2–8 pills/d in divided doses. Bisacodyl may cause abdominal cramps and electrolyte abnormalities.
Osmotic	Lactulose Magnesium sulfate Sorbitol Polyethylene glycol	Increase small bowel secretions and draw/hold water in bowel lumen	Lactulose may cause acid-base disturbance, hypokalemia, lactic acidosis, colic, bloating. Avoid magnesium in patients with renal insufficiency/cardiac disease; abuse can cause bradycardia, hypomagnesemia, hypocalcemia, hypokalemia. Sorbitol can cause abdominal cramping, bloating. Polyethylene glycol can cause diarrhea; nausea; aspiration, which can cause pulmonary edema.
Lubricants	Mineral oil Glycerin suppositories Petroleum	Soften and lubricate passage of stool	Mineral oil can cause pneumonitis if aspirated and interfere with absorption of fat-soluble vitamins.
Peripherally acting mu-opioid receptor antagonists (PAMORAs)	Methynaltrexone Naloxegol	Selective peripheral opioid antagonist, counteracts opioid intestinal side effect	Methynaltrexone require SC injection; not for daily use. Naloxegol can be taken daily. Both can cause diarrhea, abdominal cramping; contraindicated in bowel obstruction.
Surfactants	Docusate	Lubricate and soften stool	Studies have shown lack of efficacy.
Chloride channel activator Guanylate cyclase-C agonist	Lubiprostone Linaclotide	Increase intestinal secretions and improves fecal transit Increase intestinal secretions and improve fecal transit	Lubiprostone is for chronic constipation, OIC, irritable bowel syndrome with constipation (IBS-C); patient may experience headache, nausea, and diarrhea. Linaclotide may decrease intestinal pain; for chronic constipation or IBS-C, can cause diarrhea.
Enemas	Tap water Mineral oil Soapsuds Sodium phosphate	Facilitate peristalsis by causing colonic distention Draw water in to bowel lumen	Excessive use of tap water enemas can cause electrolyte abnormalities (i.e., hyponatremia). Avoid sodium phosphate enema in renal failure; can cause hyperphosphatemia.

TABLE 11.6 Adapted MASCC Recommendation on Management of Constipation in Patient With Advanced Cancer[37]

- All patients with advanced cancer should be regularly assessed for constipation (suggestion).
- The management of constipation should be individualized (suggestion).
- Patients should be offered adequate privacy and appropriate equipment (e.g., commode, foot stool) to promote defecation (suggestion).
- Lifestyle changes (e.g., dietary fiber, exercise) have a limited role in patients with advanced cancer (suggestion).
- Reversible causes of constipation should be treated, and potential aggravating factors should be minimized (suggestion).
- Conventional laxatives should be considered as first-line treatment in patients with functional constipation (level of evidence I; recommendation).
- Conventional laxatives should be considered first-line treatment in patients with secondary constipation (suggestion).
- PAMORAs should always be considered in patients with opioid-induced constipation (level of evidence I; recommendation).
- Patients prescribed opioid analgesics should be routinely co-prescribed laxatives (or a PAMORA) (suggestion).
- Suppositories/enemas should only be used in patients with evidence of stool in the rectum and/or descending colon that have not responded to other interventions (suggestion).
- Other interventions should generally only be used in patients with "resistant" constipation (level of evidence (suggestion).
- All patients with constipation should be regularly re-assessed (suggestion).
- Patients with ongoing "resistant" constipation should be referred to a specialist for further investigation/management (suggestion).
- If patients with functional constipation/secondary constipation do not respond to first-line conventional laxatives, then re-assess the patient and consider adding or switching to another conventional laxative or specialist medication (suggestion).

Level of evidence: I = recommendation; IV–V = suggestion.

depression. Diarrhea can cause some patients to develop aversion to food, resulting in anorexia and unintended weight loss.[54] See Table 11.7 for diarrhea alarm symptoms.

When evaluating a patient's diarrhea, a detailed history and physical should be performed. Diarrhea should be evaluated for quantity, quality, and duration of symptoms. A dietary and medication history should be obtained, including over-the-counter medications and nutritional supplements. Patients should be assessed for recent hospitalizations (*Clostridium difficile* exposure) and illnesses that could give clues to an etiology. Patients showing signs of pain, fever, dizziness, nausea, emesis, or bleeding should trigger an urgent evaluation.[1]

The National Institute for Cancer uses a diarrhea grading system to determine severity for cancer patients undergoing therapy.[56]

- Mild diarrhea: grade 1: two or three stools above normal per day
- Mild to moderate: grade 2: four to six stools above normal per day,
- Moderate to severe: grade 3: seven to nine stools above normal, possibly with severe cramps, incontinence
- Severe: grade 4 is severe: 10 or more stools above normal, hemodynamic instability, bloody diarrhea

There are several treatment agents that can cause diarrhea in cancer patients. Irinotecan and 5-fluorouracil have the potential to cause severe diarrhea. In fact, one of irinotecan's dose-limiting toxicities is diarrhea.[1,57] Patients treated with it require strict adherence to a loperamide dosing plan (Table 11.8).[2,57] Patients need to be evaluated for dehydration and electrolyte

TABLE 11.7 Diarrhea Alarm Symptoms[54,55]

Etiology	Alarm Symptom
Neuroendocrine tumor	Weight loss, abdominal mass, fatigue, night sweats
Carcinoid syndrome	Flushing, wheezing, heart murmur, abdominal pain, widen blood vessels on facial skin, shortness of breath
Inflammatory bowel disease	Bloody stools, abdominal pain, fever, fatigue, malnutrition, or weight loss
Mastocytosis	Urticaria pigmentosa, dermatographism
Hyperthyroidism	Tremor, lid lag, tachycardia
Food protein-induced enterocolitis syndrome Parasite	Intermittent vomiting, watery diarrhea with blood or mucus
Celiac disease	Dermatitis herpetiformis, weight loss
Malnutrition	Muscle wasting, weight loss, dependent edema

TABLE 11.8 Antidiarrheal Agents[29,30,50,52,54]

Agent	Mechanism	Dosing	Side Effects
Loperamide - Acts through opioid receptor	Inhibits gastric motility, reduces fecal volume, antisecretory activity, increases tone in anal sphincter	4 mg and 2–4 mg after each stool; 16 mg maximum daily dose	US black box warning: torsade de pointes and sudden death if taking more than maximum daily dose; dizziness, abdominal cramps, nausea
Diphenoxylate and atropine - Act through opioid receptor - Related to meperidine	Inhibit GI (gastrointestinal) motility and propulsion	2.5–5 mg oral four times daily; maximum daily dose 24 mg	Uncommon significant side effects: flushing, tachycardia, dizziness, confusion, depression, euphoria, sedation, hallucination Medication is controlled Can potentiate barbiturates and tricyclic antidepressants Monitor for atropinism Overdose can cause respiratory depression, coma, and death; risk of addiction
Octreotide - Octapeptide analogue of somatostatin	Reduces intestinal secretions, inhibit GI serotonin release, gastrin, vasoactive intestinal polypeptide, insulin, secretin, motilin, and pancreatic peptide; antispasmodic	100 µg SC every 8 h for 48 h and then 10 µg/h if needed	Abdominal cramping Uncommon significant side effects: sinus bradycardia, hypertension, fatigue, abdominal distension, low B_{12} level, cholethiasis, hypothyroidism, pancreatitis, glucose dysregulation
Bismuth - subsalicylate	Antisecretory and antimicrobial	30 mL or 2 tablets orally every 30 min (maximum 240 mL or 16 tablets in 24 h)	Blackens tongue and stool Neurotoxicity with large doses Uncommon significant side effects: anxiety, confusion, muscle spasm, headache

abnormalities frequently when receiving these chemotherapies. Colitis and diarrhea are common side effects associated with immune checkpoint inhibitors such as pembrolizumab or nivolumab.[58] If a patient experiences these symptoms, the immune checkpoint inhibitor is held, and a course of steroids is given in hopes the patient may resume therapy. If gastrointestinal side effects are severe or grade 4, this will indicate cessation of immune checkpoint inhibitor therapy after steroid treatment.[1,58,59]

For treatment of patients with diarrhea, start with antidiarrheal agents (Table 11.8), a BRAT (bananas, rice, applesauce, toast) diet, other dietary modification, and hydration if needed. If possible, hold or treat the offending agent. If not improved and the patient has grade 2–4 diarrhea, consider hospitalization and evaluate for electrolyte abnormalities. Patients may require aggressive hydration with close management of vital signs and output to maintain euvolemia.

If a patient is on an immune checkpoint inhibitor, start steroids.[58,59] If infection is suspected or proven, treat according to culture. If diarrhea remains refractory, consider instituting octreotide. Octreotide is used for refractory diarrhea because it slows intestinal motility, decreases intestinal secretions, and stimulates intestinal absorption of water and electrolytes. Octreotide's primary side effects are abdominal cramping, fatty stools, and flatulence.[1] It is also useful for partial small bowel obstruction to decrease cramping and may even reverse it by decreasing intestinal secretions.

Bowel Obstruction

Palliative care providers must be skilled at the identification and management of bowel obstructions. There are two types of bowel obstruction:

1. Functional: Functional bowel obstruction/paralytic ileus is usually a temporary interruption of gastrointestinal peristalsis, without evidence of mechanical obstruction
2. Structural: Structural bowel obstruction can be full or partial mechanical obstruction preventing bowel motility.[60]

Patients receiving palliative care may present with a functional bowel obstruction secondary to

1. Medications: opioid, anticholinergics, antidiarrhea agent
2. Neurologic disorders
3. Advanced diabetes: gastroparesis secondary to neurological damage to gut
4. Severe electrolyte abnormalities
5. End of life, actively dying[16]

In these cases, except for active dying and some neurologic disorders, conservative management consisting of bowel decompression, rest, electrolyte correction, hydration, and increased mobility (if possible) may resolve symptoms back to baseline. Strategic use of metoclopramide and careful reintroduction of a bowel regimen once the patient starts to recover may be helpful. However, patients are likely to have recurrence. Inpatient and outpatient hospices should be able to manage functional and partial bowel obstruction outside of the acute care setting.[10]

One widely used treatment for constipation in partial bowel obstruction is oral petroleum jelly "Vaseline balls." The theory is that patients freeze small balls of petroleum jelly covered in confectioners' sugar and swallow two or three of them to lubricate the stool to produce a bowel movement. Although used routinely in hospice care, the reports of efficacy are still anecdotal.[61]

Structural bowel obstructions can be secondary to direct invasion or compression of the bowel wall (i.e., malignant bowel obstruction, hernia, strictures, adhesions, diverticulitis, postradiation fibrosis, radiation enteritis, and extrinsic compression). If the obstruction is partial, the patient may respond to conservative measures, including bowel rest, symptom management, and decompression with a nasal gastric tube. If the obstruction is full based on the etiology, the patient may respond to conservative management if surgery is not aligned with goals of care. However, if the patient has good performance status, adequate nutrition, and acceptable prognosis, consultation for surgical intervention is recommended.[60,62]

Palliative management goals for malignant bowel obstruction in patients with advanced disease is to control pain and nausea/vomiting, decrease secretions, and clarify goals of care. Malignant bowel obstructions are commonly seen in ovarian and gastrointestinal cancers[63] and usually signify poor prognosis. Surgical resection, debulking, diversion (ostomy) are the standard of care, but not all patients are appropriate candidates. The goals of surgery have to be well defined. For patients with advanced disease and poor performance status, surgery may be palliative. For nonsurgical candidates, stenting and medical management may be interventions that can improve a patient's quality of life.[1,2,64]

Use a stepwise approach to conservatively manage a bowel obstruction. The medical management should initially include the following:[2,65]

1. Advance care planning and goals-of-care discussion; malignant bowel obstruction has a higher rate of hospital mortality regardless of intervention.[64,66,67]
2. If patients are having significant vomiting and abdominal pain from distention, place a nasogastric tube for decompression if appropriate; bowel rest.
3. Intravenous fluid hydration, electrolyte replacement with bowel rest.
4. Intravenous steroids (i.e., 6–16 mg of dexamethasone daily to decrease bowel wall edema).
5. Analgesia with opioids; haloperidol for nausea; avoid prokinetic agents.
6. Somastatin analogues (octreotide) can be beneficial in reducing the release of gastrointestinal hormones resulting in decreased gut secretion and can be introduced early in treatment if the patient is not a surgical candidate.
7. May consider other anticholinergics to reduce secretion (scopolamine, hyoscyamine); use with caution in the elderly since the anticholinergics may cause or worsen delirium; glycopyrrolate may be preferable since it does not cross the blood-brain barrier.

If the obstruction does not resolve with conservative management or the patients are not candidates for surgical intervention or a stent, then it is necessary to review the entire palliative care plan:

1. Prognosis and disease trajectory.
2. Long-term management of symptoms, including duration of intravenous hydration, decision concerning parental nutrition, decision concerning candidacy for venting gastrostomy tube, which relieves symptoms by decompressing stomach and small bowel.
3. Discussion concerning hospice care and disposition secondary to high clinical need and symptom burden that these patients suffer.
4. Hospice referral so that management of these symptoms in the home or inpatient setting is optimized.[2,63–65]

Patients with serious illness often have gastrointestinal symptoms that require aggressive management. Addressing these symptoms appropriately can result in improved quality of life and significant reduction in morbidity for patients. A stepwise evidence-based approach is required to successfully manage these symptoms in patients undergoing curative, maintenance, and/or palliative therapy.

References

1. Anthony LB, Chauhan A. Diarrhea, constipation, and obstruction in cancer management. In: Olver I, ed. *The MASCC Textbook of Cancer Supportive Care and Survivorship*. Cham, Germany: Springer International; 2018:421–436.
2. Curseen KA. Palliative care for gastrointestinal cancer patients. In: Bekaii-Saab T, El-Reyes BF, Pawlik TM, eds. *Handbook of Gastrointestinal Cancers: Evidence-Based Treatment and Multidisciplinary Patient Care*; 2019:451.
3. Ide K, Seto K, Usui T, Tanaka S, Kawakami K. Correlation between dental conditions and comorbidities in an elderly Japanese population: a cross-sectional study. *Medicine*. 2018;97(24):e11075.
4. Murtaza B, Hichami A, Khan AS, Ghiringhelli F, Khan NA. Alteration in taste perception in cancer: causes and strategies of treatment. *Frontiers in Physiology*. 2017;8:134.
5. Devi S, Singh N. Dental care during and after radiotherapy in head and neck cancer. *National Journal of Maxillofacial Surgery*. 2014;5(2):117.
6. Felton D, Cooper L, Duqum I, et al. Evidence-based guidelines for the care and maintenance of complete dentures: a publication of the American College of Prosthodontists. *Journal of Prosthodontics: Implant, Esthetic and Reconstructive Dentistry*. 2011;20:S1–S12.
7. Viljoen J, Azie N, Schmitt-Hoffmann A-H, Ghannoum M. A phase 2, randomized, double-blind, multicenter trial to evaluate the safety and efficacy of three dosing regimens of isavuconazole compared with fluconazole in patients with uncomplicated esophageal candidiasis. *Antimicrobial Agents and Chemotherapy*. 2015;59(3):1671–1679.
8. Saxby C, Ackroyd R, Callin S, Mayland C, Kite S. How should we measure emesis in palliative care? *Palliative Medicine*. 2007;21(5):369–383.
9. Glare P, Miller J, Nikolova T, Tickoo R. Treating nausea and vomiting in palliative care: a review. *Clinical Interventions in Aging*. 2011;6:243.
10. Reuben DB, Mor V. Nausea and vomiting in terminal cancer patients. *Archives of Internal Medicine*. 1986;146(10):2021–2023.

11. Kumar G, Hayes KA, Clark R. Efficacy of a scheduled IV cocktail of antiemetics for the palliation of nausea and vomiting in a hospice population. *American Journal of Hospice and Palliative Medicine.* 2008;*25*(3):184–189.

12. Del Fabbro E, Bruera E, Savarese D. Assessment and management of nausea and vomiting in palliative care:. *UpToDate.* 2017. Accessed on March 2016.

13. Smith HS, Smith EJ, Smith AR. Pathophysiology of nausea and vomiting in palliative medicine. *Annals of Palliative Medicine.* 2012;*1*(2):87–93.

14. Garrett K, Tsuruta K, Walker S, Jackson S, Sweat M. Managing nausea and vomiting: current strategies. *Critical Care Nurse.* 2003;*23*(1):31–50.

15. Ni Chroinin D, Montalto A, Jahromi S, Ingham N, Beveridge A, Foltyn P. Oral health status is associated with common medical comorbidities in older hospital inpatients. *Journal of the American Geriatrics Society.* 2016;*64*(8):1696–1700.

16. Goldstein NE, Morrison RS. *Evidence-Based Practice of Palliative Medicine E-Book.* Elsevier Health Sciences; 2012.

17. Roscoe JA, Morrow GR, Aapro MS, Molassiotis A, Olver I. Anticipatory nausea and vomiting. *Supportive Care in Cancer.* 2011;*19*(10):1533–1538.

18. Mahendraratnam N, Farley JF, Basch E, Proctor A, Wheeler SB, Dusetzina SB. Characterizing and assessing antiemetic underuse in patients initiating highly emetogenic chemotherapy. *Supportive Care in Cancer.* 2019;*27*(12):4525–4534.

19. Anderson WD III, Strayer SM. Evaluation of nausea and vomiting: a case-based approach. *American Family Physician.* 2013;*88*(6):371–379.

20. Bruera E, Belzile M, Neumann C, Harsanyi Z, Babul N, Darke A. A double-blind, crossover study of controlled-release metoclopramide and placebo for the chronic nausea and dyspepsia of advanced cancer. *Journal of Pain and Symptom Management.* 2000;*19*(6):427–435.

21. Navari RM, Qin R, Ruddy KJ, Liu H, Powell SF, Bajaj M, Dietrich L, Biggs D, Lafky JM, Loprinzi CL. Olanzapine for the Prevention of Chemotherapy-Induced Nausea and Vomiting. *New England Journal of Medicine.* 2016 Jul 14;*375*(2):134–142. doi:10.1056/NEJMoa1515725. PMID: 27410922; PMCID: PMC5344450.

22. Kumar A, Solanki SL, Gangakhedkar GR, Shylasree T, Sharma KS. Comparison of palonosetron and dexamethasone with ondansetron and dexamethasone for postoperative nausea and vomiting in postchemotherapy ovarian cancer surgeries requiring opioid-based patient-controlled analgesia: a randomised, double-blind, active controlled study. *Indian Journal of Anaesthesia.* 2018;*62*(10):773.

23. Abrams DI, Guzman M. Cannabis in cancer care. *Clinical Pharmacology & Therapeutics.* 2015;*97*(6):575–586.

24. Hall W, Christie M, Currow D. Cannabinoids and cancer: causation, remediation, and palliation. *Lancet Oncology.* 2005;*6*(1):35–42.

25. Meeks TW, Jeste DV. Beyond the black box: what is the role for antipsychotics in dementia? *Current Psychiatry.* 2008;*7*(6):50.

26. Ralph SJ, Espinet AJ. Use of antipsychotics and benzodiazepines for dementia: time for action? What will be required before global de-prescribing? *Dementia.* 2019;*18*(6):2322–2339.

27. 2019 American Geriatrics Society Beers Criteria® Expert Update Panel. American Geriatrics Society 2019 updated AGS Beers Criteria for potentially inappropriate medication use in older adults. *Journal of the American Geriatrics Society.* 2019;*67*(4):674–694.

28. Chiu L, Chow R, Popovic M, et al. Efficacy of olanzapine for the prophylaxis and rescue of chemotherapy-induced nausea and vomiting (CINV): a systematic review and meta-analysis. *Supportive Care in Cancer.* 2016;*24*(5):2381–2392.

29. Navari RM, Qin R, Ruddy KJ, et al. Olanzapine for the prevention of chemotherapy-induced nausea and vomiting. *New England Journal of Medicine.* 2016;*375*(2):134–142.

30. Harris D. Safe and effective prescribing for symptom management in palliative care. *British Journal of Hospital Medicine.* 2019;*80*(12):C184–C189.

31. Navari RM, Reinhardt RR, Gralla RJ, et al. Reduction of cisplatin-induced emesis by a selective neurokinin-1–receptor antagonist. *New England Journal of Medicine.* 1999;*340*(3):190–195.

32. Parker LA, Rock EM, Limebeer CL. Regulation of nausea and vomiting by cannabinoids. *British Journal of Pharmacology.* 2011;*163*(7):1411–1422.

33. Muldrew DH, Hasson F, Carduff E, et al. Assessment and management of constipation for patients receiving palliative care in specialist palliative care settings: a systematic review of the literature. *Palliative Medicine.* 2018;*32*(5):930–938.

34. Sykes N. Constipation and diarrhoea. *Management of Advanced Disease.* 2004:94.

35. Librach SL, Bouvette M, De Angelis C, et al.; Canadian Consensus Development Group for Constipation in Patients With Advanced Progressive Illness. Consensus recommendations for the management of constipation in patients with advanced, progressive illness. *Journal of Pain and Symptom Management.* 2010;*40*(5):761–773.

36. Larkin PJ, Sykes N, Centeno C, et al. The management of constipation in palliative care: clinical practice recommendations. *Palliative Medicine.* 2008;*22*(7):796–807.

37. Davies A, Leach C, Caponero R, et al. MASCC recommendations on the management of constipation in patients with advanced cancer. *Supportive Care in Cancer.* 2020;*28*(1):23–33.

38. Dhingra L, Shuk E, Grossman B, et al. A qualitative study to explore psychological distress and illness burden associated with opioid-induced constipation in cancer patients with advanced disease. *Palliative Medicine.* 2013;*27*(5):447–456.

39. Ducrotté P, Caussé C. The Bowel Function Index: a new validated scale for assessing opioid-induced constipation. *Current Medical Research and Opinion.* 2012;*28*(3):457–466.

40. Russo M, Strisciuglio C, Scarpato E, Bruzzese D, Casertano M, Staiano A. Functional chronic constipation: Rome III criteria versus Rome IV criteria. *Journal of Neurogastroenterology and Motility.* 2019;*25*(1):123.

41. Clemens KE, Klaschik E. Management of constipation in palliative care patients. *Current Opinion in Supportive and Palliative Care.* 2008;*2*(1):22–27.

42. Alame AM, Bahna H. Evaluation of constipation. *Clinics in Colon and Rectal Surgery.* 2012;*25*(1):5.

43. Andrews CN, Storr M. The pathophysiology of chronic constipation. *Canadian Journal of Gastroenterology.* 2011;*25*(Suppl B):16B–21B.

44. Lever E, Cole J, Scott S, Emery P, Whelan K. Systematic review: the effect of prunes on gastrointestinal function. *Alimentary Pharmacology & Therapeutics.* 2014;*40*(7):750–758.

45. Ishihara M, Ikesue H, Matsunaga H, et al. A multi-institutional study analyzing effect of prophylactic medication for prevention of opioid-induced gastrointestinal dysfunction. *Clinical Journal of Pain.* 2012;*28*(5):373–381.

46. Etropolski M, Kelly K, Okamoto A, Rauschkolb C. Comparable efficacy and superior gastrointestinal tolerability (nausea, vomiting, constipation) of tapentadol compared with oxycodone hydrochloride. *Advances in Therapy.* 2011;*28*(5):401–417.

47. Radbruch L, Sabatowski R, Loick G, et al. Constipation and the use of laxatives: a comparison between transdermal fentanyl and oral morphine. *Palliative Medicine.* 2000;*14*(2):111–119.

48. Haazen L, Noorduin H, Megens A, Meert T. The constipation-inducing potential of morphine and transdermal fentanyl. *European Journal of Pain.* 1999;*3*(S1):9–15.

49. Wirz S, Wittmann M, Schenk M, et al. Gastrointestinal symptoms under opioid therapy: a prospective comparison of oral sustained-release hydromorphone, transdermal fentanyl, and transdermal buprenorphine. *European Journal of Pain.* 2009;*13*(7):737–743.

50. Emanuel LL, Librach SL. *Palliative Care E-Book: Core Skills and Clinical Competencies.* Elsevier Health Sciences; 2011.

51. Thomas J, Karver S, Cooney GA, et al. Methylnaltrexone for opioid-induced constipation in advanced illness. *New England Journal of Medicine.* 2008;*358*(22):2332–2343.

52. Candy B, Jones L, Larkin PJ, Vickerstaff V, Tookman A, Stone P. Laxatives for the management of constipation in people receiving palliative care. *Cochrane Database of Systematic Reviews.* 2015;*2015*(5):CD003448.

53. Nee J, Zakari M, Sugarman MA, et al. Efficacy of treatments for opioid-induced constipation: systematic review and meta-analysis. *Clinical Gastroenterology and Hepatology.* 2018;*16*(10):1569–1584. e1562.

54. Chu C, Rotondo-Trivette S, Michail S. Chronic diarrhea. *Current Problems in Pediatric and Adolescent Health Care.* 2020;*50*(8):100841.

55. Schiller LR, Pardi DS, Sellin JH. Chronic diarrhea: diagnosis and management. *Clinical Gastroenterology and Hepatology.* 2017;*15*(2):182–193.e183.

56. Maroun JA, Anthony LB, Blais N, et al. Prevention and management of chemotherapy-induced diarrhea in patients with colorectal cancer: a consensus statement by the Canadian Working Group on Chemotherapy-Induced Diarrhea. *Current Oncology.* 2007;*14*(1):13.

57. Abigerges D, Armand J-P, Chabot GG, et al. Irinotecan (CPT-11) high-dose escalation using intensive high-dose loperamide to control diarrhea. *JNCI: Journal of the National Cancer Institute.* 1994;*86*(6):446–449.

58. Yanai S, Nakamura S, Matsumoto T. Nivolumab-induced colitis treated by infliximab. *Clinical Gastroenterology and Hepatology.* 2017;*15*(4):e80–e81.

59. Robert C, Long GV, Brady B, et al. Nivolumab in previously untreated melanoma without BRAF mutation. *New England Journal of Medicine.* 2015;*372*(4):320–330.

60. Bicanovsky LK, Lagman RL, Davis MP, Walsh D. Managing nonmalignant chronic abdominal pain and malignant bowel obstruction. *Gastroenterology Clinics.* 2006;*35*(1):131–142.

61. Tavares CN, Kimbrel JM, Protus BM, Grauer PA. Petroleum jelly (Vaseline balls) for the treatment of constipation: a survey of hospice and palliative care practitioners. *American Journal of Hospice and Palliative Medicine.* 2014;*31*(8):797–803.

62. Ripamonti C, Bruera E. Palliative management of malignant bowel obstruction. *International Journal of Gynecologic Cancer.* 2002;*12*(2):135–143.

63. Chakraborty A, Selby D, Gardiner K, Myers J, Moravan V, Wright F. Malignant bowel obstruction: natural history of a heterogeneous patient population followed prospectively over two years. *Journal of Pain and Symptom Management.* 2011;*41*(2):412–420.

64. Franke AJ, Iqbal A, Starr JS, Nair RM, George Jr TJ. Management of malignant bowel obstruction associated with GI cancers. *Journal of Oncology Practice.* 2017;*13*(7):426–434.

65. Goldberg J, Goldman D, McCaskey S, Koo D, Epstein A. Illness understanding, prognostic awareness and end of life care after drainage percutaneous endoscopic gastrostomy for malignant bowel obstruction in metastatic gastrointestinal cancer (FR481C). *Journal of Pain and Symptom Management.* 2018;*55*(2):633.

66. Hardy J, Haberecht J. Palliative care: core skills and clinical competencies.—by LL Emanuel and SL Librach. *Internal Medicine Journal.* 2008;*38*(12):933.

67. Mercadante S, Chen W. Palliative care of bowel obstruction in cancer patients. 2017.

12

Cardiopulmonary System

Kimberly Angelia Curseen and Jabeen Taj

Introduction

According to the World Health Organization, heart disease is the leading cause and chronic lower respiratory disease the fourth leading cause of death. Over 600,000 die from heart disease each year.[1] It is estimated that 328 million people worldwide have chronic obstructive pulmonary disease (COPD). In 15 years, it will surpass cardiac disease as the leading cause of death.[2] It is not surprising that heart and lung diseases are also the third and fourth leading diagnoses for hospice admission, respectively.[3] Patients with these chronic illnesses are managed by interprofessional teams that include physician assistants, and they provide primary palliative care (Table 12.1).[4]

The broad range of palliative care needs are similar in cardiopulmonary disease as in other forms of serious illness. Patients require symptom management for total pain and suffering; serious illness conversations; and holistic support for the patient and their caregivers through the interdisciplinary team (physician, advanced practice provider, nurse, chaplain, and social worker). For a description of some of the common diseases that fall in the purview of cardiopulmonary palliative care, please refer to Box 12.1.[5]

Physical Symptoms in Cardiopulmonary Disease

Whenever a patient with cardiopulmonary disorders is able to self-report symptoms, a robust history and physical examination are the best tools to implement accurate symptom management. This approach is the most likely to achieve patient comfort.

In cardiopulmonary diseases, patients have classic versus nonclassic symptoms. Classic symptoms tend to respond to primary disease management performed by primary teams or primary palliative care management. The nonclassic symptoms may or may not respond to disease-directed therapy and may require a more individualized symptom-focused approach.

TABLE 12.1 Primary Versus Specialty Palliative Care Cardiopulmonary Disease[4]

Primary Palliative Care	Secondary Palliative Care
- Basic symptom management	- Complex symptom management
- Prognosis diagnosis	- Conflict resolution
- Shared decision-making: goals of treatment; treatment preferences	- Complex decision-making
	- Psychological, social, spiritual distress
- Advance care planning	- Transition to hospice

BOX 12.1 Common Cardiopulmonary Diseases Leading to Palliative Care Referrals

Obstructive lung disease-
Chronic obstructive pulmonary disease (COPD)/emphysema
Restrictive lung disease
Interstitial lung disease, idiopathic pulmonary fibrosis, amyotrophic lateral sclerosis
Advanced heart failure
Cystic fibrosis
Adult congenital heart disease
Primary pulmonary hypertension

For example, management of nausea in advanced heart failure differs from management of nausea secondary to chemotherapy and is based on the pathophysiology: gut congestion >> delayed gastric emptying, acid reflux >> proton pump inhibitors/H_2 blockers. This is helpful in management of nausea and vomiting in end-stage heart failure. These kinds of symptoms are often appropriately managed by specialty palliative care (Table 12.2).[6]

TABLE 12.2 Commonly Seen Symptoms in Cardiopulmonary Disease[6]

Classic (Respond to Disease-Directed Therapy)	Nonclassic (May or May Not Respond to Disease-Directed Therapy)
Fatigue	Anorexia, thirst
Dyspnea	Nausea
Edema	Pain (25%–75%)
	Anxiety
	Depression
	Insomnia
	Delirium
	Refractory dyspnea

Pain Management

The principles of pain management remain the same as in any serious or chronic illness. A good pain history requires time and a focused interview, including location, intensity, quality, and radiation of pain and relieving and exacerbating factors. This includes temporal patterns (i.e., worse during the day or night, relationship to meals, sleep disruption). For example, if a patient reports waking up in pain every single morning, the prescription of a long-acting pain medicine at bedtime provides more restful sleep, and the patient will awaken more refreshed and in less pain.

Effective treatment of pain is dependent on an accurate pain assessment. For example, management of neuropathic pain is quite different from that of visceral pain, which is seen in reduced end-organ perfusion. Generally, the lowest dose of opioids with low-to-moderate potency—such as oxycodone or low-dose morphine—is a good starting point in agents for patients with cardiopulmonary disease and chronic pain issues. Unlike cancer pain, visceral pain may have a variable response to opioids, and it tends to improve with treatment of the underlying disease state. As the disease becomes progressively more refractory to therapy, pain becomes severe and poorly controlled. In this situation, it is reasonable to titrate opioids to more pure preparations, such as morphine sulfate, including long-acting morphine, fentanyl, and hydromorphone. We do not recommend combination agents (acetaminophen-codeine or acetaminophen-hydrocodone) due to the ceiling doses of acetaminophen that are reached before opioids can be effectively titrated.

The nonsteroidal anti-inflammatory drugs are contraindicated in congestive heart failure and in patients with renal disease or risk of bleeding.[7] Although infrequently seen in a disease with cardiac problems, amyotrophic lateral sclerosis (ALS) causes pain related to spasm, which responds well to nonopioid antispasmodics such as baclofen, cyclobenzaprine, or diazepam. Nonopioid pain medications such as acetaminophen are recommended prior to opioids/adjuvant.[8]

Dyspnea

Dyspnea is defined as the subjective awareness of one's breathing.[9] There are several scales that can be used to grade dyspnea as a symptom, such as the Respiratory Distress Observation Scale (RDOS), which can also be useful in the assessment of a patient who cannot self-report (Table 12.3).[10]

Guidelines for use:

1. RDOS is not a substitute for patient self-report if able.
2. RDOS is an adult assessment tool.
3. RDOS cannot be used when the patient is paralyzed with a neuromuscular blocking agent.
4. Count respiratory and heart rates for 1 minute; auscultate if necessary.
5. Grunting may be audible with intubated patients on auscultation.[10]

TABLE 12.3 Objective Scales to Assess Respiratory Distress: Respiratory Distress Observation Scale (RDOS)

Variable	0 Points	1 Point	2 Points	Total
Heart rate per minute	<90 beats	90–109 beats	≥110 beats	
Respiratory rate per minute	≤18 breaths	19–30 breaths	>30 breaths	
Restlessness/nonpurposeful movements	None	Occasional, slight movements	Frequent movements	
Paradoxical breathing pattern: abdomen moves in on inspiration	None		Present	
Accessory muscle use: rise in clavicle on inspiration	None	Slight rise	Pronounced rise	
Grunting: guttural sound at the end of inspiration	None		Present	
Nasal flaring: involuntary movement of nares	None		Present	
Look of fear	None		Eyes wide open, facial muscles tense, brow furrowed, mouth open, teeth together	
Total				

Management of dyspnea in a patient with advanced refractory cardiopulmonary illness is a complicated task that requires both knowledge and expertise, which facilitates careful medication selection and adjustments. Nonpharmacological modalities are often more useful to manage dyspnea than pharmacological means. These include bedside fan, elevation of the head of the bed, pursed-lip breathing, or different positions, especially if pleural effusion is involved. These are interventions that can be employed for better control of dyspnea that reduce anxiety and instill a sense of control of one's body functions.[9]

Dyspnea in advanced life-limiting diseases responds well to opioid therapy, and the starting doses are generally much lower than those used for pain. Generally, a low dose such as 2.5–5 mg of oral morphine solution every 2–4 hours as needed for breathlessness is a good starting dosage for patients with severe dyspnea. Total morphine dosage over 24 hours can be used to calculate the lowest but most effective long-acting form. This may require a frequency of three times daily for sustained control of symptoms.[11]

Severe respiratory distress or a dyspnea crisis—which was defined by the American Thoracic Society (2009) as "sustained and severe resting breathing discomfort that occurs in patients with advanced, often life-limiting illness and overwhelm the patient and caregivers 'ability to achieve symptom relief'"—requires rapid treatment with periodic adjustments to alleviate the crisis. For the hospitalized terminally ill patient, it is reasonable to consider intravenous opioids titrated to effect to achieve comfort. Systemic opioids are effective medications to manage severe dyspnea and associated anxiety in these situations. Benzodiazepines are not first-line therapy for dyspnea but they may be useful when there is an associated

---

BOX 12.2 Modified Medical Research Council (MRC) Scale

1- I only get breathless with strenuous exercise.

2- I get short of breath when hurrying on a level or walking up a slight hill.

3- I walk slower than people of the same age on the level because of breathlessness or have to stop for breath when walking at my own pace on the level.

4- I stop for breath after walking about 100 yards or after a few minutes on the level.

5- I am too breathless to leave the house or I am breathless when dressing.

---

element of anxiety.[12] Refer to Box 12.2 for a subjective measurement scale that is useful to evaluate patients' dyspnea severity.[13]

Cough

Evaluation and management of cough is similar to the management of dyspnea. The most appropriate first step for patients with cardiopulmonary illnesses is identification and treatment of the underlying comorbidities. For patients with heart failure, this may mean diuresis; for patients with COPD, a trial of bronchodilators and/or steroids may be beneficial. It is also important to consider that patients who are chronically ill may have developed gastroparesis, which can increase gastric reflux; this can also trigger a nonproductive cough. When managing cough, first-line agents should be antitussives such as dextromethorphan and benzonatate alone or with the addition of an antitussive opioid. In order to mitigate risk of adverse events, in this instance it is important to take into consideration other concomitant opioids that are being used for pain management. Expectorants such as guaifenesin can be useful as well. Many medications used for pain and symptom management—such as nonsteroidal anti-inflammatories and opiates—can potentiate reflux. Patients treated with proton pump inhibitors or H_2 blockers to alleviate gastric reflux will show improvement of their cough. For refractory cough, there is some evidence for use of nebulized lidocaine, and there is mixed evidence for use of nebulized morphine and fentanyl.[14]

Fatigue

Fatigue management can be challenging for cardiopulmonary disease patients. Fatigue in heart failure with a reduced ejection fraction is associated with poor prognosis and depression.[15] In a study evaluating patients with New York Heart Association (NYHA) class III–IV heart failure, 60% reported fatigue as their worst symptom or combined with dyspnea. This led to reductions in self-care and poor prognosis. Optimization of heart failure management is an important strategy. If fatigue is acute, the heart failure team should consider cardiac medication adjustments.[16] Palliative care providers should treat fatigue in these patients by using a multimodal approach that focuses first on education and then on nonpharmacological strategies, which include good sleep hygiene for the patient, including avoiding technology in the bedroom, no caffeine in the afternoon or evening, and minimizing naps during the day. Strategies such as energy conservation and problem-solving group therapy have been proposed as interventions. These empower patients to manage their symptoms by learning to live within the limitations of the illness and make appropriate accommodations (i.e., *adjust to the new normal*). Palliative interdisciplinary teams that provide support in person or through telehealth (virtual medicine) can be helpful in improving quality of life for patients who struggle with this symptom.[17] Management of comorbid conditions, including depression and insomnia, are essential. Side-effect burden related to pharmacological interventions such as steroids and psychostimulants must be carefully balanced.

Insomnia

Insomnia should be managed nonpharmacologically. It is imperative to address sleep hygiene. Evaluation of insomnia should include nocturnal hypoxia, orthopnea, obstructive sleep apnea, restless leg syndrome, and anxiety. All of these conditions contribute to restlessness. If possible, focus treatment on the underlying condition and minimize nocturnal dosing of medications such as diuretics. Insomnia may be an appropriate response to physiologic distress. Patients who have suffered a cardiopulmonary arrest, intubations, and episodes of severe respiratory distress can develop post-traumatic stress or severe anxiety around sleeping for fear of dying or awakening unable to breath. In those cases, management of the anxiety with counseling, selective serotonin reuptake inhibitors (SSRIs), and/or low-dose benzodiazepines may be appropriate. Sedative hypnotics have addictive side effects and are recommended only for short-term use. There is a further risk of side effects in these patients because of compromised liver and kidney function and reduced metabolism. There is some data supporting the use of trazodone for anxiety in patients with COPD, and this may be an acceptable sleeping agent.[18,19]

Cardiopulmonary Cachexia

Anorexia and cachexia syndrome is defined as the decrease in body weight and food intake followed by a compensatory increase in appetite or decreased energy expenditure. Anorexia cachexia syndrome has been identified in several chronic conditions including cancer, COPD, congestive heart failure, chronic kidney disease, and aging.[20] Cardiopulmonary cachexia is a negative prognostic indicator; there is a 50% mortality rate at 18 months. These patients have low prealbumin, which is the best biomarker for cachexia. Patients have increased urinary albumin, which is also a poor prognostic sign. Increases in baseline dyspnea also decrease oral intake.[21,22] Treatment of this condition is not going to affect prognosis, but its presence is distressing to patients and families. Early patient and family counseling concerning this helps with understanding and setting realistic expectations. Evaluation for other causes of weight loss and anorexia is important (i.e., nausea, constipation, dysgeusia, depression, and medication effects). It is important that food is not viewed as a source of anxiety for patients or caregivers and to understand and validate rather than place undue pressure on them to increase oral intake. Physiologically, the natural disease progression incorporates a decreased oral intake. Development of nonpharmacological strategies for patients to enjoy food includes but is not limited to expansion of food choices; incorporation of several small meals a day; and choices that include favorite or "comfort" foods with high caloric value. This can be liberating for patients and caregivers alike. Management of this symptom requires shared decision-making surrounding goals of care. Pharmacological therapy may have limited benefit.

Delirium

Delirium is an acute, transient, fluctuating state of confusion resulting in inattentiveness and decreased awareness of one's surroundings. Delirium can be hypoactive (decreased physical and mental activity, inattention); hyperactive (combativeness, agitation); or mixed.[23] The first line of management of delirium is to identify and treat the underlying cause(s), and this includes optimization of medical therapy of underlying conditions; look for simple but easily overlooked causes like hypoglycemia or hypoxemia (Table 12.4).[24] However, once delirium has developed in end-stage cardiac or pulmonary disease, it is a poor prognostic sign. If the delirium is irreversible, this presents a diagnosis for hospice in addition to an opportunity to revisit the overall goals of care.[25]

Clinical tools to assess delirium include the Confusion Assessment Method and confusion assessment Method in Intensive Care Unit (CAM-ICU) Nursing Delirium Screening Scale score, Richmond Agitation and Sedation Scale, among others. An additional screening tool for differentiating delirium from dementia (cognition impaired) is the Montreal Cognitive Assessment.[23,24]

TABLE 12.4 Management of Delirium Is Dependent on Managing the Cause and Appropriate Workup

Etiology	Workup
Drugs	Toxicology, vitamin levels, heavy metal screening.
Electrolyte abnormalities	Complete blood count, serum chemistries, liver function tests, renal function tests, thyroid function tests.
Lack of drugs (withdrawal)	History and physical examination. No specific test is diagnostic; hence, all organ systems should be evaluated for pathology.
Infection	C-reactive protein, erythrocyte sedimentation rate, HIV, syphilis, urinalysis, and culture.
Reduced sensory input (hearing aids, glasses)	Elderly patients, particularly those in the intensive care unit are at risk of sensory deprivation.
Intracranial problems	Computed tomographic scan head/neck, brain magnetic resonance imaging, lumbar puncture.
Urinary retention and fecal impaction	Polypharmacy such as anticholinergic agents, benzodiazepines, opioids, dopaminergic agents.
Myocardial problems	Electrocardiogram, chest x-ray.

Concurrent strategies include reorienting patients, restoration of normal sleep-wake cycles, de-prescribing medications that potentiate or exacerbate delirium, provision of hearing aids/glasses, and removal of invasive devices and restraints, whenever possible. If pharmacological therapy is used, benzodiazepines should be avoided in favor of antipsychotics such as haloperidol (2 to 5 mg every 6 to 12 hours). It is appropriate to start with 50% of the recommended dose in patients aged 75 or older. However, for patients with advanced cardiac or pulmonary disease secondary to organ dysfunction, delirium may not be reversible and can transition to terminal delirium, which is irreversible.[1,26]

Psychological Distress

Anxiety is the most common psychological symptom in cardiopulmonary disease. This is directly influenced by the severity of dyspnea and vice versa, and it tends to improve as dyspnea improves. Undiagnosed and untreated pervasive anxiety is common in any serious illness and should be adequately managed as part of comprehensive supportive care. Anxiety may be related to physical distress as described above or psychological disorders such as major depression or adjustment disorder (Table 12.5).[27]

Understanding the underlying cause(s) of anxiety is an integral part of its effective management. Refractory dyspnea can be treated with opioids. Validation of anticipatory grief; education about breathing exercises; and guided imagery, music therapy, and pet therapy are all valuable approaches to treatment. When sporadic flares or significant triggers are seen, as in post-traumatic stress disorder, additional counseling is invaluable.[27,28]

TABLE 12.5 Common Psychological Disorders in Patients in Cardiopulmonary Disease

Anticipatory grief	Mourning the loss of a loved one before they have died; similar stages of grief intermingled with information gathering; difficulty processing complex emotions (guilt, regret, shame); need for validation; sadness; tearfulness; anxiety.
Grief	Mourning loss of functionality, vitality, life, life-changing event. Stages of grief include shock/denial, anger, bargaining, depression, acceptance (Kubler-Ross).
Seasonal affective disorder (SAD)	Depression related to changes in seasons: beginning and ending at the same time every year.
Adjustment disorder	Emotional and/or behavioral changes commence within 3 months of a specific stressor or trigger event.
Dysthymia	Persistent depressive disorder/chronic "mild" depression. May be triggered by major trauma, life-changing event, loss of a loved one, life stresses (e.g., financial worries).
Major depression	Depressed mood, anhedonia, significant weight change/appetite disturbance, psychomotor agitation/retardation, sleep disturbance (insomnia or hypersomnia), fatigue, feelings of worthlessness, difficulty concentrating, indecisiveness, suicidal thoughts/ideation.

It is important to distinguish temporal physiological responses such as sadness, grief, and anticipatory grief from mood disorders such as seasonal affective disorder, adjustment disorder, dysthymia, and major depression.[28] Pharmacological management of anxiety is primarily via utilization of SSRIs or serotonin-norepinephrine reuptake inhibitors, which affect the brain neurochemistry to stabilize mood. Benzodiazepines are used only in situations of panic attacks but do not play a significant role in long-term management of anxiety unless as short-term ancillary agents to SSRIs.[29]

Prognostication in Cardiopulmonary Disease

One of the findings in the SUPPORT study was that 54% of patients with advanced heart failure who died within 3 days were estimated by providers to have a prognosis of 6 months.[30] This general pattern of uncertainty makes prognostication difficult to communicate to patients, caregivers, and other providers because it can be variable depending on the individual patient and interventions. In a follow-up study to the SUPPORT trial, Dr. Muriel Gillick identified that barriers to effective communication, lack of cultural competence, and expansion of medical interventions that can be offered for patients at the end of life all result in more challenging decisions for patients, surrogates, and healthcare providers.[31]

In advanced cardiac disease, half of patients diagnosed with heart failure will live greater than 5 years. Patients with NYHA class III heart failure have a 4-year mortality rate of 40%, and class IV has a 1-year mortality rate of 64%.[32] Patients with COPD with stages 3–4 have a life expectancy between 8.5 and 5.8 years.[33,34] Mortality may not be impacted by hypercapnia or frequency of exacerbations.[33] These patients and families are living with chronic illness for a prolonged period of time. This provides an opportunity for ongoing goals-of-care discussions to develop over time, and this allows for advanced care planning to evolve based on the clinical course. These discussions need to include not only the goals of care and end-of-life planning, but also social planning. Social planning includes how a patient and family will manage with progressive disability—physical, emotional, psychosocial/spiritual, and financial. Patients and providers should participate in shared decision-making that takes into account these four aspects of patient care.[4]

Several prognostic tools exist to guide and help determine prognosis in patients with heart failure and COPD. These tools can help identify patients who have a poor prognosis and may benefit from specialty palliative care. Despite their inherent limitations, they can be useful starting points (Tables 12.6 and 12.7).[4,6,30,32–34]

The basics of communication with the seriously ill cardiac or pulmonary patient remain the same: compassionate truth telling while balancing empathy and hope.[4,35] Table 12.8 outlines the framework of goals-of-care and end-of-life care discussions with more complex and nuanced conversations that may need to happen with progressive illness.[4,35,36]

TABLE 12.6 Heart Failure

Model	Characteristics	Limitations
Seattle heart failure model	Online calculator of projected survival at baseline and after interventions for patients with heart failure; provides an accurate estimate of 1-, 2-, and 3-year survival (http://depts.washingtone.edu/shfm)	Model was based on stable outpatients, which may limit generalizability.
Heart Failure Risk Score	Online calculator for projecting 1- and 3-year all-cause mortality estimates for people with heart failure (http://www.heartfailurerisk.org).	Limited utility in patients with serious comorbidities.
Heart Failure Survival Score	Includes peak oxygen uptake (VO_2).	Does not risk stratify adults with congenital heart disease; requires cardiopulmonary testing patients may not have access to.
Congestion score	- Assesses patient with NYHA IV. - Gives points for orthopnea, diuretic increase, weight increase, edema, and jugular venous pressure. - 41% 2-year survival for scores 3–5	Relies on patient report for symptoms and physicians preforming consistent outpatient examinations 4–6 weeks posthospitalization.

TABLE 12.7 COPD Prognostication Tools

Model	Characteristics	Limitations
Body mass index, airflow obstruction, dyspnea, exercise capacity (BODE)	- Higher scores have greater number of COPD-related hospitalizations and increased risk of death from all causes. - Gives points based on forced expiratory volume in first second of expiration (FEV1), 6-minute walk, dyspnea scale, and body mass index. - Score between 7 and 10 = 18% 4-year survival rate. - https://www.mdcalc.com/bode-index-copd-survival	Not useful for guiding treatment; developed to predict prognosis
Global Initiative for Obstructive Lung Disease (GOLD)	- Clinically used to determine severity of expiratory airflow obstruction. - Categorize clinical severity. - Stage B may predict higher mortality than stage C. - Stages B, C, and D do not accurately reflect patient's functional status. - Measures symptom burden, exacerbation history, and FEV_1 percentage. - https://www.mdcalc.com/global-initiative-obstructive-lung-disease-gold-criteria-copd	Should not be used for diagnosis or during acute exacerbations
Pulmonary arterial hypertension	6MWT, 6MWD (Minimum Walk Distance).	Measured before initiating disease-directed therapies and as a marker of progress while titrating therapy; 6MWD of < 300 m heralds poor prognosis.

TABLE 12.8 Palliative Communication Framework in Cardiopulmonary Disease

Goals-of-Care Discussions	Reframing Goals With Progressive Illness
Knowing what you know about your illness, what's most important to you?	Have you thought about what your life goals would be as you got sicker?
What are you most proud of? What do you define as your legacy?	You have been so strong through this journey. You did everything that was asked of you.
What are you hopeful for? What are you worried about?	I hear what you are hoping for. I am worried that you are getting sicker from this disease faster than we thought.
How do you like to receive information? (simple, straightforward, no negative messages, piecemeal)	I'm afraid I don't have very positive news. You are feeling worse because your lungs are worse.
If time were short, what would you hope to accomplish?	Have you discussed with your loved ones what your wishes would be if you are unlikely to get better? (advance directive, living will, healthcare power of attorney)

Respiratory Support

Advanced respiratory support devices can be used to improve and prolong the length and quality of life. Understanding these interventions and how patients view them in their care is vital for the healthcare interdisciplinary teams. These interventions are also tools to help patients reach specific goals in the context of their serious illness progression. Even patients in hospice may continue with respiratory support if it improves their quality of life. Thus, any conversations surrounding discontinuation of these interventions are focused on whether or not they are continuing to support the goals of the patient. Consideration should also be given regarding whether these measures are still able to alleviate versus contribute to unintended suffering.

For patients with ALS who have elected to receive ongoing respiratory support, use of a bilevel positive airway pressure (BiPAP) machine or ventilator can provide an acceptable quality of life. By the time they are using these interventions regularly, they may also be appropriate for hospice care according to their prognosis. Use of these interventions is not counter to the hospice philosophy, if a patient has a prognosis of 6 months or less, which is based on the illness and not the intervention they are using (Table 12.9).[37–40]

Discontinuation of these interventions is prompted either by the patient's expressed wishes or the patient's cognitive and physical decline. Advance care planning conversations should cover this specific topic with patients/families early and should be revisited during the course of the patient's illness. Careful documentation is also important to help relay to healthcare providers and family members how these decisions were made so that patient wishes are followed. Advanced directives and Physician Orders for Life-Sustaining Treatments, Medical Orders for Life-Sustaining Treatments, and the like are intended to express explicit goals of care; however, the documentation process of these serious illness conversations is key to expressing the nuances of these decisions. This process will help "fill in the blanks."[39,40]

TABLE 12.9 Respiratory Support Interventions

Respiratory Device	Mechanism	Uses
CPAP: continuous positive airway pressure	Set continuous pressure throughout respiratory cycle, nocturnal/nap support.	- Primary use for obstructive sleep apnea
BIPAP: bilevel positive airway pressure	Present inspiratory and expiratory pressures; patient initiates breath; can set a backup respiratory rate; primary nocturnal/nap or short-course support.	- Chronic obstructive lung disease acute/chronic - Sleep apnea - Nocturnal support for respiratory weakness - Helpful in congestive heart failure exacerbations
Trilogy: noninvasive positive pressure ventilation	Noninvasive ventilator; volume control and pressure control ventilator rolled into one system; can be used for both invasive and noninvasive ventilation.	- Respiratory weakness in ALS - Neuromuscular d/o affecting respiration - Spinal cord injury affecting respiration - Can be used for other respiratory d/o requiring ventilator support
High-flow nasal cannula	Therapy is an oxygen supply system capable of delivering up to 100% humidified and heated oxygen at a flow rate of up to 60 liters per minute.	- Infants with bronchiolitis - Postextubation - Interstitial lung disease - Respiratory illness requiring high-flow oxygen

It is important to contact hospice providers whenever transitioning patients who are using respiratory support devices to determine if these providers can support this request. There is no criteria barring the use of these interventions, but based on cost and their availability, access can be limited. Prior discussion allows for a smooth transition to hospice services.

Advanced Cardiac Therapies

Patients who are potential candidates for a left ventricular assist device (LVAD) implantation require palliative care consultation/assessments, as is now included in the preassessment guidelines in concert with cardiology. For patients who choose not to receive this therapy, transitioning to in-home palliative care and hospice is appropriate. The *Colorado Program for Patient Center Decisions* has developed a decision aid tailored to patients and providers to guide discussions concerning the LVAD and also implantable cardioverter-defibrillators. It is a valuable resource.[41]

For the patients who will have an LVAD as destination therapy, there are important statistics to convey in the conversation with the patient, caregivers, and team members. The 1-year survival was 89.5%; 2-year was 81.4%; 3-year was 60.8%; and 5-year was 29.8%. This was compared to the survival rates of patients using an LVAD as a bridge to heart transplantation.[42] For patients who have had transplants, 85%–95% survive 1 year, and the 10-year survival rate is approximately 50%.[43]

Palliative care team members must also be able to assess and manage the symptoms that can result from the device, which may include pain and psychosocial and existential suffering. Furthermore, an important end-of-life issue for palliative care providers and hospices is LVAD discontinuation. This requires close consultation with cardiology teams to develop and utilize appropriate protocols. Conversations related to the eventual discontinuation of an LVAD should be part of advance care planning prior to consideration of LVAD implantation as an option.[44,45]

Patients with advanced systolic heart failure receive intravenous inotrope therapy—most commonly dobutamine and milrinone.[46] This is an ongoing therapy that is used for acute heart failure and can now be transitioned in the palliative medicine arena. Its goal is to improve heart failure symptoms and quality of life for patients in the short term. However, even for patients who do have an LVAD, these infusions may be part of end-of-life care. Palliative care providers will need to work closely with heart failure/cardiology teams to safely discontinue these medications while continuing to relieve symptoms.

Although some providers may struggle with this choice, deactivation of automated implantable cardioverter-defibrillator (AICD) at the end of life is appropriate for patients who choose this option. For many patients and families, the fear of receiving shocks from a defibrillator is frightening, and the option for deactivation is comforting. Furthermore, it may be ethically appropriate for patients and caregivers to choose this option. It is vital to have the discussion regarding the timing of deactivating an AICD prior to placement and during advance care planning. This allows patients and families/caregivers to ask questions, understand the procedure, and review symptoms. Once this decision is made and documented, the AICD unit is usually deactivated by technicians. In an emergency, the device can be deactivated by holding a strong magnet over it until a technician can be summoned.[47]

Deactivation of pacemakers has been more challenging for the medical community to reconcile. There is no ethical difference with regard to deactivation of the pacemaker versus other life-sustaining therapies. Some providers can be concerned that the deactivation of the pacemaker is different and more akin to medical or physician aid in dying. For some providers, the deactivation causes moral distress, which can be difficult to alleviate. In patients who had an atrioventricular nodal ablation, a provider may feel by deactivation of the pacemaker they are causing the death of the patient. However, patients are not obligated to continue life-sustaining therapies if they are contrary to their wishes at the end of life. Despite this, it still can be difficult for providers to accept they are not culpable in the death of the patient. As with other procedures, patients considering this option should be counseled concerning process, clinical implications, benefits, and risk. It is also important to review the protocols within your own institution to fully assess what barriers may exist and provide education for patients, families, and team members about them. If there is internal conflict, one should consider an ethics consultation to assist in the shared decision-making.[47,48] Palliative care teams can support healthcare providers and staff who may struggle with a deactivation decision by providing a safe debriefing space.

BOX 12.3 Hospice LCD[a,49,50]

Advanced heart failure: Ejection fraction ≤ 20%, NYHA class IV despite traditional heart failure therapies and noncandidacy for advanced heart failure therapies; cardiorenal syndrome.

Amyotrophic lateral sclerosis: Declining vital capacity (less than 30%); recurrent upper urinary tract infections such as pyelonephritis and sepsis; rapid decline of functional status and activities of daily living

Pulmonary disease: Disabling dyspnea as defined by FEV_1 < 30% of predicted, severe hypoxemia with PO_2 consistently ≤ 88% and hypercapnia PCO_2 ≥≥ 55 mm Hg from recent hospitalizations (past 3 months). This may be supported by further diagnoses, such as pulmonary hypertension, cor pulmonale, right-sided heart failure.

[a] LCDs are regional in their distribution and may differ based on coverage for those regions.

Referrals to Hospice

Patients are eligible for hospice when they have a life-limiting illness with a prognosis of 6 months or less. However, the uncertainty of prognosis can be a barrier to referral in cardiopulmonary illnesses (i.e., *How soon is too soon?*). In addition to attestation from two physicians about the terminal diagnosis and prognosis, hospice agencies use local coverage determinations (LCDs) and national coverage determinations to assess eligibility for hospice care.[49,50] Knowing these can help provide the needed supporting documentation required when making appropriate referrals. See Box 12.3 for some pertinent LCDs.

References

1. Benjamin EJ, Blaha MJ, Chiuve SE, et al. American Heart Association statistics committee and stroke statistics subcommittee. Heart disease and stroke statistics—2017 update: a report from the American Heart Association. *Circulation*. 2017;*135*(10):e146–e603.
2. Quaderi S, Hurst J. The unmet global burden of COPD. *Global Health, Epidemiology and Genomics* 2018;*3*:e4.
3. Mahler DA, Cerasoli F, Della L, Rudzinski M. Internet health behaviors of patients with chronic obstructive pulmonary disease and assessment of two disease websites. *Chronic Obstructive Pulmonary Diseases*. 2018;*5*(3):158.
4. Chuzi S, Pak ES, Desai AS, Schaefer KG, Warraich HJ. Role of palliative care in the outpatient management of the chronic heart failure patient. *Current Heart Failure Reports*. 2019;*16*(6):220–228.
5. Feder SL, Jean RA, Bastian L, Akgün KM. National trends in palliative care use among older adults with cardiopulmonary and malignant conditions. *Heart & Lung*. 2020;*49*(4):370–376.

6. Celli BR. Predictors of mortality in COPD. *Respiratory Medicine.* 2010;*104*(6):773–779.

7. Klinedinst R, Kornfield ZN, Hadler RA. Palliative care for patients with advanced heart disease. *Journal of Cardiothoracic and Vascular Anesthesia.* 2019;*33*(3):833–843.

8. Nicholson K, Murphy A, McDonnell E, et al. Improving symptom management for people with amyotrophic lateral sclerosis. *Muscle & Nerve.* 2018;*57*(1):20–24.

9. Crisafulli E, Clini EM. Measures of dyspnea in pulmonary rehabilitation. *Multidisciplinary Respiratory Medicine.* 2010;*5*(3):202.

10. Zhuang Q, Yang GM, Neo SH-S, Cheung YB. Validity, reliability, and diagnostic accuracy of the Respiratory Distress Observation Scale for assessment of dyspnea in adult palliative care patients. *Journal of Pain and Symptom Management.* 2019;*57*(2):304–310.

11. Sood A, Dobbie K, Tang WW. Palliative care in heart failure. *Current Treatment Options in Cardiovascular Medicine.* 2018;*20*(5):43.

12. Mularski RA, Reinke LF, Carrieri-Kohlman V, et al. An official American Thoracic Society workshop report: assessment and palliative management of dyspnea crisis. *Annals of the American Thoracic Society.* 2013;*10*(5):S98–106 doi:10.1513/AnnalsATS.201306-169ST

13. Cheng S-L, Lin C-H, Wang C-C, et al. Comparison between COPD Assessment Test (CAT) and modified Medical Research Council (mMRC) dyspnea scores for evaluation of clinical symptoms, comorbidities and medical resources utilization in COPD patients. *Journal of the Formosan Medical Association.* 2019;*118*(1):429–435.

14. Morice AH, Shanks G. Pharmacology of cough in palliative care. *Current Opinion in Supportive and Palliative Care.* 2017;*11*(3):147–151.

15. Diamant MJ, Keshmiri H, Toma M. End-of-life care in patients with advanced heart failure. *Current Opinion in Cardiology.* 2020;*35*(2):156–161.

16. Kim YJ, Radloff JC, Crane PA, Bolin LP. Rehabilitation Intervention for individuals with heart failure and fatigue to reduce fatigue impact: a feasibility study. *Annals of Rehabilitation Medicine.* 2019;*43*(6):686.

17. Wallström S, Ali L, Ekman I, Swedberg K, Fors A. Effects of a person-centred telephone support on fatigue in people with chronic heart failure: subgroup analysis of a randomised controlled trial. *European Journal of Cardiovascular Nursing* 2020;*11*(5):393–400.

18. Naqvi SS, Pollok J, van Agteren JE, et al. Pharmacological interventions for the treatment of depression in chronic obstructive pulmonary disease. *Cochrane Database of Systematic Reviews.* 2016;*2016*(9).

19. Xiang Y-T, Wong T-S, Tsoh J, et al. Insomnia in older adults with chronic obstructive pulmonary disease (COPD) in Hong Kong: a case-control study. *COPD: Journal of Chronic Obstructive Pulmonary Disease.* 2014;*11*(3):319–324.

20. Engineer DR, Garcia JM. Leptin in anorexia and cachexia syndrome. *International Journal of Peptides* 2012;*2012*:287457.

21. Treece J, Chemchirian H, Hamilton N, et al. A review of prognostic tools in heart failure. *American Journal of Hospice and Palliative Medicine.* 2018;*35*(3):514–522.

22. Yoshida T, Delafontaine P. Mechanisms of cachexia in chronic disease states. *American Journal of the Medical Sciences.* 2015;*350*(4):250–256.

23. Bush SH, Tierney S, Lawlor PG. Clinical assessment and management of delirium in the palliative care setting. *Drugs.* 2017;*77*(15):1623–16243.

24. Miranda F, Arevalo-Rodriguez I, Díaz G, et al. Confusion Assessment Method for the intensive care unit (CAM-ICU) for the diagnosis of delirium in adults in critical care settings. *Cochrane Database of Systematic Reviews.* 2018;*2018*(9):CD013126.

25. Hosker CM, Bennett MI. Delirium and agitation at the end of life. *BMJ.* 2016;*353*:i3085.

26. Fink AM, Gonzalez RC, Lisowski T, et al. Fatigue, inflammation, and projected mortality in heart failure. *Journal of Cardiac Failure.* 2012;*18*(9):711–716.

27. Usmani ZA, Carson KV, Heslop K, Esterman AJ, De Soyza A, Smith BJ. Psychological therapies for the treatment of anxiety disorders in chronic obstructive pulmonary disease. *Cochrane Database of Systematic Reviews.* 2017;*2017*(3):CD010673.

28. Moser DK, Arslanian-Engoren C, Biddle MJ, et al. Psychological aspects of heart failure. *Current Cardiology Reports.* 2016;*18*(12):119.

29. Sharfman G, Braun UK. *Palliative and End-of-Life Issues in Patients With Advanced Respiratory Diseases. Depression and Anxiety in Patients With Chronic Respiratory Diseases.* Springer; 2017:183–194.

30. Connors AF, Dawson NV, Desbiens NA, et al. A controlled trial to improve care for seriously ill hospitalized patients: the Study to Understand Prognoses and Preferences for Outcomes and Risks of Treatments (SUPPORT). *JAMA.* 1995;*274*(20):1591–1598.

31. Gillick MR. Decision making near life's end: a prescription for change. *Journal of Palliative Medicine.* 2009;*12*(2):121–125 doi:10.1089/jpm.2008.0240

32. Taylor CJ, Ordóñez-Mena JM, Roalfe AK, et al. Trends in survival after a diagnosis of heart failure in the United Kingdom 2000–2017: population based cohort study. *BMJ.* 2019;*364*:I223.

33. Casanova C, de Torres JP, Aguirre-Jaíme A, et al. The progression of chronic obstructive pulmonary disease is heterogeneous: the experience of the BODE cohort. *American Journal of Respiratory and Critical Care Medicine.* 2011;*184*(9):1015–1021.

34. Shavelle RM, Paculdo DR, Kush SJ, Mannino DM, Strauss DJ. Life expectancy and years of life lost in chronic obstructive pulmonary disease: findings from the NHANES III Follow-up Study. *International Journal of Chronic Obstructive Pulmonary Disease.* 2009;*4*:137.

35. Schallmo MK, Dudley-Brown S, Davidson PM. Healthcare providers' perceived communication barriers to offering palliative care to patients with heart failure: an integrative review. *Journal of Cardiovascular Nursing.* 2019;*34*(2):E9–E18.

36. Back A, Arnold R, Tulsky J. *Mastering Communication With Seriously Ill Patients: Balancing Honesty With Empathy and Hope*: Cambridge University Press; 2009.

37. Daly FN, Lugassy MM. Correction to: Hospice and end of life care in neurologic disease. *Neuropalliative Care.* 2019;*105*:304.

38. Niedermeyer S, Murn M, Choi PJ. Respiratory failure in amyotrophic lateral sclerosis. *Chest.* 2019;*155*(2):401–408.

39. Coradazzi AL, Inhaia CL, Santana M, et al. Palliative withdrawal ventilation: why, when and how to do it? *Hospice & Palliative Medicine International Journal.* 2019;*3*:10–14.

40. Venkatnarayan K, Khilnani GC, Hadda V, et al. A comparison of three strategies for withdrawal of noninvasive ventilation in chronic obstructive pulmonary disease with acute respiratory failure: randomized trial. *Lung India.* 2020;*37*(1):3.

41. Thompson JS, Matlock DD, McIlvennan CK, Jenkins AR, Allen LA. Development of a decision aid for patients with advanced heart failure considering a destination therapy left ventricular assist device. *JACC: Heart Failure.* 2015;*3*(12):965–976.

42. Dhaliwal B, Becnel M, Merced-Ortiz F, et al. LVAD as bridge to transplant leads to better outcomes when compared to transplant-only strategy. *Journal of Cardiac Failure.* 2019;*25*(8):S156.

43. Anyanwu A, Treasure T. Prognosis after heart transplantation: transplants alone cannot be the solution for end stage heart failure: *BMJ.* 2003;*326*(7388):509–510.

44. Brush S, Budge D, Alharethi R, et al. End-of-life decision making and implementation in recipients of a destination left ventricular assist device. *Journal of Heart and Lung Transplantation* 2010;*29*(12):1337–1341.

45. McLean S, Dhonnchu TN, Mahon N, McQuillan R, Gordijn B, Ryan K. Left ventricular assist device withdrawal: an ethical discussion. *BMJ Supportive & Palliative Care.* 2014;*4*(2):193–195.

46. López-Candales A, Carron C, Schwartz J. Need for hospice and palliative care services in patients with end-stage heart failure treated with intermittent infusion of inotropes. *Clinical cardiology* 2004;*27*(1):23–28.

47. Farley MA, Goldstein NE, Hamilton RM, Wiegand DL, Richard Zellner J. HRS expert consensus statement on the management of cardiovascular implantable electronic devices (CIEDs) in patients nearing end of life or requesting withdrawal of therapy. 2010;*7*(7):1008–1026.

48. Bevins MB. The ethics of pacemaker deactivation in terminally ill patients. *Journal of Pain and Symptom Management.* 2011;*41*(6):1106–1110.
49. Medicare Cf, Services M. Medicare Coverage Database. LCD (local coverage determination) for hospice: determining terminal status (L25678).
50. Oberoi-Jassal R, Pope J, Jassal N. *Hospice Care.* Springer; 2019:937–939.

13

Genitourinary Issues in Palliative Care

Min Ji Kim and Kimberson Tanco

Voiding Issues and Incontinence
Urinary Retention

Etiology

Voiding properly requires the passage of urine to be unobstructed and for bladder structure and function to be intact. Activation of the parasympathetic system by cholinergic receptors leads to bladder contraction and bladder neck sphincter relaxation to allow voiding, while the sympathetic system controls the mechanisms necessary to store urine. Neurological impairment, such as compression of the spinal cord or injury to nerve roots due to tumor involvement, subsequently leads to difficulty with voiding. Decrease or interruption in urine output can also be due to an anatomical obstruction, usually in the lower urinary tract at the level of the bladder neck, prostate, or urethra[1] or in the upper urinary tract when both ureters are affected, such as in malignancy.[2,3] Obstruction in the lower urinary tract due to urethral stricture or scarring should be considered, especially in the setting of prior urethral instrumentation or injury, as well as evaluation for prostatic enlargement or cancer. Infectious causes for urinary retention in men and women include cystitis and urethritis.[3] Additional neurologic, obstructive, and infectious or inflammatory causes for urinary retention are listed in Table 13.1.

Medications that have an anticholinergic effect also cause voiding impairment due to relaxation of the bladder wall and contraction of the bladder neck sphincter.[4] Such medications frequently used in the palliative care setting include haloperidol, phenothiazines, antihistamines, and tricyclic antidepressants such as amitriptyline,[3] as seen in Table 13.2. Opioid use is also considered a risk factor, though most likely to occur along with concurrent factors such as preexisting early bladder outlet obstruction, advanced age, immobility, combination

TABLE 13.1 Obstructive, Neurologic, Infectious/Inflammatory Causes of Urinary Retention

Obstructive	Neurologic	Infectious/Inflammatory
Lower urinary tract • Urethral strictures • Transitional cell carcinoma (bladder) • Blood clot • Calculi/stones • Posterior urethral valves • Neurogenic bladder • Benign prostatic hypertrophy	Peripheral central nervous system (CNS) • Autonomic neuropathy • Diabetes mellitus • Guillain-Barré • Lyme disease • Herpes zoster • Pernicious anemia • Poliomyelitis • Tabes dorsalis	Men • Balantitis • Prostatitis • Cystitis • Periurethral abscess • Urethritis
Upper urinary tract • Ureteral calculi or strictures • Kidney stones • External mass/tumor • Transitional cell carcinoma (ureter, kidney) • Retroperitoneal fibrosis • Infection • Obstructed stent • Blood clot • Trauma	Central CNS • Cerebral vascular disease • Intervertebral disk disease • Multiple sclerosis • Parkinson disease • Shy-Drager syndrome • Spinal cord trauma • Spinovascular disease • Transverse myelitis • Neoplasm or tumor	Women • Acute vulvovaginitis • Vaginal lichen planus • Vaginal lichen sclerosis • Vaginal pemphigus • Cystitis • Periurethral abscess • Urethritis

use with anticholinergic or α-adrenergic drugs, or ongoing fecal impaction, which can add to pressure on the urethra.

Urinary retention should be first addressed by identification of causal or contributing factors. This includes ruling out potential upper or lower urinary tract obstruction, review of medications, and assessment for constipation and metabolic abnormalities, such as hyperglycemia and hypercalcemia. In the appropriate clinical scenario, ruling out a potential spinal cord injury or nerve root damage is needed.

Lower Urinary Tract Obstruction

Patients with progressively worsening urinary retention due to a lower urinary tract obstruction may initially have symptoms such as increasing urinary hesitancy, weak urinary stream, waking up to urinate at night, and difficulty with emptying their bladder fully, sometimes

TABLE 13.2 Commonly Used Medications in Palliative Care Associated With Urinary Retention

Anticholinergics	Atropine, belladonna, dicyclomine, glycopyrrolate, homatropine, hyoscyamine, oxybutynin, scopolamine
Antidepressants	Amitriptyline, doxepin, imipramine, nortriptyline
Antihistamines	Chlorpheniramine, cyproheptadine, diphenhydramine, hydroxyzine
Antipsychotics	Chlorpromazine, haloperidol, prochlorperazine
Muscle relaxants	Baclofen, cyclobenzaprine, diazepam
Other agents	Amphetamines, opioids

leading to incontinence. Severe bladder outlet obstruction or urinary retention can lead to pain and restlessness from lower abdominal or suprapubic discomfort and often confusion or changes in mental status. Especially in the elderly population, confusion is a common presentation and is often due to metabolic or electrolyte abnormalities in the setting of renal impairment or infectious complications. The discomfort related to urinary retention may be masked in some patients receiving opioids for pain or medications with sedating effects such as neuroleptics. In contrast to acute urinary obstruction, chronic urinary obstruction is usually gradual and painless, with overflow incontinence being seen in acute or chronic urinary retention. Bladder volume greater than 300 mL on ultrasound is indicative of urinary retention, requiring intervention.[5]

Treatment of lower urinary tract obstruction is insertion of a urinary catheter to relieve the obstruction. The anatomy of the patient determines the appropriate size and type of urinary catheter used. If passage of a catheter into the urethra is impossible, such as in the presence of a urethral stricture or mass, a suprapubic catheter will be needed to drain the bladder until further evaluation can be performed with endoscopy by a urologist.[6,7]

In men with urinary obstruction due to prostatic enlargement, medical treatments include an α-blocker such as tamsulosin and 5-α-reductase inhibitors such as finasteride.[8] These may not be effective in refractory urinary retention, in which case procedural intervention or a temporary catheter may be needed to relieve obstructive symptoms. Palliative transurethral prostatectomy (TURP) may be considered in patients with prostatic enlargement or advanced prostate cancer causing symptoms.[9] However, chance for treatment failure after TURP is not insignificant.[10] Also, due to an increased risk for bleeding, clots, infection, and persistent voiding difficulty, urologic intervention may not be appropriate in certain at-risk patients.

Potential complications following relief of bladder obstruction include transient hypotension, hematuria, and postobstructive diuresis. Hypotension usually resolves without intervention, and hematuria is rarely clinically significant, occurring in 11% of patients with acute urinary retention.[11,12] Once the obstruction is relieved, urine output per hour should be monitored as large volumes of urine output can indicate postobstructive diuresis. Large-volume diuresis can lead to metabolic or electrolyte derangements. While some patients can be managed by increasing oral fluid intake, those unable to tolerate oral intake or have excessive urine output can be managed with intravenous fluid repletion. Usually, half-normal saline is given to replace half the volume of urine output, but choice and rate of fluid administration can change based on whether or not the patient is hyponatremic or hypernatremic.

Upper Urinary Tract Obstructions

Upper urinary tract obstructions due to bilateral ureteral blockage or unilateral ureteral blockage in the setting of a single kidney can occur in the setting of cancer, such as compression of the ureter by a tumor mass or encasement of the ureter by lymph nodes or metastatic involvement. Hydronephrosis caused by extrinsic compression is often seen in advanced cancer, with the majority being urologic, gastrointestinal, or gynecologic malignancies in origin. Periureteral fibrosis following prior radiation or chemotherapy may also be contributing factors.[13]

Patients with acute upper urinary tract obstruction present with decreased urine output, abdominal pain, flank pain, and colic. Unlike patients with lower urinary tract obstructions, bladder distension is not present. In laboratory work, evidence of acute kidney injury with elevated serum creatinine, elevated potassium, and metabolic acidosis can be seen. Chronic obstruction can present with subtle or no symptoms but will be apparent via evidence of hydronephrosis or blunting and atrophy of the renal cortex on imaging. Renal ultrasonography is useful for assessing the severity of obstruction as well as identifying the cause, which may be obstructing stones in the kidney or the ureter or a mass. A computed tomographic (CT) scan may also be helpful and can provide more information than an ultrasound.

If imaging shows bilateral ureteric obstruction, management includes a cystoscopy to evaluate the bladder for tumor involvement and bilateral retrograde pyelograms to outline the ureter and identify the level of the obstruction. In the case of an extrinsic malignant ureteral obstruction, a retrograde ureteric stent can then be placed or a percutaneous nephrostomy tube if a ureteric stent cannot be placed. Periodic endoscopic stent changes or nephrostomy changes are usually performed every 3 to 6 months,[14] though this may be difficult in the case of tumor invasion of the distal ureteral or trigone. Alternatively, permanent indwelling metallic stents also have specific advantages and may be options.[13] These are considerations that may need to be determined in conjunction with the patient's prognosis, functional status, and caregiver support. If the obstruction is able to be relieved, for example by treatment of the tumor by radiation or chemotherapy, the stent or nephrostomy tube may eventually be removed.

In the setting of unilateral ureteric involvement, the same workup with laboratory tests and imaging is pursued. If the involved side is symptomatic, cystoscopic placement of a ureteric stent or nephrostomy tube can relieve the obstruction. However, if the contralateral kidney is functioning well and the side with the obstruction is not causing symptoms, intervention is usually not required.

Urinary Incontinence

Involuntary urine loss can be due to total urethral incontinence, overflow incontinence, urgency incontinence, stress incontinence, or extraurethral incontinence from urinary fistulas. Management can help to prevent complications such as perineal rashes and infections and reduce patient discomfort and symptom burden.

Total urethral incontinence is due to sphincter dysfunction from tumor involvement, loss of nervous system function from injury to the spinal cord or nerve roots, or postsurgical complications. Sphincter function can be investigated with urodynamic studies, and an endoscopic examination by a urologist can also help to identify the underlying cause for sphincter dysfunction.[15] Management involves use of an indwelling Foley catheter or, in men, an external condom catheter or penile clamp. However, there are inherent safety risks with use of the penile clamp, which acts as a compression device on the urethra, in the long term.[16] In patients with urinary incontinence following TURP, biofeedback-assisted pelvic floor muscle training was shown to have some benefit.[17,18] More invasive procedures such as placement of an artificial sphincter in the setting of advanced malignancy or in the palliative care setting is usually not pursued.

Overflow incontinence is due to bladder outlet obstruction or urethral obstruction. Acute or chronic urinary retention can present as overflow incontinence. Voiding is impaired and occurs in small amounts, causing bladder distension that may be palpable on examination or obvious in imaging studies. Immediate treatment is insertion of a catheter to help relieve the obstruction. Depending on the cause and potential for surgical treatment as well as patient prognosis, an indwelling catheter, intermittent catheterization, or an intraurethral stent may be longer term solutions.

Stress incontinence is due to faulty urethral support, leading to urinary leakage in the setting of increased intra-abdominal pressure caused by activities such as laughing, sneezing, coughing, straining, or even walking. This type of incontinence is usually less of an issue in the palliative care setting, and while surgical management is an option, it is not usually appropriate in patients with advanced illness. Less invasive procedures such as cystoscopic injection of intraurethral bulking agents, such as collagen, may be considered appropriate in some patients. Electroacupuncture of the lumbosacral area is also being studied as a noninvasive treatment to reduce leakage of urine in patients with stress incontinence.[19] Another solution may be medications that constrict the urethra. Phenylpropanolamine, an α-agonist, was used in the past but is currently off market. Duloxetine is a serotonin and norepinephrine reuptake inhibitor that can increase sphincter contraction and help with the management of stress incontinence.[20] If symptoms are severe, a long-term indwelling or external catheter can be placed.

Urge incontinence is due to increased spontaneous bladder muscle wall activity causing a sudden urge to urinate. Causes include irritation of the bladder wall due to either intrinsic or extrinsic tumor involvement or inflammatory changes to the bladder from radiation, medications (i.e., cyclophosphamide), or a urinary tract infection (UTI). Lack of inhibition from the central nervous system, such as due to deficiencies in the cerebrovascular system, can also lead to urge incontinence. In the palliative care setting, a patient's ability to reach the toilet in time during sudden urges to urinate is often impaired, exacerbating the situation. Utilizing bedside devices such as a bedside commode or urinal bottle for males in accordance with appropriate fall precautions are helpful in promoting quality of life. Urge incontinence can be treated with anticholinergic medications, such as oxybutynin or tolterodine, that control bladder overactivity by relaxing the bladder muscle.[20] In elderly patients at increased risk for adverse side effects, cautious incorporation of medications with avoidance of polypharmacy and lower doses or "as needed" dosing may be more appropriate. However, some patients may be unable to tolerate anticholinergic medications due to side effects that impair quality of life. Intradetrusor injection of onabotulinum A toxin has also been found to reduce incontinence due to overactive bladder syndrome,[21-23] although higher rates of UTI and transient retention were also seen.[21]

Alternative treatment options for the management of urinary incontinence are important to consider in situations where one wishes to avoid pharmacological treatment, such as anticholinergics in the elderly population. Behavioral modifications such as bladder retraining and pelvic floor exercises are noninvasive options.[24,25] In the frail and elderly, prompted voiding (being reminded to make toilet visits) and timed voiding have been shown to reduce episodes of incontinence, in addition to physical exercise, which can reduce time to toilet.[24] Acupuncture has also been studied as an alternative treatment for patients with overactive bladder syndrome in reducing incontinence episodes,[26] although further studies are needed and its use in palliative care patients is unclear. If urinary incontinence is severe or if there is lack of improvement with treatment, additional options include placement of an indwelling urinary catheter connected to a urine-collecting bag or an external urinary collection device. For female patients, an external urine-collecting device covering the perineum and the urethral opening can be used,[27] while in male patients, an external urinary catheter with a condom-like sheath covering the penis[28] is an alternative to an indwelling urinary catheter. A summary of management of urinary incontinence based on type of incontinence can be seen in Table 13.3.

TABLE 13.3 Management of Urinary Incontinence

Type of Incontinence	Suggested Management	Notes
Total urethral incontinence	Indwelling catheter External condom catheter Penile clamp	
Overflow incontinence	Indwelling catheter Intermittent catheterization Intraurethral stent	
Stress incontinence	Medications • Duloxetine	Selective serotonin and norepinephrine reuptake inhibitor; increases urethral sphincter contraction
	• α-Adrenergic stimulants	For instance, phenylpropanolamine; not approved by Food and Drug Administration in the United States and no strong evidence for efficacy
	Cystoscopic intraurethral bulking agents	For instance, collagen; high short-term benefit but limited long-term effect
	Behavioral therapy • Pelvic floor exercises, biofeedback • Prompted voiding, timed voiding, decreasing time to toilet Indwelling or external catheter or urine-collecting device	For highly motivated female patients able to contract pelvic muscles
Urge incontinence	Medications • Oxybutynin • Tolterodine	Possible anticholinergic side effects (constipation, dry mouth, worsened cognitive function); use with caution in dementia patients Risk for urinary tract infection, transient retention
	Intradetrusor onabotulinum A toxin Acupuncture	Some studies indicate benefit[24]
	External urinary collection device or catheter Behavioral modifications • Prompted voiding, timed voiding, physical exercise to decrease time to toilet	Especially for elderly patients unable to tolerate anticholinergic side effects of medication

Fistulas

A fistula refers to a nonanatomic connection between two organs. Fistulas involving the genitourinary system are most commonly uroenteric (connection between the urinary tract and gastrointestinal tract), vesicovaginal (connection between the bladder and vagina), urethrocutaneous (connection between the urethra and the outer skin), and rectourethral (connection between the rectum and the urethra). These abnormal connections lead to urinary leakage and incontinence and can be very physically and psychologically distressing to the patient and family.

A uroenteric fistula usually forms in the setting of colonic malignancy and inflammation involving the bowel wall and rarely from the bladder. Patients will present with gas in the urine and dysuria, and many will also have UTIs due to the abnormal connection to the bowel. In most cases, a cystoscopy and CT of the abdomen with oral and rectal contrast will identify the fistula. Magnetic resonance imaging (MRI) is also sensitive enough to detect the fistula. Management depends on the degree of bowel disease and patient comorbidities. In a healthy patient, resection of the involved bowel and closure of the bladder connection could be pursued.[29,30] In the palliative care setting, the patient may not be able to tolerate this type of surgical approach, and a less invasive surgery for fecal diversion and/or urinary diversion with bilateral percutaneous nephrostomy may be other options.

A vesiculovaginal fistula occurs following gynecological surgery or local trauma, causing urine to pass from the bladder into the vagina. Investigation with CT urography to assess ureteric involvement and cystoscopy and vaginoscopy can lead to diagnosis. Small fistulas unrelated to malignancy may close on their own after urinary diversion via urethral or suprapubic drainage. If possible, a corrective approach with surgery will be pursued, with risk for recurrent fistula formation or stress/urge incontinence.[31] If the patient has extensive disease or is too frail for surgery, then an indwelling catheter, suprapubic catheterization, or nephrostomy tubes can be used to divert and reduce leakage.

A rectourethral fistula can occur as a complication following radical prostatectomy or in the setting of locally invasive prostate or rectal cancer. Urine will pass through the rectum or feces will pass through the urethra. Diagnosis is obtained via cystourethroscopy or proctoscopy. A temporary diverting colostomy and bladder catheterization, along with treatment of underlying cancer, can lead the fistula to close. Surgical management may be carefully considered in the appropriate context.[32]

Pain

Renal Colic

Pain due to urinary tract abnormalities is very distressing and must be addressed promptly. Renal colic or flank pain occurs due to obstruction of the ureter by a stone or blood clot, leading to capsular distension. Colicky-type pain extending from the costovertebral angle along the ureters down to the testis or labium is due to ureteric muscle spasm from stones or clots. Intravenous fluid and α-blockers are given to help with passage of stones that are small enough to be passed (generally those with diameter less than 10 mm). Pain can also be relieved by opiates or nonsteroidal anti-inflammatory drugs (NSAIDs) such as ketorolac or diclofenac. However, caution is advised in the use of NSAIDs in palliative care patients due to risk for renal failure, bleeding, and platelet dysfunction with their use, especially in the setting of urinary tract obstruction. Treatment of the obstruction may involve placement of a ureteric stent or nephrostomy or extra-anatomic diversion, depending on the scenario. Some patients may have stent-related pain, for which α-blockers such as tamsulosin have been shown to improve pain.[33]

Bladder Pain and Spasms

The mechanism of bladder spasms is severe contractions of the detrusor muscle. As the bladder expands, the trigone sends signals to the brain that the bladder needs to be emptied, and contraction occurs. Bladder pain is classified as either obstructive or irritative.

Obstructive bladder pain is usually due to acute rather than chronic obstruction. Acute obstruction manifests as severe lower abdominal pain, restlessness, anxiety and/or delirium, increased urinary frequency, and overflow incontinence, while chronic obstruction is associated with a sense of fullness but usually is painless. First, assessment of adequate bladder emptying should be performed; measurement of a postvoid residual may be needed. Acute obstruction and bladder distension should be relieved with placement of a catheter.

Irritative bladder pain is due to inflammation and manifests as dysuria, UTI, urge incontinence, and increased urinary frequency. Irritation of the bladder wall leads to spasms that are felt as a painful sensation in the suprapubic area and may be accompanied by leakage of urine. Common irritants include diet soda or caffeine, external radiation causing radiation cystitis, chemotherapy agents (cyclophosphamide), tumors that are intrinsic or external, and bladder calculi. The presence of an indwelling catheter can further irritate the bladder wall due to the inflated intravesical balloon; deflating the balloon or using a catheter with a smaller balloon may be helpful. Other reversible causes should be addressed, such as discontinuing offending agents or treating a UTI that is present.

As for palliation of symptoms, use of medications such as low-dose oxybutynin 2.5 mg twice a day can help relieve bladder spasms in patients with overactive bladder.[34] However, the potential for dry mouth, constipation, or delirium potentiated by anticholinergics such as oxybutynin, tolterodine, solifenacin, dicyclomine, and hyoscyamine should be noted. Mirabegron is another agent that acts as a bladder muscle-relaxing agent as a β-3-agonist. Studies combining the use of anticholinergics such as solifenacin with mirabegron have shown both good efficacy and safety in patients with symptoms related to overactive bladder.[35-37] Belladonna and opium suppositories have also been used to alleviate bladder pain, and some studies support use in the perioperative setting to reduce urologic procedure–related pain as well.[38-40] Systemic opioid therapy may also be needed to treat intermittent, sudden onset bladder spasm–related pain, with as-needed dosing given via the intravenous route being preferred due to its rapid onset of action, in contrast to oral pain medications. Medications that may be used for bladder pain and spasms are shown in Table 13.4.

Intravesical therapy, or bladder instillation of medications following insertion of a urethral catheter, and other procedural interventions are additional options that can relieve bladder or urinary tract–related pain. Intravesical injection of bupivacaine, baclofen, or opioids such as diamorphine and oxycodone have been shown to reduce bladder pain.[41,42] Intravesical onabotulinum toxin A injections have also been shown to improve bladder pain symptoms in patients who do not respond to other treatments, though with the possibility of urinary

TABLE 13.4 Medications for Treatment of Bladder Pain and Spasms

Drug Class	Drug Name and Dosing	Notes
Bladder muscle relaxants	Oxybutynin 5 mg two or three times daily	Extended-release option also available
	Tolterodine 2–4 mg twice daily	Extended-release option also available
	Solifenacin 5–10 mg daily	Use lower dose for CrtCl < 30
	Dicyclomine 10–20 mg four times daily	Not officially approved for bladder spasticity
	Hyoscyamine 0.125–0.25 mg every 4 hours as needed	
	Flavoxate 100–200 mg twice daily	
	Mirabegron 25–50 mg daily	Use lower dose for CrtCl < 30; avoid use in end-stage renal disease
Bladder muscle analgesic	Phenazopyridine 100–200 mg three times daily	Use three times a day for 2 days; give after meals
Rectal opioids	Belladonna/opium suppository 16.2 mg/30 mg daily or twice daily	Maximum 4 suppositories every 24 hours
Bladder-emptying agents	Tamsulosin 0.4 mg daily Terazosin 1–10 mg daily	May cause orthostatic hypotension

retention following treatment.[43–45] Nerve blocks such as an intrathecal saddle block or lumbar sympathetic blockade can be considered for relief of pain or recurrent bladder spasms.[46,47] Other treatment modalities include lithotripsy in the setting of urolithiasis, while pain related to bladder mass or cancer may be addressed with intravesical chemotherapy or surgical resection in the appropriate clinical scenario. When deciding between nonpharmacological or pharmacological agents for palliation of symptoms, generally the least invasive approach should be attempted, with imaging or a urology referral being potentially necessary steps, especially in urgent or emergent situations such as acute urinary obstruction.

Infections

Classic signs of UTI include fever, dysuria, increased urinary frequency and urgency, pelvic or suprapubic pain, and hematuria. Altered mental status may also be present. Choice of initial empiric antibiotic therapy should be based on probability of UTI and results of urinalysis and antibiotic susceptibility of the identified organism. The hospital antibiogram should be used to assist in antibiotic selection.

Among UTIs acquired in the hospital, urinary catheter–related UTIs are the most common. Having an indwelling or suprapubic catheter increases the risk for UTIs. Incidence of bacteriuria or UTIs increases with longer duration of catheterization. Bacteriuria occurs at a rate of 5%–10% per day once the catheter is placed, with 50% of patients having bacteriuria by 10 to 14 days, and almost all patients having bacteriuria at 6 weeks.[48] If the patient is not having symptoms of a UTI, meaning they are with asymptomatic bacteriuria or funguria, treatment with antimicrobials is not necessary and may be treated initially with catheter exchange or removal if possible.[49,50] In an attempt to decrease the incidence of UTI, the practice of exchanging chronic indwelling catheters at scheduled intervals such as every 4 weeks is common but not supported by sufficient data as an effective strategy. The duration of antibiotic treatment for catheter-associated UTI is also under debate and is generally considered to be between 3 and 14 days.[51,52] One strategy that has been proposed to reduce the incidence of UTIs is regular intermittent clean catheterization if patients are able to perform this on their own or have necessary assistance. However, in the palliative care setting and especially at end of life, an indwelling catheter may be necessary for the comfort of the patient or befitting the clinical circumstances of the patient.

Hematuria

Hematuria, or blood in the urine, can present as dark-colored or red urine (gross hematuria) or may be invisible to the naked eye (microscopic hematuria) but detected by microscopy to reveal the presence of red blood cells or hemoglobin in urine studies. Symptoms such as fever or chills, dysuria, and increased urinary frequency and urgency may indicate a UTI, while lower abdominal pain or flank pain may indicate problems in the bladder, kidneys, ureters, or prostate, such as cystitis, pyelonephritis, bladder or kidney stones, or tumor involvement. Use of aspirin, NSAIDs, or blood thinners can also predispose to blood in the urine. Patients with advanced cancer may also have coagulopathy. Treatment of hematuria depends on the etiology; for example, a UTI should be treated with antibiotics, while hemorrhagic cystitis may require intravesical agents. Addressing hematuria becomes more urgent in the setting of brisk bleeding causing severe anemia or formation of clots that can obstruct parts of the urinary tract such as the ureters or the bladder outlet.

Lower Urinary Tract

In the lower urinary tract system, hematuria is caused by abnormalities or inflammation in the bladder, prostate, or urethra due to malignancy, stones, radiation, infection, traumatic catheterization, or procedures. Hemorrhagic cystitis is another cause of significant or recurrent hematuria and is a result of chemotherapy (cyclophosphamide) or radiation in cancer patients.

In the setting of brisk bleeding, risk for urinary tract obstruction from blood clots, or rarely hypotension and shock, are of immediate concern. Blood clots must be evacuated, usually with placement of a large-bore catheter (≥22 French) that allows for vigorous irrigation of the bladder until clots are no longer obtained with clear backflow. Placement of a three-way indwelling catheter allows for continuous bladder irrigation in the case of severe hematuria, although continuous irrigation also raises risk for bladder perforation, and monitoring for catheter obstruction is needed.[53] If a urethral catheter cannot be placed or there is intractable hematuria or obstruction of the irrigating catheter, a cystourethroscopy is used to identify and treat the cause of bleeding through cauterization, endoscopic resection of lesions or masses, or removal of blood clots.[53] If bleeding continues to be refractory, other treatment measures include bladder irrigation with formalin, 1% silver nitrate, 1% to 2% alum, or prostaglandin.[54–57]. Formalin instillation has greater risk for perforation and bladder fibrosis but is also effective.[56] In the case of radiation cystitis or cyclophosphamide-related hemorrhagic cystitis, treatment measures also include hyperbaric oxygen.[58] In extreme cases, embolization of the bleeding source or urinary diversion with or without palliative cystectomy may be options. However, as cystectomy with urinary diversion is associated with the greatest morbidity, it should only be considered if all other options have not been successful, and the benefits are considered to outweigh the risks in each clinical scenario.[56]

Trauma to the urinary tract can also cause gross hematuria, and treatment can be complicated depending on the anatomical structures involved. Urethral trauma due to catheterization or catheter removal is commonly seen and can be addressed with replacement or manipulation of the catheter. Men with benign prostatic hyperplasia (BPH) or patients on anticoagulation are at greater risk for catheter-related traumatic hematuria.

Prostate-related bleeding can be due to prostatitis, BPH, or advanced prostate cancer. A 5-α-reductase inhibitor such as finasteride should be considered in the setting of BPH and hematuria. Patients with advanced prostate cancer can also present with hematuria, and surgical treatment such as a limited TURP, radiation, or androgen deprivation treatment can be considered in the appropriate context.

Upper Urinary Tract

Hematuria can also occur due to upper urinary tract pathology such as a renal mass, kidney or ureteral stones, or strictures. Diagnostic studies such as renal ultrasound, CT of the abdomen, or cystoscopy and ureteroscopy would help determine the cause of bleeding. Rarely, a cause for bleeding may not be apparent despite these diagnostic modalities, and additional studies such as a renal arteriography may be needed to help identify vasculature issues, such as arteriovenous malformations or renal vein varices, which can be treated with embolization.[59]

For managing kidney stones, recognizing when nephrolithiasis requires surgical versus medical management is important. Hemodynamic instability and infection, stone greater than 10 mm in size, bilateral ureteral stones or high-grade unilateral obstruction, presence of stone in the setting of a solitary kidney, or worsened renal dysfunction are all indications for urology consultation for possible procedural involvement such as stent or percutaneous nephrostomy. The location of the kidney stone is also important, as distal ureteral stones are more likely to pass on their own rather than proximal stones.[60] Medical management includes use of intravenous fluids, pain control with opioids, and an α-1-agonist such as tamsulosin.

The presence of a tumor involving the kidney, such as renal cell carcinoma, can lead to hematuria. If bleeding is persistent in the setting of a renal mass with metastasis, a radical nephrectomy could be performed. In the setting of metastatic disease, palliative cytoreductive nephrectomy may still be considered, although a shift in current treatment paradigms appears to be occurring with the advent of immunotherapy.[61] Palliative embolization of the renal artery is another option to control bleeding and pain due to inoperable renal tumors in select patients with inoperable or unresectable renal carcinoma who are thought to be appropriate for this treatment by specialists.[62–65]

Pediatric Issues

In the pediatric population at end of life, urinary tract problems such as urinary retention and urinary obstruction can be due to a number of reasons, some of which are specific for the pediatric population. For example, posterior urethral valves, which are congenital valves located in the prostatic urethra, are the most common obstructing lesions in male infants and children and should be suspected when anuria is seen in a newborn or infant. A rare tumor such as rhabdomyosarcoma of the bladder may also be the cause of acute urinary retention in the pediatric population. Other pediatric causes for urinary retention include urethral polyps, urethral atresia, ectopic ureteroceles, and pelvic tumors.[66]

Urinary retention can occur due to neurologic issues such as spinal cord compression, UTI, locally invasive masses or lesions, or constipation.[67] Urinary retention can also be seen as an adverse effect of medications, such as opioids. Usually, urinary retention from opioids is seen when it is given rapidly via the epidural or spinal route.

Symptoms of urinary obstruction or retention include pain, restlessness, or agitation, and prompt management is needed. Ureteral obstruction can be addressed by a stent. For urinary obstruction, a urinary catheter may be needed to relieve symptoms while addressing the underlying cause. If urinary retention is thought to be a result of opioids, substituting pain medication to an alternative opioid, using a cholinomimetic agent such as bethanechol to stimulate bladder contraction, or intermittent catheterization may be necessary.[68ff]

Considerations at End of Life

Low urine output at end of life is also seen in the setting of progressively worsening kidney function and multiorgan failure. Providers should assist in preparing families for these potential urinary issues at the end of life and the fact that urine output will decrease during the final days of life. Increasing weakness and debility can also lead to urinary incontinence, which can be stressful for both the patient and the family. The use of a urinary catheter at end of life would be appropriate to help avoid pain and discomfort with frequent cleaning or changing of clothing or linens and can help prevent bedsores caused by wet diapers or clothes.

In the palliative care setting, factors such as symptom burden, premorbid health status, and functional capacity should be considered in determining the appropriate treatment or intervention. More invasive or complex procedures may increase symptom burden rather than be of benefit in a frail, ill, or dying patients. Less aggressive or conservative measures may be more appropriate in keeping with a focus on quality of life. For example, complicated surgeries involving resection of bowel and bladder may be the appropriate treatment in a healthy patient with an enterovesical fistula, but in the palliative care setting, the patient may not be able to tolerate invasive surgery. A less invasive procedure such as diverting colostomy can be a better option in this situation.

At end of life, certain complications may not materialize due to limitation of time for it to develop. Therefore, choice of an intervention is dependent on the patient's prognosis. For example, in a patient with advanced disease or during the dying process, the risk and benefit of a bladder catheter must be considered. A bladder catheter may increase risk for infection but will also reduce the stress associated with getting up to urinate, decrease fall risks, preserve the dignity of the patient, and reduce caregiver burden. If the patient does develop a catheter-associated UTI, however, removal of the catheter may then be considered.

In patients experiencing genitourinary issues, the healthcare team needs to properly assess the impact of certain symptoms, such as dysuria, frequency, and incontinence, as well as interventions, such as catheters and tubes, on the quality of life of the patient, including body image issues. Most of these patients will also be on multiple medications and risks of drug interactions, and toxicities should also be evaluated. Finally, these patients may be experiencing significant symptom burden such as fatigue, drowsiness, dryness, and confusion. Choice of medications and interventions should be personalized based on potential of reducing or exacerbating these symptoms.

References

1. Choong S, Emberton M. Acute urinary retention. *BJU International*. 2000;*85*(2):186–201.
2. Feng MI, Bellman GC, Shapiro CE. Management of ureteral obstruction secondary to pelvic malignancies. *Journal of Endourology*. 1999;*13*(7):521–524.
3. Serlin DC, Heidelbaugh JJ, Stoffel JT. Urinary Retention in Adults: Evaluation and Initial Management. *American Family Physician*. 2018;*98*(8):496–503.
4. Curtis LA, Dolan TS, Cespedes RD. Acute urinary retention and urinary incontinence. *Emergency Medicine Clinics of North America*. 2001;*19*(3):591–619.
5. Billet M, Windsor TA. Urinary Retention. *Emergency Medicine Clinics of North America*. 2019;*37*(4):649–660.
6. Wu JN, Meyers FJ, Evans CP. Palliative care in urology. *Surgical Clinics of North America*. 2011;*91*(2):429–444, x.
7. Sinclair CT, Kalender-Rich JL, Griebling TL, Porter-Williamson K. Palliative Care of Urologic Patients at End of Life. *Clinics in Geriatric Medicine*. 2015;*31*(4):667–678.
8. Thomas K, Chow K, Kirby RS. Acute urinary retention: a review of the aetiology and management. *Prostate Cancer and Prostatic Diseases*. 2004;*7*(1):32–37.
9. Crain DS, Amling CL, Kane CJ. Palliative transurethral prostate resection for bladder outlet obstruction in patients with locally advanced prostate cancer. *Journal of Urology*. 2004;*171*(2 Pt 1):668–671.
10. Gnanapragasam VJ, Kumar V, Langton D, Pickard RS, Leung HY. Outcome of transurethral prostatectomy for the palliative management of lower urinary tract symptoms in men with prostate cancer. *International Journal of Urology*. 2006;*13*(6):711–715.
11. Boettcher S, Brandt AS, Roth S, Mathers MJ, Lazica DA. Urinary retention: benefit of gradual bladder decompression—myth or truth? A randomized controlled trial. *Urologia Internationalis*. 2013;*91*(2):140–144.
12. Nyman MA, Schwenk NM, Silverstein MD. Management of urinary retention: rapid versus gradual decompression and risk of complications. *Mayo Clinic Proceedings*. 1997;*72*(10):951–956.
13. Sountoulides P, Mykoniatis I, Dimasis N. Palliative management of malignant upper urinary tract obstruction. *Hippokratia*. 2014;*18*(4):292–297.
14. Hyams ES, Shah O. Malignant extrinsic ureteral obstruction: a survey of urologists and medical oncologists regarding treatment patterns and preferences. *Urology*. 2008;*72*(1):51–56.
15. Hester AG, Kretschmer A, Badlani G. Male Incontinence: The Etiology or Basis of Treatment. *European Urology Focus*. 2017;*3*(4–5):377–384.
16. Anderson CA, Omar MI, Campbell SE, Hunter KF, Cody JD, Glazener CM. Conservative management for postprostatectomy urinary incontinence. *Cochrane Database Systematic Reviews*. 2015;*1*:CD001843.

17. Hsu LF, Liao YM, Lai FC, Tsai PS. Beneficial effects of biofeedback-assisted pelvic floor muscle training in patients with urinary incontinence after radical prostatectomy: A systematic review and metaanalysis. *International Journal of Nursing Studies.* 2016;*60*:99–111.

18. Kondo K, Noonan KM, Freeman M, Ayers C, Morasco BJ, Kansagara D. Efficacy of Biofeedback for Medical Conditions: an Evidence Map. *Journal of General Internal Medicine.* 2019;*34*(12):2883–2893.

19. Liu Z, Liu Y, Xu H, et al. Effect of Electroacupuncture on Urinary Leakage Among Women With Stress Urinary Incontinence: A Randomized Clinical Trial. *JAMA.* 2017;*317*(24):2493–2501.

20. Weiss BD. Selecting medications for the treatment of urinary incontinence. *American Family Physician.* 2005;*71*(2):315–322.

21. Visco AG, Brubaker L, Richter HE, et al. Anticholinergic therapy vs. onabotulinumtoxina for urgency urinary incontinence. *New England Journal of Medicine.* 2012;*367*(19):1803–1813.

22. Nitti VW, Dmochowski R, Herschorn S, et al. OnabotulinumtoxinA for the Treatment of Patients with Overactive Bladder and Urinary Incontinence: Results of a Phase 3, Randomized, Placebo Controlled Trial. *Journal of Urology.* 2017;*197*(2S):S216–S223.

23. Sievert KD, Chapple C, Herschorn S, et al. OnabotulinumtoxinA 100U provides significant improvements in overactive bladder symptoms in patients with urinary incontinence regardless of the number of anticholinergic therapies used or reason for inadequate management of overactive bladder. *International Journal of Clinical Practice.* 2014;*68*(10):1246–1256.

24. Stenzelius K, Molander U, Odeberg J, et al. The effect of conservative treatment of urinary incontinence among older and frail older people: a systematic review. *Age and Ageing.* 2015;*44*(5):736–744.

25. Hersh L, Salzman B. Clinical management of urinary incontinence in women. *American Family Physician.* 2013;*87*(9):634–640.

26. Zhao Y, Zhou J, Mo Q, Wang Y, Yu J, Liu Z. Acupuncture for adults with overactive bladder: A systematic review and meta-analysis of randomized controlled trials. *Medicine (Baltimore).* 2018;*97*(8):e9838.

27. Beeson T, Davis C. Urinary Management With an External Female Collection Device. *Journal of Wound, Ostomy, and Continence Nursing.* 2018;*45*(2):187–189.

28. Walton A. Managing overactive bladder symptoms in a palliative care setting. *Journal of Palliative Medicine.* 2014;*17*(1):118–121.

29. Gill HS. Diagnosis and Surgical Management of Uroenteric Fistula. *Surgical Clinics of North America.* 2016;*96*(3):583–592.

30. Cochetti G, Del Zingaro M, Boni A, et al. Colovesical fistula: review on conservative management, surgical techniques and minimally invasive approaches. *Il Giornale di chirurgia.* 2018;*39*(4):195–207.

31. Malik MA, Sohail M, Malik MT, Khalid N, Akram A. Changing trends in the etiology and management of vesicovaginal fistula. *International Journal of Urology.* 2018;*25*(1):25–29.

32. Chen S, Gao R, Li H, Wang K. Management of acquired rectourethral fistulas in adults. *Asian Journal of Urology.* 2018;*5*(3):149–154.

33. Lamb AD, Vowler SL, Johnston R, Dunn N, Wiseman OJ. Meta-analysis showing the beneficial effect of α-blockers on ureteric stent discomfort. *BJU International.* 2011;*108*(11):1894–1902.

34. De E, Gomery P, Rosenberg LB. Palliation of Bladder Spasms #337. *Journal of Palliative Medicine.* 2017;*20*(10):1158–1159.

35. Mueller ER, van Maanen R, Chapple C, et al. Long-term treatment of older patients with overactive bladder using a combination of mirabegron and solifenacin: a prespecified analysis from the randomized, phase III SYNERGY II study. *Neurourology and Urodynamics.* 2019;*38*(2):779–792.

36. Yamaguchi O, Kakizaki H, Homma Y, et al. Long-term safety and efficacy of antimuscarinic add-on therapy in patients with overactive bladder who had a suboptimal response to mirabegron monotherapy: a multicenter, randomized study in Japan (MILAI II study). *International Journal of Urology.* 2019;*26*(3):342–352.

37. Gratzke C, Chapple C, Mueller ER, et al. Efficacy and Safety of Combination Pharmacotherapy for Patients with Overactive Bladder: A Rapid Evidence Assessment. *European Urology.* 2019;*76*(6):767–779.

38. Fetzer SJ, Goodwin L, Stanizzi M. Effectiveness of a Pre-emptive Preoperative Belladonna and Opium Suppository on Postoperative Urgency and Pain After Ureteroscopy. *Journal of Perianesthesia Nursing.* 2019;*34*(3):594–599.

39. Lee FC, Holt SK, Hsi RS, Haynes BM, Harper JD. Preoperative Belladonna and Opium Suppository for Ureteral Stent Pain: A Randomized, Double-blinded, Placebo-controlled Study. *Urology.* 2017;*100*:27–32.

40. Lukasewycz S, Holman M, Kozlowski P, et al. Does a perioperative belladonna and opium suppository improve postoperative pain following robotic assisted laparoscopic radical prostatectomy? Results of a single institution randomized study. *Canadian Journal of Urology.* 2010;*17*(5):5377–5382.

41. Wallace E, Twomey M, Victory R, O'Reilly M. Intravesical baclofen, bupivacaine, and oxycodone for the relief of bladder spasm. *Journal of Palliative Care.* 2013;*29*(1):49–51.

42. McCoubrie R, Jeffrey D. Intravesical diamorphine for bladder spasm. *Journal of Pain and Symptom Management.* 2003;*25*(1):1–3.

43. Dellis A, Papatsoris AG. Intravesical treatment of bladder pain syndrome/interstitial cystitis: from the conventional regimens to the novel botulinum toxin injections. *Expert Opinion on Investigative Drugs.* 2014;*23*(6):751–757.

44. Chiu B, Tai HC, Chung SD, Birder LA. Botulinum Toxin A for Bladder Pain Syndrome/Interstitial Cystitis. *Toxins (Basel).* 2016;*8*(7).

45. LeClaire EL, Duong J, Wykes RM, Miller KE, Winterton TL, Bimali M. Randomized controlled trial of belladonna and opiate suppository during intravesical onabotulinum toxin A injection. *American Journal of Obstetrics and Gynecology.* 2018;*219*(5):488.e481–488.e487.

46. Tsushima T, Miura T, Hachiya T, et al. Treatment Recommendations for Urological Symptoms in Cancer Patients: Clinical Guidelines from the Japanese Society for Palliative Medicine. *Journal of Palliative Medicine.* 2019;*22*(1):54–61.

47. Gulati A, Khelemsky Y, Loh J, Puttanniah V, Malhotra V, Cubert K. The use of lumbar sympathetic blockade at L4 for management of malignancy-related bladder spasms. *Pain Physician.* 2011;*14*(3):305–310.

48. Sedor J, Mulholland SG. Hospital-acquired urinary tract infections associated with the indwelling catheter. *Urology Clinics of North America.* 1999;*26*(4):821–828.

49. Iacovelli V, Gaziev G, Topazio L, Bove P, Vespasiani G, Finazzi Agrò E. Nosocomial urinary tract infections: A review. *Urologia.* 2014;*81*(4):222–227.

50. Yoshikawa TT, Nicolle LE, Norman DC. Management of complicated urinary tract infection in older patients. *Journal of the American Geriatrics Society.* 1996;*44*(10):1235–1241.

51. Hooton TM, Bradley SF, Cardenas DD, et al. Diagnosis, prevention, and treatment of catheter-associated urinary tract infection in adults: 2009 International Clinical Practice Guidelines from the Infectious Diseases Society of America. *Clinical Infectious Diseases.* 2010;*50*(5):625–663.

52. Trautner BW. Management of catheter-associated urinary tract infection. *Current Opinion in Infectious Diseases.* 2010;*23*(1):76–82.

53. Avellino GJ, Bose S, Wang DS. Diagnosis and Management of Hematuria. *Surgical Clinics of North America.* 2016;*96*(3):503–515.

54. Goel AK, Rao MS, Bhagwat AG, Vaidyanathan S, Goswami AK, Sen TK. Intravesical irrigation with alum for the control of massive bladder hemorrhage. *Journal of Urology.* 1985;*133*(6):956–957.

55. Donahue LA, Frank IN. Intravesical formalin for hemorrhagic cystitis: analysis of therapy. *Journal of Urology.* 1989;*141*(4):809–812.

56. Ok JH, Meyers FJ, Evans CP. Medical and surgical palliative care of patients with urological malignancies. *Journal of Urology.* 2005;*174*(4 Pt 1):1177–1182.

57. Abt D, Bywater M, Engeler DS, Schmid HP. Therapeutic options for intractable hematuria in advanced bladder cancer. *International Journal of Urology.* 2013;*20*(7):651–660.

58. Shilo Y, Efrati S, Simon Z, et al. Hyperbaric oxygen therapy for hemorrhagic radiation cystitis. *Israel Medical Association Journal.* 2013;*15*(2):75–78.

59. Eom HJ, Shin JH, Cho YJ, Nam DH, Ko GY, Yoon HK. Transarterial embolisation of renal arteriovenous malformation: safety and efficacy in 24 patients with follow-up. *Clinical Radiology.* 2015;*70*(11):1177–1184.

60. Morse RM, Resnick MI. Ureteral calculi: natural history and treatment in an era of advanced technology. *Journal of Urology.* 1991;*145*(2):263–265.

61. Psutka SP, Chang SL, Cahn D, Uzzo RG, McGregor BA. Reassessing the Role of Cytoreductive Nephrectomy for Metastatic Renal Cell Carcinoma in 2019. *American Society of Clinical Oncology Education Book*. 2019;*39*:276–283.

62. Maxwell NJ, Saleem Amer N, Rogers E, Kiely D, Sweeney P, Brady AP. Renal artery embolisation in the palliative treatment of renal carcinoma. *British Journal of Radiology*. 2007;*80*(950):96–102.

63. Ginat DT, Saad WE, Turba UC. Transcatheter renal artery embolization for management of renal and adrenal tumors. *Techniques in Vascular and Interventional Radiology*. 2010;*13*(2):75–88.

64. Guziński M, Kurcz J, Tupikowski K, Antosz E, Słowik P, Garcarek J. The Role of Transarterial Embolization in the Treatment of Renal Tumors. *Advances in Clinical and Experimental Medicine*. 2015;*24*(5):837–843.

65. Jaganjac S, Schefe L. Palliative embolization of renal tumors. *Vojnosanitetski pregled*. 2015;*72*(12):1105–1110.

66. Curtis LA, Dolan TS, Cespedes RD. Acute urinary retention and urinary incontinence. *Emergency Medicine Clinics of North America*. 2001;*19*(3):591–619.

67. Gatti JM, Perez-Brayfield M, Kirsch AJ, Smith EA, Massad HC, Broecker BH. Acute urinary retention in children. *Journal of Urology*. 2001;*165*(3):918–921.

68. Davies D. Care in the final hours and days. In: Goldman A, Hain R, Liben S, eds. Oxford textbook of palliative care for children, 2nd ed. Oxford: Oxford University Press; 2012: 368–374.

14

Assessment and Management of Pain

Russell K. Portenoy, Ebtesam Ahmed, and Calvin Krom

Introduction

Pain is highly prevalent in most populations with serious chronic illness. In those with cancer, the most studied group, persistent pain is experienced by almost two-thirds with advanced metastatic disease, more than half of those receiving antineoplastic therapy, and about one-third of cancer survivors.[1] Although data are more limited in other patient populations, studies have revealed high prevalence rates for persistent pain among those with advanced heart failure, chronic obstructive pulmonary disease, chronic kidney disease, and other disorders.[2]

Patients who experience chronic pain in association with serious chronic illness pose complex issues in assessment and management. This complexity calls for a clinical approach that addresses pain management as part of comprehensive care that aims to prevent and relieve multiple sources of distress and illness burden.

Pain, Suffering, and Illness Burden

According to the International Association for the Study of Pain, pain is "an unpleasant sensory and emotional experience associated with actual or potential tissue damage or described in terms of such damage."[3] This definition, which underscores the common observation that both pain intensity and distress are only loosely associated with observable tissue injury, may be illuminated by the meanings attached to other terms—nociception and suffering.[3] Nociception refers to the physiological processes activated by potentially tissue-damaging stimuli, which may ultimately reach consciousness as pain. *In contrast, pain itself is not a sensation, but rather a perception—a human experience that reflects both sensory activity in the nervous system and a complex interplay of thoughts, feelings, and relationships.*

Suffering is a set of complex and multidimensional perceptions associated with distress and loss. Suffering may or may not be tied to significant changes in health. A 2015 systematic review of 128 empirical and theoretical papers concerning suffering among those with cancer may be related to disturbances in the physical, cognitive, psychological, social, functional, and existential or spiritual domains of experience.[4] Pain may or may not be an important contributor. When pain exists in the context of serious illness, the importance of suffering is highlighted by the concept of *total pain*, a term coined in the 1960s by Dame Cicely Saunders, a pioneer in the modern hospice movement.[5] Total pain described the experience of patients with advanced cancer whose distress could only be explained by the interaction between physical pathology and disturbances in other experiential domains, including the psychological and emotional, social, and spiritual. The term raised awareness of the need to assess pain and provide analgesic therapy within a broader therapeutic framework, one that that considers the contribution of pain to suffering and manages pain as part of a more comprehensive approach to care.

Pain Management and Palliative Care

The complex connections between pain and suffering underscore the need for a patient-centered approach to the assessment and management of pain in serious illness. This approach is exemplified by palliative care. Palliative care is a model appropriate for all populations with serious chronic illness; this care aims to prevent and relieve suffering and illness burden experienced by the patient and family from the time of diagnosis forward.[6] Among its core values are respect for patient autonomy and dignity, support for the family as the unit of care, and commitment to medically appropriate care aligned with the values and preferences of the patient and family. Among its clinical objectives are repeated goal setting and care planning that addresses the burden of illness related to both the physical aspects of the disease, such as the burden imposed by pain and other symptoms, and the psychological, social, and spiritual needs of the patient and family.

Specialists in palliative care typically focus on the care of those with advanced illness and limited prognosis. Seriously ill patients with pain who have access to specialist palliative care an acute illness are more likely to experience relief than those who do not.[7] Although specialists endorse the view that palliative care is needed to sustain or enhance the quality of life throughout the course of illness, they typically focus on interventions at the end of life to help ensure that pain does not stand in the way of the "good death."[8]

Pain Assessment

The management of chronic pain is grounded in a comprehensive pain assessment. This assessment targets the pain while addressing other objectives of palliative care.

Pain Characteristics

The evaluation of specific pain characteristics may clarify specific phenomena, like severity or location, that can be used to monitor the course of treatment. Equally important, this evaluation may identify a pain syndrome, reveal a disease-related etiology for the pain, or clarify the pain pathophysiology. Important pain characteristics include (1) severity, (2) temporal features, (3) location, (4) quality, (5) factors that increase or decrease the pain, (6) impact on the patient's daily life and functioning, and (7) and present and past pain management strategies and their outcomes.

The repeated measurement and documentation of pain severity are essential. The most common bedside approaches employ a unidimensional pain severity scale, such as a five-level verbal rating scale (none, mild, moderate, severe, excruciating); an 11-point numerical scale (where 0 is no pain and 10 is the worst pain imaginable); or a 10-cm visual analog scale (anchored at one end by the words "no pain" or "least possible pain" and at the other end by "worst possible pain"). Other validated scales are pictorial (e.g., a faces scales) and are used for younger children and patients who cannot manage other tools. Importantly, interpretation of a pain score depends on the question asked, which must be documented along with the score. For example, the patient may be asked to rate the severity of pain "right now" or "on average during the past day" or "at its worst during the past week."

Validated multidimensional pain measures are generally used in research. The widely used Brief Pain Inventory (BPI) is a self-rating scale that assesses pain intensity and pain interference in various areas of function.[9] A short-form version of the BPI (BPI-SF) and translations in multiple languages are available.

The temporal features of the pain include onset (rapid or gradual); duration; course (stable, improving, worsening, or fluctuating); and the presence of periodic flares of pain known as "breakthrough pain." Studies in cancer populations have confirmed that breakthrough pain is independently associated with adverse outcomes and may be managed using an analgesic drug that specifically targets episodic pains.[10,11] Although the epidemiology, assessment, and treatment of breakthrough pain in other types of chronic illness have not been studied, treatment often is provided depending on the pain severity, frequency, and impact.

Questions about pain location first clarifies whether the pain is focal, multifocal, or generalized, noting that some therapies, such as nerve blocks, become possible when pain is limited in extent. Other questions probe the possibility of referred pain. Pain may be referred following injury to neural structures, somatic structures, or viscera.[12] There are numerous examples. Peripheral nerve injury may cause pain anywhere along the course of the nerve or anywhere in the dermatome or myotome it innervates. Pain in the thigh or knee may reflect a lumbar plexus lesion, and pain in the foot or toe may be caused by damage to the L1 nerve root (known as radicular pain). Similarly, injury to somatic or visceral structures yield common pain referral patterns. A lesion affecting the lower cervical vertebrae may refer pain between the scapulae, and hip pathology often refers pain to the knee. Shoulder pain may occur from ipsilateral diaphragmatic irritation, scapula pain may indicate disease of the gallbladder or nearby structures, and midback pain may be a harbinger of a lesion in the rostral retroperitoneum.

Knowledge of pain referral patterns influences decisions about evaluation. For example, the cause of progressive knee pain in a patient with metastatic disease may be a somatic lesion affecting the knee joint or hip or neural injury at the level of the peripheral nerve (femoral neuropathy from a lesion in thigh or pelvis), plexus (proximal lumbosacral pain from a pelvic sidewall lesion), or root (L2 or L3 radicular pain from a lesion in the lumbar spine). For the patient with cancer and progressive knee pain, the evaluation therefore may include plain radiography of knee and hip, computed tomographic scanning of the pelvis or magnetic resonance imaging evaluation of the lumbar spine. Knowledge of these possibilities guides the physical examination in the hope of finding signs that point to one or another potential etiology and guide the radiographic workup.

Pain Syndrome, Etiology, and Pathophysiology

The history, physical findings, and data from the patient's chart or initial workup may allow description of the pain in terms of syndrome, etiology, and pathophysiology. These characterizations strongly influence further assessments and pain management approaches.

Pain Syndromes. The utility of syndrome identification has been most clearly demonstrated in the cancer population. Numerous syndromes have been identified, some related to the disease itself and others to antineoplastic therapies.[13] Recognition of a treatment-related syndrome, such as chemotherapy-induced painful polyneuropathy, may obviate the need for additional workup or suggest a targeted treatment approach. Alternatively, recognition of a potential syndrome that may herald a catastrophic outcome, such as band-like thoracic pain as a harbinger of impending spinal cord compression, indicates the need for prompt workup and urgent treatment.

Although empirical information about pain syndromes in other chronic illnesses is limited, syndrome identification still may be useful. For example, the diabetic patient with advanced heart failure who develops worsening bilateral foot pain may have clinical findings that strongly suggest the syndrome of diabetic distal symmetrical neuropathy. This recognition may suggest the need for laboratory testing to exclude other causes of peripheral neuropathy and eliminate the need for imaging or electrophysiological studies.

Pain Etiology. The etiology of pain refers to the existence of a lesion or disorder that is directly responsible for the pain. If the etiology of chronic pain can be identified, treatment directed against this etiology may be feasible and yield analgesia. A common example is the use of radiation to treat focal bone pain due to a metastasis. The importance of etiology justifies an approach to pain assessment that routinely evaluates the relationship between the pain and the primary illness and/or comorbidities.

Pain Pathophysiology. Pain assessment provides the information necessary to draw inferences about the types of mechanisms that may be sustaining the pain. Although these inferences greatly simplify a complex biology, they are widely used to guide analgesic treatment. Pain is labeled *nociceptive* if it is inferred that the sustaining mechanisms involve ongoing injury to either somatic or visceral structures. This classification is suggested based on the quality of the pain and the finding of tissue injury. Somatic nociceptive pain is typically described as aching, stabbing, throbbing, or pressure-like. Visceral nociceptive pain varies with the structures involved; obstruction of hollow viscus is usually associated with gnawing or crampy pain, whereas injury to organ capsules or mesentery is described as aching or stabbing.

Pain is labeled *neuropathic* if the evaluation suggests that it is sustained by abnormal somatosensory processing in the peripheral or the central nervous system and there is some identifiable neurologic injury. Patients with neuropathic pain may use any of a variety of verbal descriptors, but some descriptors—such as "burning," "numbness," "prickling," "shock-like," or "electrical"—are particularly suggestive of neuropathic pain.[3,14] These descriptors are called paresthesias when they are not very uncomfortable or painful, and dysesthesias when they are. Further evidence of a neuropathic mechanism may be found on the neurological examination, which may elicit sensory disturbances in or around the area of the pain. These disturbances include hypesthesia (decreased sensation of a nonnoxious stimulus) or hyper-esthesia (increased sensation of a nonnoxious stimulus); hypalgesia (decreased sensation of a noxious stimulus) or hyperalgesia (increased sensation of a noxious stimulus); or allodynia (pain induced by a nonnoxious stimulus) or hyperpathia (exaggerated pain response to a noxious or nonnoxious stimulus).

Psychogenic pain is a generic term that conventionally refers to pain resulting from psychopathology. Psychiatric disorders that prominently include pain are described in the *Diagnostic and Statistical Manual of the American Psychiatric Association*.[15] Psychogenic pain appears to be rare in populations with serious illness, and the label should not be applied unless there is positive evidence that the pain is primarily due to psychological factors.

Although psychogenic pain may be rare, the impact of psychological, psychosocial, and spiritual factors on the pain experience is universal. Pain that is inferred to be due primarily to nociceptive or neuropathic mechanisms may be substantially caused or exacerbated and modified by these factors—a concept inherent in the term *total pain*. Pain severity or pain-related distress may be amplified or attenuated, and the ability to cope with pain or retain function despite pain may be profoundly influenced. An accurate assessment of these factors defines and determines the comprehensive treatment plan.

Some patients with chronic pain may not be easily classified according to the mechanisms that are inferred based on the history, examination findings, and objective data. If the pain cannot be described as nociceptive, neuropathic, mixed, or psychogenic, it should be labeled *idiopathic*.

General Principles of Pain Management

If chronic pain is associated with a treatable pathology, an etiology-focused intervention may be an important part of pain management. When pain is due to a neoplasm, for example, radiation therapy, and occasionally chemotherapy or surgery, may be used to achieve local control of the tumor and reduce pain.[16,17] Similarly, more effective management of fluid status in patients with heart failure may lessen lower extremity pain associated with swelling. Other conditions associated with advanced illness also may provide an opportunity for etiology-focused treatments; for example, pain associated with pressure injury may be diminished by primary treatments that promote healing and protect the affected area.

Although etiology-focused interventions should be routinely considered, they seldom obviate the need for primary analgesic therapies. Analgesic drug therapy is the mainstay approach, and opioid therapy is no longer seen as the first-line treatment when pain is moderate or severe. On the other hand, the lack of opioid availability in low- and middle-income countries has been called an "access abyss" and is considered a major issue in global health.[18,19]

Opioid therapy in the treatment of pain associated with serious illness does not conflict with the continuing imperative in the United States and other countries to address the rise in opioid abuse and mortality that has occurred during the past three decades. More judicious and integrative use of opioids for all types of pain is an appropriate response to these problems. At the same time, however, greater caution should not lead to undertreatment when the clinical context supports the use of opioids. Unfortunately, definitive clinical trials of opioid therapy are lacking, and the worldwide acceptance of opioid therapy for pain in serious and advanced illness is not based on high-quality evidence of safety and effectiveness.[20] Nonetheless, the role of opioid therapy gains support from evidence of short-term safety and efficacy,[20] prospective surveys that suggest favorable outcomes in more than 70% of patients,[21,22] and extensive worldwide clinical experience.

The Analgesic Ladder

In the mid-1980s, the World Health Organization published an influential guideline for cancer pain management that included an "analgesic ladder" approach to the selection of drug therapy.[23] According to this approach, patients with mild-to-moderate cancer-related pain may be treated with drugs on the first rung of the ladder, specifically acetaminophen or a nonsteroidal anti-inflammatory drug (NSAID), plus an adjuvant drug to augment analgesia (i.e., an adjuvant analgesic) or treat a side effect, as needed. The second rung was intended for both opioid-naïve patients with generally moderate-to-severe pain and those with generally mild pain that did not respond to a trial of acetaminophen or a NSAID. For these patients, the guideline recommended opioids that were used conventionally to treat moderate pain; these opioids were labeled "weak" in the guideline. The third rung of the analgesic ladder was indicated for patients with generally severe pain or pain that did not respond to a drug used for moderate pain. It included opioids conventionally used for severe pain—designated the "strong" opioids. The guideline also suggested that acetaminophen or a NSAID, or an adjuvant drug, be considered whenever administering an opioid.

The analgesic ladder is still widely used as an educational tool, one that underscores the essential nature of opioid drugs for the management of pain due to active cancer and other serious illnesses. There are several important caveats to consider: (1) Designations "weak" and "strong" should not be used because they do not reflect the clinical pharmacology of the drugs involved; (2) the approach should never be generalized to the treatment of patients with so-called chronic noncancer pain, such as low back pain or headache; (3) the analgesic ladder is *not* an evidence-based guideline and should *not* be considered a set of best practices. For example, for opioid therapy clinicians should rely on up-to-date evidence-based guidelines that have been developed by many organizations in varied countries.[24,25]

These guidelines have common features related to drug selection, dosing, and side-effect management.

Nonsteroidal Anti-inflammatory Drugs

In populations with chronic pain due to serious illness, the use of a nonopioid analgesic—acetaminophen or one of the NSAIDs—is informed by studies in cancer pain [26,27] and experience in the management of acute pain and chronic inflammatory conditions. In the cancer population, these drugs are typically considered if pain is relatively mild and the risk of side effects is tolerable. NSAIDs appear to be especially useful in cancer patients with bone pain or pain related to grossly inflammatory lesions.

Acetaminophen, which is commercially available in multiple oral formulations and an intravenous formulation, is widely used for its analgesic and antipyretic effects.[28] It has no significant anti-inflammatory effects but may be preferred due to a side-effect profile that lacks gastrointestinal and platelet toxicity. Hepatotoxicity is the major concern but can be minimized by avoiding use in those with known liver disease, limiting the maximum total daily dose (recommended to be 3.2 g/d in the United States), and educating patients about the need to avoid over-the-counter medications that also contain this drug.

The NSAIDs reduce production of peripheral and central prostaglandins through inhibition of the enzyme cyclooxygenase (COX). The favorable effects on pain and inflammation produced by COX inhibition must be balanced against the associated toxicities. The subtype COX-1, for example, helps maintain the protective mucous lining of the stomach, and COX-1 inhibition therefore increases the risk of peptic ulcer disease. Although the subtype COX-2 is mostly induced through activation of the inflammatory cascade, it is involved constitutively in kidney function and some other physiologic systems.

The NSAIDs vary in their selectivity for COX-1 and COX-2, and those drugs that are relatively more selective for COX-2 have a lower risk of upper gastrointestinal adverse effects.[29] Although celecoxib is the only drug marketed in the United States as a COX-2-selective drug, several other NSAIDs are relatively COX-2 selective, such as nabumetone, meloxicam, and etodolac.[29]

The gastrointestinal toxicity induced by NSAIDs includes both ulcer formation and gastrointestinal hemorrhage from the upper and lower tracts. Patients at high risk of ulcer disease and those with a bleeding diathesis have strong relative contraindications to NSAID therapy. If NSAID therapy is pursued, it is prudent to use a relatively COX-2-selective drug. Risk of upper gastrointestinal toxicity is further reduced by co-administration of a proton pump inhibitor, such as omeprazole.[30] The prostaglandin analogue misoprostol also can reduce this risk.[30]

The effects of NSAIDs on coagulation are complicated and associated with varied toxicities. All these drugs interfere with platelet function, and patients with a bleeding diathesis have a strong relative contraindication to the use of these drugs. Paradoxically, all NSAIDs also are prothrombotic as a result of the effect of COX-2 inhibition on the clotting cascade. Drugs that are relatively COX-2 selective are more likely to produce toxicities that include symptomatic peripheral vascular disease, myocardial infarction, transient ischemic attacks, and stroke.[31-33]. A high risk of symptomatic vascular disease is therefore another strong relative contraindication to the use of the NSAIDs. There is some evidence that naproxen is relatively safer than other NSAIDs from a cardiovascular perspective,[34] and this drug may be preferred in those patients who may be at high risk from the prothrombotic effects of NSAIDS.

All NSAIDs cause adverse renal effects, including fluid overload, acute nephritis, and chronic kidney disease. Effects on fluid balance may explain the risk of worsening symptoms when NSAIDs are given to patients with congestive heart failure. NSAIDs should be used very cautiously in those with renal insufficiency or heart failure. The risk of hepatotoxicity, which is also shared by all NSAIDs, also suggests caution when these drugs are considered for use in populations with varied hepatopathies.

Given this risk profile, a careful evaluation of risk and benefit for the individual patient should inform the decision to offer NSAID treatment. There is substantial individual variation in the response to different drugs, and the response to NSAID trials in the past also should guide drug selection in the present. If treatment is undertaken, a COX-2-selective drug or naproxen usually is preferred, the lowest effective dose should be used, and the duration of treatment should be limited, if possible. If consistent with the goals of care, NSAID-treated patients should be evaluated periodically for occult fecal blood, changes in blood pressure, and effects on renal or hepatic function.

Adjuvant Analgesics

The term *adjuvant analgesics* was first used to describe drugs that were approved for nonpain indications but could be added to opioid therapy to enhance analgesia. Although the term is a misnomer now—some of these drugs are now approved primary analgesics in specific conditions—palliative care specialists continue to use them as opioid co-analgesics in most situations. There are numerous drugs in many drug classes; a simple classification divides them into several large categories, including multipurpose analgesics and drugs used for neuropathic pain (Table 14.1). Given the risks associated with polypharmacy, it is prudent to consider trials of all these medications after opioid response is ascertained.

Multipurpose Analgesics

Some adjuvant analgesics may be considered for diverse pain syndromes. These include glucocorticoids, antidepressants, alpha-2 adrenergic agonists, cannabinoids, topical therapies, botulinum toxin, neuroleptics, and N-methyl-D-aspartate (NMDA) inhibitors.

Glucocorticoids. The glucocorticoids are extensively used in the management of symptoms associated with advanced cancer, including pain, nausea, anorexia, and fatigue.[35,36] Although there is weak evidence of analgesic efficacy,[37] clinical experience supports a trial of one of these drugs for bone pain, neuropathic pain, pain from bowel or duct obstruction or organ capsule expansion, headache caused by increased intracranial pressure, and pain caused by lymphedema. There is no evidence favoring one glucocorticoid

TABLE 14.1 Adjuvant Analgesics

Category	Class	Types	Examples	Comment
Multipurpose analgesics	Glucocorticoids	—	Dexamethasone, prednisone, methylprednisolone	Commonly used in advanced illness for pain/other symptoms.
	Antidepressants	Secondary amine tricyclics	Desipramine, nortriptyline	Established analgesics, which are better tolerated than the tertiary amine drugs, and with the SNRIs, used in the medically ill for opioid-refractory pain, including neuropathic pain.
		Tertiary amine tricyclics	Amitriptyline, imipramine	Established analgesics, generally with a more problematic side-effect profiles than the secondary amine tricyclics.
		SNRIs	Duloxetine, minalcipran, venlafaxine, desvenlafaxine	Established analgesics, often selected first for opioid-refractory pain because of relatively good side-effect profile compared to the tricyclic compounds. abrupt cessation can cause discontinuation syndrome.
		SSRIs	Paroxetine, citalopram, escitalopram	Poor evidence of analgesia but ability to mitigate chronic or recurrent anxiety can have a positive effect on pain.
	Alpha-2 adrenergic agonists	—	Tizanidine, clonidine, dexmedetomidne	Tizanidine is best tolerated and may be tried for opioid-refractory pain. Clonidine is used neuraxially as an analgesic.
	Cannabinoids	Pharmaceutical	Nabiximols, nabilone, delta(9)-tetrahydrocannabinol	Evidence of analgesic efficacy is evolving. Available drugs may be considered if other adjuvant analgesics are ineffective.
		Nonpharmaceutical	Medical cannabis	Available in many states but cannot be prescribed. Laws and regulations vary by state and should be consulted.
	Topical agents	Local anesthetics	Patch, cream, gels	5% patch is convenient and used for regional neuropathic and musculoskeletal pain syndromes.
		Capsaicin	8% patch, 0.075% patch or cream	8% patch approved for postherpetic neuralgia; may provide months of benefit after short exposure in a monitored setting. Low-concentration capsaicin may be useful for neuropathic or musculoskeletal pain syndromes.
		Compounds, others	Ketamine, amitriptyline, menthol, others	—
	Botulinum toxin		Botulinum A, B	Potentially useful for many types of focal or regional pain.
	Neuroleptics	First/second generation	Haloperidol, olanzapine	Poor evidence of efficacy.
	NMDA receptor antagonists	—	Ketamine	Evidence is mixed, but ketamine is used by palliative care specialists for severe opioid-refractory pain syndromes. Evidence of efficacy in refractory depression may increase use.

	Drug class	Mechanism	Drugs	Comments
Drugs used for neuropathic pain	All multipurpose analgesics	—	—	—
	Gabapentinoids	—	Pregabalin, gabapentin	Extensive evidence of analgesia in many types of neuropathic pain. Patients may respond to gabapentin, pregabalin, both, or neither. Use first for neuropathic pain, unless prominent depression is comorbid, in which case an antidepressant is used first.
	Other anticonvulsants	—	Oxcarbazepine, lacosamide, lamotrigine, topiramate	—
	GABA agonists	$GABA_A$	Clonazepam	Poor evidence of analgesia.
		$GABA_B$	Baclofen	Poor evidence of analgesia.
Drugs used for bone pain in cancer	Glucocorticoids	—	Dexamethasone, prednisone, methylprednisolone	—
	Osteoclast inhibitors	Bisphosphonates	Zolendronate, alendronate, ibandronate, pamidronate, risendronate, clodronate, others	Used to prevent and treat skeletal-related events due to cancer, including pain.
		RANKL inhibitor	Denosumab	Used to prevent and treat skeletal-related events due to cancer, including pain.
		Calcitonin	—	Poor evidence of efficacy.
	Radioisotopes	—	Samarium 153, strontium 89, phosphorus 32, others	—
Drugs used for pain and other symptoms in malignant bowel obstruction	Glucocorticoids	—	Dexamethasone, prednisone, methylprednisolone	—
	Antiemetics	Dopamine antagonist	Metoclopramide, haloperidol	—
		$5\text{-}HT_3$ antagonist	Ondansetron, granisetron	—
	PPI or H_2 blocker	—	Omeprazole, ranitidine	—
	Anticholinergic drug	—	Hyoscine (scopolamine) butylbromide or hydrobromide, glycopyrrolate	Risk of cognitive side effects probably lessened by using glycopyrrolate or, in some countries, hyoscine butylbromide.
	Somatostatin analogue	—	Octreotide, lanreotide	Evidence of efficacy is mixed and should not be considered a first-line approach for this reason.

GABA, γ-aminobutyric acid; NMDA, *N*-methyl-D-aspartate; PPI, proton pump inhibitor; RANKL, receptor activator of nuclear factor–κB ligand; SNRIs, serotonin norepinephrine reuptake inhibitors; SSRIs, selective serotonin reuptake inhibitors.

over another. In the United States, experience is greatest with dexamethasone, but predni-sone and methylprednisolone are acceptable alternatives. A typical low-dose regimen starts with a loading dose of dexamethasone 10–20 mg, followed by 1–2 mg twice daily, which is continued until clinical events warrant a change. Some clinicians also use a short-term, high-dose regimen for very severe pain; a loading dose or dexamethasone 20–100 mg is followed by 32–96 mg per day in divided doses, which are tapered over weeks as other analgesic approaches are implemented.

Acute glucocorticoid risks include hyperglycemia and neuropsychiatric symptoms that range from anxiety and insomnia to frank psychosis. Long-term use is also associated with osteoporosis, myopathy, and immune suppression. These risks increase with the dose of the drug and predisposing factors associated with the medical condition of the patient.[38] Given the risks, ineffective regimens should be tapered and discontinued.

Analgesic Antidepressants. Antidepressants have been used as analgesics for decades and can be considered for any type of chronic pain.[39–41] Drugs and drug classes vary in the potential for analgesic effects and the risks of side effects.[42,43] The tricyclic antidepressants are analgesic and include tertiary amine drugs, such as amitriptyline and imipramine, and secondary amine drugs, such as desipramine and nortriptyline. The serotonin-norepinephrine reuptake inhibitors (SNRIs) also are analgesic; the evidence is strongest for duloxetine, but there is support as well for milnacipran, venlafaxine, and desvenlafaxine.[41,42–46] There is very little evidence of analgesic efficacy for the selective serotonin reuptake inhibitors (SSRIs), such as fluoxetine, paroxetine, and sertraline, and these drugs are not preferred when pain is the primary indication for therapy.

Both the SNRIs and the SSRIs have more favorable side-effect profiles than the tricyclic compounds.[43] When pain is a target of therapy, the preferred drugs are the SNRIs; duloxetine is usually selected first given the number of positive trials. Commonly reported side effects include fatigue, nausea or other gastrointestinal problems, dizziness, sleep disturbances, and both somnolence and agitation. Although tricyclic drugs may be considered, they should be used cautiously in patients with significant heart disease, including those with heart failure, arrhythmia, or QTc prolongation; similar caution is appropriate in those with cognitive impairment, high fall risk, or urinary retention. Desipramine and nortriptyline have a better safety profile than the tertiary amine drugs and are preferred in medically fragile populations. If a tertiary amine drug, such as amitriptyline, is offered to a patient who has not responded to other antidepressants, side-effect risk should be minimized by the use of a low starting dose and slow dose titration.

Dosing of the SNRIs when the target symptom is pain mirrors the approach used when the indication is depression. Initial doses of the tricyclic drugs should be low when treating pain (e.g., 10 to 25 mg of either desipramine or nortriptyline), and doses should be increased every few days until treatment-limiting side effects occur or the dose is at the upper range for antidepressant effects. If a favorable outcome is not observed, one or more trials of alternative SNRIs or tricyclic antidepressants may be considered.

Dose tapering is recommended when stopping or switching antidepressants to avoid the antidepressant discontinuation syndrome.[47] This syndrome, which is characterized by flu-like symptoms, nausea, dizziness, insomnia, and hyperarousal, is relatively common, particularly when the antidepressant regimen has involved relatively high doses and a long treatment period. The symptoms are usually tolerated and resolve within several weeks, but some patients are severely affected and require re-institution of therapy followed by tapering using smaller decrements and longer intervals between dose reductions.

Alpha-2 Adrenergic Agonists. The alpha-2 adrenergic agonists include clonidine, tizanidine, and dexmedetomidine. Analgesic effects have been demonstrated for all three.[48-50] Tizanidine is available orally and may be better tolerated than clonidine. It is considered a second-line adjuvant analgesic, potentially useful for any type of chronic pain. It is relatively sedating and may be a preferred second-line drug when pain is accompanied by insomnia. Treatment is usually initiated with a nighttime dose of 2–4 mg, and the dose is gradually increased to as high as 24 mg per day in two or three divided doses.

The side effects associated with the alpha-2 adrenergic agonists include mental clouding and somnolence, dry mouth, dizziness, and orthostasis with increased risk of falls. Clonidine commonly causes constipation. These side effects may interfere with treatment, particularly in medically fragile patients with advanced illness.

Cannabinoids. Cannabinoids bind to endogenous cannabinoid receptors and produce an array of effects, among which is analgesia.[51,52] Nabiximols, an oromucosal spray containing mostly delta-(9)-tetrahydrocannabinol (THC) and cannabidiol, is approved in some countries for opioid-refractory cancer pain and spasticity related to multiple sclerosis.[53-55] Single-entity THC and single-entity nabilone also are commercially available in the United States but have minimal evidence of analgesic efficacy[56-58]; these drugs are rarely considered in the setting of pain that has been refractory to other treatments. Cannabis itself has analgesic efficacy in some studies.[59] In those countries and regions that have legal access to cannabis, pain appears to be a common reason for use. Research into a variety of possible indications for the cannabinoids, and cannabis specifically, include a number of conditions—such as mood disorders, post-traumatic stress, and sleep disorders—that would be important for populations with serious chronic illness. The role of these drugs is likely to evolve as this work unfolds.

Topical Analgesics. Topical therapies have a very low risk of adverse effects and should be considered for local or regional pains. A 2017 overview of Cochrane reviews aggregated the results of 13 systematic reviews of controlled trials[60] and found strong evidence of analgesic efficacy for selected NSAIDs (including diclofenac and ketoprofen) in musculoskeletal pain, moderate-quality evidence of limited efficacy for high-concentration capsaicin in postherpetic neuralgia, and limited evidence for other NSAIDs, salicylate, low-concentration capsaicin, lidocaine, clonidine, and herbal remedies. The most widely used topical analgesics contain local anesthetics; available formulations include lidocaine 5% patches and varied gels or creams. Lidocaine patches are approved in the United States for a 12-h/d dosing regimen. With very limited systemic absorption from this patch,[61] however, around-the-clock application may be used, if beneficial, and two or three patches may be applied, if necessary, to cover the painful region.

Topical capsaicin is available in a low-concentration (0.075%) cream or patch, which may be useful for regional neuropathic pains and joint pains.[60] A high-concentration (8%) patch also is approved for postherpetic neuralgia in the United States and peripheral neuropathic pain in the European Union.[62] The high-concentration patch is applied for a short time in a monitored setting and, when effective, can yield several months of pain relief.

Other topical drugs, such as amitriptyline, doxepin, baclofen, ketamine, gabapentin, and menthol, have been used empirically in compounded creams or gels, despite a lack of evidence and no data evaluating dose, additive effects, or formulation differences. One controlled trial found a strong trend supporting the efficacy of a gel containing baclofen 10 mg, amitriptyline 40 mg, and ketamine 20 mg for neuropathic symptoms associated with chemotherapy-induced peripheral neuropathy,[63] and another small study suggested benefit from menthol 1% in cancer-related neuropathic pain.[64]

Botulinum Toxin. There is growing evidence that diverse pain syndromes can respond favorably to the local injection of botulinum toxin, including peripheral neuropathic pain, plantar fasciitis, piriformis syndrome, postsurgical pain, joint pain, low back pain, and pain due to osteoarthropathy.[65,66] There has been favorable experience in cancer patients with chronic post-treatment pain syndromes.[67] If cost and availability are not prohibitive, it may be considered for diverse types of opioid-refractory regional pain syndromes.

Neuroleptics. A systematic review of controlled trials found limited evidence of analgesic efficacy for selected neuroleptics.[68] The potential for adverse effects, however, suggests that these drugs should not be routinely considered for pain unless this symptom is accompanied by another indication for neuroleptic therapy.

NMDA Receptor Antagonists. The NMDA receptor antagonists include ketamine, memantine, amantadine, dextromethorphan, and methadone. Evidence of analgesic efficacy for memantine, amantadine, and dextromethorphan is very limited, and these drugs are rarely considered for trials as adjuvant analgesics. Methadone, as described previously, is commercially available in most countries as a racemate of two optical isomers; it is the d-isomer that interacts with the NMDA receptor, and it is this interaction that may explain the unexpectedly high potency of this drug when substituted for another opioid. There is no evidence that this pharmacology makes methadone a more effective analgesic, either overall or for neuropathic pain.

Ketamine is a dissociative anesthetic and has attained some acceptance as a potentially useful analgesic, notwithstanding conflicting data.[69-72] Palliative care specialists may consider this drug for severe opioid-refractory pain in the setting of advanced illness.[73,74] This usage may grow with emerging evidence of an important therapeutic effect on depression.[75]

Although there is anecdotal experience with oral ketamine,[76] it is generally administered by the intravenous or subcutaneous route using continuous infusion, repeated brief infusion, or repeated bolus injection. Brief infusion—sometimes called "burst" therapy—has been used to manage episodes of severe pain; this approach, which may start with 100 mg/d, escalating by 100-mg/d increments, for 2–5 days,[77,78] is likely to be less safe than approaches employing continuous infusion. Infusions may start with a loading bolus, such as 0.1–0.5 mg/kg, followed by 0.05–0.2 mg/kg/h, which is then gradually titrated until benefits occur or side effects supervene.[73,74,79] An alternative approach starts with 50–100 mg/d, irrespective of weight, and increases the dose by 25%–50% every day, depending on effects. Regardless of the approach, side effects must be anticipated, including hypertension, tachycardia, and psychotomimetic effects that may manifest as intense dysphoria, dissociation, nightmares, or hallucinations. It is common practice to coadminister a benzodiazepine or a neuroleptic to reduce the risk of psychotomimetic effects.[73,74] Some clinicians also preemptively reduce the opioid dose by 25%–50% when initiating therapy.

Drugs Used for Neuropathic Pain

Patients with opioid-refractory neuropathic pain may be treated with the multipurpose adjuvant analgesics or a group of adjuvant analgesics that are conventionally used only for neuropathic pain. Among the latter drugs, the gabapentinoids—gabapentin and pregabalin—are prioritized in evidence-based guidelines.[40,80–82] Patients with opioid-refractory pain and depressed mood often receive an analgesic antidepressant first, whereas others are initially treated with a gabapentinoid. Patients with advanced cancer are usually considered for an initial trial of a glucocorticoid.

Gabapentinoids. Gabapentin and pregabalin have multiple actions, among which is reducing the likelihood of depolarization of nociceptive neurons through binding to the alpha-2 delta protein modulator of the N-type, voltage-gated calcium channel.[83] Although evidence of analgesic efficacy in some types of acute pain[84] suggest that these drugs are multipurpose analgesics, efficacy in chronic pain has been established for only some neuropathic pain syndromes.[85,86] Limited observations suggest that patients may be responders to gabapentin, to pregabalin, to both, or to neither.[87] One trial in cancer-related neuropathic pain suggested that pregabalin was superior to gabapentin,[88] but this finding has not been replicated. Pregabalin may be preferred, however, given pharmacokinetics that support easier and more rapid titration.[89]

The gabapentinoids are not hepatically metabolized, and drug-drug interactions do not occur. Side effects, such as mental clouding, occur commonly, however.[90] For this reason, a low starting dose and dose titration are recommended. In the medically frail, the starting doses of pregabalin and gabapentin are 25–50 mg/d and 100–200 mg/d, respectively. The lowest doses are used in those with severe renal disease. The effective doses vary, and if the initial dose is tolerated, dose escalation every few days usually is needed to determine whether the drug will be beneficial.[86] The effective pregabalin dose is usually between 150 mg/d and 600 mg/d in two divided doses, and the effective gabapentin dose is usually between 900 and 3600 mg/d in two or three divided doses.

Other Anticonvulsants. A review of Cochrane reviews found no high-quality evidence that other anticonvulsant drugs are analgesic in neuropathic pain.[91] The extant data, and clinical experience, nonetheless suggest that several may be considered when opioid-refractory neuropathic pain has not responded to trials of antidepressants and gabapentinoids.

Carbamazepine is an older drug approved for trigeminal neuralgia in the United States; it has some evidence of analgesic efficacy[92] but is not favored because of its adverse effect profile and the need to monitor blood counts during treatment. Phenytoin and valproate also are older drugs with limited supporting data and adverse effect profiles worse than newer drugs. Among the more recently approved drugs, oxcarbazepine was analgesic in a study of peripheral neuropathic pains,[93] and both lacosamide and topiramate have limited evidence of efficacy in painful diabetic neuropathy.[94,95] Lamotrigine has been efficacious in some neuropathic pains, but not chemotherapy-induced painful neuropathy.[96] There is no evidence for other anticonvulsant drugs, including levetiracetam, zonisamide, and tiagabine.

GABA Agonists. GABA (γ-aminobutyric acid) agonists lead to neuronal hyperpolarization by enhancing GABA-induced chloride ion flux. The benzodiazepines are $GABA_A$ agonists approved for the treatment of anxiety and other conditions; baclofen is a $GABA_B$ agonist used for the management of spasticity. Anecdotal reports suggest that clonazepam may be analgesic[97] and is favored by some clinicians when pain is accompanied by severe anxiety. All benzodiazepines should be used very cautiously in opioid-treated patients, however, due to concern about potentiated risks of respiratory depression, cognitive impairment, and falls. Baclofen may be efficacious in trigeminal neuralgia,[98] and based on anecdotal experience, this drug is occasionally offered for refractory neuropathic pain. A starting dose of 5 mg twice daily can be gradually escalated to doses that may exceed 200 mg per day in some patients; tapering should precede discontinuation to avoid withdrawal seizures.

Drugs Used for Bone Pain

Cancer-related bone pain that does not respond adequately to an opioid may be managed using a variety of bone-specific interventions. When focal pain is related to a metastasis, radiation is highly effective. Percutaneous invasive techniques, such as radio-frequency ablation and cementoplasty (including vertebroplasty/kyphoplasty), and magnetic resonance–guided focused ultrasound, also are considered in selected cases, when available.[99,100] For patients with multiple metastases and multifocal pain, an NSAID or an opioid usually is supplemented first with a glucocorticoid and/or a bone-targeting therapy. The most important of these bone-targeted therapies, specifically those that inhibit osteoclast function, are also widely used prophylactically in patients with metastatic disease to reduce the risk of adverse skeletal-related events (SREs), including pain, pathological fracture, spinal cord compression, hypercalcemia, necessity for radiation to address impending fracture, and need for bone surgery.[101,102]

Osteoclast Inhibitors. The osteoclast inhibitors include the bisphosphonates, denosumab, and calcitonin. The bisphosphonates are most often used and include zolendronate, alendronate, ibandronate, pamidronate, risendronate, clodronate, neridronate, and olpadronate. A recent systematic review of 13 bisphosphonate studies concluded that these drugs reduce pain, have a rapid onset, and provide relief for 1–3 months; a positive effect on quality of life was not demonstrated.[103] The most common adverse effects are a transitory flu-like syndrome and, with oral therapy, upper gastrointestinal symptoms.[104] Renal insufficiency can occur and contraindicates treatment in those with moderate-to-severe renal dysfunction. Ocular inflammation and severe musculoskeletal pain are rare, and the potential for hypocalcemia should be recognized. Periodic monitoring of renal function and serum calcium levels should be performed during treatment. With treatment for months or years, rare but serious adverse events include osteonecrosis of the jaw and atypical femoral fracture; predisposing factors include dental pathology, diabetes, and long-term glucocorticoid therapy.[104]

Denosumab is a human monoclonal antibody that binds to receptor activator of nuclear factor–κB ligand (RANKL), a molecule secreted by osteoblasts that activates osteoclasts through binding to its receptor, RANK. It is effective for metastatic bone pain, and a recent systematic review of studies comparing denosumab and a bisphosphonate found that denosumab was more effective in terms of time to SREs and the need for radiation.[105] Although cost and availability favor selection of a bisphosphonate in most situations, an economic analysis suggests that denosumab's efficacy and adverse event profile can make it a cost-effective option in multiple myeloma patients.[106]

Calcitonin also inhibits osteoclast activity. A 2006 systematic review found only two trials assessing pain-related outcomes, however, and concluded that there is no support for the use of this drug for the primary indication of pain.[107] Given the abundant evidence supporting the use of other drug classes, calcitonin cannot be recommended for this indication.

Radioisotopes. Numerous compounds have been developed that link a bone-seeking phosphonate to a radioisotope, including phosphorus 32 (^{32}P), strontium 89 (^{89}Sr), yttrium 90 (^{90}Y), tin 117m (^{117m}Sn), samarium 153 (^{153}Sm), holmium 166 (^{166}Ho), thulium 170 (^{170}Tm), lutetium 177 (^{177}Lu), rhenium 186 (^{186}Re), rhenium 188 (^{188}Re), and radium 223 (^{223}Ra).[108,109] Systematic reviews confirm that the most studied drugs, which contain strontium 89 or samarium 153, provide meaningful pain relief to about 75% of patients with pain due to bone metastases, and approximately 10%–25% experience complete pain relief.[110,111] Initial response occurs in 1 to 3 weeks, peak response can require more than a month, and duration of response can be at least several months. The major adverse effects are transitory pain flare and bone marrow toxicity, which is clinically relevant in as many as one-third of patients and may continue for months after treatment. Patients with preexisting bone marrow suppression and those with renal insufficiency are at increased risk of toxicity.

The clinical use of a radioisotope as an adjuvant analgesic requires production or sourcing of the compound and the availability of skilled personnel and facilities. Given the cost and complexity of the treatment and the lack of data demonstrating advantages over the osteoclast inhibitors, the use of radioisotopes has been limited to a highly selected subset of patients.

Drugs Used for Pain and Other Symptoms in Bowel Obstruction

The management of bowel obstruction includes short-term or long-term nasogastric suctioning and decompression through surgery, percutaneous venting, or stenting. The last procedures are generally favored over prolonged nasogastric suctioning, which may be uncomfortable for the patient, produce symptomatic irritation of nasopharyngeal or oropharyngeal tissues, or cause injury to the nares. In populations with bowel obstruction associated with advanced gastrointestinal or pelvic neoplasms, medical treatments also are used for pain, distension, and nausea and vomiting. These medical treatments may become the sole therapy for patients who eschew decompression in the setting of advanced cancer or are not candidates for these interventions.

Treatment of pain associated with malignant bowel obstruction usually includes an opioid, notwithstanding the risk of worsening bowel dysmotility. If increased colic or distention occurs when an opioid is added, a different opioid should be tried or treatment should proceed while minimizing or eliminating the opioid. Laxatives may be coadministered with the opioid, but based on clinical observations, drugs that stimulate peristalsis, including the stimulant cathartics (e.g., senna) and the opioid antagonists (e.g., methylnaltrexone), should be avoided; an osmotic drug such as polyethylene glycol may be preferred.

Other drugs may enhance symptom control. A glucocorticoid is usually administered, typically in a low-dose regimen, and there is some evidence that this treatment can mitigate the obstruction, presumably by reducing peritumoral edema.[112] Antiemetics should be provided to reduce nausea. Metoclopramide has prokinetic properties, which might be helpful in partial obstruction but worsen colic in severe obstruction. For this reason, other dopamine antagonists, such as haloperidol, and the 5-HT$_3$ (5-hydroxytryptamine-3) antagonists, such as ondansetron, are preferred. If pyrosis occurs, it is managed with a proton pump inhibitor, such as omeprazole, or an H$_2$ blocker, such as ranitidine. A systematic review of seven studies confirmed that the latter drugs can reduce the volume of gastric secretions, which also may have a beneficial effect on symptoms.[113]

Patients who have persistent colicky pain may be offered a trial of an anticholinergic drug or a somatostatin analogue. The anticholinergic drugs have antisecretory effects in the bowel. Despite very limited evidence,[114,115] hyoscine butylbromide, hyoscine hydrobromide (also called scopolamine hydrobromide), and glycopyrrolate are employed for this indication. Given their relatively lower penetration into the central nervous system, glycopyrrolate and hyoscine butylbromide may be preferable. Anticholinergic side effects, such as tachycardia, must be anticipated.

The somatostatin analogues octreotide and lanreotide inhibit gastrointestinal secretions and motility. A recent systematic review, which evaluated six controlled trials of octreotide and one trial of lanreotide, found mixed results,[116] with only low-level evidence of benefit. Nonetheless, palliative care specialists continue to endorse a trial of octreotide in malignant bowel obstruction.[115,117,118] Some clinicians, however, recommend a trial only after other therapies fail.[119] Octreotide treatment may be provided using two or three injections per day or continuous infusion; a long-acting formulation requires monthly injection. Lanreotide is administered by biweekly injection. The optimal dose of octreotide varies; most patients respond at a dose of 600–800 µg/d. Side effects include nausea, diarrhea, steatorrhea, and changes in blood glucose levels.

Opioids

Based on receptor interactions, opioid drugs can be divided into pure µ-receptor agonists, partial agonists, agonist-antagonists, and the pure antagonists. Drugs in another group have mixed mechanisms and are considered with the opioids because of a mode of action that combines pure µ-receptor agonism with other mechanisms (Table 14.2).

The pure µ-agonists, such as morphine, vary in potency, kinetics, and other characteristics. They produce dose-dependent effects without a clinically relevant ceiling dose for analgesia; the maximum dose is determined by the occurrence of treatment-limiting adverse

TABLE 14.2 Opioid Drugs

Drug	Approximate Equianalgesic Doses		Elimination Half-Life (h)	Comment
	Oral	IV		
Morphine	30 mg	10 mg	2–4	Available in multiple formulations, including once-daily and twice-daily extended-release formulations.
Codeine	200 mg	100 mg	2–4	Prodrug, metabolized in the liver to the active compound, morphine. As a result of large genetically determined variation in the cytochrome P 450 enzyme responsible for conversion to morphine (2D6), effects are unpredictable. As a result, it is no longer recommended.
Oxycodone	20 mg	—	2–4	Available in a twice-daily controlled-release formulation.
Hydromorphone	7.5 mg	1.5 mg	2–4	Available in a once-daily controlled-release formulation.
Oxymorphone	10 mg	1 mg	2–4	Available in a twice-daily controlled-release formulation.
Fentanyl transdermal system	—	—	—	Consult prescribing information for guideline related to converting other opioids to the transdermal fentanyl patch. Based on clinical experience, a 100-µg/h patch is roughly equianalgesic to morphine 4 mg/h. Dosing interval for patches is 48–72 hours. One to three doses are needed to approach steady state. Cachexia can change the pharmacokinetics unpredictably, and external heat can result in unintended overdose.
Fentanyl	—	0.1 mg	3–12	
Methadone	20 mg	10 mg	8 to ≥ 100	Safe use requires familiarity with unique pharmacology, including long and variable half-life, potential for drug-drug interactions, and possibility of QTc prolongation. Potency varies depending on the extent of opioid treatment prior to a switch to methadone. Opioid-naïve patients should receive no more than 7.5 mg/d in divided doses; opioid-treated patients should receive 10%–25% of the calculated equianalgesic dose, but no more than 40 mg per day when starting therapy. Long half-life allows long dosing interval in most patients (every 6 to 8 hours).
Levorphanol	4 mg	2 mg	12–15	Relatively long half-life may allow a long dosing interval in most patients.
Hydrocodone	30 mg	—	2–4	Available combined with a nonopioid analgesic in immediate-release formulations and in twice-daily extended-release formulations.
Tramadol	—	120 mg	5–6	Available in an immediate-release formulation and a once-daily extended-release formulation.
Tapentadol	—	—	4–5	Available in an immediate-release formulation and in a twice-daily extended-release formulation.
Buprenorphine transdermal system	—	—	—	Low-dose patches, changed weekly, can be used to initiate opioid therapy.

effects. Partial μ-receptor agonists may have a ceiling effect for μ-receptor-mediated analgesia and can induce abstinence if administered to an animal made physically dependent on a pure μ-receptor agonist. The agonist-antagonist drugs are weak antagonists at the μ-receptor and agonists at another opioid receptor subtype; they have an analgesic ceiling effect and also can induce abstinence when administered to someone who is physically dependent on an opioid drug. Pure μ-receptor antagonists reverse both analgesic and nonanalgesic effects associated with μ-receptor activation. Finally, the mixed mechanism drugs are both μ-receptor agonists and reuptake inhibitors at monoamine receptors (serotonin, norepinephrine, or dopamine). The last drugs have a ceiling effect imposed by the potential for monoaminergic toxicity.

Pure μ-Agonists. As described by the analgesic ladder, persistent pain in a patient with a serious chronic illness that is generally moderate in severity or has not responded to a nonopioid drug should be treated with an opioid. There have been no comparative effectiveness studies of the opioids used for this indication, and drug selection generally reflects experience, availability, and cost. Combination products containing acetaminophen plus either hydrocodone or oxycodone are often used, but a single-entity pure μ-agonist, such as low-dose morphine, could be equally effective.[120] Although codeine was historically considered the prototype "weak" opioid for the analgesic ladder, it is associated with highly variable effects due to genetically determined metabolic variation and is no longer recommended for this reason.[121] Similarly, propoxyphene was prescribed commonly in the past but is no longer available due to a relatively high risk of serious complications. Tilidine is available in some countries other than the United States.

When persistent pain is generally severe or has not responded to an appropriate dose of a drug administered conventionally for moderate pain, a single entity, pure μ-receptor agonist conventionally used for severe pain is generally preferred. The analgesic ladder designated morphine as the prototype, but any of the pure μ-agonist drugs, such as hydromorphone, oxycodone, oxymorphone, fentanyl, levorphanol, or methadone, may be used. Drug selection usually considers the patient's prior experience with any of the specific drugs, availability on formularies, cost, and the prescriber's experience.

A long-acting formulation may be preferred when pain is constant or nearly so, or when there is a need to improve convenience or adherence. Modified-release oral formulations are available for many of these drugs, such as morphine, oxycodone, oxymorphone, hydrocodone, or hydromorphone. These oral formulations are administered once or twice a day. Transdermal formulations of fentanyl (administered every 2 or 3 days) also are long acting. Additionally, two opioids, levorphanol and methadone, may be long-acting due to long elimination half-lives (Table 14.2), which usually supports dosing intervals of at least every 6 hours to maintain stable effects.

Some of the pure μ-agonist drugs have characteristics that influence decisions about drug selection. Meperidine is not preferred because an active metabolite, normeperidine, can accumulate with repetitive dosing, particularly in the setting of renal insufficiency, and produce neurotoxicity.[122,123] Morphine may not be preferred in patients with significant renal insufficiency, or changing renal function, because of the potential risk associated with accumulation of two renally excreted active metabolites, morphine-3-glucuronide and morphine-6-glucuronide.[124,125] Hydromorphone or fentanyl may be preferred.[123,126,127]

Methadone is used to manage opioid addiction and is also an effective treatment for chronic pain. It may be considered a preferred option because it is relatively low cost and theoretically less likely to be abused by those with a history of substance use disorder. It is, however, a challenging drug to use safely and should not be prescribed by clinicians who are unfamiliar with its pharmacology and safe prescribing practices.[128] The half-life of methadone is both long and variable, and this characteristic creates uncertainty about the time required to approach steady state when treatment is initiated or the dose increased. Most patients require 4–7 days to approach steady state, but some patients require several weeks. As the blood level rises toward steady state, there is a potential for delayed onset of adverse effects, and this necessitates close monitoring for a prolonged period after a change in therapy.

Equally important, methadone can produce unexpectedly potent effects when it is substituted for another opioid. This phenomenon may have a number of causes, one of which is related to the fact that commercially available methadone in most of the world is a racemic mixture of two optical isomers. One of the isomers, l-methadone, is a pure μ-receptor agonist and the other, the d-isomer, is an NMDA receptor antagonist. NMDA antagonists may be associated with nonopioid analgesia and the reversal of opioid tolerance. When a patient who is receiving another pure μ-receptor agonist is switched to methadone, the potency of methadone may be much higher than expected. Higher potency due to interaction with the NMDA receptor means that a relatively lower methadone dose would produce effects, including potential side effects. Guidelines for safe switching from another opioid to methadone must be followed to reduce the risk of unintended overdose.[128] Methadone also can prolong the QTc interval,[129,130] necessitating a baseline electrocardiogram in most patients and, if appropriate, monitoring of the electrocardiogram during dose titration.

Other Opioids. Buprenorphine, the partial agonist, is used for the treatment of chronic pain and the treatment of addiction. It is available for pain in a 7-day transdermal patch. There is uncertainty about the extent to which it demonstrates a ceiling effect for analgesia in the clinical setting, but the potential to induce withdrawal if administered to a patient who is physically dependent on another opioid is well recognized. Although experience with buprenorphine in the management of chronic pain associated with serious illness is relatively limited, it also may be considered, particularly in those patients who develop persistent moderate or severe pain and are opioid naïve or have limited opioid exposure.

The agonist-antagonist drugs, such as butorphanol and nalbuphine, are rarely considered for the management of chronic pain. They are not viewed favorably because of their analgesic ceiling effect, potential to induce abstinence if administered to a physically dependent patient, and limited dosage forms.

The opioid antagonist drugs include naloxone, naltrexone, and nalmefene. Naloxone is generally administered to acutely reverse opioid effects, and the last two drugs are used clinically in the management of selective addictive disorders.

The mixed-mechanism drugs tramadol and tapentadol are used for both acute and chronic pain, and the older drug, tramadol, has achieved wide usage in some countries. Both drugs are available in immediate-release and long-acting formulations. In the United States, however, neither of these opioids has gained popularity in the treatment of persistent pain associated with cancer or other serious illnesses. Like buprenorphine, tramadol and tapentadol are occasionally considered as alternatives to the use of conventional pure μ-agonist drugs. Additional favorable studies of these drugs in the medically ill, and additional experience, may increase their use.

Routes of Administration

The oral and transdermal routes are preferred in the management of chronic pain. The transdermal route is available for the highly lipophilic opioids fentanyl and buprenorphine. Although evidence is limited, observational data suggest that transdermal fentanyl may be associated with relatively less constipation than oral formulations and may therefore have value when constipation has been difficult to manage.[131,132] Transdermal patches should be used cautiously in patients with cachexia; the literature is again very limited, but some studies suggest transdermal fentanyl may produce fentanyl concentrations that are higher or lower than expected in this context.[133,134] Patients at risk for recurrent fever should not receive transdermal systems due to the potential for increases in drug concentration associated with enhanced absorption caused by ambient heat.[135]

Although most patients with serious chronic illness can be managed with oral and transdermal formulations throughout the course of the illness, alternative routes are required by some. Rectal formulations of oxymorphone, hydromorphone, and morphine are commercially available in the United States, and there is anecdotal experience with rectal administration of controlled-release morphine or oxycodone tablets. The potency of rectal opioids approximates oral dosing,[136] and absorption is variably affected by a variety of factors, including location of the suppository (low in the rectum, where the blood drains into the systemic circulation, or high in the rectum, where blood drains through the liver via the portal circulation) and contents of the rectum at the time of dosing.[137,138] For these reasons, the rectal route usually is considered when patients receiving relatively low opioid doses have a temporary inability to take oral medications.

Opioids that are both lipophilic and highly potent may be clinically useful when administered through the oral or nasal mucosa. This approach has been explored to create formulations that have a rapid onset of effect. The most notable examples are the transmucosal formulations of fentanyl—known collectively as transmucosal immediate-release formulations (TIRFs)—which have been approved for the treatment of cancer-related breakthrough pain. These formulations include an intraoral lozenge, an effervescent buccal tablet, a buccal patch, a sublingual tablet, sublingual spray, and a nasal spray. The TIRFs are efficacious and have an onset of action faster than orally administered drugs.[139–142] The few comparative trials do not allow definitive conclusions about the appropriate positioning of these drugs against relatively less-costly oral drugs for cancer-related breakthrough pain, but clinical experience would support a trial when the response to a short-acting oral opioid is inadequate or when breakthrough pain has a very rapid onset. There are insufficient data to recommend one formulation over another, and in the United States, all these drugs require adherence to a mandatory federal risk evaluation and mitigation strategy, the purpose of which is to reduce the risk of abuse and unintentional overdose.

In some clinical situations, the sublingual use of an injectable opioid formulation may be considered for a therapeutic trial. Although there is considerable experience in the use of sublingual administration of concentrated oral morphine solution during the care of patients at the end of life, this drug is poorly absorbed through mucous membranes, and it is likely that much of its effects reflect enteral absorption after swallowing.[143]

Patients who are unable to swallow or absorb opioid drugs are candidates for long-term parenteral dosing. Repetitive intramuscular injections are painful and associated with variable absorption; they are not preferred. Repetitive injection or infusion may be safely accomplished with subcutaneous or intravenous access. Subcutaneous access may be provided using a "butterfly" needle or a catheter placed under the skin. Numerous studies have demonstrated the efficacy and safety of subcutaneous administration,[144] and clinical experience suggests that the needle or catheter may be left in place for a week or more without the development of local pain or infection. Continuous subcutaneous or intravenous infusion requires the availability of an infusion device, and in developed countries, options included ambulatory devices with programmable features that permit coadministration of a continuous infusion and patient-controlled dosing to address episodic pains.

A small proportion of patients respond poorly to systemic opioid therapy and may be considered for neuraxial therapy. Many methods are in use,[145] and the ability to try one or another typically depends on local availability of the clinical expertise, resources to cover the cost, and clinical factors such as prognosis. Among the approaches employed are a percutaneous epidural catheter tunneled to the anterior abdominal wall; a totally implanted epidural catheter connected to a subcutaneous portal; and an intrathecal catheter connected to a totally implanted continuous infusion device. If the resources exist, an implantable pump system, which is refilled percutaneously, is usually considered for patients with life expectancies of 3 or more months. A systematic review,[146] which included one randomized trial comparing neuraxial analgesia via an implanted pump against usual analgesic therapy, concluded that intraspinal therapy is effective and can yield analgesia with relatively fewer side effects than systemic analgesic therapy. The preferred opioids for neuraxial analgesia are morphine and hydromorphone, but others are used empirically; other drugs, such as a local anesthetic or clonidine, often are combined with the opioid.[147] Ziconotide, a unique calcium channel blocker, also is available for use in neuraxial analgesia and has been shown to be effective in controlled trials; if available, it may be considered for first-line therapy in some situations.[148]

Opioid Administration

In the opioid-naïve patient, treatment usually is initiated with a short-acting drug. Although a low dose of an oral modified-release opioid (e.g., morphine 20–30 mg per day) or transdermal fentanyl (12 µg/d) may be used, the short-acting formulation allows relatively quick evaluation of the effects produced by the initial dose. If a patient is receiving a short-acting opioid but pain is not controlled despite dose titration and multiple doses per day, it is customary to switch to a single-entity pure µ-agonist opioid in a long-acting oral or transdermal formulation. Some patients prefer to remain on a short-acting drug, however, and in the absence of evidence showing better outcomes for the long-acting formulations, this preference should be considered.

Dose Titration. Effective opioid therapy requires individualization of the dose through a process of dose titration.[24,25] The objective of dose titration is to identify the dose associated with a favorable balance between analgesia and side effects. Although there is a concern that the development of analgesic tolerance will inevitably lead to the need for continual dose increases, the reality is far more complex. For unclear reasons, dose titration to a favorable balance between analgesia and side effects usually is followed by a prolonged period of stability unless there is progression in the pain-producing pathology. Indeed, should a chronically ill patient receiving opioid therapy experience a resurgence of pain after successful dose titration, this should be followed by an evaluation of the underlying pain-producing pathology and other factors that may drive pain complaints, such as anxiety or delirium. Although dose escalation may be needed in the absence of these factors, in which case it may be appropriate to ascribe it to analgesic tolerance, this is an uncommon scenario.

Most patients with persistent pain due to serious chronic illness experience periodic events that increase pain and may necessitate opioid dose escalation. When an increase in opioid dose is indicated, an increment of 30%–50% of the total daily dose is usually safe and effective. Alternatively, the daily dose can be escalated by an amount equivalent to the average daily use of rescue medication during the past several days. If the pain-producing event is transitory, it is appropriate to attempt dose reduction after it resolves.

Most patients experience satisfactory analgesia at a total daily dose equivalent to less than several hundred milligrams of morphine per day.[149] There is no ceiling dose for analgesia, however, and occasional patients benefit from much higher doses—sometimes equivalent to grams of morphine per day. As the dose rises, it is important to reassess the nature of the pain, ensure that expressed need for treatment is not related to other factors (e.g., so-called chemical coping—the use of the opioid to self-manage a mood disturbance or a comorbid psychiatric condition—or the possibility of addiction) and repeatedly establish that the benefits of therapy clearly outweigh the side effects and burdens.

Rescue dosing. Given the high prevalence of breakthrough pain,[10,11,149] all patients who are receiving a long-acting opioid also should be evaluated for the presence of episodic pains and considered for coadministration of a short-acting analgesic—the so-called rescue dose. Based on clinical experience, the effective dose of the oral rescue drug usually is between 5% and 15% of the total daily opioid dose.

As noted, the transmucosal immediate-release fentanyl formulations are important alternatives for breakthrough pain. The appropriate starting doses for these drugs are controversial. Although some experts support using a dose that is proportionate to the baseline opioid dose, the use of the lowest doses available is recommended by the manufacturers and is a safer approach.

Poorly Responsive Pain. If opioid dose escalation produces treatment-limiting side effects, the patient should be designated "poorly responsive" to the specific therapy. A change in treatment is then indicated. As a corollary to this observation, a patient who reports that an opioid has been ineffective but who, on questioning, denies having experienced adverse effects should not be labeled as poorly responsive. Continued treatment with appropriate dose titration may yet be successful.

Varied approaches may be considered for patients who are poorly responsive to an opioid regimen. These approaches include opioid "rotation," more aggressive management of the problematic side effects, or the addition of a pharmacological or nonpharmacological therapy that may reduce the need for the opioid.

Opioid Rotation. Opioid rotation is the switch from one opioid to another to improve opioid-related outcomes. This technique is widely used, despite guidelines based on experience rather than research.[150,151] Switching drugs first requires information about relative potency—the difference in doses required to produce effects. Relative potency information has been collated and presented in many well-known equianalgesic dose tables (Table 14.2).

When switching from one opioid drug to another, the first step involves calculation of the total daily dose of the new drug that would be equianalgesic to the current drug, using the figures in the equianalgesic table. With one exception, this calculated equianalgesic dose then must be reduced to ensure the safety of the approach. For most switches, a reduction of 25% to 50% in the calculated equianalgesic dose is implemented. If the new drug is methadone, however, a larger reduction—75% to 90%—is necessary, and the maximum daily starting dose should not exceed 40 mg.[128] Another exception is transdermal fentanyl; no reduction in the calculated equianalgesic dose is needed when changing to the transdermal patch because a safety factor is already built in to the recommended equianalgesic ratios.

Opioid Side Effects

Treatment-limiting side effects are common during opioid therapy.[20] Although all pure μ-agonist opioids have the same profile of nonanalgesic effects, individual variation is very substantial. For this reason, common side effects should be anticipated, regularly evaluated, and managed as they occur.

Gastrointestinal Effects. Opioids inhibit propulsive gastrointestinal motility and reduce secretions; both actions contribute to constipation. Constipation also may be worsened by advanced age, reduced physical activity, limited oral nutrition, dehydration, and many comorbid conditions. Given the high prevalence and severity of constipation, most experts strongly consider prophylactic laxative therapy, initiated at the start of opioid therapy and before clinically significant constipation occurs.

Numerous treatments are available, but the evidence needed to inform care is very limited. Based on clinical experience, management usually begins with the elimination of nonessential constipating drugs and, if possible, an increase in fluid intake. Supplemental fiber may be helpful but should be avoided in debilitated patients because of the potential for bowel obstruction.

Available laxatives include bulk-forming agents, osmotic agents, lubricants, surfactants, contact cathartics, secretagogues, prokinetic drugs, and opioid antagonists.[152] The conventional first-line approach is a combination of a stool softener, usually docusate, and a cathartic agent, such as senna. The osmotic agents, propylethylene glycol, lactulose, and sorbitol, offer another well-tolerated and usually effective approach. There have been no studies of dose-response or combination therapy, and based on experience, most clinicians will explore dose escalation and varied combinations of these first-line approaches if necessary.

New treatments should be considered if routine conventional therapy yields an unsatisfactory outcome.[152–156] Opioid antagonists with selective peripheral effects can reverse the bowel effects of opioids with minimal risk of induced withdrawal. These drugs include oral and parenteral methylnaltrexone; naloxegol; and naldemedine. Relatively high oral doses of oral naloxone (more than 8 mg/d) may be an alternative. The secretagogues include lubiprostone, which is approved for opioid-induced constipation in the United States, and both linaclotide and plecanatide. These drugs act on electrolyte channels in the gut wall to increase chloride or sodium secretion.[152]

The prokinetic drugs have varied mechanisms. Prucalopride is a selective 5-HT$_4$ receptor agonist recently approved for chronic constipation, and metoclopramide is a dopamine (D$_2$) antagonist that is rarely used for refractory constipation based on limited clinical observations.

There also is limited evidence that probiotic therapy may mitigate constipation.[156] Information about the specific constituents, dosing, or the duration required to realize benefit is lacking. The probiotic products are generally considered to be safe, however, and in those who can manage the therapy, a trial of a commercially available product at the dosage recommended is reasonable. Given the availability of multiple new agents for constipation, a small number of other drugs that possess minimal evidence of efficacy and a side-effect liability that may be problematic in the chronically ill, such as misoprostol and colchicine, are not favored for opioid-induced constipation.

Opioids also produce upper gastrointestinal side effects, including pyrosis and nausea. Although nausea often is transitory, occurring at initiation of treatment or after dose increases, it can be highly distressing and often requires treatment.[157] Conventional antiemetic therapy usually involves a dopamine antagonist, such as prochlorperazine, metoclopramide, or haloperidol, or a 5-HT antagonist, such as ondansetron or dolasetron.[157,158] If nausea is movement-induced or associated with vertigo, empirical treatment with an anticholinergic drug, such as meclizine, should be considered. Similarly, metoclopramide may be preferred if nausea is accompanied by early satiety or bloating, both suggestive of gastroparesis. If pyrosis is experienced, treatment with a proton pump inhibitor may be helpful. Occasional patients with refractory nausea are managed using other drugs with known antiemetic effects, such as a glucocorticoid such as dexamethasone, a commercially available cannabinoid such as tetrahydrocannabinol or nabilone, or a benzodiazepine such as lorazepam.

Somnolence and Cognitive Impairment. Opioid drugs often cause somnolence or cognitive impairment, which may be transitory or persistent. When these symptoms compromise the benefits of therapy, the first step is treatment of other potential etiologies and thoughtful de-prescribing of centrally acting drugs, if possible. A trial of opioid dose reduction of 25% to 50% usually can determine whether pain relief would be compromised at a dose that may produce fewer adverse effects.

Symptomatic Therapies Also Should Be Considered. Methylphenidate has been shown to decrease opioid-induced somnolence in cancer patients.[159,160] A low starting dose, such as 5 mg at breakfast and at lunchtime, may be up-titrated, while monitoring for potential side effects, including anorexia, jitteriness, anxiety, and insomnia. Other psychostimulants also have been used empirically, including dextroamphetamine, amphetamine, modafinil, and armodafinil; experience in the United States is greatest with modafinil.[161]

Other Side Effects. Opioid therapy may be associated with many other adverse effects. Two appear to be relatively common and potentially serious. Opioid-induced sleep-disordered breathing is a well-established phenomenon, which may result in adverse consequences due to sleep apnea.[162] Clinical recognition is the key to management and may be particularly challenging in highly symptomatic, seriously ill populations. Daytime sleepiness, fatigue, or mood disorder that appears insufficiently explained by other factors may initiate questions about sleep abnormalities. History from a bed partner may be very useful. Selected patients may be considered for referral to a sleep specialist for further evaluation and management.

Opioids also affect multiple endocrine pathways. Hypogonadism appears to be a relatively common effect, and some patients experience a clinically relevant increase in prolactin or decrease in serum cortisol.[163] The clinical manifestations of hypogonadism are manifold and include fatigue, mood disturbances, decreased libido, infertility, and adverse effects on bone. If consistent with the goals of care, measurement of sex hormones may offer the opportunity to treat symptoms through hormone replacement. In particular, clinical experience suggests that appropriately selected men with low testosterone may experience symptomatic benefit with testosterone repletion.

Opioid Abuse and Addiction

In the United States, concern about a historically high rate of opioid abuse and rising opioid-related mortality has led to a reduction in prescribing opioids for chronic pain unassociated with serious illness. Although there is no intent to drive prescribing lower among populations with pain associated with serious illness, the societal focus on the risks of opioid therapy has raised the consciousness of all clinicians about the obligation to assess and manage so-called drug abuse outcomes. To do so, the phenomenology of abuse and addiction must be appreciated. and a standard approach to opioid-related decision-making and adherence monitoring is needed.[164]

Abuse-Related Phenomenology. To manage the risks of abuse and addiction, clinicians must have a working knowledge of the definitions and characteristics of the related phenomena.

Tolerance is a neurophysiologic process defined by declining drug effects induced by exposure to the drug. It should never be equated with addiction and may not be evident in those who are diagnosed with opioid use disorder or addiction. Tolerance potentially affects any opioid effect, and there is very large variation in the occurrence and manifestations of this process. From the clinical perspective, tolerance to analgesic effects could reduce analgesic efficacy and is therefore a potential concern, whereas tolerance to side effects, such as respiratory depression, improves safety and allows the dose titration necessary to obtain favorable effects. Although the reduction in analgesic effects over time suggests that analgesic tolerance may be occurring, worsening pain also may be due to other causes, such as progression of the underlying disease. For this reason, a decline in analgesia cannot be considered strong evidence of tolerance unless there is no alternative explanation.

Most patients achieve a favorable balance between analgesia and side effects during opioid dose titration and then stabilize. In the absence of worsening disease, this stable period can be very prolonged. This observation, combined with the variation in the development and characteristics of tolerance, suggests that concerns about tolerance should never be used to delay appropriate opioid therapy.

Physical dependence is another neurophysiological process, this one defined by the occurrence of an abstinence syndrome following abrupt dose reduction or administration of an antagonist. It also should never be equated with addiction, may or may not manifest in those who are diagnosed with an addictive disorder, and should never be the reason to delay or avoid opioid therapy to treat pain in the seriously ill.

There is large individual variation in the development of physical dependence, and it is prudent to assume that patients receiving daily doses of an opioid for even a few days have the potential for signs of withdrawal. Patients who are perceived to have this potential should be labeled "physically dependent" and not "dependent," which is a term used synonymously with addiction. If a patient is assumed to be physically dependent, efforts should be made to prevent the occurrence of abstinence. Sudden discontinuation of the drug should be avoided if possible, and the use of antagonist drugs, including the agonist-antagonist opioids, should be undertaken with great caution. In those assumed to have substantial physical dependence, naloxone should be used only to reverse symptomatic respiratory depression—not to reverse somnolence—and it is prudent to use a dilute solution (e.g., 0.4 mg in 10 mL saline) administered in small boluses while monitoring effects.

If opioid dose reduction is needed, a decrement of 25% to 33% is usually tolerated. There are exceptions, however, and some patients develop severe symptoms at far smaller dose reductions. The symptoms that occur also are variable. For example, some patients develop anxiety and jitteriness, with no gastrointestinal or other symptoms, whereas others experience only nausea, vomiting, and diarrhea. It is important to educate patients and families about the potential for abstinence and the varied ways it may present and prepare to intervene to mitigate symptoms if they become distressing.

Drug abuse refers to either the use of an illicit drug or the nonmedical use of a prescribed drug with addictive potential. In the clinical setting, alternative terms are also used, including nonadherence, misuse, and aberrant drug-related behavior. Although it is certainly true in the United States that a clinician may come under scrutiny by the authorities when patients engage in prescription drug abuse, the management of this type of abuse is usually best approached as a clinical issue and not a legal one. The major exception to this focus on the clinical imperative—to base further treatment decisions on a careful assessment of benefit and risk—is the perceived occurrence of diversion.

Diversion, the transfer of abusable prescription drugs into the illicit marketplace, is always illegal and must be managed accordingly. A health professional perceived by the authorities to be abetting this process can be charged with a felony, and for this reason, the suspicion of diversion usually leads to discontinuation of therapy.

Addiction is an illness that results from complex interactions between a genetic predisposition, access to an abusable drug, and a variety of psychological and environmental factors that predispose to the development of an addictive pattern of use.[164] It is a biopsychosocial syndrome diagnosed through assessment of drug-related behaviors. Diagnostic criteria are described in the fifth edition of the American Psychiatric Association's *Diagnostic and Statistical Manual of Mental Disorders*.[15] These criteria highlight the importance of aberrant drug-related behaviors that are consistent with drug craving, loss of control over drug use, compulsive use of the drug, and continued use despite harm to the patient or others.

Aberrant drug-related behaviors (also described as abuse, misuse, and non-adherence behaviors) are highly variable. The clinician may view them as more or less serious, and they may occur transiently or more persistently. They often do not fulfill the diagnostic requirements for addiction. As noted, if aberrant behaviors suggest diversion of the drug into the illicit marketplace, the clinician should strongly consider discontinuing prescribing. If the behaviors do not suggest diversion, however, and the evaluation does not clearly indicate a level of opioid risk that exceeds benefit, the clinician may choose to continue prescribing with new measures to monitor adherence and reduce the risk of recurrence. If the evaluation suggests a new psychological process, such as the use of the medication to self-manage a mood disorder[165] or a psychiatric comorbidity such as generalized anxiety, treatment may include interventions that target these processes. Of course, aberrant behaviors may raise the possibility of de novo or recurrent addiction, the diagnosis of which may similarly suggest targeted treatments.

Pseudoaddiction is a descriptive term indicating that the stress of unrelieved pain may be contributing to the development of aberrant drug-related behaviors. The term does not exclude a diagnosis of addiction or another psychiatric disorder, and care must be taken lest its use in the clinical setting unintentionally distract from the need to diagnose and manage another problem. At the same time, the need to treat a presumptive diagnosis of addiction or another disorder does not eliminate the possibility that the stress associated with poorly controlled pain is an impediment. A careful pain history, institution of more controls over prescribing, the use of nonopioid and nonpharmacological therapies for pain, and monitoring should allow these distinctions to be clarified.

Risk Management. Although the risk of iatrogenic addiction is low, patients who lack a prior history of abuse or addiction, particularly if the patient has a serious chronic illness, the risk can never be entirely excluded, and clinicians who prescribe opioids or other potentially abusable drugs should adhere to practices designed to minimize the risk of outcomes related to drug abuse or addiction. The best approach incorporates a model of "universal precautions" that is adaptable to all types of patients and clinical scenarios. This approach includes risk stratification and specific steps that the clinician may follow to structure therapy and assess outcomes (Table 14.3).

Nonpharmacological Approaches for Pain Management

There are numerous nonpharmacological approaches that may reduce pain in populations with serious chronic illness. They include interventions such as neural blockade and implant therapies, which are considered for highly selected opioid-refractory patients, and many types of noninvasive therapies—categorized as psychological, rehabilitative, or integrative.

TABLE 14.3 Five-Step "Universal Precautions" Approach to Safe Opioid Prescribing

Steps	Considerations	Comment
1. Assess and stratify risk	Assess risk of opioid misuse/abuse based on history, examination findings, review of records, and check of prescription drug–monitoring program; obtaining a urine or saliva drug screen also provides information relative to risk assessment. Stratify risk into categories that inform next steps. A bed-bound patient with advanced illness may be considered to have nil or extremely low risk. Others may be categorized as "moderate" or "high."	All patients should be assessed for risk of opioid misuse/abuse. Higher risk of misuse/abuse is associated with (1) past or present history of alcohol or drug abuse; (2) family history of alcohol or drug abuse; and (3) any type of major psychiatric disorder. Younger age and history of physical/sexual abuse are also associated. Validated measures of opioid risk are available but seldom used in the clinical setting.
2. Decision: Prescribe or not	If diversion is occurring or is likely to occur, prescribing should not be done unless controls can be implemented to eliminate the risk. If drug abuse is occurring, a risk-to-benefit evaluation is needed. If the risks cannot be managed because the patient cannot control drug use, then prescribing should not be done.	Diversion is illegal, and prescribing a controlled substance when diversion is occurring places the clinician at risk. Other types of problematic drug-related behavior can be addressed medically, through understanding of risk and benefit, best practices, and standards of care.
3. Structure prescribing to minimize risk	Treatment requirements should be matched to the level of risk to allow appropriate monitoring of adherence and to help the patient maintain control over drug use. Options include small number of tablets and frequent refills, use of one pharmacy, pill counts, no use of short-acting drugs, required consultation with psychiatry or addiction medicine, urine or saliva drug testing.	"Structuring" therapy means implementing strategies for adherence monitoring. Based on anecdotal observations, the use of methadone or buprenorphine may be preferred if risk of abuse is high. Consider obtaining the input of a specialist in addiction medicine.
4. Monitor drug-related behaviors	Monitor drug-related behaviors (i.e., treatment adherence) throughout the course of therapy	Monitoring drug-related behaviors should be part of routine outcome monitoring. Outcomes are described as the "four As": analgesia (effectiveness); adverse effects (side effects); activity (impact of treatment on function); and aberrant drug-related behavior.
5. Respond to aberrant behaviors	If aberrant drug-related behavior occurs, reassessment is needed to determine diagnosis. Management is guided by diagnosis and may include discontinuation of therapy or increased adherence monitoring. Always document aberrant behaviors, their assessment, and management.	The differential diagnosis of aberrant drug-related behavior includes recreational abuse, addiction, so-called pseudoaddiction, psychiatric disorders associated with impulsive drug taking, patient confusion about instructions for dosing, organic brain syndrome associated with confusion or impulsivity, family or caregiver issues, or criminal activity.

Interventional Therapies

The simplest interventional therapy is local anesthetic or glucocorticoid injection into muscle or related soft tissue or into joints. The most common type targets myofascial pains related to trigger points in muscle or connective tissue. These injections typically employ a local anesthetic and usually can be provided by the treating clinician, without referral to specialists. Injection into a trigger point usually is followed by massage or stretching, which may prolong the immediate benefit. Injections are avoided in those with a bleeding diathesis.

Other interventional therapies are typically implemented by specialists in pain management or interventional radiology. Neural blockade, for example, involves administration of a local anesthetic or a neurolytic solution near a peripheral nerve. Local anesthetic injections may be diagnostic, prognostic, or therapeutic. Diagnostic blocks elucidate the neural pathway involved in the experience of pain, prognostic blocks are used to evaluate the safety of a planned neurolytic block, and a therapeutic block is undertaken with the intent to attain rapid relief of pain. The benefit provided by a successful therapeutic block with local anesthetic may be prolonged in some cases through subsequent neurolysis or in other cases by repeated local anesthetic injections or by infusion of a local anesthetic near the nerve (perineural or epidural).

Neurolytic procedures using alcohol or phenol have been developed for spinal nerves, peripheral nerves transmitting only sensory fibers, and autonomic ganglia.[167] All of these procedures carry risk related to the use of a tissue-damaging substance, and with one exception, they have been largely supplanted by other approaches to pain. The exception is celiac plexus blockade for the management of epigastric pain due to neoplastic invasion of the celiac axis, particularly pain caused by pancreas cancer. The response to neurolytic celiac plexus blockade has been observed to be so satisfactory that it is often performed if the patient's pain does not promptly respond to an initial opioid trial.[168–170]

Neuromodulation

The term *neuromodulation* may be used to characterize interventions that deliver either drugs or electrical stimulation to specific regions of the peripheral or central nervous system. The delivery of drugs may employ a pump external to the body, which is connected to a percutaneous catheter whose distal end is positioned near the target tissue, or an implanted pump and catheter system. As described previously, neuraxial infusion of opioids, local anesthetics, and other drugs are well-established approaches that comprise a variety of epidural and subarachnoid therapies.

Electrical neuromodulation of peripheral nerves has been used for many decades to alter neural processing and potentially relieve pain. The best known treatment is noninvasive: transcutaneous electrical nerve stimulation (TENS).[171] A trial of TENS may be considered whenever chronic pain is limited to an area that can be stimulated through electrode placement on the skin or over the sensory nerve that supplies the painful region. There is wide variation in the individual's response to specific stimulation parameters, and the clinician who oversees a trial of TENS should instruct the patient to try various electrode placements, high-frequency and low-frequency stimulation, and timing of stimulation.

When a painful area lies within the innervation of a sensory nerve, stimulation of the nerve also can be accomplished by implanting an electrode nearby. This technique is known as percutaneous electrical nerve stimulation. It is rarely considered for the management of pain in populations with serious chronic illness.

A newer form of noninvasive peripheral nerve stimulation is called scrambler therapy. It employs surface electrodes to stimulate multiple primary afferents simultaneously. It has been evaluated through case series, surveys, and small trials involving patients with chronic noncancer neuropathic pain or chemotherapy-induced peripheral neuropathy. Two recent randomized, sham-controlled pilot trials in patients with chemotherapy-induced peripheral neuropathy yielded conflicting results.[172,173] Surveys have reported successful use in those with varied types of cancer pain.[174] Further trials are needed to determine whether this approach has broader utility.

Electrical stimulation also can be delivered to the central nervous system. Dorsal column stimulation, which is an implanted system comprising a generator connected to an electrode placed in the epidural space, has a long history and may be effective for diverse chronic pain syndromes.[175] There is evidence that it may be useful in the treatment of refractory angina,[176] and occasionally, it is considered for a seriously ill patient with opioid-refractory pain below the midchest.

Invasive brain stimulation—both deep-brain stimulation and motor cortex stimulation—has been used for chronic pain, but experience in the treatment of patients with serious chronic illness is minimal, and it is rarely considered. In contrast, the advent of noninvasive transcranial stimulation approaches—transcranial direct current stimulation or transcranial magnetic stimulation—offers new opportunities to explore neuromodulatory therapies for pain and other symptoms, such as mood disorders, cognitive impairment, and fatigue. Further studies are needed to determine the role that these therapies can play in the management of chronic pain.[177]

Rehabilitative Approaches

Although the primary aim of rehabilitative therapies may be functional improvement, these diverse approaches often are considered as part of a plan to address pain in populations with chronic serious illness. The therapies, which usually are implemented in collaboration with physical and occupational therapists, include therapeutic exercise, hydrotherapy, devices, and physical modalities such as heat and cold, vibration, and ultrasound. Physical modalities or place TENS in the list with heat and cold, vibration, ultrasound and TENS.

Therapeutic Exercise. Therapeutic exercise involves the systematic use of movements, postures, or activities for the purpose of mitigating symptom distress or functional impairment by improving flexibility, stability, range of motion, or motor functioning. The exercises may be active or passive (e.g., mobilization of joints by the therapist). The type, frequency, and duration of exercise is determined by the therapist and the ordering physician based on the patient's capacity to benefit, goals of the intervention, and patient preferences based on the goals of care.

There is a paucity of evidence related to the use of therapeutic exercise in the chronically ill. Studies in related contexts have been positive, however. For example, a systematic review of 18 randomized studies found that physical therapy is an effective approach for postoperative pain and range of motion after breast cancer treatment,[178] and two randomized trials in patients with chemotherapy-induced peripheral neuropathy also yielded positive results.[179,180]

Hydrotherapy. Hydrotherapy involves submersion in water for therapeutic purposes. It is intended to enhance muscle relaxation and facilitate physical therapy through so-called aquatic exercise. Evidence of positive outcomes is limited, particularly in populations with serious chronic illnesses, and availability varies. Nonetheless, hydrotherapy may be offered to patients with pain and specific functional goals based on anecdotal observations of favorable outcomes.

Devices. Numerous devices are available to support functional outcomes and provide symptomatic benefit. Although evidence of efficacy is very limited, the potential for benefit gains support from clinical observations. Ambulation aides, such as canes and walkers, may reduce the load on joints, pelvis, and spine and be valued for their effects on pain. Arm and shoulder pain associated with malignant plexopathy and wrist or ankle pain related to arthropathy or local nerve injury may be reduced by orthoses that constrain arm mobility or the mobility of the distal limbs, respectively. In those with amputation, the fitting of a prosthesis may be followed by reduced stump pain. Patients with chronic focal or regional pain associated with functional impairment, or pain exacerbations related to movement, may benefit from an evaluation by an occupational therapist focused on the potential utility of devices for symptom management.

Physical Modalities. The so-called physical modalities include heat or cold, ultrasound, and electrical nerve stimulation. One or more may be applied to focal areas of pain as part of a rehabilitative approach to pain and impairment. Studies are limited, particularly those directly relevant to persistent pain associated with serious illness. Nonetheless, these approaches are widely used in self-management strategies taught to patients with pain and their families or as part of a care plan implemented by physical therapists.

Cold or heat can be applied to a painful area and the effects with respect to pain and function quickly evaluated. Cold is applied with ice packs, chemical gel packs, or vapocoolant sprays. Superficial heating is performed with hot packs, medicated heat patches, heating pads, or warm baths. Given the local vasoconstriction that occurs, there is a theoretical concern about the application of cold on areas of the body affected by ischemia. Concern about skin injury should be appreciated when either modality is used to treat a patient with cognitive impairment or the modality is applied to a denervated area of the body. Generally, however, these modalities are considered safe and worthy of a trial in those with focal pain syndromes.

Ultrasound and TENS also are widely used despite limited evidence of efficacy in any type of chronic pain.[181] Clinical observations suggest that some patients with focal musculoskeletal or neuropathic pain benefit, and one or the other approach is commonly tried.

Neuroablative Approaches

Procedures designed to surgically denervate a painful area have been developed for every level of the neuraxis, from peripheral nerves to cortex.[182] Historically, the most useful approach has been cordotomy.[183] Like neurolytic blocks, however, these procedures are rarely considered now, largely due to the development of interventions such as neuraxial infusion.

Psychologic Approaches

Numerous cognitive and behavioral approaches have been adapted to the treatment of pain and other conditions in populations with cancer.[184–186] The principles and best practices are likely to apply to other populations with serious chronic illness.

For patients with chronic pain associated with serious illness, cognitive interventions may include education-based approaches and mind-body approaches such as relaxation training, distraction (imagery) techniques, mindfulness training, hypnosis, and biofeedback. These approaches offer self-management tools to patients or family caregivers, which may be used to mitigate distress and buttress coping, adaptation, and resilience.

Although there is abundant literature suggesting that both education-based approaches[187] and the mind-body approaches[188] are beneficial in populations with chronic pain, including those with cancer, there are relatively few high-quality trials of interventions in the diverse populations with serious illness. More research is needed, particularly in populations with advanced illness. Nonetheless, the overall experience supports the conclusion that the systematic use of an education-based or mind-body therapy can be beneficial for a subset of patients with chronic pain due to serious illness.

In addressing the problem of chronic pain, the mind-body approaches are considered to be adjunctive to pharmacotherapy-based therapy. They are therefore usually considered for patients with mild or moderate pain, particularly if pain is associated with distress or pain-related functional impairment. A clinician who is overseeing the treatment for pain should assess whether a patient may benefit from one of these approaches and is physically able to participate. If access to treatment is possible (a trained professional is available and the patient is able to afford the treatment), the clinician should be able to explain the rationale for the use of these techniques to the patient and family, make a referral, and support the therapeutic goals.

Unfortunately, many of these interventions cannot be routinely provided to patients or caregivers because the availability of professionals with these skills is limited, insurance coverage has been historically poor, and patients often lack the resources necessary to participate. Accordingly, access to these therapies depends on clinicians whose primary focus is on medical management. Fortunately, some approaches can be implemented by the nonspecialist as part of the routine care plan for pain and related conditions. Most clinicians, for example, can plan and implement a structured psychoeducational intervention. This may focus on improving adherence to analgesic medications or on helping patients or caregivers recognize internal or environmental triggers that may incite pain or pain-related anxiety.[187] Nonspecialists also may able to teach patients simple relaxation exercises, such as deep breathing or guided imagery.

Relaxation and Imagery. Relaxation therapies induce a so-called relaxation response characterized by decreased arousal and diminished sympathetic activity. Typically, the patient is trained in an approach to achieving relaxation that may involve breathing techniques or progressive muscle relaxation. Breathing techniques may involve training in so-call diaphragmatic breathing[189] or a simple controlled breathing approach (e.g., the "4-7-8" technique—slow inhalation for a count of 4, breath holding for a count of 7, and slow exhalation for a count of 8). Progressive muscle relaxation involves training in a systematic approach to contracting and relaxation muscles.[190]

Rarely, patients who are being taught relaxation experience an adverse reaction, such as anxiety or a fear of losing control. Clinicians should be aware of the possibility and abort the procedure if distress occurs.

Imagery can be combined with a relaxation approach[190] or taught to the patient separately. The patient is taught to recall pleasant images or perceptions to create a positive emotional state. When training is provided by a qualified professional, the approach may include phases during which images are selected and rehearsed.

Integrative Medicine Approaches

Integrative medicine refers to the combined use of conventional medical care along with interventions that have historically been termed *complementary* or *alternative*. The alternative label may no longer be favored, however, given the growing acceptance of an integrated approach that always considers the appropriateness and value of conventional treatments. In the United States, the preferred approach may be called "complementary and integrative medicine."

Among the numerous complementary therapies used in pain management are (1) mind-body therapies that overlap or supplement those that are also considered as psychological approaches for pain management; (2) treatments that are part of alternative medical systems, such as traditional Chinese medicine (TCM), Ayurveda, homeopathy, or naturopathy; (3) biological-based therapies, such as herbal therapies or specialized diets; (4) body-based therapies, such as massage, yoga, Pilates, tai chi, and chiropractic; and (5) energy therapies, such as therapeutic touch and reiki. All of these treatments can be considered a concomitant component of optimal pharmacotherapy-based treatment in populations with pain associated with serious chronic illness.

As described previously, some of the mind-body therapies—relaxation training, imagery, mindfulness training, hypnosis, and biofeedback—have sufficient evidence of benefit for the treatment of pain to warrant consideration as conventional psychological treatments.[188] Other mind-body therapies—training in meditation techniques, encouragement of prayer, and the therapeutic use of music[191] and art—are often considered complementary and offered, when available, as part of an integrative medicine approach to pain management.

When a complementary therapy is considered for patients with pain due to serious illness, the clinician must evaluate the evidence of benefit weighed against the potential for risk and burden, as would be expected in selecting any therapy. The published literature describing some of these treatments, like the mind-body approaches and acupuncture,[192] is substantial, includes evidence of higher quality and generally establishes safety; these treatments are often recommended. In contrast, some treatments—such as cervical spinal manipulation in the setting of multifocal bone metastases and herbal remedies with unknown ingredients—lack high-quality evidence of benefit and have inherent risks. Patients should be discouraged from pursuing these approaches.

Most complementary therapies lack high-quality evidence of efficacy,[193,194] and the extent to which the treatment may be beneficial for pain is based on the limited evidence that has been published and accumulated clinical experience. Most of these approaches, which include many body-based interventions and the so-called energy therapies, are not associated with adverse effects if prudently administered. If a patient is interested in a complementary therapy that is both available and affordable, the therapy is likely to be safe, and the approach is reasonable given the severity of the underlying disease and goals of care, clinicians who are open to an integrative model will generally attempt to support the patient in obtaining the treatment while continuing conventional treatments.

Selected Complementary and Integrative Therapies. Several types of complementary therapies are relatively accepted for the management of pain in the seriously ill. The mind-body therapies and acupuncture are the most important. Massage therapy, which includes varied manual techniques that apply superficial or deep pressure to soft tissues, such as lymphedema therapy, may lack evidence of efficacy[195] but has been widely used; a large clinical experience in the cancer population suggests that some patients with pain may benefit.[196]

Other body-based therapies, such as tai chi and other movement therapies, have limited to no evidence of efficacy for pain associated with chronic illness. Nonetheless, some studies suggest a positive effect on functioning and other symptoms.[197] Patients who have the capacity to participate in therapies that support movement and balance definitely benefit, particularly with reduction in fall risk.

The energy therapies, such as therapeutic touch and reiki, are not associated with adverse effects and have been shown to improve overall quality of life. There is no high-quality evidence supporting efficacy, but some clinical trials have demonstrated positive short-term effects on pain in patients with cancer.[198]

Conclusion

Pain is highly prevalent among populations with serious chronic illness. Pain assessment and management should be considered a component of palliative care, a patient-centered and family-focused approach predicated on a multidimensional assessment and a care plan that can address multiple sources of distress and burden. The most effective strategy for chronic pain in those with serious chronic illness is opioid-based pharmacotherapy, and well-accepted guidelines for treatment hold the promise of satisfactory pain relief for most patients. The knowledge necessary to provide this therapy safely and effectively, and to address the challenge posed by the minority with pain that is poorly responsive to an opioid, is fundamental to the practice of palliative care. As integrative medicine becomes increasingly more important and relevant for the patient with serious illness, it is essential to have knowledge of the ways in which these modalities can indeed become more integrated and therefore more effective. Physician assistants must have this compendium of knowledge to provide a comprehensive approach to the management of their patients.

References

1. Van den Beuken-van Everdingen, de Rijke JM, Kessels AG, et al. Prevalence of Pain in Patients with Cancer: A Systematic Review of the Past 40 Years. *Annals of Oncology.* 2007;*18*(9):1437–1449.

2. Moens K, Higginson IJ, Harding R, EURO IMPACT. are there differences in the prevalence of palliative care-related problems in people living with advanced cancer and eight non-cancer conditions? A systematic review. *Journal of Pain and Symptom Management.* 2014;*48*(4):660–677.

3. International Association for the Study of Pain. IASP taxonomy Washington DC2017. November 30, 2017. https://www.iasp-pain.org/Taxonomy

4. Best M, Aldridge L, Butow P, Olver I, Webster F. Conceptual analysis of suffering in cancer: a systematic review. *Psychooncology.* 2015;*24*(9):977–986.

5. Clark D. "Total pain," disciplinary power and the body in the work of Cicely Saunders, 1958–1967. *Social Science and Medicine.* 1999;*49*(6):727–736.

6. National Consensus Project for Quality Palliative Care. *Clinical Practice Guidelines for Quality Palliative Care.* 4th ed. Richmond, VA: National Coalition for Hospice and Palliative Care; 2018. https://www.nationalcoalitionhpc.org/ncp

7. El Mokhallalati Y, Woodhouse N, Farragher T, Bennett MI. Specialist palliative care support is associated with improved pain relief at home during the last 3 months of life in patients with advanced disease: analysis of 5-year data from the national survey of bereaved people (VOICES). *BMC Medicine.* 2019;*17*(1):50. doi:10.1186/s12916-019-1287-8

8. Meier EA, Gallegos JV, Thomas LP, Depp CA, Irwin SA, Jeste DV. Defining a good death (successful dying): literature review and a call for research and public dialogue. *American Journal of Geriatric Psychiatry.* 2016;*24*(4):261–271.

9. Daut RL, Cleeland CS, Flanery RC. Development of the Wisconsin Brief Pain Questionnaire to assess pain in cancer and other diseases. *Pain.* 1983;*17*:197.

10. Deandrea S, Corli O, Consonni D, et al. Prevalence of breakthrough cancer pain: a systematic review and a pooled analysis of published literature. *Journal of Pain and Symptom Management.* 2014;*47*:57.

11. Mercadante S, Portenoy R. Breakthrough cancer pain: 25 years of study. *Pain.* 2016;*157*:2657–2663.

12. Gerwin RD. Myofascial and visceral pain syndromes: visceral-somatic pain representations. *Journal of Musculoskeletal Pain.* 2002;*10*:165–175.

13. Portenoy RK, Ahmed E. Cancer pain syndromes. *Hematology/Oncology Clinics of North America.* 2018; *32*(3):371–386.

14. Haanpaa M, Attal N, Backonja M, et al. NeuPSIG guidelines on neuropathic pain assessment. *Pain.* 2011;*152*(1):14 27.

15. American Psychiatric Association. *Diagnostic and Statistical Manual of Mental Disorders.* 5th ed. Washington, DC: American Psychiatric Association; 2013.

16. Schrijvers D. Disease modifying therapies in advanced cancer. In: Cherny NI, Fallon MT, Kaasa S, Portenoy RK, Currow DC, eds. *Oxford Textbook of Palliative Medicine.* 5th ed. Oxford University Press; 2015:765–770.

17. Rich SE, Chow R, Raman S, et al. Update of the systematic review of palliative radiation therapy fractionation for bone metastases. *Radiotherapy and Oncology.* 2018 Mar;*126*(3):547–557.

18. Knaul FM, Farmer PE, Krakauer EL, et al. Lancet Commission on Palliative Care and Pain Relief Study Group. Alleviating the access abyss in palliative care and pain relief—an imperative of universal health coverage: The Lancet Commission Report. *Lancet.* 2018;*391*(10128):1391–1454.

19. Bhadelia A, De Lima L, Arreola-Ornelas H, Kwete XJ, Rodriguez NM, Knaul FM. Solving the global crisis in access to pain relief: lessons from country actions. *American Journal of Public Health.* 2018 Nov 29:e1–e3.

20. Wiffen PJ, Wee B, Derry S, Bell RF, Moore RA. Opioids for cancer pain—an overview of Cochrane reviews. *Cochrane Database of Systematic Reviews.* 2017 Jul 6;7:CD012592.

21. Greco MT, Roberto A, Corli O. Quality of cancer pain management: an update of a systemic review of undertreatment of patients with cancer. *Journal of Clinical Oncology.* 2014 Dec 20;*32*(36):4149–4154.

22. Deandrea S, Montanari M, Moja L, Apolone G. Prevalence of undertreatment in cancer pain. A review of published literature. *Annals of Oncology.* 2008;*19*(12):1985–1991.

23. World Health Organization. Palliative care. https://www.who.int/cancer/palliative/painladder/en/ May 6, 2019.

24. National Comprehensive Cancer Network (NCCN). NCCN Clinical practice guidelines in oncology. http://www.nccn.org/professionals/physician_gls/f_guidelines.asp. Accessed May 6, 2019.

25. European Association of Palliative Care. National guidelines in palliative care. http://www.eapcnet.eu/publications/national-guidelines. Accessed May 6, 2019.

26. Vardy J, Agar M. Nonopioid drugs in the treatment of cancer pain. *Journal of Clinical Oncology.* 2014;*32*(16);1677–1690.

27. Derry S, Wiffen PJ, Moore RA, et al. Oral nonsteroidal anti-inflammatory drugs (NSAIDs) for cancer pain in adults. *Cochrane Database of Systematic Reviews.* 2017;*12*(7):CD012638.

28. Graham GG, Davies MJ, Day RO, Mohamudally A, Scott KF. The modern pharmacology of paracetamol: therapeutic actions, mechanism of action, metabolism, toxicity and recent pharmacological findings. *Inflammopharmacology.* 2013;*21*(3):201–232.

29. Yang M, Wang HT, Zhao M, et al. Network meta-analysis comparing relatively selective COX-2 inhibitors versus coxibs for the prevention of NSAID-induced gastrointestinal injury. *Medicine (Baltimore).* 2015;*94*(40):e1592.

30. Yuan JQ, Tsoi KK, Yang M, et al. Systematic review with network meta-analysis: comparative effectiveness and safety of strategies for preventing NSAID-associated gastrointestinal toxicity. *Alimentary Pharmacology and Therapeutics.* 2016;*43*(12):1262–1275.

31. Waksman JC, Brody A, Phillips SD. Nonselective nonsteroidal antiinflammatory drugs and cardiovascular risk: are they safe? *Annals of Pharmacotherapy.* 2007;*41*:1163–1173.

32. Hinz B, Renner B, Brune K. Drug insight: cyclo-oxygenase-2 inhibitors—a critical appraisal. *Nature Clinical Practice. Rheumatology.* 2007;*3*:552–560.

33. Trelle S, Reichenbach S, Wandel S, et al. Cardiovascular safety of non-steroidal anti-inflammatory drugs: network meta-analysis. *BMJ.* 2011; *342*:c7086.

34. Angiolillo DJ, Weisman SM. Clinical pharmacology and cardiovascular safety of naproxen. *American Journal of Cardiovascular Drugs.* 2017;*17*(2): 97–107.

35. Paulsen O, Klepstad P, Rosland JH, et al. Efficacy of methylprednisolone on pain, fatigue, and appetite loss in patients with advanced cancer using opioids: a randomized, placebo-controlled, double-blind trial. *Journal of Clinical Oncology.* 2014;*32*(29):3221–3228.

36. Yennurajalingam S, Frisbee-Hume S, Palmer JL, et al. Reduction of cancer-related fatigue with dexamethasone: a double-blind, randomized, placebo-controlled trial in patients with advanced cancer. *Journal of Clinical Oncology.* 2013;*31*(25):3076–3082.

37. Haywood A, Good P, Khan S, et al. Corticosteroids for the management of cancer-related pain in adults. *Cochrane Database of Systematic Reviews.* 2015;*24*(4):CD010756.

38. Huscher D, Thiele K, Gromnica-Ihle E, et al. Dose-related patterns of glucocorticoid-induced side effects. *Annals of the Rheumatic Diseases.* 2009 Jul;*68*(7):1119–1124.

39. Chan HN, Fam J, and Ng BY. Use of antidepressants in the treatment of chronic pain. *Annals of the Academy of Medicine, Singapore.* 2009;*38*(11):974–979.

40. Finnerup NB, Attal N, Haroutounian S, et al. Pharmacotherapy for neuropathic pain in adults: a systematic review and meta-analysis. *Lancet Neurology.* 2015;*14*(2):162–173.

41. Watson CPN, Gilron I, Pollock BG, et al. Antidepressant analgesics. In: McMahon JR, Koltzenburg M, Tracey I, Turk DC, eds. *Wall and Melzack's Textbook of Pain.* 6th ed. London: Churchill Livingstone; 2013:465–490.

42. Griebeler ML, Morey-Vargas OL, Brito JP, et al. Pharmacologic interventions for painful diabetic neuropathy: an umbrella systematic review and comparative effectiveness network meta-analysis. *Annals of Internal Medicine.* 2014;*161*(9):639–649.

43. Wang, SM, Han C, Bahk WM, et al. Addressing the side effects of contemporary antidepressant drugs: a comprehensive review. *Chonnam Medical Journal.* 2018;*54*(2):101–112.

44. Dharmshaktu P, Tayal V, Kalra BS. Efficacy of antidepressants as analgesics: a review. *Journal of Clinical Pharmacology.* 2012;*52*(1):6–17.

45. Lee YC, Chen PP. A review of SSRIs and SNRIs in neuropathic pain. *Expert Opinion on Pharmacotherapy.* 2010;*11*(17):2813–2825.

46. Saarto T, Wiffen PJ. Antidepressants for neuropathic pain. *Cochrane Database of Systematic Reviews.* 2007;*17*(4):CD005454.

47. Wilson E, Lader M. A review of the management of antidepressant discontinuation symptoms. *Therapeutic Advances in Psychopharmacology.* 2015;*5*(6):357–368.

48. Eisenach JC, DuPen S, Dubois M, Miguel R, Allin D. Epidural clonidine analgesia for intractable cancer pain. The Epidural Clonidine Study Group. *Pain.* 1995;*61*(3):391–399.

49. Yazicioğlu D, Caparlar C, Akkaya T, Mercan U, Kulacoglu H. Tizanidine for the management of acute postoperative pain after inguinal hernia repair: a placebo-controlled double-blind trial. *European Journal of Anaesthesiology.* 2016;*33*(3):215–222.

50. Arain SR, Ruehlow RM, Uhrich TD, Ebert TJ. The efficacy of dexmedetomidine versus morphine for postoperative analgesia after major inpatient surgery. *Anesthesia and Analgesia.* 2004 Jan;*98*(1):153–158.

51. Russo EB, Guy GW, Robson PJ. Cannabis, pain, and sleep: lessons from therapeutic clinical trials of Sativex, a cannabis-based medicine. *Chemistry & Biodiversity.* 2007;*4*(8):1729–1743.

52. Whiting PF, Wolff RF, Deshpande S, et al. Cannabinoids for medical use: a systematic review and meta-analysis. *JAMA.* 2015;*313*(24):2456–2473.

53. Johnson JR, Burnell-Nugent M, Lossignol D, Ganae-Motan ED, Potts R, Fallon MT. Multicenter, double-blind, randomized, placebo-controlled, parallel-group study of the efficacy, safety, and tolerability of THC:CBD extract and THC extract in patients with intractable cancer-related pain. *Journal of Pain and Symptom Management.* 2010;*39*(2):167–179.

54. Lichtman AH, Lux EA, McQuade R, et al. Results of a double-blind, randomized, placebo-controlled study of nabiximols oromucosal spray as an adjunctive therapy in advanced cancer patients with chronic uncontrolled pain. *Journal of Pain and Symptom Management.* 2018;*55*(2):179–188.

55. Portenoy RK, Ganae-Motan ED, Yanagihara R, et al. Nabiximols for opioid-treated cancer patients with poorly controlled chronic pain: a randomized, placebo-controlled, graded-dose trial. *Journal of Pain.* 2012;*13*(5):438–449.

56. Skrabek RQ, Galimova L, Ethans K, Perry D. Nabilone for the treatment of pain in fibromyalgia. *Journal of Pain.* 2008 Feb;*9*(2):164–173.

57. Wissel J, Haydn T, Muller J, et al. Low dose treatment with the synthetic cannabinoid nabilone significantly reduced spasticity-related pain: a double-blind placebo-controlled crossover trial. *Journal of Neurology.* 2006 Oct;*253*(10):1337–1341.

58. Maida V, Ennis M, Irani S, Corbo M, Dolzhykov M. Adjunctive nabilone in cancer pain and symptom management: a prospective observational study using propensity scoring. *Journal of Supportive Oncology.* 2008;*6*(3):119–124.

59. Aviram J, Samuelly-Leichtag G. Efficacy of cannabis-based medicines for pain management: a systematic review and meta-analysis of randomized controlled trials. *Pain Physician.* 2017;*20*(6):E755–E796.

60. Derry S, Wiffen PJ, Kalso EA, et al. Topical analgesics for acute and chronic pain in adults—an overview of Cochrane reviews. *Cochrane Database of Systematic Reviews.* 2017;*12*(5):CD008609.

61. Gammaitoni AR, Alvarez NA, Galer BS. Pharmacokinetics and safety of continuously applied lidocaine patches 5%. *American Journal of Health-Systemy Pharmacy.* 2002;*59*(22):2215–2220.

62. Burness CB, McCormack PL. Capsaicin 8% patch: a review in peripheral neuropathic pain. *Drugs.* 2016;*76*(1):123–134.

63. Barton DL, Wos EJ, Qin R, et al. A double-blind, placebo-controlled trial of a topical treatment for chemotherapy-induced peripheral neuropathy: NCCTG trial N06CA. *Supportive Care in Cancer.* 2011;*19*(6):833–841.

64. Fallon MT, Storey DJ, Krishan A, et al. Cancer treatment-related neuropathic pain: proof of concept study with menthol—a TRPM8 agonist. *Supportive Care in Cancer.* 2015;*23*(9):2769–2777.

65. Safarpour Y, Jabbari B. Botulinum toxin treatment of pain syndromes—an evidence based review. *Toxicon.* 2018;*147*:120–128.

66. Sandrini G, De Icco R, Tassorelli C, Smania N, Tamburin S. Botulinum neurotoxin type A for the treatment of pain: not just in migraine and trigeminal neuralgia. *Journal of Headache Pain.* 2017;*18*(1):38.

67. Rostami R, Mittal SO, Radmand R, Jabbari B. Incobotulinum toxin—a improves post-surgical and post-radiation pain in cancer patients. *Toxins (Basel)*. 2016;*8*(1):22.

68. Seidel S, Aigner M, Ossege M, Pernicka E, Wildner B, Sycha T. Antipsychotics for acute and chronic pain in adults. *Cochrane Database of Systematic Reviews*. 2013 ;*29*(8):CD004844.

69. Michelet D, Brasher C, Horlin AL, et al. Ketamine for chronic non-cancer pain: a meta-analysis and trial sequential analysis of randomized controlled trials. *European Journal of Pain*. 2018;*22*(4):632–646.

70. Bell RF, Eccleston C, Kalso EA. Ketamine as an adjuvant to opioids for cancer pain. *Cochrane Database of Systematic Reviews*. 2017;*6*:CD003351.

71. Zhao J, Wang Y, Wang D. The effect of ketamine infusion in the treatment of complex regional pain syndrome: a systemic review and meta-analysis. *Current Pain and Headache Reports*. 2018;*22*(2):12.

72. Ghate G, Clark E, Vaillancourt C. Systematic review of the use of low-dose ketamine for analgesia in the emergency department. *CJEM*. 2018;*20*(1):36–45.

73. Okun T. Ketamine: an introduction for the pain and palliative medicine physician. *Pain Physician*. 2007;*10*(3):493–500.

74. Quibell R, Fallon, M, Mihalyo M, Twycross R, Wilcock A. Ketamine. *Journal of Pain and Symptom Management*. 2015;*50*(2):268–278.

75. Fond G, Loundou A, Rabu C, et al. Ketamine administration in depressive disorders: a systematic review and meta-analysis. *Psychopharmacology (Berlin)*. 2014;*231*(18):3663–3676.

76. Marchetti F, Coutaux, A, Bellanger A, Magneux C, Bourgeois P, Mion G. Efficacy and safety of oral ketamine for the relief of intractable chronic pain: a retrospective 5-year study of 51 patients. *European Journal of Pain*. 2015;*19*(7):984–993.

77. Jackson K, Ashby M, Howell D, et al. The effectiveness and adverse effects profile of "burst" ketamine in refractory cancer pain: the VCOG PM 1-00 study. *Journal of Palliative Care*. 2010;*26*(3):176–183.

78. Mercadante S, Caruselli A, Casuccio A. The use of ketamine in a palliative-supportive care unit: a retrospective analysis. *Annals of Palliative Medicine*. 2018 Apr;*7*(2):205–210.

79. Loveday BA, Sindt J. Ketamine protocol for palliative care in cancer patients with refractory pain. *Journal of the Advanced Practitioner in Oncology*. 2015;*6*(6):555–561.

80. Attal N, Cruccu G, Baron R, et al. EFNS guidelines on the pharmacological treatment of neuropathic pain: 2010 revision. *European Journal of Neurology*. 2010;*17*(9):1113–e88.

81. National Institute for Health and Care Excellence (NICE). Neuropathic pain: the pharmacological management of neuropathic pain in adults in non-specialist settings. 2013. https://pathways.nice.org.uk/pathways/neuropathic-pain. Accessed May 9, 2019.

82. Moulin D, Boulanger A, Clark AJ, et al. Pharmacological management of chronic neuropathic pain: revised consensus statement from the Canadian Pain Society. *Pain Research and Management*. 2014;*19*(6):328–335.

83. Alles SRA, Smith PA. Etiology and pharmacology of neuropathic pain. *Pharmacological Reviews*. 2018;*70*(2):315–347.

84. Zhai L, Song Z, Liu K. The effect of gabapentin on acute postoperative pain in patients undergoing total knee arthroplasty: a meta-analysis. *Medicine (Baltimore)*. 2016;*95*(20):e3673.

85. Moore RA, Straube S, Wiffen PJ, Derry S, McQuay HJ. Pregabalin for acute and chronic pain in adults. *Cochrane Database of Systematic Reviews*. 2009;*8*(3):CD007076.

86. Wiffen PJ, Derry S, Bell RF, et al. Gabapentin for chronic neuropathic pain in adults. *Cochrane Database of Systematic Reviews*. 2017;*9*(6):CD007938.

87. Toth C. Substitution of gabapentin therapy with pregabalin therapy in neuropathic pain due to peripheral neuropathy. *Pain Medicine*. 2010;*11*(3):456–465.

88. Mishra S, Bhatnagar S, Goyal GN, Rana SP, Upadhya SP. A comparative efficacy of amitriptyline, gabapentin, and pregabalin in neuropathic cancer pain: a prospective randomized double-blind placebo-controlled study. *American Journal of Hospice and Palliative Care*. 2012;*29*(3):177–182.

89. Bockbrader HN, Wesche D, Miller R, Chapel S, Janiczek N, Burger P. A comparison of the pharmacokinetics and pharmacodynamics of pregabalin and gabapentin. *Clinical Pharmacokinetics*. 2010;*49*(10):661–669.

90. Bennett MI. Effectiveness of antiepileptic or antidepressant drugs when added to opioids for cancer pain: systematic review. *Palliat Medicine*. 2011;*25*(5):553–559.

91. Wiffen PJ, Derry S, Moore RA, et al. Antiepileptic drugs for neuropathic pain and fibromyalgia—an overview of Cochrane reviews. *Cochrane Database of Systematic Reviews.* 2013;*11*(11):CD010567.

92. Wiffen PJ, Derry S, Moore RA, Kalso EA. Carbamazepine for chronic neuropathic pain and fibromyalgia in adults. *Cochrane Database of Systematic Reviews.* 2014;*10*(4):CD005451.

93. Demant DT, Lund K, Vollert J, et al. The effect of oxcarbazepine in peripheral neuropathic pain depends on pain phenotype: a randomised, double-blind, placebo-controlled phenotype-stratified study. *Pain.* 2014;*155*(11):2263–2273.

94. Hearn L, Derry S, Moore RA. Lacosamide for neuropathic pain and fibromyalgia in adults. *Cochrane Database of Systematic Reviews.* 2012;*15*(2):CD009318.

95. Wiffen PJ, Derry S, Lunn MP, Moore RA. Topiramate for neuropathic pain and fibromyalgia in adults. *Cochrane Database of Systematic Reviews.* 2013;*30*(8):CD008314.

96. Wiffen PJ, Rees J. Lamotrigine for acute and chronic pain. *Cochrane Database of Systematic Reviews.* 2007;*18*(2):CD006044.

97. Hugel H, Ellershaw JE, Dickman A. Clonazepam as an adjuvant analgesic in patients with cancer-related neuropathic pain. *Journal of Pain and Symptom Management.* 2003;*26*(6):1073–1074.

98. Fromm GH, Terrence CF, Chattha AS. Baclofen in the treatment of trigeminal neuralgia: double-blind study and long-term follow-up. *Annals of Neurology.* 1984;*15*(3):240–244.

99. Chiras J, Shotar E, Cormier E, Clarencon F. Interventional radiology in bone metastases. *European Journal of Cancer Care (England).* 2017;*26*(6).

100. Lee HL, Kuo CC, Tsai JT, Chen CY, Wu MH, Chiou JF. Magnetic resonance-guided focused ultrasound versus conventional radiation therapy for painful bone metastasis: a matched-pair study. *Journal of Bone and Joint Surgery. American Volume.* 2017;*99*(18):1572–1578.

101. Brodowicz T, Hadji P, Niepel D, Diel I. Early identification and intervention matters: a comprehensive review of current evidence and recommendations for the monitoring of bone health in patients with cancer. *Cancer Treatment Reviews.* 2017;*61*:23–34.

102. Kimura T. Multidisciplinary approach for bone metastasis: a review. *Cancers (Basel).* 2018;*10*(6):E156.

103. Hendriks LE, Hermans BC, van den Beuken-van Everdingen MH, Hochstenbag MM, Dingemans AM. Effect of bisphosphonates, denosumab, and radioisotopes on bone pain and quality of life in patients with non-small cell lung cancer and bone metastases: a systematic review. *Journal of Thoracic Oncology.* 2016;*11*(2):155–173.

104. Orozco CK, Maalouf NM. Safety of bisphosphonates. *Rheumic Disease Clinics of North America.* 2012;*38*(4):681–705.

105. Menshawy A, Mattar O, Abdulkarim A, et al. Denosumab versus bisphosphonates in patients with advanced cancers-related bone metastasis: systematic review and meta-analysis of randomized controlled trials. *Supportive Care in Cancer.* 2018;*26*(4):1029–1038.

106. Raje N, Roodman GD, Willenbacher W, et al. A cost-effectiveness analysis of denosumab for the prevention of skeletal-related events in patients with multiple myeloma in the United States of America. *Journal of Medical Economics.* 2018;*21*(5):525–536.

107. Martinez-Zapata MJ, Roqué M, Alonso-Coello P, Catala E. Calcitonin for metastatic bone pain. *Cochrane Database of Systematic Reviews.* 2006;*19*(3):CD003223.

108. Das T, Banerjee S. Radiopharmaceuticals for metastatic bone pain palliation: available options in the clinical domain and their comparisons. *Clinical & Experimental Metastasis.* 2017;*34*(1):1–10.

109. Lange R, Ter Heine R, Knapp RF, de Klerk JM, Bloemendal HJ, Hendrikse NH. Pharmaceutical and clinical development of phosphonate-based radiopharmaceuticals for the targeted treatment of bone metastases. *Bone.* 2016;*91*:159–179.

110. Guerra Liberal FDC, Tavares AAS, Tavares JMRS. Palliative treatment of metastatic bone pain with radiopharmaceuticals: a perspective beyond strontium-89 and samarium-153. *Applied Radiation and Isotopes.* 2016;*110*:87–99.

111. Roqué I Figuls M, Martinez-Zapata MJ, Scott-Brown M, Alonso-Coello P. Radioisotopes for metastatic bone pain. *Cochrane Database of Systematic Reviews.* 2011;*6*(7):CD003347.

112. Feuer DJ, Broadley KE. Corticosteroids for the resolution of malignant bowel obstruction in advanced gynecological and gastrointestinal cancer. *Cochrane Database of Systematic Reviews.* 2000;(2):CD001219.

113. Clark K, Lam L, Currow D. Reducing gastric secretions—a role for histamine 2 antagonists or proton pump inhibitors in malignant bowel obstruction? *Supportive Care in Cancer.* 2009;*17*(12):1463–1468.

114. Longford E, Scott A, Fradsham S, et al. Malignant bowel obstruction—a systematic literature review and evaluation of current practice. *BMJ Supportive and Palliative Care.* 2015;*5*(1):119.

115. Mercadante S, Casuccio A, Mangione S. Medical treatment for inoperable malignant bowel obstruction: a qualitative systematic review. *Journal of Pain and Symptom Management.* 2007;*33*(2):217–223.

116. O'Connor B, Creedon B. Pharmacological treatment of bowel obstruction in cancer patients. *Expert Opinion in Pharmacotherapy.* 2011;*12*(14):2205–2214.

117. Obita GP, Boland EG, Currow DC, Johnson MJ, Boland JW. Somatostatin analogues compared with placebo and other pharmacologic agents in the management of symptoms of inoperable malignant bowel obstruction: a systematic review. *Journal of Pain and Symptom Management.* 2016;*52*(6):901–919.

118. Laval G, Marcelin-Benazech B, Guirimand F, et al. Recommendations for bowel obstruction with peritoneal carcinomatosis. *Journal of Pain and Symptom Management.* 2014;*48*(1):75–91.

119. Mercadante S, Porzio G. Octreotide for malignant bowel obstruction: twenty years after. *Critical Reviews in Oncology/Hematology.* 2012;*83*(3):388–392.

120. Klepstad P, Kaasa S, Jystad A, Hval B, Borchgrevink PC. Immediate- or sustained-release morphine for dose finding during start of morphine to cancer patients: a randomized, double-blind trial. *Pain.* 2003;*101*:193.

121. Tobias JD, Green TP, Coté CJ. Section on Anesthesiology and Pain Medicine Committee on Drugs. Codeine: time to say "no." *Pediatrics.* 2016;*138*(4): e20162396.

122. Quigley C. Opioids in people with cancer-related pain. *BMJ Clinical Evidence.* 2008;*2008*:2408.

123. Dean M. Opioids in renal failure and dialysis patients. *Journal of Pain and Symptom Management.* 2004;*28*(5):497–504.

124. Penson RT, Joel SP, Gloyne A, Clark S, Slevin ML. Morphine analgesia in cancer pain: role of the glucuronides. *Journal of Opioid Management.* 2005;*1*:83.

125. Quigley C, Joel S, Patel N, Baksh A, Slevin M. Plasma concentrations of morphine, morphine-6-glucuronide and morphine-3-glucuronide and their relationship with analgesia and side effects in patients with cancer-related pain. *Palliative Medicine.* 2003;*17*:185.

126. Launay-Vacher V, Karie S, Fau JB, Izzedine H, Deray G. Treatment of pain in patients with renal insufficiency: the World Health Organization three-step ladder adapted. *Journal of Pain.* 2005;*6*:137.

127. Murtagh FE, Chai MO, Donohoe P, Edmonds PM, Higginson IJ. The use of opioid analgesia in end-stage renal disease patients managed without dialysis: recommendations for practice. *Journal of Pain & Palliative Care Pharmacotherapy.* 2007;*21*(2):5–16.

128. McPherson ML, Walker KA, Davis MP, et al. Safe and appropriate use of methadone in hospice and palliative care: expert consensus white paper. *Journal of Pain and Symptom Management.* 2019;*57*(3):635–645.e4.0.

129. Reddy S, Hui D, El Osta B, et al. The effect of oral methadone on the QTc interval in advanced cancer patients: a prospective pilot study. *Journal of Palliative Medicine.* 2010;*13*:33.

130. Cruciani RA, Sekine R, Homel P, et al. Measurement of QTc in patients receiving chronic methadone therapy. *Journal of Pain and Symptom Management.* 2005;*29*:385–391.

131. Van Seventer R, Smit JM, Schipper RM, Wicks MA, Zuurmond WW. Comparison of TTS-fentanyl with sustained-release oral morphine in the treatment of patients not using opioids for mild-to-moderate pain. *Current Medical Research and Opinion.* 2003;*19*:457.

132. Tassinari D, Sartori S, Tamburini E, et al. Adverse effects of transdermal opiates treating moderate-severe cancer pain in comparison to long-acting morphine: a meta-analysis and systematic review of the literature. *Journal of Palliative Medicine.* 2008;*11*:492.

133. Suno M, Endo Y, Nishie H, Kajizono M, Sendo T, Matsuoka J. Refractory cachexia is associated with increased plasma concentrations of fentanyl in cancer patients. *Therapeutics and Clinical Risk Management.* 2015;*11*:751–757.

134. Heiskanen T, Mätzke S, Haakana S, Gergov M, Vuori E, Kalso E. Transdermal fentanyl in cachectic cancer patients. *Pain.* 2009;*144*(1–2):218–222.

135. Carter KA. Heat-associated increase in transdermal fentanyl absorption. *American Journal of Health-System Pharmacy*. 2003;60:191.

136. Wilkinson TJ, Robinson BA, Begg EJ, Duffull SB, Ravenscroft PJ, Schneider JJ. Pharmacokinetics and efficacy of rectal versus oral sustained-release morphine in cancer patients. *Cancer Chemotherapy and Pharmacology*. 1992;31:251.

137. Walsh D, Tropiano PS. Long-term rectal administration of high-dose sustained-release morphine tablets. *Supportive Care in Cancer*. 2002;10:653.

138. Moolenaar F, Meijler WJ, Frijlink HW, Visser J, Proost H. Clinical efficacy, safety and pharmacokinetics of a newly developed controlled release morphine sulphate suppository in patients with cancer pain. *European Journal of Clinical Pharmacology*. 2000;56:219.

139. Rauck R, Reynolds L, Geach J, et al. Efficacy and safety of fentanyl sublingual spray for the treatment of breakthrough cancer pain: a randomized, double-blind, placebo-controlled study. *Current Medical Research and Opinion*. 2012;28:859.

140. Jandhyala R, Fullarton JR, Bennett MI. Efficacy of rapid-onset oral fentanyl formulations vs. oral morphine for cancer-related breakthrough pain: a meta-analysis of comparative trials. *Journal of Pain and Symptom Management*. 2013;46:573.

141. Portenoy RK, Burton AW, Gabrail N, et al. A multicenter, placebo-controlled, double-blind, multiple-crossover study of fentanyl pectin nasal spray (FPNS) in the treatment of breakthrough cancer pain. *Pain*. 2010;151:617.

142. Kosugi T, Hamada S, Takigawa C, et al. A randomized, double-blind, placebo-controlled study of fentanyl buccal tablets for breakthrough pain: efficacy and safety in Japanese cancer patients. *Journal of Pain and Symptom Management*. 2014;47:990.

143. Coluzzi PH. Sublingual morphine: efficacy reviewed. *Journal of Pain and Symptom Management*. 1998;16:184–192.

144. Caccialanza R, Constans T, Cotogni P, Zaloga GP, Pontes-Arruda A. Subcutaneous infusion of fluids for hydration or nutrition: a review. *JPEN Journal of Parenteral and Enteral Nutrition*. 2018;42(2):296–307.

145. Swarm RA, Karanikolas M, Cousins MJ. Interventional approaches for chronic pain. In: Cherny NI, Fallon MT, Kaasa S, Portenoy RK, Currow DC (eds). *Oxford Textbook of Palliative Medicine*. 5th ed. Oxford University Press; 2015:589–598.

146. Myers J, Chan V, Jarvis V, Walker-Dilks C. Intraspinal techniques for pain management in cancer patients: a systematic review. *Supportive Care in Cancer*. 2010;18(2):137–149. doi:10.1007/s00520-009-0784-2

147. Deer TR, Pope JE, Hayek SM, et al. The Polyanalgesic Consensus Conference (PACC): recommendations on intrathecal drug infusion systems best practices and guidelines [published correction appears in *Neuromodulation*. 2017;20(4):405–406]. *Neuromodulation*. 2017;20(2):96–132.

148. Clarke CFM. Neuraxial drug delivery for the management of cancer pain: cost, updates, and society guidelines. *Current Opinion in Anaesthesiology*. 2017;30(5):593–597.

149. Caraceni A, Bertetto O, Labianca R, et al. Episodic (breakthrough) pain prevalence in a population of cancer pain patients. Comparison of clinical diagnoses with the QUDEI—Italian Questionnaire for Intense Episodic Pain. *Journal of Pain and Symptom Management*. 2012;43(5):833–841.

150. Reddy A, Yennurajalingam S, Pulivarthi K, et al. Frequency, outcome, and predictors of success within 6 weeks of an opioid rotation among outpatients with cancer receiving strong opioids. *Oncologist*. 2013;18(2):212–220.

151. Fine PG, Portenoy RK; Ad Hoc Expert Panel on Evidence Review and Guidelines for Opioid Rotation. Establishing "best practices" for opioid rotation: conclusions of an expert panel. *Journal of Pain and Symptom Management*. 2009;38(3):418–425.

152. Bharucha AE, Lacy BE. Mechanisms, evaluation, and management of chronic constipation. *Gastroenterology*. 2020;158(5):1232–1249.e3.

153. Ford AC, Brenner DM, Schoenfeld PS. Efficacy of pharmacological therapies for the treatment of opioid-induced constipation: systematic review and meta-analysis. *American Journal of Gastroenterology*. 2013;108:1566.

154. Candy B, Jones L, Vickerstaff V, Larkin PJ, Stone P. Mu-opioid antagonists for opioid-induced bowel dysfunction in people with cancer and people receiving palliative care. *Cochrane Database of Systematic Reviews.* 2018;6:CD006332.

155. Nee J, Zakari M, Sugarman MA, et al. Efficacy of treatments for opioid-induced constipation: systematic review and meta-analysis. *Clinical Gastroenterology and Hepatology.* 2018;16(10):1569–1584.e2.

156. Ford AC, Quigley EM, Lacy BE, et al. Efficacy of prebiotics, probiotics, and synbiotics in irritable bowel syndrome and chronic idiopathic constipation: systematic review and meta-analysis. *American Journal of Gastroenterology.* 2014;109(10):1547–1562.

157. Smith HS, Laufer A. Opioid-induced nausea and vomiting. *European Journal of Pharmacology.* 2014;722:67–78. doi:10.1016/j.ejphar.2013.09.074

158. Laugsand EA, Kaasa S, Klepstad P. Management of opioid-induced nausea and vomiting in cancer patients: systematic review and evidence-based recommendations. *Palliative Medicine.* 2011;25:442.

159. Bruera E, Driver L, Barnes E, et al. Patient controlled methylphenidate for cancer related fatigue: a preliminary report. *Journal of Clinical Oncology.* 2003;21(23):4439–4443.

160. Kerr CW, Drake J, Milch RA, et al. Effects of methylphenidate on fatigue and depression: a randomized, double-blind, placebo-controlled trial. *Journal of Pain and Symptom Management.* 2012;43(1):68–77.

161. Webster L, Andrews M, Stoddard G. Modafinil treatment of opioid-induced sedation. *Pain Medicine.* 2003;4:135.

162. Cao M, Javeheri S. Effects of chronic opioid use on sleep and wake. *Sleep Medicine Clinics.* 2018;13(2):271–281.

163. Gudin JA, Laitman A, Nalamachu S. Opioid-related endocrinopathy. *Pain Medicine.* 2015;16(Suppl 1):S9–S15.

164. Portenoy RK. Acute and chronic pain. In: Ruiz P, Strain E, eds. *Lowinson & Ruiz's Substance Abuse: A Comprehensive Textbook.* 5th ed. Philadelphia, PA: Lippincott, Williams and Wilkins; 2011:695.

165. Kwon JH, Hui D, Bruera E. A pilot study to define chemical coping in cancer patients using the Delphi method. *Journal of Palliative Medicine.* 2015;18(8):703–706. doi:10.1089/jpm.2014.0446

166. Higgins C, Smith BH, Matthews K. Incidence of iatrogenic opioid dependence or abuse in patients with pain who were exposed to opioid analgesic therapy: a systematic review and meta-analysis. *British Journal of Anaesthesiology.* 2018;120(6):1335–1344.

167. Jackson TP, Gaeta R. Neurolytic blocks revisited. *Current Pain and Headache Reports.* 2008;12(1):7–13.

168. Mercadante S, Catala E, Arcuri E, Casuccio A. Celiac plexus block for pancreatic cancer pain: factors influencing pain, symptoms and quality of life. *Journal of Pain and Symptom Management.* 2003;26(6):1140–1147.

169. Arcidiacono PG, Calori G, Carrara S, McNicol ED, Testoni PA. Celiac plexus block for pancreatic cancer pain in adults. *Cochrane Database of Systematic Reviews.* 2011;16(3):CD007519.

170. Wyse JM, Carone M, Paquin SC, Usatii M, Sahai AV. Randomized, double-blind, controlled trial of early endoscopic ultrasound-guided celiac plexus neurolysis to prevent pain progression in patients with newly diagnosed, painful, inoperable pancreatic cancer. *Journal of Clinical Oncology.* 2011;29(26):3541–3546.

171. Hurlow A, Bennett MI, Robb KA, Johnson MI, Simpson KH, Oxberry SG. Transcutaneous electric nerve stimulation (TENS) for cancer pain in adults. *Cochrane Database of Systematic Reviews.* 2012;(3):CD006276.

172. Loprinzi C, Le-Rademacher JG, Majithia N, et al. Scrambler therapy for chemotherapy neuropathy: a randomized phase II pilot trial. Supportive Care in Cancer. 2020;28:1183.

173. Smith TJ, Razzak AR, Blackford AL, et al. A pilot randomized sham-controlled trial of MC5—a scrambler therapy in the treatment of chronic chemotherapy-induced peripheral neuropathy (CIPN). *Journal of Palliative Care.* 2020;35:53.

174. Ricci M, Fabbri L, Pirotti S, Ruffilli N, Foca F, Maltoni M. Scrambler therapy: what's new after 15 years? The results from 219 patients treated for chronic pain. *Medicine (Baltimore).* 2019;98(2):e13895.

175. Verrills P, Sinclair C, Barnard A. A review of spinal cord stimulation systems for chronic pain. *Journal of Pain Research.* 2016;9:481–492.

176. Taylor RS, De Vries J, Buchser E, Dejongste MJ. Spinal cord stimulation in the treatment of refractory angina: systematic review and meta-analysis of randomized controlled studies. *BMC Cardiovascular Disorders*. 2009;9:13.

177. Terranova C, Rizzo V, Cacciola A, et al. Is there a future for non-invasive brain stimulation as a therapeutic tool? *Frontiers in Neurology*. 2019;9:1146.

178. De Groef A, Van Kampen M, Dieltjens E, et al. Effectiveness of postoperative physical therapy for upper-limb impairments after breast cancer treatment: a systematic review. *Archives of Physical Medicine and Rehabilitation*. 2015;96:1140.

179. Kleckner IR, Kamen C, Gewandter JS, et al. Effects of exercise during chemotherapy on chemotherapy-induced peripheral neuropathy: a multicenter, randomized controlled trial. *Supportive Care in Cancer*. 2018;26:1019.

180. Dhawan S, Andrews R, Kumar L, et al. A randomized controlled trial to assess the effectiveness of muscle strengthening and balancing exercises on chemotherapy-induced peripheral neuropathic pain and quality of life among cancer patients. *Cancer Nursing*. 2020;43(4):269–280.

181. Gibson W, Wand BM, Meads C, et al. Transcutaneous electrical nerve stimulation (TENS) for chronic pain—an overview of Cochrane reviews. Cochrane Database of Systematic Reviews. 2019;2:CD011890.

182. Burchiel KJ, Raslan AM. Contemporary concepts of pain surgery. *Journal of Neurosurgery*. 2019;130(4):1039–1049. doi:10.3171/2019.1.JNS181620

183. Javed S, Viswanathan A, Abdi S. Cordotomy for intractable cancer pain: a narrative review. *Pain Physician*. 2020;23(3):283–292.

184. Brothers BM, Thornton LM, Anderson B. Cognitive and behavioral interventions. In: Holland JC, ed. *Psychooncology*. New York: Oxford University Press; 2010:415–421.

185. Phianmongkhol Y, Thongubon K, Woottiluk P. Effectiveness of cognitive behavioral therapy techniques for control of pain in lung cancer patients: an integrated review. *Asian Pacific Journal of Cancer Prevention*. 2015;16(14):6033–6038.

186. Carlson LE, Zelinski E, Toivonen K, et al. Mind-body therapies in cancer: what is the latest evidence? *Current Oncology Reports*. 2017;19(10):67. doi:10.1007/s11912-017-0626-1

187. Bennett MI, Bagnall AM, José Closs S. How effective are patient-based educational interventions in the management of cancer pain? Systematic review and meta-analysis. *Pain*. 2009;143(3):192–199. doi:10.1016/j.pain.2009.01.016

188. Garland EL, Brintz CE, Hanley AW, et al. Mind-body therapies for opioid-treated pain: a systematic review and meta-analysis. *JAMA Internal Medicine*. 2019;180(1):91–105. doi:10.1001/jamainternmed.2019.4917

189. Ma X, Yue ZQ, Gong ZQ, et al. The effect of diaphragmatic breathing on attention, negative affect and stress in healthy adults. *Frontiers in Psychology*. 2017;8:874. doi:10.3389/fpsyg.2017.00874

190. De Paolis G, Naccarato A, Cibelli F, et al. The effectiveness of progressive muscle relaxation and interactive guided imagery as a pain-reducing intervention in advanced cancer patients: a multicentre randomised controlled non-pharmacological trial. *Complementary Therapies in Clinical Practice*. 2019;34:280–287. doi:10.1016/j.ctcp.2018.12.014

191. Bradt J, Dileo C, Magill L, Teague A. Music interventions for improving psychological and physical outcomes in cancer patients. Cochrane Database of Systematic Reviews 2016;(8):CD006911.

192. He Y, Guo X, May BH, et al. Clinical evidence for association of acupuncture and acupressure with improved cancer pain: a systematic review and meta-analysis. *JAMA Oncology*. 2019;6(2):271–278. doi:10.1001/jamaoncol.2019.5233

193. Greenlee H, Balneaves LG, Carlson LE, et al. Clinical practice guidelines on the use of integrative therapies as supportive care in patients treated for breast cancer. *Journal of the National Cancer Institute. Monographs*. 2014;2014:346.

194. Bao Y, Kong X, Yang L, et al. Complementary and alternative medicine for cancer pain: an overview of systematic reviews. *Evidence-Based Complementary and Alternative Medicine*. 2014;2014:170396. doi:10.1155/2014/170396

195. Shin ES, Seo KH, Lee SH, et al. Massage with or without aromatherapy for symptom relief in people with cancer. *Cochrane Database of Systematic Reviews.* 2016;(6):CD009873.

196. Cassileth BR, Vickers AJ. Massage therapy for symptom control: outcome study at a major cancer center. *Journal of Pain and Symptom Management.* 2004;28:244.

197. Chen YW, Hunt MA, Campbell KL, Peill K, Reid WD. The effect of Tai Chi on four chronic conditions—cancer, osteoarthritis, heart failure and chronic obstructive pulmonary disease: a systematic review and meta-analyses. *British Journal of Sports Medicine.* 2016;*50*(7):397–407. doi:10.1136/bjsports-2014-094388

198. So PS, Jiang Y, Qin Y. Touch therapies for pain relief in adults. Cochrane Database of Systematic Reviews 2008;(4):CD006535.

15

Psychological and Psychiatric Aspects of Care

Scott A. Irwin, Jeremy Hirst, Manuel Trachsel,
Chase Samsel, Joshua Briscoe, and Nicole Bates

Introduction

Serious psychological and emotional symptoms frequently accompany a progressive and/or life-threatening illness. *Total pain* is distress with not only physical but also social, spiritual, and emotional sources. The World Health Organization definition of palliative care makes specific reference to this important component of treatment: "Palliative Care . . . integrates the psychological aspects of patient care."[1] While it is often difficult to distinguish what suffering near the end of life is caused by physical symptoms or psychosocial and existential issues (Box 15.1), it is well established that unrelieved suffering of any kind is associated with poor quality of life.

Several barriers to psychiatric involvement have been described: professional factors, for example, failure to recognize the limits of palliative care clinicians in addressing psychological distress, or lack of confidence among psychiatrists about their ability to be of value in caring for patients near the end of life. Practice pattern changes within the field of psychiatry may have played a role as well: The emergence of palliative care coincided with a movement toward increased reliance on psychopharmacology and away from psychotherapeutic modes of care; nonpsychiatrists began to use tools to treat psychological distress, at times even without formal psychotherapeutic interventions. Systems-level factors contributed as well, and this includes funding structures that have been unfamiliar with or inadequate to compensate psychiatry providers.[3,4]

However, psychiatrists and other mental health specialists, such as psychologists, social workers, marriage and family therapists, and child-life specialists, have increasingly developed ways to bring their expert skills and knowledge to the care of seriously ill patients, even

BOX 15.1 Causes of Suffering That May Benefit From Psychiatric Expertise.[2]

Anger	Abandonment
Anxiety	Fear
Bereavement	Grief
Boundary setting	Hope/hopelessness
Burden	Insomnia
Caregiving	Loneliness
Coping	Loss
Delirium	Nausea
Dementia	Pain
Denial	Personality issues
Dependence	Professional burnout/self-care
Depression	Shortness of breath
Desire for hastened death	Substance use problems
Dignity	Suicidal ideation
Distress	

as they near the final phase of life. Palliative care psychiatry, which shares some overlap with psychosomatic medicine and psychooncology, is an emerging subspecialty at the intersection of palliative care and psychiatry.[2,5,6] Effective management of psychosocial and psychiatric issues often enables improvements in other domains, as evidenced by the example of reduction in physical pain that frequently follows effective treatment of depression.

Physician assistants can contribute meaningfully to care for seriously ill patients by developing expertise in psychiatric diagnosis, pharmacology, supportive psychotherapy, behavioral and environmental management, capacity assessment, and issues of loss and grief for patients, families, and fellow health professionals. This chapter provides a practical examination of specific tools and guidelines in psychiatry and behavioral health that physician assistants can utilize in the care of seriously ill patients, their caregivers, and loved ones.

When to Consult With Mental Health Experts

A preexisting psychiatric illness can influence a patient's and family's ability to manage a progressive and/or life-threatening illness and present a significant barrier to care. When these situations exceed a team's own expertise, expert consultation with mental health professionals may be necessary.[7] Situations that may call for expert consultation include disabling and refractory signs and symptoms of anxiety, depression, delirium, insomnia, substance use disorders, challenging behaviors and personalities, dementia, and severe mental illnesses (e.g., schizophrenia and bipolar illnesses).

In addition to these specific symptom clusters, psychiatric assistance may be sought to help patients struggling with a general lack of meaning and loss of dignity. Mental health experts may assist patients in finding new ways to find hope amidst refractory symptoms, social isolation, and existential and emotional distress.[5]

Specific Psychiatric Conditions and the Palliative Care Patient

Anxiety

In palliative care settings, anxiety ranges from normal fears and worries about progressive and/or life-threatening illness and the dying process, to pathologic anxiety disorders that significantly impair function and well-being.[8] Some degree of anxiety is expected as patients face the end of life, though up to 70% of advanced cancer patients report moderate-to-severe anxiety, and up to 25% of patients meet criteria for formal anxiety disorders.[9–12] Diagnoses are varied, with common disorders and risk factors listed in Box 15.2.

Anxiety disorders carry significant consequences for patients receiving palliative care, in both experience of symptoms and their medical care. In addition to subjective psychological and cognitive symptoms, physical symptoms are common in anxiety and panic, including palpitations, dyspnea and hyperventilation, gastrointestinal distress, sweating, headaches, muscle tension, lightheadedness or dizziness, and fatigue.[9,16] Anxious patients also report less trust in physicians, impaired interactions in care discussions, more doubt about treatments, and poorer physical performance status.[13]

Diagnostic Evaluation

Similar to depression, screening for anxiety disorders is routinely recommended in palliative care settings, and the Hospital Anxiety and Depression Scale (HADS) remains the most widely studied instrument,[17] though the Edmonton Symptom Assessment Scale (ESAS) is also frequently used.[16,18] For patients screening positive for anxiety, normal fears and worries must be distinguished from pathologic anxiety (i.e., anxiety that exceeds a patient's ability to cope with stressors).[9] A more in-depth clinical interview should follow, with review of *Diagnostic and Statistical Manual of Mental Disorders, Fifth Edition* (*DSM-5*) diagnostic criteria of conditions[19] and referral to a mental health expert if diagnostic clarity is needed. Importantly, a primary anxiety disorder should not be diagnosed until medical causes of anxiety, restlessness, or agitation are ruled out (Box 15.2).

Psychotherapy

Given limited data supporting specific pharmacotherapy for anxiety, psychotherapy and psychosocial interventions for anxiety are often favored.[20] Psychotherapy can be helpful for patients with prior success in therapy, inadequate response to medications or aversion to medication use, an ability to adhere to treatment, and no current cognitive impairment.[14] As patients move closer to death, the goals of psychotherapy often narrow to a more

BOX 15.2 Potential Risk Factors and Etiologies of Anxiety, Agitation, and Restlessness in Palliative Care[9,13–15]

Risk Factors

o Female gender

o Lower social supports

o A tentative (vs. strong or nonexistent) belief in the afterlife

o Younger age

o Cancer diagnosis

o Use of psychotropic agents

o Poor caregiver coping

Psychiatric diagnoses and psychological causes

o Nonpathologic anxiety or existential distress, including death anxiety

o Generalized anxiety disorder

o Adjustment disorder with anxiety (with/without depressed mood)

o Panic disorder

o Agoraphobia

o Social anxiety disorder

o Separation anxiety disorder

o Specific phobia

o Acute stress disorder

o Post-traumatic stress disorder

o Anxiety disorder due to a general medical condition

o Obsessive-compulsive disorder

Uncontrolled pain

Respiratory distress

o Hypoxemia

o Dyspnea, including terminal dyspnea

o Pulmonary embolism

Delirium

o Metabolic derangements

o Hypoglycemia

o Infection

o Organ failure

o Malnutrition

Medications/Substances

o Respiratory agents (β-agonists, bronchodilators, theophylline)

o Antihypertensives

o Antiemetics with dopamine antagonism (i.e., metoclopramide, prochlorperazine): akathisia

o Steroids: affective lability, akathisia, insomnia

o Antipsychotics

o Psychostimulants

o Immunotherapies

o Substance intoxication or withdrawal (alcohol, benzodiazepines, opioids, caffeine, etc.)

palliative care–like approach: to maximize psychological and physical comfort by helping patients and their families emotionally and practically prepare for death.[14] Attrition rates are high due to progressive and/or life-threatening illness, so the frequency and duration of planned therapy should be carefully considered.[21] Specific modalities employed with success include[10,14,21,22]

- Psychoeducation
- Supportive psychotherapy
- Skill-based therapy (progressive muscle relaxation, hypnosis, music therapy, meditation, distraction, etc.)
- Cognitive behavioral therapy
- Existential therapies, including managing cancer and living meaningfully
- Expressive therapies (music and art therapy, etc.)
- Religious/clergy support when existential distress includes religious themes

Pharmacotherapy

Several Cochrane reviews have concluded that evidence from published studies is too weak to recommend any specific pharmacology for targeting anxiety in palliative care.[20] Clinicians must therefore extrapolate from studies of anxiety treatment in the general population and other disease states, typically cancer.[13,15,17,18]

Limited available literature and expert opinions position benzodiazepines and selective serotonin reuptake inhibitors (SSRIs) as first-line treatments for many anxiety symptoms in progressive and/or life-threatening illness and cancer.[17,20] SSRIs, as in depression, have strong data for anxiety in general populations and are well tolerated, though may be inadequate for patients with life expectancies of a few months or less, given 4–5 weeks for maximal effect.[23] Benzodiazepines have advantages of rapid onset; efficacy for generalized anxiety, panic, and insomnia; as well as potential benefits in nausea.[17] Considering medical frailty in palliative care populations, medications should generally be started at lower doses, and with more gradual titration, than in healthy populations, with special care in using benzodiazepines, which may increase the risk for sedation, falls, and confusion.[14] Treating additional contributors to anxiety, chiefly pain and physical symptoms, is also essential.[20] Amid a relative lack of evidence-based medications for anxiety in palliative care, agents including ketamine, psilocybin, and medical marijuana/CBD (cannabidiol)/THC (delta-(9)-tetrahydrocannabinol)[24,25] are demonstrating some encouraging early results for anxiety near the end of life, but caution is warranted.[26–29] Cannabinoids are receiving increased attention and use in cancer and palliative care settings. However, in contrast to evidence supporting benefits for certain physical symptoms in cancer and palliative care (e.g., nausea and neuropathic pain), studies do not yet support a benefit for anxiety or mental illness generally; anxiety and agitation are in fact risks of cannabinoid use. Thus, cannabinoids cannot currently be recommended for anxiety in palliative care. Specific dosing and pharmacology are beyond the scope of this text, although common medications are summarized in Table 15.1.

TABLE 15.1 Medication Considerations for Anxiety in Palliative Care Settings[14,26-31]

Drug Class	Examples	Recommended for	Special Considerations
Benzodiazepines	Lorazepam Clonazepam Temazepam Oxazepam Diazepam Alprazolam Midazolam	- Generalized anxiety and panic (first line) - Insomnia (longer-acting agents) - Potential use in terminal dyspnea	- Lorazepam, oxazepam, temazepam advised in liver dysfunction, given lack of active metabolites - May worsen delirium and cognition - Risk of central respiratory suppression - Risk of misuse, combination with alcohol and opioids
Selective serotonin reuptake inhibitorss (SSRIs)	Sertraline Citalopram Escitalopram* Fluoxetine[a] Paroxetine[b]	- Generalized anxiety disorder, panic disorder, post-traumatic stress disorder - Patients with life expectancy > 2 months	- Requires 4–6 weeks for maximum effect - Some patients experience increased activation, restlessness, anxiety in first days–weeks of use
Other antidepressants	Mirtazapine Trazodone Venlafaxine Duloxetine	- Comorbid insomnia - Comorbid pain	- Rapid sedation, but anxiolytic effect may take 4–6 weeks - As with SSRIs, long time frame of action
Antipsychotics	Haloperidol Risperidone Olanzapine Quetiapine	- Comorbid delirium, insomnia, and/or agitation - Potentially safer with respiratory compromise - Steroid-induced symptoms	- Risk of akathisia and extrapyramidal side effects - Potential QTc impacts, especially with intravenous haloperidol - Anticholinergic side effects with olanzapine, quetiapine
Hypnotics	Zolpidem Zaleplon Eszopiclone Rozerem	- Insomnia	- Risk of grogginess, confusion, parasomnias
Antihistamines	Hydroxyzine Diphenhydramine	- Short term/as needed for anxiety relief	- May be less effective than benzodiazepines - Risks of sedation, confusion, delirium
Novel agents	Psilocybin Ketamine	- May be used with or without therapy - Existential distress, depression, anxiety	- Psilocybin in research settings only - Limited availability of ketamine - Risk of medication abuse

[a] Food and Drug Administration approved in children.
[b] Contraindicated in children.

Depression

Even in the general population, depression is the leading cause of disability worldwide, and it presents as a very common and often debilitating psychiatric complication in palliative care.[32] The prevalence of major depressive disorder in palliative care settings ranges from 9.6% to 19.3% across studies, with another 15.4%–36.3% of patients suffering from any form of depressive disorder, such as adjustment disorder.[8] Patients receiving palliative care with major depression are more likely to report comorbid pain, demonstrate poor performance status, and desire hastened death.[33] Given the clinical impact of depression near the end of life, physician assistants in palliative care must be comfortable with screening for and diagnosing depression, as well as referring for specialized mental health treatment when appropriate.

Diagnostic Evaluation

Choosing an appropriate depression screening tool is a challenge, given the large array of imperfect options in medically ill patients. The most important initial step is to invite discussion about a patient's mood. Simply asking one or two basic questions targeting core features of depression ("Are you depressed?" and "Have you lost interest or pleasure?") has documented success in identifying cases of depression, although sensitivities and specificities vary widely (54%–100% across reports).[34] The best-studied depression screen in palliative care populations remains the HADS,[35] though the ESAS and Edinburgh Postnatal Depression Scale are also frequently used in progressive and/or life-threatening illness and cancer.[8,36]

Identifying potential medical causes of depressive symptomatology, including thyroid dysfunction; poorly controlled pain; delirium; central nervous system involvement of disease (e.g., metastases, stroke); infection; and metabolic derangements (e.g., altered glucose, electrolytes, renal function), is vital to accurate diagnosis and treatment.[37] Likewise, depression must be differentiated from similar primary psychiatric conditions to ensure proper management. Adjustment disorders, anxiety disorders, post-traumatic stress disorder, persistent depressive disorder (dysthymia), and bipolar spectrum illness may all present with features of depression.[38]

Additional diagnostic challenges in the palliative care setting include distinguishing depression from demoralization and variants of normal grief, both of which overlap clinically with major depression.[39–42] Comparisons among major depression, normal grief, and demoralization are outlined in Table 15.2.[33,39,40,43]

Assessment of Lethality

While evaluating depressive symptoms, clinicians must explore whether patients are struggling with suicidality. Progressive and/or life-threatening illness, particularly advanced cancer, increases the risk of suicide by up to 11 times that of the general population.[45] Beyond this, depression and hopelessness may manifest in palliative care settings as a wish for hastened death.[46] Despite common fears, screening for suicidal risk factors among patients with signs of depression does not increase suicide risk.[47] This allows for proper stabilization and initiation of treatment interventions.[48] Moreover, research showed that failure to directly ask about suicidality may miss significant portions of people who are suicidal, especially

TABLE 15.2 Distinguishing Depression From Normal Grief and Demoralization[41,43,44]

Feature	Depression	Normal Grief	Demoralization
Core features	Low mood, lack of interest and pleasure	Psychological, physical, and social reactions to loss	Loss of hope and meaning; subjective incompetence/helplessness
Sadness	Persistent, though may be diurnal	Experienced in waves	Variable
Loss of pleasure	Anhedonia and loss of anticipatory pleasure	Not persistent	Loss of anticipatory pleasure only
Satisfaction from relationships	Diminished or absent	Preserved	Variable
View of self	Distorted, especially. guilt and worthlessness	Generally intact	Helpless, loss of dignity
Hopelessness	Present	Absent	Present
Suicidality/desire for hastened death	Increased risk	Absent	Increased risk

in adolescents and young adults, and well-validated screening forms exist, such as the Ask Suicide-Screening Questions.[49] Suicide screening should thus be part of an initial palliative care assessment, and discovering active suicidal thoughts warrants prompt referral to mental health experts as well as local crisis resources for further evaluation and to ensure safety.

Psychotherapy

Even without providing formalized psychotherapy, many healthcare providers deliver key elements of supportive psychotherapy in their daily practice: empathic listening, positive regard, validation of feelings, and encouragement of adaptive coping. Patients impaired by depressive symptoms may benefit from more structured psychotherapy, either individually or group based. There is a moderate-to-large benefit from psychotherapy targeting depression in palliative care, though no specific modality can be recommended as superior.[50] Psychotherapy at the end of life may broadly be categorized into skill building and supportive-expressive modalities, which are summarized briefly in Table 15.3.

The unpredictable course and timing of disease progression in palliative care settings may limit or halt a patient's ability to engage in the work of psychotherapy. As such, psychotherapy for depression should be undertaken as early in the medical disease process as possible and with clear goals defined to be achieved in a relatively short time frame.[53]

Pharmacotherapy

Treatment with antidepressant agents (SSRIs, SNRIs, tricyclic antidepressants, and novel antidepressants) has consistently demonstrated benefits for moderate-to-severe depressive symptoms, including in patients with progressive and/or life-threatening illness.[54] SSRIs (e.g., sertraline, escitalopram, fluoxetine) are first-line treatments for major depression in children and adults and are well tolerated and efficacious. Mirtazapine, with few drug interactions, lack of impact on platelet function, and potential benefits for insomnia and appetite, is also

TABLE 15.3 Psychotherapy Modalities in Palliative Care Settings[33,51,52]

Modality	Key Features
SKILL-BUILDING PSYCHOTHERAPIES	
Cognitive behavioral therapy (CBT)	▪ Emphasizes connections between thoughts, emotions, and behaviors ▪ Targets cognitive distortions to reduce maladaptive behaviors
Problem-solving therapy	▪ Aims to reduce distress through directly resolving identified problems for patients and caregivers
Behavior-focused therapies	▪ Include relaxation therapy, mindfulness, biofeedback, hypnosis, guided imagery
SUPPORTIVE-EXPRESSIVE PSYCHOTHERAPIES	
Supportive therapy	▪ Enhances adaptive coping and redirects from maladaptive coping to reduce immediate distress
Interpersonal psychotherapy (IPT)	▪ Formulates depression as an interpersonal struggle (grief, role transition, interpersonal dispute, interpersonal deficit) that can be resolved
Existential psychotherapy	▪ Explores meanings of, and anxieties related to, existence and death
Dignity therapy	▪ Encourages elements of dignity near death through brief, semistructured, recorded interviews ▪ Therapist creates a "generativity document" as a legacy
Life review	▪ Pursues meaning through exploring life events and engaging in activity to reminisce, resolve conflicts, and leave a legacy
Life narrative	▪ Facilitates recording life experiences, creating meaning from illness in the context of a patient's life and character
Meaning-centered psychotherapy	▪ Uses teaching, discussion, and exercises to enhance a sense of meaning and purpose in progressive and/or life-threatening illness ▪ Studied in manualized, group settings for advanced cancer
Logotherapy	▪ Acknowledges suffering and aims to reduce distress through finding meaning, purpose, positivity
Grief therapy	▪ Explores grief and loss as patients approach death; attuned to patients' emotions and affect ▪ Work with loved ones may begin before or after death

attractive in palliative care settings. No single antidepressant has emerged as superior in palliative care settings, and a full review of antidepressant pharmacology and dosing is beyond the scope of this text.[23,54] Common medications for depression are summarized in Table 15.4.

Despite the benefits of antidepressant therapy, special considerations in palliative care settings, including complex medical illness, drug interactions, short prognosis, and medical frailty, may impact both the tolerability and the efficacy of these medications. One major concern in beginning antidepressant therapy in palliative care is limited life span: while antidepressants show benefit over placebo in reducing depressive symptoms among physically ill patients, this benefit may not appear for 4–5 weeks and only in about 30% of patients being treated with first-line approaches,[55] during which patients receiving palliative care may die or markedly decline.[23] For patients facing death within several months, psychostimulants (methylphenidate and modafinil are best studied) may be recommended as appropriate first-line therapy, either as monotherapy or in addition to an SSRI, SNRI, or other antidepressant.[56]

TABLE 15.4 Pharmacotherapy for Depression in Palliative Care[23,33,54]

Class or Drug	General Comments	Examples
Selective serotonin reuptake inhibitors (SSRIs)	• First line • Generally well tolerated • Fluoxetine: long half-life can be helpful in inconsistent oral access • Sertraline: few drug-drug interactions, limited impact on QTc, well tolerated	• Sertraline • Citalopram • Escitalopram[a] • Fluoxetine[a] • Paroxetine[b]
Serotonin norepinephrine reuptake inhibitors (SNRIs)	• Potentially more complications than SSRI in kidney/liver disease • May have benefits in neuropathic or chronic pain • Venlafaxine: no interactions with tamoxifen; significant withdrawal syndrome	• Venlafaxine[a] • Duloxetine • Desvenlafaxine
Tricyclic antidepressants (TCAs)	• Higher risk due to side effect profile, lethality in overdose • May have benefits for sleep and pain	• Amitriptyline • Nortriptyline • Imipramine • Doxepin
Mirtazapine	• May be first-line • Benefits for sleep and appetite • Avoids inhibition of platelets seen with SSRIs	• Mirtazapine
Psychostimulants	• First line with short life expectancy or prominent apathy • Commonly underdosed[22]	• Methylphenidate • Modafinil
NMDA (*N*-methyl-D-aspartate) antagonists	• Rapid onset, benefit in pain • Still under study; not widely available	• Ketamine

[a] Food and Drug Administration approved in children.
[b] Contraindicated in children.

Finally, though more study is needed, ketamine shows emerging promise for treating depression in palliative care settings. Its rapid onset of action, efficacy for treating pain and availability in intravenous, oral, and intranasal formulations offer unique benefits in this setting.[57]

Delirium

Delirium is an acute change in mental status accompanied by difficulties in shifting and sustaining attention not accounted for by another neurocognitive disorder.[19] It is a prevalent condition in palliative care inpatient populations, ranging up to 60% during admissions and 80% as patients near the end of life.[58–62] Despite its prevalence, it can be missed in as many of 40% of inpatient referrals to psychiatry.[63] This can impact management, as underlying precipitating and perpetuating factors may go unaddressed. Failure to recognize delirium impairs treatment adherence and prognostication as delirium is associated with increased mortality and is a nonspecific sign of impending death.[64,65]

Delirium is not dementia, but dementia can predispose a patient to delirium. Diagnosing delirium itself can be challenging because these deficits may appear in other conditions, like depression or dementia, but these usually develop in a more insidious fashion.[63] Hypoactive delirium is less easily recognized than hyperactive delirium (agitated), possibly because hypoactive patients draw less attention to themselves; therefore, clinicians should be vigilant to monitor for acute changes in mental status that result in either increased or decreased activity. The confusion assessment method (CAM) is a straightforward screening instrument for delirium that has also been modified and validated for use in the intensive care unit and inpatient hospice.[66–68] Pediatric and preschool-aged versions exist and have been validated in critically ill populations.[69,70] The CAM will screen in delirium when both the first *and* second criteria are present with either the third *or* fourth criterion:

1. Acute change in mental status
2. Fluctuating attention
3. Disorganized thought process
4. Altered level of consciousness

While accurate diagnosis is important, identifying predisposing, precipitating, and perpetuating factors of delirium merits equal attention (Box 15.1). Some of these can be eliminated entirely, while others can be better managed to reduce their impact on quality of life and the risk for ongoing and recurrent delirium. Examples of *nonmodifiable* factors for delirium include male sex, older or younger age, developmental delay, organ failure, dementia, and the presence of chronic medical comorbidities. These factors should be taken into account when considering interventions that increase the risk for delirium (e.g., procedures, new medications). Examples of modifiable factors are listed in Table 15.5.[71,72] Specific patient populations

TABLE 15.5 Modifiable Risk Factors for Delirium and Possible Interventions

Risk Factor	Intervention
Sensory impairment	Use eyeglasses, communication devices, and hearing aids
Sleep deprivation	At night: darken room, limit stimuli, consider eye mask and ear plugs During the day: promote wakefulness, encourage mobility and activities Limit use of sedatives Avoid benzodiazepines for the management of insomnia
Substances (medications and other)	Perform medication reconciliation and review Judicious de-prescribing as indicated Avoid polypharmacy and drug-drug interactions Assess for substance intoxication or withdrawal
Acute medical illness	Perform history, physical examination, and targeted studies to discern and manage possible sources of infection, vascular insults, intracranial pathology, pain, metabolic derangements
Pain	Judicious use of opioids and opioid-sparing adjuncts Consider interventional pain modalities as indicated (e.g., nerve and plexus blocks) to limit systemic exposure to analgesics
Immobility	If possible, engage physical/occupational therapy Limit use of restraints (including "pseudorestraints" if not indicated, like urinary catheters and telemetry)
Disorders of nutrition and elimination	Promote adequate hydration and nutrition when consistent with the goals of care; if terminal anorexia, ensure adequate mouth care Monitor for and manage constipation or diarrhea Monitor for and manage urinary retention

also have unique risk factors that predispose them to delirium (e.g., organ ischemia time in transplantation, atrial fibrillation after cardiac surgery).[73,74]

Medications warrant special consideration. Individual medications can be deliriogenic and so can the interactions between medications resulting from polypharmacy. Medications with anticholinergic effects can be particularly problematic.[75] Even antipsychotics with anticholinergic properties, like olanzapine, can precipitate or perpetuate delirium (e.g., urinary retention).[76] Benzodiazepines and opioids, commonly used in palliative care settings, can precipitate and perpetuate delirium.[77] Therefore, they need to be titrated carefully to the lowest effective dose on a time-limited basis with close monitoring. A patient's medication list should be reviewed at each visit for unnecessary medications, possible drug-drug interactions, and opportunities for dose tapers to limit the risk of adverse effects.

Delirium can impact prognosis in regard to both function and mortality. In patients with dementia, hypoactive delirium may be associated with greater mortality, whereas in other populations, the severity of the delirium itself (regardless of activity level) correlates with greater mortality.[78] As previously noted, delirium is prevalent in patients approaching the end of life and can be a nonspecific harbinger for poor prognosis and impending death.[58,60,79–83] It is also associated with an increased risk for readmission to the hospital and institutionalization (i.e., discharge to another facility that is not home).[64,84] Diagnosing terminal delirium is also important for critical discussions about end of life and for appropriate management of agitation, which may differ from other delirium subtypes. Clinicians can also support families in acknowledging that delirium is often part of the dying process, helping to guide them in what to expect.[59,85]

Beyond identifying and managing those factors contributing to delirium, the symptoms of delirium itself warrant management due to the extreme distress they can cause the patient, their loved ones, and the care team. The use of antipsychotics is common in the management of hyperactive delirium but now has become more controversial, with conflicting evidence about whether they impact the duration or outcome of delirium.[86–88] Some trials may be confounded by failing to separate out those patients with symptoms that would be expected to respond to D_2 antagonism (e.g., active psychosis), as there is evidence for their use in settings where psychosis is a prominent component of delirium.[89,90] For agitated patients, a more sedating D_2 antagonist like chlorpromazine, olanzapine, or quetiapine may be indicated, taking into consideration the available routes of administration (quetiapine has no parenteral formulation) and side effects (chlorpromazine and quetiapine can cause orthostatic hypotension; several antipsychotics may have anticholinergic effects). If disturbing psychosis without agitation is the primary symptom to be addressed, haloperidol or aripiprazole can be considered as they are less sedating. It is important to obtain a baseline electrocardiogram (ECG) to screen for prolonged QTc as D_2 antagonists can variably prolong QT further and increase the risk for torsades de pointes. After initiating therapy, repeat the ECG, particularly if the patient receives intravenous haloperidol or is regularly receiving medications known to prolong the QT. Case reports and small studies exist that may support the use of methylphenidate in hypoactive delirium, but this has yet to be validated in a randomized controlled trial, so they cannot be recommended at this time.[91–93] Although benzodiazepines are traditionally avoided in managing delirium as they can be disinhibiting and may worsen mental status, they are useful in two clinical situations. γ-aminobutyric acid withdrawal (e.g., from alcohol, benzodiazepines) requires benzodiazepines, and prompt recognition is required given this unique treatment strategy. The symptoms of terminal hyperactive delirium can also be treated with benzodiazepines (typically higher doses than usually given in adults—up to 3 mg of lorazepam), with the goal of sedation, and may be used in combination with a D_2 antagonist like haloperidol in any setting.[94]

Insomnia

Insomnia is present in up to 70% of patients being seen in the palliative care setting, with negative impacts on pain, depression, anxiety, and quality of life for both patients and caregivers.[95] Insomnia may be defined as difficulty falling asleep, staying asleep, waking up before desired, or waking from sleep feeling unrestored despite having had an opportunity for sleep.

Causes of insomnia are wide ranging. Reversal of potential causes is preferable to initiating a sedative medication that may be accompanied by side effects (Table 15.6). Behavioral interventions should be a first-line treatment for insomnia. Medications for insomnia should be reserved for refractory cases (Table 15.7). Assessment for their continued need and the presence of side effects should be routine (Box 15.3).

The Challenging Patient

The concept of "the challenging (or difficult) patient" is generally applied to those patients with challenging personality traits or frank personality disorders. This concept is also applicable to parents and/or caregivers of children, elder parents, or other guardians in the family unit when these persons are critical facilitators of treatment and decision-making. This concept and these dynamics in caregivers applies not only to parents, but also to children of elderly parents and other guardians of family members. This is also an important part of the role of psychiatry in addressing the family units and as a liaison to palliative care and

TABLE 15.6 Selected Causes of Insomnia[96]

Environment	Device alarms, excessive lighting, noisy roommates, televisions, computer screens, frequent vital sign checks overnight, noisy air mattresses, transferring rooms, laboratory and imaging studies taken at night.
Pain	Frequently heightened at night when usual distractions are absent; exacerbated by weakness and being unable to reposition oneself
Respiratory symptoms	Shortness of breath, cough, hiccups, need for suctioning, positioning of oxygen cannulas, trach collars, and endotracheal tubes
Depression	Negative ruminations, restlessness, diurnal variation of symptoms leading to a surge in activity and improved mood in the evening, thus delaying sleep and over time shifting the sleep phase later
Anxiety	Anxious ruminations, frequent fear of not waking up in the setting of progressive and/or life-threatening illness
Medication side effects	Examples: frequent need for urination from diuretics, need for fluids with various treatments such as chemotherapy, stimulation from corticosteroids, impaired sleep architecture from opioids, and receiving enteral tube feeds overnight

TABLE 15.7 Selected Medications for the Treatment of Insomnia[96]

Melatonin	1. Over the counter, variable purity 2. Double-blind, placebo-controlled studies have not found consistent benefit 3. Generally thought of as safe < 3 mg/day 4. Dosing ranges from 0.3 to 5 mg
Ramelteon	1. A selective melatonin receptor antagonist 2. Significant drug-drug interactions through cytochrome P450 1A2, such as with ciprofloxacin 3. No studies in the palliative care population, but has been studied in the intensive care unit patient population 4. Initial dose of 8 mg
Mirtazapine	1. Antagonizes presynaptic alpha-2 adrenergic receptors and postsynaptic serotonin 5-HT$_2$ and serotonin 5-HT$_3$ receptors 2. Has sedative properties for many patients at 7.5–15 mg, may lose this effect at doses beyond 30 mg 3. May be an option for patients with depression, anxiety, and insomnia
Trazodone	1. Controversial in its use as a hypnotic due to inconsistent findings and risk of adverse effects, but is a commonly used medication for insomnia 2. Dosing for insomnia typically ranges from 25 to 300 mg at bedtime
Benzodiazepines	1. Perhaps the most commonly used medications for sleep despite their significant risks 2. May further predispose to delirium 3. Rapid development of tolerance to the sedating quality of benzodiazepines 4. Patients will frequently develop physical dependence on benzodiazepines 5. Increased risk of falls 6. Sedative synergism with opioids, increasing the risk for respiratory depression
Nonbenzodiazepine hypnotics	1. Examples: zolpidem, zaleplon, zopiclone, eszopiclone 2. While studies have shown a lower risk of developing tolerance than with benzodiazepines, studies of hospitalized elderly show increased risk of falls with zolpidem[97] 3. At least one study showed this class of medication was safer in patients with chronic obstructive pulmonary disease compared to benzodiazepines[98,]
Doxepin[100]	1. At low doses works primarily at the histamine H$_1$ receptor, which is thought to be how it impacts sleep. 2. While not studied in the palliative care population yet, it has been found to be safe and effective in elderly patients when used at doses of 3–6 mg. 3. Anticholinergic side effects are possible, especially at higher doses, and should be carefully monitored.

BOX 15.3. Selected Behavioral/"Sleep Hygiene" Techniques for Insomnia[96]

1. No caffeine or stimulating medications after lunch

2. No alcohol near bedtime

3. No smoking near bedtime

4. Use the bed for sleep only; get up out of bed if not sleeping or actively falling asleep

5. Regular exercise and activity, but not immediately adjacent to bedtime

6. No screens in bed (i.e., smartphones, tablets, computers)

7. Go to bed and get up at the same time every day

8. When trying to repair a delayed sleep phase, first focus on a consistent wake-up time

hospice teams. Examples of patients in this section can be read as synonymous with care-giver/guardians. Patients and caregivers with substance use disorders (see Chapter 19) are also frequently included in this category.

The *DSM5* lists criteria for the following personality disorders: paranoid, schizoid, schizotypal, antisocial (adults only), conduct disorder (children only), borderline, histrionic, narcissistic, avoidant, dependent, and obsessive-compulsive. All of these disorders can impede a patient's access to care.[101] The characteristics of a personality disorder can occur in patients and caregivers even without a baseline personality disorder due to psychological regression in times of extreme stress, such as during a progressive and/or life-threatening illness. In that case the signs observed are described as "traits." In order for a "disorder" to be diagnosed, the symptoms must be pervasive, cause impairment, and have been persistent during adolescence or early adulthood. Adolescents with convincing and persistent features of personality disorders can and should be diagnosed with traits or full disorders.

Borderline personality disorder (BPD), however, may be the most commonly identified and challenging personality disorder among medical patients and caregivers, in part because of the immense amount of energy these patients often demand from the teams caring for them. The key features of BPD include the unstable nature of interpersonal relationships (including with medical providers), their fluctuating sense of self-worth, affective lability, and significant impulsivity. Perceived abandonment and uncertainty often drive the expression of these maladaptive traits. The traits of BPD are listed in Table 15.8.

It is important for medical providers to identify the patient with BPD and BPD traits early in care and early in life in order to institute a treatment plan that will both support the patient and protect the providers from developing animosity toward the patient, which could negatively impact the care provided.[102,104] Appropriate interventions can be provided even without a definitive diagnosis, which may be impossible to determine in the crisis setting of medical illness[101–106] (Table 15.8).

Histrionic, narcissistic, and antisocial personality, as well as conduct disorders, and traits may also present with significant maladaptive behaviors in the medical setting:

1. Histrionic personality disorder may present as overly dramatic, attention seeking, and excessively emotional.
2. Antisocial personality/conduct disorders frequently show hallmark symptoms of a blatant disregard for the rights of others through manipulation, excessive demands, impulsive anger, cruelty, and frank lying. Conduct disorder will frequently have specific examples of cruelty to animals or younger children.
3. Persons with narcissistic personality disorder, while presenting with a sense of grandiosity, have an intensely fragile ego. They need frequent admiration and have an inability to tolerate criticism or therapeutic recommendations. They may demand to see the "chief medical officer" or "director" or mention names of all of the most famous experts that they have seen, often using first names to show real or feigned familiarity.[107]

Implementing a management plan for patients demonstrating these traits or disorders early is important to ensure compassionate and effective care for these frequently challenging

TABLE 15.8 Traits of Borderline Personality Disorder

Symptom/Trait	Interventions
"Splitting": Tendency to characterize people or situations as all "good" or all "bad," arising from an inability to recognize shades of gray. This can lead to patients demonizing some providers, which can lead to an ever-shrinking number of people they allow to care for them.	1. Evaluate patients as a team to highlight the unified nature of the care team directly to the patient. 2. Recognize that patients may explicitly or subtly develop "favorites" among the staff, often very quickly (example: "You are the best physician assistant"), as well as people they demonize. Proactively resist feeding into this disordered assessment of their care team. 3. Limit or disallow transfers of care between clinicians without clinical justification.
Perceived abandonment: Anger outbursts or inappropriate requests for assistance/neediness may be part of a desperate attempt to avoid abandonment or as a result of feeling abandoned.	1. Set specific times to round on the patient every day during a hospitalization; in the outpatient setting, set specific recurring appointments; and if needed, set specific times for a phone check-in between in-person appointments. This routine may allow the patient to have a sense of reliable contact and therefore reduce inappropriate attempts to get attention. While this may seem like burden for the providers, in general this type of planned contact reduces the amount of time needed to care for a patient with BPD and increases patient satisfaction.
Recurrent suicidal or self-injurious behaviors.	1. These types of behaviors necessitate referral to and collaboration with an expert mental health professional. It will be important to evaluate each act to determine level of risk and potential need for inpatient psychiatric hospitalization. In general, patients with BPD are at chronic elevated risk for self-harm and suicide due to their frequent impulsivity and periods of intense dysphoria and hopelessness. However, repetitive psychiatric hospitalization is often not beneficial. Evaluation by an expert is indicated in these instances.
Periodic intense expressions of emotion, such as anger, irritability, sadness, and anxiety, that may last minutes to hours, rarely a day, and often has an irrational trigger.	1. Recognize that these episodes are usually short-lived. Do not interpret the anger as a sustained and final evaluation of a person or situation. For example, if they are angry with a particular provider at one point, they are likely to recover from this feeling if that clinician remains neutral over time and importantly does not abandon them as a result of the rude behavior. 2. Consider setting a limit around these episodes, such as calmly letting the patient know that when or if they are acting in an aggressive fashion, staff will need to leave their room and will be back once the patient is able to interact appropriately. Proactively set this expectation during a time of calm and not during a dysregulated or agitated episode. 3. Develop a plan with the patient regarding how to manage periods of anxiety with self-soothing techniques. Complex coloring books; guided meditation (either by a provider or through a smartphone application); practicing grounding techniques (e.g., holding ice in one's hand, peeling/sniffing a frozen orange); puzzles; and other forms of distraction are often easily available and useful when preplanning for such an episode is possible.

patients and their families (Table 15.8). Remembering that these patients are suffering can be helpful. Setting clear limits that are consistent across providers is important, being careful not to miss legitimate concerns the patient may have. Tending to our own needs as providers is essential: Seeking support and supervision, as well as preventing "splitting" from colleagues can improve the quality of care and foster personal resilience.[108]

Severe and Persistent Mental Illness

Although most patients do recover from mental disorders and respond to evidence-based psychotherapeutic and psychopharmacological treatment strategies, some patients remain unresponsive and develop *severe and persistent mental illness* (SPMI) which is defined by *treatment-refractoriness*.[109] Studies have shown that about one-fifth of all patients with major depressive disorder fail to respond to several trials of adequate treatment and may die from suicide despite long-term treatment.[110] Of patients diagnosed with schizophrenia, 10%–30% show little or no response to antipsychotic treatment, including last-resort drugs such as clozapine.[111,112]

In principle, any mental disorder can develop into SPMI. Due to this inherent treatment refractoriness, patients can become demoralized due to induced false hope from many medication and other therapeutic trials, some of which may not be evidence based.[113]

Mental disorders are among the most substantial causes of death worldwide, with 14.3% of deaths attributable to mental disorders.[114] Patients with SPMI have a 10- to 25-year life expectancy reduction and significant higher *mortality rates* due to increased substance use, accidents, suicide, or chronic physical sequelae of SPMI (e.g., cardiovascular, respiratory, and infectious diseases; diabetes; and hypertension) compared to the general population.[115,116] For example, the mortality rate among patients with schizophrenia is about 2.5 times higher and among patients with depression about 1.6 times higher than in the general population.[117,118] Furthermore, patients with SPMI have a complex combination of physical, psychological, social, existential, and spiritual needs requiring highly skilled multiprofessional mental health care.[114,119] The SPMI with the highest mortality rate is anorexia nervosa, from which 5%–6% of affected patients die.[120]

Two challenging situations arise with SPMI in palliative care: (1) when patients with SPMI develop progressive and/or life-threatening *medical* illness; and (2) when the SPMI itself becomes a chronic, progressive, and life-threatening illness.

(1) When patients with SPMI develop progressive and/or life-threatening *medical* illness:

The majority of excess mortality in SPMI patients is due to chronic diseases such as cancer, heart disease, or chronic obstructive pulmonary disease, similar to the general population mortality and decreased longevity in patients with SPMI and progressive and/or life-threatening *medical* illness compared with the general population is due to higher rates of substance use, decreased engagement with preventive healthcare, and poorer access to medical care. Patients with schizophrenia, for example, have a similar incidence of most cancers as the general population, but these patients have up to a two-fold risk of dying of their disease due to underdetection and undertreatment."[121] Somatic symptoms may be overlooked, hard to assess, or misclassified. In these situations, partnerships among psychiatrists/psychotherapists and other medical specialists are necessary.[122]

Unfortunately, patients with SPMI do not always receive the same high-quality palliative care as patients without SPMI. For example, patients with schizophrenia are less likely to receive adequate opioid analgesia at the end of life.[123] To prevent such undertreatment, it is fundamental for clinicians to recognize schizophrenia and other types of SPMI.

Also, there are no guidelines to help clinicians determine the level of care necessary for patients with SPMI who are receiving hospice services. In general, inpatient hospice units (or hospices in general) will be ill-equipped to manage patients with SPMI, made even harder by issues of capacity and guardianship when applicable, while an inpatient psychiatric unit will be ill-equipped to manage progressive and/or life-threatening *medical* illness management needs (e.g., unable to provide intravenous/subcutaneous analgesia, unable to provide suctioning or supplementary oxygen). A patient's prognosis should be considered when discerning an appropriate disposition. For example, if a patient is suffering from terminal delirium, an inpatient hospice setting may be better equipped to manage the symptoms and sequelae, as well as handling the dying process.

Patients with SPMI and progressive and/or life-threatening *medical* illness will likely require higher doses of medications, with which many palliative care clinicians are familiar. For example, olanzapine is often used at a low dose for the management of nausea or hiccups and slightly higher doses for the management of agitated delirium, but patients with schizophrenia may be need even higher doses.[124] De-prescribing of any psychotropic medication in patients with SPMI should be considered in collaboration with a mental health clinician. Conversely, most psychotropic medications are protein bound, and therefore as a patient's nutritional status worsens, the patients may require less medication to manage their underlying disorder and to avoid side effects.

Some medications used for SPMI warrant special consideration. For example, lithium is a mood stabilizer used in the treatment of bipolar disorder. It may affect kidney function, and kidney injury may lead to lithium toxicity and even death. Lithium levels should continue to be monitored as indicated to avoid lithium toxicity, which can exacerbate symptoms like nausea and confusion; lithium should only be discontinued either in collaboration with a mental health clinician or as the patient is actively dying.

(2) When the SPMI itself becomes a chronic, progressive, and life-threatening illness:

Depending on the stage of illness, a more palliative approach rather than remission or cure may be appropriate. With a shift in approach to the SPMI, therapeutic relationships may improve, and patients may come to see palliative care–based approaches as a better fit to their situation.[125] Often, this approach can enhance the quality of life and diminish the risk of suicide."[122]

Based on the World Health Organization's definition of palliative care, a palliative psychiatry–based approach has been described for discussing the feasibility of palliative care approaches as an alternative clinical approach in psychiatry.[125,126] The phrase *palliative psychiatry* applies only to complicated cases of SPMI with higher than average mortality rates. According to such a definition, many established interventions in psychiatry aiming to promote quality of life rather than remission might be considered palliative, such as psychiatric long-term residential care for patients with clozapine-resistant schizophrenia or a decision to forgo involuntary refeeding severe, chronic, and refractory anorexia nervosa.[112,127]

Arguments have been raised against a palliative care approach in psychiatry based on the lack of evidence or expert consensus with regard to the definition of end-stage psychiatric disorders.[128,129] However, to qualify a mental disorder as "end stage" is not necessary in order to apply a palliative approach; the presence of treatment-refractory SPMI is sufficient for it to be considered, much like the use of palliative care for patients with chronic, progressive, and life-threatening illness who are not close to end stage. Therefore, a palliative medicine approach to psychiatric conditions should be considered in treatment planning and something to discuss with both patient and caregivers. This may lead to an enhanced team approach that also incorporates chaplains, pharmacists, and other professionals in the care of the patient.

References

1. World Health Organization. *WHO Definition of Palliative Care.* 2013. Retrieved from http://www.who.int/cancer/palliative/definition/en

2. Irwin SA, Ferris FD. The opportunity for psychiatry in palliative Care. *Canadian Journal of Psychiatry.* 2008;*53*(11):713–724.

3. Meier DE, Beresford L. Growing the interface between palliative medicine and psychiatry. *Journal of Palliative Medicine.* 2010;*13*(7):803–806.

4. JA B, SD B. Integrating psychiatry and palliative medicine: the challenges and opportunities. In: Chochinov HM, Breitbart W, eds. *Handbook of Psychiatry in Palliative Medicine.* 2nd ed. Oxford: Oxford University Press; 2009: ch. 2.

5. Fairman N, Irwin SA. Palliative care psychiatry: update on an emerging dimension of psychiatric practice. *Current Psychiatry Reports.* 2013;*15*(7):374.

6. Fairman N, Hirst JM, Irwin SA. *Clinical Manual of Palliative Care Psychiatry.* American Psychiatric Association.

7. Friedman D, Linnemann RW, Altstein LL, et al. Effects of a primary palliative care intervention on quality of life and mental health in cystic fibrosis. *Pediatric Pulmonology.* 2019;*54*(7):984–992.

8. Mitchell AJ, Chan M, Bhatti H, et al. Prevalence of depression, anxiety, and adjustment disorder in oncological, haematological, and palliative-care settings: a meta-analysis of 94 interview-based studies. *Lancet Oncology.* 2011;*12*:160–174.

9. Ford JA. The complexity of assessment and treatment for anxiety in patients with a terminal illness. *Journal of Hospice and Palliative Nursing.* 2016;*18*:131–138.

10. Horne-Thompson A, Grocke D. The effect of music therapy on anxiety in patients who are terminally ill. *Journal of Palliative Medicine.* 2008;*11*(7):582–590.

11. Wilson KG, Chochinov HM, Graham Skirko M, et al. Depression and anxiety disorders in palliative cancer care. *Journal of Pain and Symptom Management.* 2007;*33*(2):118–129.

12. Smith EM, Gomm SA, Dickens CM. Assessing the independent contribution to quality of life from anxiety and depression in patients with advanced cancer. *Palliative Medicine.* 2003;*17*(6):509–513.

13. Spencer R, Nilsson M, Wright A, Pirl W, Prigerson H. Anxiety disorders in advanced cancer patients: correlates and predictors of end-of-life outcomes. *Cancer.* 2010.

14. Roth AJ, Massie MJ. Anxiety and its management in advanced cancer. *Current Opinion in Supportive and Palliative Care.* 2007.

15. Kolva E, Rosenfeld B, Pessin H, Breitbart W, Brescia R. Anxiety in terminally ill cancer patients. *Journal of Pain and Symptom Management.* 2011.

16. Delgado-Guay M, Parsons HA, Li Z, Palmer JL, Bruera E. Symptom distress in advanced cancer patients with anxiety and depression in the palliative care setting. *Supportive Care in Cancer.* 2009.

17. Traeger E, Greer JA, Fernandez-Robles C, Temel JS, Pirl WF. Evidence-based treatment of anxiety in patients with cancer. *Journal of Clinical Oncology.* 2012;*30*(11):1197–1205.
18. Wilson KG, Chochinov HM, Skirko MG, et al. Depression and anxiety disorders in palliative cancer care. *Journal of Pain and Symptom Management.* 2007;*33*(2):118–129.
19. American Psychiatric Association. *Diagnostic and Statistical Manual of Mental Disorders.* 5th ed. Arlington, VA: American Psychiatric Association; 2013.
20. Salt S, Mulvaney CA, Preston NJ. Drug therapy for symptoms associated with anxiety in adult palliative care patients. *Cochrane Database of Systematic Reviews.* 2017;*5*(5):CD004596.
21. Moorey S, Cort E, Kapari M, et al. A cluster randomized controlled trial of cognitive behaviour therapy for common mental disorders in patients with advanced cancer. *Psychological Medicine.* 2009;*39*(5):713–723.
22. Grossman CH, Brooker J, Michael N, Kissane D. Death anxiety interventions in patients with advanced cancer: a systematic review. *Palliative Medicine.* 2018;*32*(1):172–184.
23. Rayner L, Price A, Evans A, Valsraj K, Hotopf M, Higginson IJ. Antidepressants for the treatment of depression in palliative care: systematic review and meta-analysis. *Palliative Medicine.* 2011;*25*:36–51.
24. Briscoe J, Kamal AH, Casarett DJ. Top ten tips palliative care clinicians should know about medical cannabis. *Journal of Palliative Medicine.* 2019;*22*(3):319–325.
25. Cyr C, Arboleda MF, Aggarwal SK, et al. Cannabis in palliative care: current challenges and practical recommendations. *Annals of Palliative Medicine.* 2018;*7*(4):463–477.
26. Grob CS, Danforth AL, Chopra GS, et al. Pilot study of psilocybin treatment for anxiety in patients with advanced-stage cancer. *Archives of General Psychiatry.* 2011.
27. Ross S, Bossis A, Guss J, et al. Rapid and sustained symptom reduction following psilocybin treatment for anxiety and depression in patients with life-threatening cancer: a randomized controlled trial. *Journal of Psychopharmacology.* 2016.
28. Irwin SA, Iglewicz A. Oral ketamine for the rapid treatment of depression and anxiety in patients receiving hospice care. *Journal of Palliative Medicine.* 2010;*13*(7):903–908.
29. Irwin SA, Iglewicz A, Nelesen RA, et al. Daily oral ketamine for the treatment of depression and anxiety in patients receiving hospice care: a 28-day open-label proof-of-concept trial. *Journal of Palliative Medicine.* 2013;*16*(8):958–965.
30. Irwin S, Hirst J, Fairman N, Prommer E. Ketamine for the management of depression in palliative care: an update on the science. *Journal of Pain and Symptom Management.* 2013;*45*(2):371.
31. Daud ML. Drug management of terminal symptoms in advanced cancer patients. *Current Opinion in Supportive and Palliative Care.* 2007.
32. WHO: Depression and Other Common Mental Disorders. Global Health Estimates. 3 January 2017.
33. Rayner L, Price A, Hotopf M, Higginson IJ. The development of evidence-based European guidelines on the management of depression in palliative cancer care. *European Journal of Cancer.* 2011;*47*:702–712.
34. Mitchell AJ. Are one or two simple questions sufficient to detect depression in cancer and palliative care? A Bayesian meta-analysis. *British Journal of Cancer.* 2008;*98*(12):1934–1943.
35. Mitchell AJ, Meader N, Symonds P. Diagnostic validity of the Hospital Anxiety and Depression Scale (HADS) in cancer and palliative settings: a meta-analysis. *Journal of Affective Disorders.* 2010;*126*(3):335–348.
36. Wasteson E, Brenne E, Higginson IJ, et al. Depression assessment and classification in palliative cancer patients: a systematic literature review. *Palliative Medicine.* 2009;*23*(8):739–753.
37. Marks S, Heinrich T. Assessing and treating depression in palliative care patients. *Current Psychiatry.* 2013.
38. First MB. *DSM-5˚ Handbook of Differential Diagnosis.* 2014. American Psychiatric Association.
39. Kissane DW. Demoralisation: its impact on informed consent and medical care. *Medical Journal of Australia.* 2001;*175*(10):537–539.
40. Kissane DW, Clarke DM, Street AF. Demoralization syndrome—a relevant psychiatric diagnosis for palliative care. *Journal of Palliative Care.* 2001;*17*(1):12–21.
41. Block SD, for the American College of Physicians–American Society of Internal Medicine End-of-Life Care Consensus Panel. Assessing and managing depression in the terminally ill patient. *FOCUS.* 2005;*3*:310–319.

42. Noorani NH, Montagnini M. Recognizing depression in palliative care patients. *Journal of Palliative Medicine*. 2007;*10*(2):458–464.

43. Robinson S, Kissane DW, Brooker J, Burney S. A systematic review of the demoralization syndrome in individuals with progressive disease and cancer: a decade of research. *Journal of Pain and Symptom Management*. 2015;*49*:595–610.

44. Noorani NH, Montagnini M. Recognizing depression in palliative care patients. *Journal of Palliative Medicine*. 2007;*10*:458–464.

45. Robson A, Scrutton F, Wilkinson L, MacLeod F. The risk of suicide in cancer patients: a review of the literature. *Psychooncology*. 2010;*19*:1250–1258.

46. Kelly B, Burnett P, Pelusi D, Badger S, Varghese F, Robertson M. Factors associated with the wish to hasten death: a study of patients with terminal illness. *Psychological Medicine*. 2003;*33*(1):75–81.

47. Crawford MJ, Thana L, Methuen C, et al. Impact of screening for risk of suicide: randomised controlled trial. *British Journal of Psychiatry*. 2011;*198*:379–384.

48. Mann JJ, Apter A, Bertolote J, et al. Suicide prevention strategies. *JAMA*. 2005;*294*:2064.

49. Horowitz LM, Snyder D, Ludi E, et al. Ask suicide-screening questions to everyone in medical settings: the asq'em quality improvement project. *Psychosomatics*. 2013.

50. Fulton JJ, Newins AR, Porter LS, Ramos K. Psychotherapy targeting depression and anxiety for use in palliative care: a meta-analysis. *Journal of Palliative Medicine*. 2018;*21*:1024–1037.

51. Chochinov HM, Hack T, Hassard T, Kristjianson LJ, McClement S, Harlos M. Dignity and psychotherapeutic considerations in end-of-life care. *Journal of Palliative Care*. 2004;*20*(3):134–142.

52. Breitbart W, Gibson C, Poppito SR, Berg A. Psychotherapeutic interventions at the end of life: a focus on meaning and spirituality. *Canadian Journal of Psychiatry*. 2004;*49*(6):366–372.

53. Kissane D, Levin T. *Psychothe for Depression in Cancer and Palliative Care*. Wiley: 2010;177–206.

54. Rayner L, Price A, Evans A, Valsraj K, Higginson IJ, Hotopf M. Antidepressants for depression in physically ill people. *Cochrane Database of Systematic Reviews*. 2010.

55. Trivedi MH, Rush AJ, Wisniewski SR, et al. Evaluation of outcomes with citalopram for depression using measurement-based care in STAR*D: implications for clinical practice. *American Journal of Psychiatry*. 2006;*163*(1):28–40.

56. Riordan P, Briscoe J, Kamal AH, Jones CA, Webb JA. Top ten tips palliative care clinicians should know about mental health and serious illness. *Journal of Palliative Medicine*. 2018;*21*:1171–1176.

57. Goldman N, Frankenthaler M, Klepacz L. The efficacy of ketamine in the palliative care setting: a comprehensive review of the literature. *Journal of Palliative Medicine*. 2019;*22*(9):1154–1161.

58. Hosie A, Davidson PM, Agar M, Sanderson CR, Phillips J. Delirium prevalence, incidence, and implications for screening in specialist palliative care inpatient settings: a systematic review. *Palliative Medicine*. 2013;*27*(6):486–498.

59. Moyer DD. Review article: terminal delirium in geriatric patients with cancer at end of life. *American Journal of Hospice and Palliative Care*. 2011;*28*(1):44–51.

60. de la Cruz M, Ransing V, Yennu S, et al. The frequency, characteristics, and outcomes among cancer patients with delirium admitted to an acute palliative care unit. *Oncologist*. 2015;*20*(12):1425–1431.

61. Senel G, Uysal N, Oguz G, et al. Delirium frequency and risk factors among patients with cancer in palliative care unit. *American Journal of Hospice and Palliative Care*. 2017;*34*(3):282–286.

62. Watt CL, Momoli F, Ansari MT, et al. The incidence and prevalence of delirium across palliative care settings: a systematic review. *Palliative Medicine*. 2019 Sep;*33*(8):865–877.

63. Farrell KR. Misdiagnosing delirium as depression in medically ill elderly patients. *Archives of Internal Medicine*. 1995;*155*(22):2459–2464.

64. Witlox J, Eurelings LSM, de Jonghe JFM, Kalisvaart KJ, Eikelenboom P, van Gool WA. Delirium in elderly patients and the risk of postdischarge mortality, institutionalization, and dementia. *JAMA*. 2010;*304*(4):443–451.

65. Casarett DJ, Inouye SK. Diagnosis and management of delirium near the end of life. *Annals of Internal Medicine*. 2001;*135*(1):32–40.

66. Inouye SK, van Dyck CH, Alessi CA, Balkin S, Siegal AP, Horwitz RI. Clarifying confusion: the confusion assessment method. A new method for detection of delirium. *Annals of Internal Medicine*. 1990;*113*(12):941–948.

67. Ely EW, Margolin R, Francis J, et al. Evaluation of delirium in critically ill patients: validation of the Confusion Assessment Method for the Intensive Care Unit (CAM-ICU). *Critical Care Medicine.* 2001;*29*(7):1370–1379.

68. Rao S, Ferris FD, Irwin SA. Ease of screening for depression and delirium in patients enrolled in inpatient hospice care. *Journal of Palliative Medicine.* 2011;*14*(3):275–279.

69. Smith HA, Boyd J, Fuchs DC, et al. Diagnosing delirium in critically ill children: validity and reliability of the Pediatric Confusion Assessment Method for the Intensive Care Unit. *Critical Care Medicine.* 2011;*39*(1):150–157.

70. Smith HA, Gangopadhyay M, Goben CM, et al. The Preschool Confusion Assessment Method for the ICU: valid and reliable delirium monitoring for critically ill infants and children. *Critical Care Medicine.* 2016;*44*(3):592–600.

71. Fong TG, Tulebaev SR, Inouye SK. Delirium in elderly adults: diagnosis, prevention and treatment. *Nature Reviews Neurology.* 2009;*5*(4):210–220.

72. Elie M, Cole MG, Primeau FJ, Bellavance F. Delirium risk factors in elderly hospitalized patients. *Journal of General Internal Medicine.* 1998;*13*:204–212.

73. Anderson BJ, Chesley CF, Theodore M, et al. Incidence, risk factors, and clinical implications of post-operative delirium in lung transplant recipients. *Journal of Heart and Lung Transplantation.* 2018;*37*(6):755–762.

74. Koster S, Hensens AG, Schuurmans MJ, van der Palen J. Risk factors of delirium after cardiac surgery: a systematic review. *European Journal of Cardiovascular Nursing.* 2011;*10*(4):197–204.

75. Han L, McCusker J, Cole M, Abrahamowicz M, Primeau F, Elie M. Use of medications with anticholinergic effect predicts clinical severity of delirium symptoms in older medical inpatients. *Archives of Internal Medicine.* 2001;*161*(8):1099–1105.

76. Lim CJ, Trevino C, Tampi RR. Can olanzapine cause delirium in the elderly? *Annals of Pharmacotherapy.* 2006;*40*:135–138.

77. Marcantonio ER. Delirium in hospitalized older adults. *New England Journal of Medicine.* 2017;*377*(15):1456–1466.

78. Yang FM, Marcantonio ER, Inouye SK, et al. Phenomenological subtypes of delirium in older persons: patterns, prevalence, and prognosis. *Psychosomatics.* 2009;*50*(3):248–254.

79. Beglinger LJ, Duff K, Van Der Heiden S, Parrott K, Langbehn D, Gingrich R. Incidence of delirium and associated mortality in hematopoietic stem cell transplantation patients. *Biology of Blood and Marrow Transplantation.* 2006;*12*(9):928–935.

80. Ely EW, Stephens RK, Jackson JC, et al. Current opinions regarding the importance, diagnosis, and management of delirium in the intensive care unit: a survey of 912 healthcare professionals. *Critical Care Medicine.* 2004;*32*(1):106–112.

81. Israni J, Lesser A, Kent T, Ko K. Delirium as a predictor of mortality in US Medicare beneficiaries discharged from the emergency department: a national claims-level analysis up to 12 months. *BMJ Open.* 2018;*8*(5):e021258.

82. Yasui-Furukori N, Tarakita N, Uematsu W, et al. Delirium in hemodialysis predicts mortality: a single-center, long-term observational study. *Neuropsychiatric Disease and Treatment.* 2017;*13*:3011–3016.

83. Ely EW, Shintani A, Truman B, et al. Delirium as a predictor of mortality in mechanically ventilated patients in the intensive care unit. *JAMA.* 2004;*291*(14):1753–1762.

84. Uthamalingam S, Gurm GS, Daley M, Flynn J, Capodilupo R. Usefulness of acute delirium as a predictor of adverse outcomes in patients >65 years of age with acute decompensated heart failure. *American Journal of Cardiology.* 2011;*108*(3):402–408.

85. Pandharipande PP, Ely EW. Humanizing the treatment of hyperactive delirium in the last days of life. *JAMA.* 2017;*318*(11):1014–1015.

86. Agar MR, Lawlor PG, Quinn S, et al. Efficacy of oral risperidone, haloperidol, or placebo for symptoms of delirium among patients in palliative care: a randomized clinical trial. *JAMA Internal Medicine.* 2017;*177*(1):34–42.

87. Boettger S, Friedlander M, Breitbart W, Passik S. Aripiprazole and haloperidol in the treatment of delirium. *Australia and New Zealand Journal of Psychiatry.* 2011;*45*(6):477–482.

88. Daniels LM, Nelson SB, Frank RD, Park JG. Pharmacologic treatment of intensive care unit delirium and the impact on duration of delirium, length of intensive care unit stay, length of hospitalization, and 28-day mortality. *Mayo Clinic Proceedings*. 2018;*93*(12):1739–1748.

89. Hirst JM, Vaughan CL, Irwin SA. Delirium: use antipsychotics when appropriate and appropriately. *Journal of Palliative Medicine*. 2017;*20*(8):799.

90. Breitbart W, Alici Y. Evidence-based treatment of delirium in patients with cancer. *J Clinical Oncology*. 2012.

91. Keen JC, Brown D. Psychostimulants and delirium in patients receiving palliative care. *Palliative and Supportive Care*. 2004;*2*(2):199–202.

92. Morita T, Otani H, Tsunoda J, Inoue S, Chihara S. Successful palliation of hypoactive delirium due to multi-organ failure by oral methylphenidate. *Supportive Care in Cancer*. 2000;*8*(2):134–137.

93. Gagnon B, Low G, Schreier G. Methylphenidate hydrochloride improves cognitive function in patients with advanced cancer and hypoactive delirium: a prospective clinical study. *Journal of Psychiatry & Neuroscience*. 2005;*30*(2):100–107.

94. Hui D, Frisbee-Hume S, Wilson A, et al. Effect of lorazepam with haloperidol vs. haloperidol alone on agitated delirium in patients with advanced cancer receiving palliative care: a randomized clinical trial. *JAMA*. 2017;*318*(11):1047–1056.

95. Carter PA. Caregivers' descriptions of sleep changes and depressive symptoms. *Oncology Nursing Forum*. 2002;*29*(9):1277–1283.

96. Hirst JM, Inwin SA. Overview of insomnia in palliative care. Wolters Kluwer; 2018. https://www.uptodate.com/contents/overview-of-insomnia-in-palliative-care?search=insomnia%20in%20palliative%20care&source=search_result&selectedTitle=1~150&usage_type=default&display_rank=1. Accessed June 29, 2019.

97. Kolla BP, Lovely JK, Mansukhani MP, Morgenthaler TI. Zolpidem is independently associated with increased risk of inpatient falls. *Journal of Hospital Medicine*. 2013;*8*(1):1–6.

98. Sharafkhaneh A, Jayaraman G, Kaleekal T, Sharafkhaneh H, Hirshkowitz M. Sleep disorders and their management in patients with COPD. *Thereutic Advances in Respiratory Disease*. 2009;*3*(6):309–318.

99. Roth T. Hypnotic use for insomnia management in chronic obstructive pulmonary disease. *Sleep Medicine*. 2009;*10*(1):19–25.

100. Lankford A, Rogowski R, Essink B, Ludington B, Durrance HH, Roth T. (2012). Efficacy and safety of doxepin 6 mg in a four-week outpatient trial of elderly adults with chronic primary insomnia. *Sleep Medicine*. 2012;*13*(2):133–138.

101. McLafferty L, Childers JW. Borderline personality disorder in palliative care #252. *Journal of Palliative Medicine*. 2012;*15*(1):185–186.

102. Hay JL, Passik SD. The cancer patient with borderline personality disorder: suggestions for symptom-focused management in the medical setting. *Psychooncology*. 2000;*9*(2):91–100.

103. Oldham JM. Practice guideline for the treatment of patients with borderline personality disorder [Practide guideline]. American Psychiatric Association: Psychiatryonline; 2010. https://psychiatryonline.org/pb/assets/raw/sitewide/practice_guidelines/guidelines/bpd.pdf. Accessed June 6, 2019.

104. Meyer F, Block S. Personality disorders in the oncology setting. *Journal of Supportive Oncology*. 2011;*9*(2):44–51.

105. Chochinov HM, Kristjanson LJ, Hack TF, Hassard T, McClement S, Harlos M. Personality, neuroticism, and coping towards the end of life. *Journal of Pain and Symptom Management*. 2006;*32*(4):332–341.

106. Fitzgibbon ML, Barbuto J. Approach to the medically ill borderline patient: a case study. *Psychological Reports*. 1989;*65*(3 Pt 2):1091–1096.

107. Ward RK. Assessment and management of personality disorders. *American Family Physician*. 2004;*70*(8):1505–1512.

108. Wlodarczyk J, Lawn S, Powell K, et al. Exploring general practitioners' views and experiences of providing care to people with borderline personality disorder in primary care: a qualitative study in Australia. *International Journal of Environmental Research and Public Health*. 2018;*15*(12):2763.

109. Ruggeri M, Leese M, Thornicroft G, Bisoffi G, Tansella M. Definition and prevalence of severe and persistent mental illness. *British Journal of Psychiatry*. 2000;*177*:149–155.

110. Rush AJ, Trivedi MH, Wisniewski SR, et al. Acute and longer-term outcomes in depressed out-patients requiring one or several treatment steps: a STAR*D report. *American Journal of Psychiatry.* 2006;*163*(11):1905–1917.

111. Hasan A, Falkai P, Wobrock T, et al. World Federation of Societies of Biological Psychiatry (WFSBP) guidelines for biological treatment of schizophrenia, part 1: update 2012 on the acute treatment of schizophrenia and the management of treatment resistance. *World Journal of Biological Psychiatry.* 2012;*13*(5):318–378.

112. Miyamoto S, Jarskog LF, Fleischhacker WW. Schizophrenia: when clozapine fails. *Current Opinion in Psychiatry.* 2015;*28*(3):243–248.

113. Berk M, Singh A, Kapczinski F. When illness does not get better: do we need a palliative psychiatry? *Acta Neuropsychiatrica.* 2008;*20*(3):165–166.

114. Walker E, McGee R, Druss BG. Mortality in mental disorders and global disease burden implications: a systematic review and meta-analysis. *JAMA Psychiatry.* 2015;*72*(4):334–341.

115. Barber S, Thornicroft G. Reducing the mortality gap in people with severe mental disorders: the role of lifestyle psychosocial interventions. *Frontiers in Psychiatry.* 2018;*9*:463.

116. Walker ER, McGee RE, Druss BG. Mortality in mental disorders and global disease burden implications: a systematic review and meta-analysis. *JAMA Psychiatry.* 2015;*72*(4):334–341.

117. Saha S, Chant D, McGrath J. A systematic review of mortality in schizophrenia: is the differential mortality gap worsening over time? *Archives of General Psychiatry.* 2007;*64*(10):1123–1131.

118. Cuijpers P, Vogelzangs N, Twisk J, Kleiboer A, Li J, Penninx BW. Comprehensive meta-analysis of excess mortality in depression in the general community versus patients with specific illnesses. *American Journal of Psychiatry.* 2014;*171*(4):453–462.

119. Reininghaus U, Dutta R, Dazzan P, et al. Mortality in schizophrenia and other psychoses: a 10-year follow-up of the SOP first-episode cohort. *Schizophrenia Bulletin.* 2015;*41*(3):664–673.

120. Arcelus J, Mitchell AJ, Wales J, Nielsen S. Mortality rates in patients with anorexia nervosa and other eating disorders. A meta-analysis of 36 studies. *Archives of General Psychiatry.* 2011;*68*(7):724–731.

121. Shalev D, Brewster K, Arbuckle MR, Levenson JA. A staggered edge: end-of-life care in patients with severe mental illness. *General Hospital Psychiatry.* 2017;*44*:1–3.

122. Swiss Academy of Medical Sciences (SAMS). *Medical-Ethical Guidelines and Recommendations on Palliative Care.* Basel, Switzerland: 2013.

123. Chochinov HM, Martens PJ, Prior HJ, Kredentser MS. Comparative health care use patterns of people with schizophrenia near the end of life: a population-based study in Manitoba, Canada. *Schizophrenia Research.* 2012;*141*(2–3):241–246.

124. Riordan PA, Briscoe J, Uritsky TJ, Jones CA, Webb JA. top ten tips palliative care clinicians should know about psychopharmacology. *Journal of Palliative Medicine.* 2019;*22*(5):572–579.

125. Trachsel M, Irwin SA, Biller-Andorno N, Hoff P, Riese F. Palliative psychiatry for severe persistent mental illness as a new approach to psychiatry? Definition, scope, benefits, and risks. *BMC Psychiatry.* 2016;*16*:260.

126. World Health Organization (WHO). WHO definition of palliative care. 2014. https://www.who.int/cancer/palliative/definition/en/. Accessed July 29, 2019.

127. Trachsel M, Wild V, Krones T, Biller-Andorno N. Compulsory treatment in chronic anorexia nervosa by all means? Searching for a middle ground between a curative and a palliative approach. *American Journal of Bioethics.* 2015;*15*(7):55–56.

128. Geppert C. Futility in chronic anorexia nervosa: a concept whose time has not yet come. *American Journal of Bioethics.* 2015;*15*:34–43.

129. Lopez A, Yager J, Feinstein RE. Medical futility and psychiatry: palliative care and hospice care as a last resort in the treatment of refractory anorexia nervosa. *International Journal of Eating Disorders.* 2010;*43*(4):372–377.

Special Populations and Communities

16

Pediatric Population

Stefan J. Friedrichsdorf, Farah Khalid, and
Noelle Noah

Introduction Pediatric Palliative Care

More than 21 million children would benefit from a palliative care approach worldwide, and around 8 million children 0–19 years old do require specialized pediatric palliative care (PPC).[1] Defined by the World Health Organization (WHO) as active total care of a child's mind, body and spirit,[2] palliative care for children is an all-encompassing specialized medical care aimed at providing the best possible quality of life for infants, children and adolescents with illnesses that are serious enough to be potentially incurable and likely to result in premature death. While there are different definitions to describe PPC, its tenets remain the same across these definitions. PPC is individualized care, is introduced at diagnosis along with curative treatment, and continues throughout the child's life. Children with serious illnesses and their families have been shown to have greater physical, emotional, and psychosocial distress, thus potentially requiring palliative care interventions throughout their illness trajectories.[3-6] This being said, these needs have also been identified in children at the end of life from an acute event such as trauma and in bereaved families. This strengthens the point that palliative care needs are not illness specific but rather are determined by the impact of the illness on the child and family.[5] From diagnosis to death, a child with serious illness typically encounters the following: disease progression from stable to deteriorating to terminal, a change in treatment goals from curative to palliative, acute illnesses or exacerbations, deteriorating function, and increasing symptom burden. Hence, children's palliative care needs and the intensity of palliative care interventions are not only individualized, but also vary throughout each child's illness trajectory.

There have been ongoing discussions on the specific diagnoses of serious illnesses that may require palliative care. Terms such as "life-limiting and life-threatening illnesses" describe illnesses with typical trajectories that can be categorized into four groups (please refer to the Associate for Children's Palliative Care and the Royal College of Paediatrics and Child Health categories).[3,7]

Complex chronic conditions is another term used to describe illnesses that may require palliative care. Complex chronic conditions are defined as medical conditions that can be reasonably expected to last at least 12 months and to involve either several different organ systems or one organ system severely enough to require specialty pediatric care and probably some period of hospitalization in a tertiary care center.[8]

Using these definitions, inpatient and mortality research data have shown a wide range of diagnoses that will require palliative care. These diagnoses are found throughout most of the *International Statistical Classification of Diseases, Tenth Revision (ICD-10)* categories. Diagnoses from *ICD-10* categories of "congenital malformations, deformations and chromo-somal abnormalities," "neoplasms," and "diseases of the nervous system" remain the more common.[8–11]

The heterogeneity of illnesses that potentially require palliative care is one of the key features distinguishing adult and children's palliative care, both of which otherwise share the same philosophy and principles. An understanding of the natural history of the wide range of conditions along with a thorough understanding of children's developmental stages is imperative in anyone providing palliative care for children. Children with serious illnesses not only present at different developmental stages, but also continue to develop physically, emotionally, cognitively, and spiritually throughout their illness trajectory.[12] Their understanding of the impact of the underlying illness on their life changes as they progress through the developmental milestones, so does their understanding of death and dying. It must be stressed that children's capacity to deal with the complexities of their illness and everything it entails is not necessarily age specific. Younger children with chronic illnesses, through their illness experience, may show or have a greater resilience than their healthier counterparts.

The PPC clinicians require skill sets that are unique to pediatrics to explore the child's understanding and values and to provide information in a timely manner using developmentally appropriate language, to carry out effective triadic communication (family meetings that involve other members of the family or friends, considered "family" by the child in the sense of importance with children and their parents), and to balance between parental autonomy and the child's views and wishes in decision-making and goal setting.

Following the illness trajectories of most incurable pediatric illnesses and considering the advancement in medical technology, including increasing pharmacological and surgical treatment options, it is not uncommon for children with serious illness to live much longer than adults with illnesses that require palliative care. Hence, unlike adult services that predominantly focus on the end-of-life care that is usually of a shorter time frame, pediatric services are known to care for children over much longer periods, sometimes from infancy into adulthood.[9]

Symptom management in children with serious illnesses can be challenging. The different diagnoses that potentially require PPC can result in a wide range of symptoms, especially during the end-of-life period.[10,13–16] Factors that lead to these symptoms being underrecognized and managed suboptimally include the lack of expertise among palliative care providers in assessing symptoms in children, especially in those who have yet to acquire verbal skills, and in designing a comprehensive symptom management plan that includes both pharmacological and nonpharmacological options. PPC providers need to be sensitive to the patients' and families' cultural and religious beliefs and views on the symptom-alleviating interventions.

Another feature that is unique to PPC is the necessity of providing care for siblings of children with serious illness.[17,18] Research has shown that siblings of children with serious illness experience adverse psychological and emotional reactions, including post-traumatic stress symptoms and an overall lower quality of life.[19-21] There is also increasing evidence that siblings of children with serious illnesses want to be involved in discussions about their siblings' health and impending death and to help with the care that is needed.[18,22] Being mindful of the presence of siblings during consultations, engaging them in discussions regarding the illness and care plans, encouraging their participation in caregiving tasks, and facilitating their access to support groups or supportive teams such as child life specialists have been shown to result in better psychological and emotional outcomes for siblings of children with serious illness.[22,23]

Palliative care provision requires a broad spectrum of disciplines working together to meet the needs of children with serious illness and their families. Palliative care teams made up of physicians; advanced practice providers (physician assistants [PAs], clinical nurse specialists, or nurse practitioners); medical social workers; psychologists; and child life specialists assess physical, psychosocial, emotional, and spiritual needs of the patients and their families/caregivers and design care plans that support these needs. The roles of the PPC team include (1) symptom management, (2) addressing patient and family's beliefs and concerns about the illness; (3) initiating and revisiting goals-of-care decisions as the illness progresses by taking into consideration the benefits and harm of medical interventions and the patient and family's wishes and hopes; (4) facilitating access to and coordinating the different teams involved in supporting the needs of the patient and family; (5) maintaining normality by optimizing the patient's function and enhancing the patient's role within the family and community; (6) assessing the patient's spiritual needs, (7) promoting discussions about end-of-life preferences and providing anticipatory guidance regarding what to expect at the end of life; and (8) assessing pathological grief in bereaved families.[24-26]

Concurrent Care in the United States

The palliative care terminology used in the United States is at times different from the rest of the planet, and this fact may cause confusion for the international reader. Whereas *hospice* worldwide usually describes either a physical location (like a house) that provides respite and end-of-life care or the philosophy of providing end-of-life care at home, in the United States hospice describes a health insurance benefit. Unlike for adults, children in the United States may receive potentially curative treatment (e.g., chemotherapy) and services from a hospice agency at the same time.

The *Concurrent Care for Children* requirement of the US Affordable Care Act was put in place under President Obama in 2010. The 2016 briefing of the Mary J. Labyak Institute for Innovation at the National Center for Care at the End of Life[27] described concurrent care for children with serious illness as follows:

Until 2010, parents in all but a few states in the United States were faced with forgoing curative treatments for their children to be eligible for hospice services. Or conversely, they were not eligible for beneficial interdisciplinary hospice services while getting curative treatment. The Patient Protection and Affordable Care Act (ACA) changed that situation. It requires all state Medicaid programs to pay for both curative and hospice services for children under age 21 who qualify. On March 23, 2010, President Obama signed ACA into law enacting a new provision, Section 2302, termed the "Concurrent Care for Children" Requirement (CCCR). Section 2302 states that a child who is eligible for and receives hospice care must also have all other services provided, or have payment made for, services that are related to the treatment of the child's condition. This provision affects children who are eligible for Medicaid or the Children's Health Insurance Program (CHIP). In its simplest form, implementation of this provision could be accomplished by the state Medicaid agency eliminating any provider claims that deny or delay concurrent curative care and hospice claims.[27]

Conceptually, this model represents an excellent paradigm for palliative care.

Pain Pathophysiologies in Pediatric Palliative Care

Infants, children, and adolescents living with or dying from serious illnesses commonly experience pain, which is among the most distressing and prevalent symptoms.[28–30] Nearly all studies of such symptoms in PPC were undertaken in children with malignancies and showed a significant symptom burden to this population.[31–34] A prospective study describing patient-reported outcomes in pediatric patients with advanced cancer showed that 39% of all children were self-reporting high distress from pain, increasing to 58% at end of life.[34]

Pain in the largest group of PPC patients, children with progressive neurologic, metabolic, or chromosomal conditions with impairment of the central nervous system, has been shown to be common, underrecognized, and undertreated.[35] In this group of children, the majority experience daily pain, with nearly 22% experiencing pain nearly all the time.[35]

The majority of patients with serious illnesses experience different distinct and at times overlapping entities of pain pathophysiology concurrently and/or subsequently, explaining the need of advanced protocols providing multimodal analgesia. The most common pain entities palliative care patients are experiencing include acute somatic pain, procedural pain, neuropathic pain, psycho-spiritual-emotional pain, chronic postsurgical pain, and/or chronic persistent pain.

Pain Assessment

The measurement of pain intensity is important and required to titrate and evaluate analgesics; however, it is a necessary oversimplification. To quote Carl L. von Baeyer, "Measuring pain by its intensity alone is like describing music only in terms of its loudness."[36]

BOX 16.1 Examples of Pain Pathophysiologies

(1) Nociceptive Pain: arises from the activation of peripheral nerve endings (nociceptors) that respond to noxious stimulation (e.g., localized, sharp, squeezing, stabbing, or throbbing)

   Somatic (e.g., muscles, joints)

   Chronic somatic pain typically well localized and often results from degenerative processes (e.g., arthritis)

(2) Visceral (internal organs) (poorly localized, dull, crampy, or achy)

(3) Neuropathic Pain: resulting from injury to, or dysfunction of, the somatosensory system (burning, shooting, electric, or tingling)

   Central pain: caused by a lesion or disease of the central somatosensory nervous system

(4) Total Pain: suffering that encompasses all of a child's physical, psychological, social, spiritual, and practical struggles

(5) Persistent (Chronic) Pain

   Pain beyond expected time of healing

For example, a child scoring 8 out of 10 on a pain scale would be treated very differently according to its underlying pain pathology (see Text Box 1). While for severe cancer pain morphine is likely to be appropriate, it would be not be indicated for chronic pain or total[37] (psychosocial) pain. Of course, many children experience different kinds of pain at the same time.

A recent comprehensive review consistently reported an underestimation of pediatric pain by nurses and physicians, and the extent of underestimation tended to increase with pain severity.[38] There are many validated pediatric pain scales. An example of commonly used tools are listed next.

Multidimensional Observational Rating Scales

For nonverbal and/or children younger than 4 years, pain is measured using observation rating scales. Examples include the following:

- *Infants:* For example, CRIES (Crying; Requires increased oxygen administration; Increased vital signs; Expression; Sleeplessness)[39] or the Infant FLACC (Face, Leg, Activity, Cry, Consolability) scale (Table 16.1).[40]
- *Toddlers:* FLACC pain scale (0–10).[41]
- *Intubated:* COMFORT[42] or FLACC.[41]
- *Nonverbal, intellectually impaired:* r-FLACC,[43] Pediatric Pain Profile,[44] or Noncommunicating Children's Pain Checklist–Revised.[45]

TABLE 16.1 Infant FLACC Scale[a].

Category	Scoring		
	0	1	2
Face	No particular expression or smile	Occasional grimace or frown, withdrawn, disinterested	Frequent-to-constant quivering chin, clenched jaw
Legs	Normal position or relaxed	Uneasy, restless, tense	Kicking or legs drawn up
Activity	Lying quietly, normal position, moves easily	Squirming, shifting back and forth, tense	Arched, rigid, or jerking
Cry	No cry (awake or asleep)	Moans or whimpers, occasional complaint	Crying steadily, screams or sobs, frequent complaints
Consolability	Content, relaxed	Reassured by occasional touching, hugging, or being talked to, distracted	Difficult to console or comfort

Instructions: Each of the 5 categories is scored from zero to two, which results in a total score between 0-10

[a] From Reference 40. Reprinted with permission

Self-Assessment

- *4- to 6-year-olds*: Simplified Faces Pain Scale (S-FPS) or Simplified Concrete Ordinal Scale (S-COS) (Figure 16.1).[46]
- *6–12 years*: Faces Pain Scale–Revised (Figure 16.2).[47]
- *>10 years*: Visual Analogue Scale (VAS) (Figure 16.3)[48] or Numerical Rating Scale (NRS-11) (Figure 16.4).

Prevention and Treatment of Procedural Pain

Untreated needle pain in children with serious illness, caused by procedures such as blood draws, injections, venous cannulation, and more, can have long-term consequences, including needle phobia, preprocedural anxiety, hyperalgesia, and avoidance of healthcare, resulting in increased morbidity and mortality (see Text Box 2).[50,51] Current evidence strongly suggests that four bundled modalities should be offered for elective needle procedures in order to reduce or eliminate pain experienced by children.[51-54] Offering four simple steps (and not just some of them) for all needle procedures for all children has now been implemented systemwide in children's hospitals and pediatricians' offices on several continents.[52,55]

Failure to prevent or minimize treatable procedural pain in children is now considered both inappropriate and unethical.[57]

(1) *Topical anesthesia* should be applied to all term infants (36 weeks corrected gestational age and older) and children for every elective needle procedure every time. Older verbal children and teenagers may of course decline if they prefer the needle poke without numbing cream.

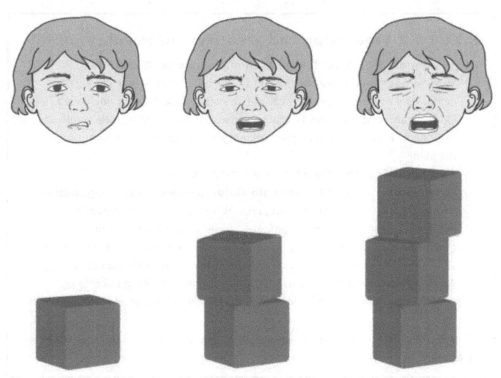

FIGURE 16.1 Simplified Faces Pain Scale (S-FPS) or Simplified Concrete Ordinal Scale (S-COS) for 4- to 6-year-old children. (Reprinted with permission from Reference 46.) Instruction: Ask child whether or not in pain. If yes, show Faces or building blocks to evaluate for "mild," "medium," or "severe" pain.

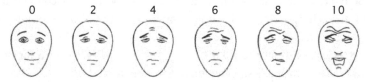

FIGURE 16.2 Faces Pain Scale–Revised (FPS-R) for children 7 years and older. (Reprinted with permission from Reference 47.) The instructions and translations into more than 60 languages are available at http://www.iasp-pain.org/Education/Content.aspx?ItemNumber=1519.

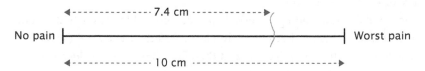

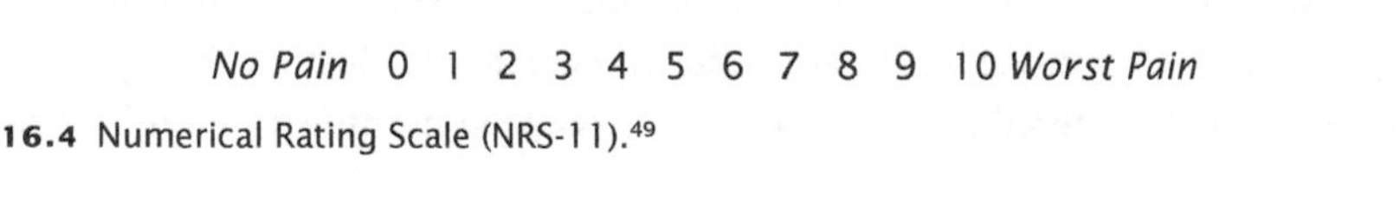

FIGURE 16.3 Visual Analogue Scale (VAS). (Reprinted with permission from Reference 48.)

No Pain 0 1 2 3 4 5 6 7 8 9 10 *Worst Pain*

FIGURE 16.4 Numerical Rating Scale (NRS-11).[49]

BOX 16.2 Prevention and Treatment of Needle Pain[52,56]

Offer a bundle of four evidence-based modalities to all children:

(1) **Topical anesthesia "numb the skin"** (for children 36 weeks corrected gestational age and older). Topical anesthetics include 4% lidocaine cream, EMLA-cream, or needle-less lidocaine application via a J-tip (sterile, single-use, disposable injector that uses pressurized gas to propel medication through the skin).

(2) **Sucrose or breastfeeding** for infants 0–12 months.

(3) **Comfort positioning "Do not hold children down."** Restraining children for procedures is never supportive, creates a negative experience, and increases anxiety and pain. For infants, consider swaddling, warmth, skin-to-skin contact, or facilitated tucking. For children 6 months and older, offer sitting upright with parents holding them on their laps or sitting nearby.

(4) **Age-appropriate distraction**, such as toys, books, blowing bubbles or pinwheels, stress balls, and using apps, videos, or games on electronic devices.

Of note: If above ineffective or not feasible, consider nitrous gas analgesia and sedation.

Topical anesthetics include the following:

- A 4% liposomal (currently all 4% lidocaine cream available over the counter in the United States and Canada is liposomal) lidocaine cream[58] is effective after 30 minutes and may be on skin up to 2 hours.[59,60]
- EMLA (lidocaine 2.5% and prilocaine 2.5%) cream may be on the skin for up to 4 hours and provides maximum analgesia after at least 60 minutes.
- Needle-less lidocaine application (e.g., via a J-tip®; sterile, single-use, disposable injector that uses pressurized gas to propel medication through the skin).[61,62]

Contrary to a common myth, topical anesthetics do *not* constrict veins and do *not* decrease the chance of venous cannulation.[52,62,63]

Other modalities, including vapocoolants, ice, cool/cold packs, vibrating devices, and others, might also be helpful but currently have insufficient evidence for or against their use to reduce pain at time of injection and therefore should be considered in addition to numbing cream, but not instead of topical anesthetics.[64]

(2) For term infants 0–12 months,[65] *breastfeeding* prevents or decreases procedural pain and has been shown to be equally effective to administering sucrose.[66] *Sucrose* reduces pain and crying during painful procedures, such as venipunctures.[67,68] The minimally effective dose of 24% sucrose for procedural pain relief in neonates is "just a drop" (0.1 mL)[69] and therefore can be administered to infants who are receiving nothing by mouth. It should be

administered about 2 minutes prior to the painful procedure and may be repeated during the intervention.

(3) *Comfort positioning*: For elective needle procedures, children should *not* be held down (this might be different in a life-saving intervention). For infants, consider primarily skin-to-skin contact (if not feasible, use swaddling, warmth, facilitated tucking, co-bedding for twins).[70-77]

For children 6 months and older, offer sitting upright, with parents holding them on their laps or sitting nearby. Restraining children for procedures is never supportive, creates a negative experience, and increases their anxiety and pain. In fact, children with cancer who have been restrained for procedures report that it makes them feel ashamed, humiliated, and powerless, and they report having lost their right to control their own body.[78]

(4) *Age-appropriate distraction* includes the use of toys, books, blowing bubbles or pinwheels, stress balls, and using apps, videos, or games on electronic devices.[79-81] A recent Cochrane review identified sufficient evidence for the effectiveness of cognitive behavioral therapy (CBT), breathing interventions, distraction, and hypnosis for reducing children's pain and/or fear due to needles.[82]

Offering these four simple modalities (or three to children older than 12 months) and not just some of them for all needle procedures for all children has now been implemented systemwide in children's hospitals and pediatricians' offices on several continents.[52,55]

In addition to these four modalities, it is recommended that healthcare professionals and parents use neutral words and avoid language that can increase fear and may be falsely reassuring (e.g., "It will be over soon"; "You will be OK").[50]

(5) *Deferral Process* (or *"Plan B"*): If adequate procedural analgesia and anxiolysis is not feasible with the above bundled modalities alone (e.g., because the child has been held down in the past and as a result has become too anxious or it was difficult to draw blood in the past, etc.), consider adding a child life specialist, referral to a child psychologist to overcome needle phobia, and/or consider sedation, especially by offering nitrous gas.[83]

Nitrous gas analgesia and sedation: Data reveal that children receiving nitrous gas before and during painful procedures have lower levels of distress, had lower pain scores, were more relaxed, and many had no recollection of the procedure afterward.[84-86] Nitrous gas concentrations between 40% and 70% can be titrated to achieve minimal sedation only, avoiding moderate sedation.[87,88] Children receiving minimal sedation are able to respond to verbal commands, maintain and protect their airway, have spontaneous ventilation, and have unaffected cardiovascular functions.[89]

Multimodal Analgesia

Advanced pain management for children with serious illness often requires multimodal analgesia. This describes an approach of utilizing multiple analgesic agents (e.g., basic analgesia, opioids, adjuvant analgesia); regional anesthesia (e.g., nerve blocks or neuroaxial analgesia); rehabilitation (e.g., physical therapy, motor graded imagery); psychological (e.g., CBT) and integrative (formally known as "nonpharmacological") therapies (e.g., massage, hypnosis), which usually act synergistically for more effective pediatric pain control with fewer side

Multimodal (Opioid-Sparing) Analgesia

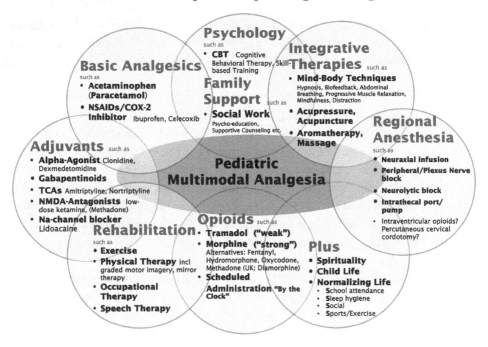

FIGURE 16.5 Multimodal analgesia for children in palliative care. (Used with permission: Stefan Friedrichsdorf, Benioff Children's Hospitals in Oakland and San Francisco, University of California at San Francisco [UCSF].)

effects than a single analgesic or modality[90,91] (see Figure 16.5). Treating complex pain in seriously ill children exclusively with medications (the "pharmacology-only approach") will often fail to provide adequate analgesia.

Case Part 1

Emma is a 9-year-old girl recently diagnosed with a bone tumor (Ewing sarcoma) who is now undergoing cancer-directed chemotherapy, surgery, and radiation.

She rates her pain on the Faces Pain Scale–Revised as 8/10. The pain appears to be acute, nociceptive cancer and postoperative pain.

Weight: 18 kg

She requires a **blood draw**. For every elective needle procedure,

Apply 4% lidocaine cream (30 minutes before) or EMLA-cream (60 minutes before). Comfort positioning (never hold her down); she likes to sit on her parent's lap. Offer distraction (she likes blowing bubbles).

Lumbar puncture: Under nitrous gas (or propofol or ketamine)
Bone marrow aspiration: Deep sedation (e.g., propofol or ketamine)

Basic Analgesia

The WHO Step 1 basic analgesia[92] includes the nonopioid analgesics acetaminophen (paracetamol), nonsteroidal anti-inflammatory drugs (NSAIDs), and cyclooxygenase 2 (COX-2) inhibitors. Of note, ibuprofen sodium (available over the counter in many countries) requires only half the dose, has an analgesic effect within 10 minutes, and lasts longer.[93] In some countries, dipyrone (Metamizole; not available in the United States) is included under basic analgesia.[94] For dosing recommendations, see Table 16.2.

Paracetamol (acetaminophen) is generally well tolerated by children and lacks gastrointestinal and hematological side effects. Significant hepatoxicity[95] is rare, but careful attention to dosing is paramount.

TABLE 16.2 Basic Analgesia for Children: Dosing Recommendations[a]

Drug	Route	Age	Pediatric Dose	Maximal Dose	Dosing Interval
Ibuprofen	Oral	>3–6 months[b]	5–10 mg/kg	400–600 mg/dose	6–8 h
Ibuprofen sodium[c] 256 mg tablet = 200 mg ibuprofen	Oral	>6 months	5–(10) mg/kg	200–(400) mg/dose	6–8 h
Acetaminophen (paracetamol)	Oral, rectal	Neonates 0–30 days	5–10 mg/kg	20–40 mg/kg/d	4–6 h (maximum 4 doses/d)
	Oral, rectal	Infants 1–3 months	10 mg/kg	40 mg/kg/d	4–6 h (maximum 4 doses/d)
	Oral, rectal	4 months–2 years	10–15 mg/kg	40–60 mg/kg/d	4–6 h (maximum 4 doses/d)
	Oral, rectal	>2 years	10–15 mg/kg	90 mg/kg/d or 650 mg every 6 h	4–6 h
	IV[d]	<1 year	<10 kg = 7.5 mg/kg	30 mg/kg/d	6 h
	IV[d]	1–2 years	15 mg/kg	60 mg/kg/d	6 h
	IV[d]	>2 years (<50 kg)	15 mg/kg	75 mg/kg/d	6 h
	IV[d]	>13 years (>50 kg)	1000 mg	4000 mg/d	6 h
Ketorolac[e]	IV	6 months–2 years[b]	0.25 mg/kg	30 mg/dose	6–8 h
	IV	>2 years	0.5 mg/kg	30 mg/dose	6–8 h
Celecoxib[f]	Oral	>6 months	1–2 mg/kg	100 mg/dose	12–24 s

[a]Used with permission: Stefan Friedrichsdorf, Benioff Children's Hospitals in Oakland and San Francisco, University of California at San Francisco (UCSF))
[b] For NSAIDs in infants less than 3–6 months, consult the pediatric pain service.
[c] Fast acting, compared to standard ibuprofen: onset of analgesia after 10 minutes, last longer, and only half the dose required.
[d] Due to high cost, only if rectal or oral administration contraindicated; reevaluate daily.
[e] Recommend dosing no longer than 5 days.
[f] If classical NSAIDs contraindicated; safety and efficacy has been established in children 2 years of age or older for a maximum of 6 months of treatment in juvenile rheumatoid arthritis.

Ibuprofen has the fewest gastrointestinal side effects among NSAIDs that are nonselective for COX-2. It should be used with caution in individuals with hepatic or renal impairment or a history of gastrointestinal bleeding or ulcers, and it inhibits platelet aggregation. Ketorolac has the advantage of intravenous administration, but it should be rotated to oral ibuprofen as soon as tolerated. Celecoxib (a COX-2 inhibitor) might be considered if classical NSAIDs are contraindicated (e.g., owing to bleeding risks or gastrointestinal side effects). It may not display less renal toxicity compared to classic NSAIDs. Safety and efficacy have been established only in children 2 years of age or older and for a maximum of 6 months of treatment in juvenile rheumatoid arthritis.

Opioids

For medium-severe acute pain WHO Step 2, opioid morphine will be added.[92] Other equally effective "strong" opioids include fentanyl, hydromorphone, and oxycodone (in the United Kingdom only: diamorphine). A switch from one opioid to another is often accompanied by a change in the balance between analgesia and side effects.[96] The most frequently used opioid and gold standard in pediatrics for moderate-to-severe pain remains morphine. Opioid-associated side effects (e.g., constipation, pruritus, and nausea) should be anticipated and treated accordingly. For recommended starting doses, see Tables 16.3, 16.4 and 16.5.

Two potentially particularly effective multimechanistic opioids include the "weak" tramadol (for mild-to medium-pain) and "strong" methadone (for medium-severe pain).[97] Tramadol appears to play a key role not only in outpatient surgery (due to its relative respiratory safety, more than 6000 pediatric tramadol scripts were filled at Children's Minnesota in 2018) but especially in treating episodes of inconsolability in children with progressive neurologic, metabolic, or chromosomally based condition with impairment of the central nervous system.[97] However, the recent 2017 US Food and Drug Administration warning against pediatric use of tramadol does not seem to be based on clinical evidence (three children died worldwide in 49 years, and therefore it appears far safer than any other opioid), and unfortunately puts children at risk for unrelieved pain or distressing symptoms.[97]

Methadone, due to its multimechanistic action profile, is possibly among the most effective and most underutilized opioid analgesics in children with severe unrelieved pain, especially in children receiving palliative care. *However, methadone should not be prescribed by those unfamiliar with its use: Its effects should be closely monitored for several days, particularly when it is first started and after any dose changes.*[98–101]

TABLE 16.3 Opioid Analgesics: Usual Starting Doses for Children With Acute Pain (>6 Months)[a]

Medication (Route of Administration)	Starting Intravenous Dose	Intravenous/Oral Ratio	Starting Oral Dose (or Transdermal)
Morphine (Oral, SL, IV, SC, rectal)	**Bolus dose:** 0.05–0.1 mg/kg (maximum 5 mg) every 2–4 h **Continuous infusion:** 0.01–0.02 mg/kg/h (maximum 0.5–1 mg/h)	1:3 (i.e., 1 mg IV = 3 mg oral)	**0.15–0.3 mg/kg (maximum 7.5–15 mg) every 4 h**
Fentanyl (IV, SC, SL, transdermal, buccal)	**Bolus dose:** 0.5–1 µg/kg (maximum 25–50 µg) (slowly over 3–5 min; fast bolus of high doses, especially > 5–10 µg /kg may cause thorax rigidity) **Continuous infusion: 0.5-**1 µg/kg/h (maximum 25–50 µg/h)	1:1 (IV to transdermal)	**12 µg/h patch** (must be on the equivalent of at least 30 mg oral morphine/24 h before switching to patch)
Hydromorphone (Oral, SL, IV, SC, rectal)	**Bolus dose:** 15–20 µg/kg (maximum 1 mg) every 4 h **Continuous infusion:** 2–5 µg/kg/h (maximum 100–250 µg/h)	1:5	**60 µg/kg (maximum 2000–3000 µg or 2–3 mg) every 3–4 h**
Oxycodone (PO, SL, PR)	**Intravenous not available in USA**	**Intravenous not available in USA**	0.1–0.2 mg/kg (maximum 5–10 mg) every 4 h *or* 0.15–0.3 mg/kg (maximum 7.5–15 mg) every 6 h
Tramadol (Oral, rectal)	**Intravenous not available in USA** *(Bolus dose: 1 mg/kg every 3–4 h; continuous Infusion: 0.25 mg/kg/h]*	1:1	1–2 mg/kg every 3–4 h, maximum of 8 mg/kg/d (>50 kg: maximum of 400 mg/d)
Methadone (Oral, rectal, SL, IV)	0.04–0.08 mg/kg (maximum 2–4 mg) IV every 8 h	**1:1 to 1:2** (in adults usually IV, usually 50% of oral dose; in pediatrics, usually IV = 80% of oral dose)	0.05–0.1 mg/kg (maximum 2.2–5 mg) oral every 8 h

IV, intravenous; n/a, not applicable; SC, subcutaneous; SL, sublingual.

Above doses represent starting doses, which then need to be titrated to effect and may be significantly higher. Maximum per kilogram dose capped at 50 kg body weight. Calculated rescue (breakthrough) dose: 10%–16% of 24-hour opioid dose to be given every 1–2 hours as needed. Methadone should not be prescribed without proper training about dosing and potential side effects. Prescribing clinicians should closely observe the child for potential side effects from the time he or she receives the first dose and following medication changes, such as tapering, titration, or adding other potentially sedating medications.

[a] Used with permission: Stefan Friedrichsdorf, Benioff Children's Hospitals in Oakland and San Francisco, University of California at San Francisco (UCSF).

TABLE 16.4 Opioid Analgesia for Neonates and Infants 0–6 Months of Age[92]

Opioids

Morphine	Oral/rectal/SL	0.075–0.15 mg (neonates 0–30 days) 0.08–0.2 mg (infants 1–12 months)	6 h
		0.08–0.2 mg (infants 1–6 months)	4–6 h
Morphine[a]	IV/SC[b]	0.025–0.05 mg/kg (neonates 0–30 days) 0.08–0.2 mg (infants 1–12 months)	6 h
		0.1 mg/kg (infants 1–6 months) 0.1 mg (infants 1–6 months) 1.1 0.1 mg (infants 1–6 months)	6 h
		Infusion (with PCA bolus of same dose): 0.005–0.01 mg/kg/h (neonates 0–30 days) 0.01–0.03 mg/kg/h (infants 1–6 months)	
Fentanyl[a]	IV/SC[b]	1–2 µg/kg (neonates and infants 0–12 months) 0.08–0.2 mg (infants 1–12 months)	2–4 h
		Infusion (with PCA bolus of same dose): 0.5–1 µg/kg/h (neonates and infants 0–6 months)	
Oxycodone	Oral/rectal/SL	0.05–0.125 mg/kg (infants 1–6 months)	4 h–

[a] The intravenous doses for neonates are based on acute pain management and sedation dosing information. Lower doses are required for nonventilated neonates.
[b] Administer intravenously slowly over at least 5 minutes.

TABLE 16.5 Usual Starting Doses for Patient (or Nurse) –Controlled Analgesia (PCA) Pumps for Children in Acute Pain (>6 Months)[a]

	Continuous Infusion (µg/kg/h)	PCA bolus (µg)	Lockout time (minutes)	Maximum Number of Boluses/Hour
Morphine	10–20 (maximum 500–1000)	10–20 (maximum 500–1000)	5–10	4–6
Hydromorphone	2–5 (maximum 100–250)	2–5 (maximum 100–250)	5–10	4–6
Fentanyl	0.5–1 (maximum 25–50)	0.5–1 (maximum 25–50)	5	4–6

Dose escalation usually in 50% increments for both continuous and PCA bolus dose (Department of Pain Medicine, Palliative Care and Integrative Medicine, Children's Hospitals and Clinics of Minnesota, USA). Doses for children > 6 months of age and are capped at 50 kg body weight.
[a] Used with permission: Stefan Friedrichsdorf, Benioff Children's Hospitals in Oakland and San Francisco, University of California at San Francisco (UCSF).

Case Part 2

You start the following medications according the WHO pain ladder (Figure 16.6) approach for Emma:

Paracetamol (acetaminophen): 15 mg × 18 kg = 270 mg every 6 hours by mouth

Ibuprofen 10 mg × 18 kg = 180 mg every 6 hours by mouth

If NSAIDs are contraindicated (e.g., due to bleeding risk or neutropenia), consider the COX-2 inhibitor **celecoxib** instead: 2 mg × 18 kg = 36 mg orally twice daily.

Since she is in severe acute cancer and postoperative pain, a strong opioid will be started immediately (and we will NOT wait on the effect of the basic analgesia).

Oral morphine 0.3 mg × 18 kg = 5.4 mg every 4 hours by mouth (= 32.4 mg/d) plus 10% of total daily dose = 3.2 mg orally every 1–2 hours as needed for breakthrough pain *or*

Intravenous morphine 0.1 mg × 18 kg = 1.8 mg IV every 4 hours (= 10.8 mg/d) plus 10% of total daily dose = 1.1 mg IV every 1–2 hours as needed for breakthrough pain *or*

Morphine continuous intravenous or subcutaneous infusion plus PCA: 20 μg × 18 kg = 360 μg *or* 0.36 mg/h IV plus 0.36 mg PCA bolus (lockout time 5–10 minutes, maximum 4–6 boluses/h)

If inadequate analgesia (and no severe opioid-induced side effects, titrate to effect in 50% steps (e.g., from 5.4 mg to 8.1 mg morphine every 4 hours orally plus 4.9 mg every 1–2 hours as needed), carefully observing for oversedation or respiratory depression.

Of note: Intravenous morphine can be swallowed by mouth.

IV, intravenous; PCA, patient- (or nurse-) controlled analgesia;

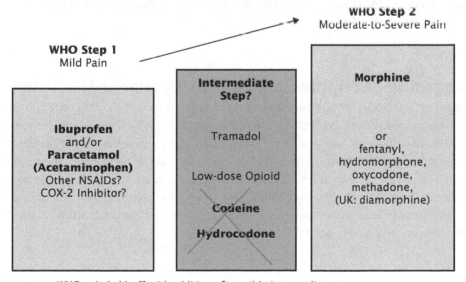

FIGURE 16.6 WHO pain ladder,[92] with addition of possible intermediate step.

Case Part 3

Three years later: Emma is now a 12-year-old girl with a 3-year history of Ewing sarcoma, which unfortunately did not respond well to cancer-directed chemotherapy, surgery, and radiation. Most recent imaging revealed several metastases in her lung and liver and a large primary tumor in her left hip infiltrating the spinal cord and compressing her left sciatic nerve. For the last few days, she reported constant acute background pain rated up to 5/10 and adequately controlled on oral morphine.

When asked in more detail, she reports, "Shooting pain hundreds of times per day from my buttock into my feet." She displays significant allodynia on examination in parts of her left lower extremity. She presents to clinic today with a sudden loss of some bladder control and sudden inability to walk on both legs.

Identify and Treat Underlying Disease Process

As always, when a child presents with a distressing symptom, we need to try to identify and treat the underlying disease process if this is feasible and within the goals of care for this particular child and family. A medical examination and history are paramount.

Case Part 4

Symptomatically, Emma's presentation is suggestive of metastatic spinal cord compression, a true palliative care emergency, which requires prompt action within hours. This diagnosis was confirmed by imagery. The new symptoms of lower extremity weakness and urinary incontinence could be resolved by repeated palliative radiation therapy aimed at the spinal metastasis and the administration of dexamethasone. Her neuropathic leg pain (likely due to her sciatic nerve compression) continued but was improved by using a corticosteroid.

Integrative (Nonpharmacological) Treatment Modalities

Integrative modalities (sometimes referred to as complementary or alternative medicine) that have been described as effective in the management of pediatric pain include hypnosis, yoga, acupuncture, and massage.[102–111] Active mind-body techniques, such as guided imagery, hypnosis, biofeedback, yoga, and distraction each and all evoke pain modulation by engaging a number of mechanisms within the analgesic neuraxis. These techniques may have heightened importance in low- and middle-income countries where there is lack of diversity of pain management drugs or the costs do not allow access to them and a clinician must be even more creative to fight against pain.

Case Part 5

For Emma, it was most important to learn *active* strategies and "to be in control," although she enjoyed the *passive* modalities (massage, aromatherapy) as well. Physical therapy and occupational therapy started working with her. She and her parents were able to follow the daily exercises as spelled out by her therapist, whom she saw once per week. Emma enthusiastically learned deep breathing, biofeedback, and self-hypnosis and also used some relaxation "apps" on her smartphone. She felt all of these modalities helped to reduce her pain, and they helped her feel more in control. After a few days, she would usually go daily "to her happy place" in her imagination using deep breathing as an induction technique.

Biofeedback is a method of treatment that uses monitors to feed back to patients physiological information of which they are normally unaware. By watching the monitor, patients can learn by trial and error to adjust their thinking and other mental processes in order to control "involuntary" bodily processes such as blood pressure, temperature, gastrointestinal functioning, and brain wave activity. Biofeedback requires trained instructors and specialized equipment.

Relaxation therapy might include progressive muscle relaxation and is used to help patients recognize any lower body tension associated with pain and anxiety. Children can be taught how to tense and relax different muscle groups in a relaxed and quiet setting or to visualize a happy or peaceful scene and reduce body tensions that way.

Hypnosis involves the cultivation of an altered state of awareness, leading to heightened suggestibility, which allows for changes in a child's perception and experience, bypassing conscious effort. In hypnosis, the clinician enters the child's world, engaging the child's imagination as the agent of change and creating alternate experiences to promote therapeutic change. In trance, the child addresses distressing symptoms utilizing suggestions by the clinician for altering sensations and perceptions and increasing comfort.[112] Teaching hypnosis to children and adolescents is an extremely versatile skill that can be acquired by pediatric clinicians through formalized training workshops and practice.[113]

Cognitive and behavioral methods include comfort measures such as pacifiers, massage, touch, music; distraction methods such as bubbles, counting, toys, video games; suggestion methods such as magic glove (see, e.g., Leora Kuttner, PhD, at https://www.youtube.com/watch?v=cyApK8Z_SQQ) techniques; breathing techniques such as patterned, shallow, or deep breathing; guided imagery; muscle relaxation and hypnosis. A counseling relationship that supports coaching and problem-solving is an important component of these approaches.

Transcutaneous electrical nerve stimulation (TENS) can be used independently or with other pain treatment modalities. TENS uses stimulation pulses delivered to skin electrodes around the area of pain. It is thought that electrical stimulation delivered by a TENS unit reduces pain through nociceptive inhibition at the presynaptic level in the dorsal horn, thus limiting its central transmission. The electrical stimuli on the skin preferentially activate low-threshold, myelinated nerve fibers. The afferent input from these fibers inhibits propagation of nociception carried in the small, unmyelinated C fibers by blocking transmission along these fibers to the target or T cells located in the dorsal horn. The TENS unit is compact, portable, and easily managed by many children.

Acupressure or acupuncture is an approach based on traditional Chinese medicine and has been used for thousands of years. Its utility in reducing postoperative nausea and vomiting is well documented. There are few studies in children.

Psychological Interventions

Anxiety, depressive, and behavioral disorders are early risk factors of chronic pain in children and adolescents (rather than vice versa).[114] At low levels of anxiety, higher pain is predictive of greater disability; however, highly anxious adolescents tend to function poorly regardless of level of pain.[115] Psychological treatments significantly reduce pain intensity that is reported by children and adolescents with headache, abdominal pain, and musculoskeletal/joint pain.[116,117] CBT led to significant improvements in pain coping, catastrophizing, and efficacy that were sustained over time in adolescents with chronic pain.[118] CBT has been shown to increase gray matter in the prefrontal cortex of patients with chronic pain, and this increase in prefrontal cortical gray matter has been associated with reduced pain catastrophizing.[119]

Physical Therapy/Rehabilitation

Physical therapy and exercise are key modalities in the treatment of patients with chronic pain and primary pain disorder, including in children with serious illness.[120–127] Patients with chronic pain usually have a lower physical activity level,[128] and physical activity has been shown to reduce the risk for depression.[129] In patients participating in a rehabilitative pain program, the rate of improvement in function was significantly more rapid than the decrease in pain.[124] Graded motor imagery, including mirror therapy, is the process of thinking about moving without actually moving.[130]

Spirituality

Religion, spirituality, or life philosophy play an important role in the life of most parents whose children are receiving PPC,[131] and screenings tools, such as FICA (Faith, Import, Community, Address), have been successfully implemented in clinical PPC.[132] A link between spiritual coping and quality of life in adolescents with serious illness has been described.[133,134]

Case Part 6

Emma (current weight 30 kg) has been on *scheduled oral morphine* 6 mg every 4 hours plus 3.6 mg (10% of daily dose) once every 1 to 2 hours as needed. She required five as-needed doses of the morphine in the last 24 hours. However, she also continued to experience medium-to-severe neuropathic leg pain (VAS 6–8/10). The dose was increased by 50% to scheduled oral morphine 9 mg every 4 hours plus 5.4 mg once every 1–2 hours as needed. This improved her analgesia somewhat, and she did not display any opioid-induced side effects. Therefore, the dose was increased by another 50% to 13.5 mg every 4 hours. On the following day, she reported being sick of taking so many tablets and liquids. She said, "It takes too long for the extra dose to work" and complained they made her sleepy. Her parents were distressed to see her in pain and also expressed worries that she might get nauseous if she was taking too much oral medication.

A decision was made to *rotate her opioid and route of administration to intravenous hydromorphone* to achieve a better effect/side-effect profile. Since she had displayed pruritus with fentanyl in the past, hydromorphone was chosen. She went home with a portable pump delivering hydromorphone 0.15 mg/h plus 0.15 mg PCA bolus every 10 minutes with a maximum of five boluses per hour. On the following day, she reported an average pain of 4–6/10, which was an improvement and that the PCA boluses were helpful "for a short while." She initially used about two PCA boluses per hour (thereby tripling the continuous infusion) over 24 hours without any side effects, so the dose was escalated by 50% to 0.22 mg/h plus 0.22 mg PCA bolus. She now reported improved analgesia. She stated, "For me 4–5/10 is ok because then I can sleep." Emma then used about four to eight PCA boluses/day.

Emma started seeing a *physical therapist* and daily exercises as an inpatient and then at home increased her activity level significantly. She started seeing a *psychologist* once a week who was experienced in CBT. The hospital chaplain connected with the *spiritual leader* of her faith community to arrange for home visits.

Adjuvant Analgesia

Adjuvant analgesics are *medications that, when added to primary analgesics, further improve pain control*. Occasionally, they may also be primary analgesics, especially in pediatric patients with neuropathic and/or visceral pain (Table 16.6). They can be added at any step in the WHO ladder.

Corticosteroids are potent anti-inflammatory agents useful in both nociceptive and neuropathic pain. Reducing inflammation and peritumor edema can relieve pressure on a nerve or the spinal cord, decreasing intracranial pressure from a brain tumor or decreasing obstruction of a hollow viscus.

In advanced disease, dexamethasone is the corticosteroid of choice because of its minimal mineralocorticoid effects and thus decreased risk of salt and fluid retention. Corticosteroids may also enhance pain control through the creation of a sense of euphoria. Most of the complications of steroid use (proximal muscle weakness, osteoporosis, and immunosuppression) are long-term sequelae and are therefore not a concern at the end of life. Steroid psychosis is occasionally a problem that may require rotation to another corticosteroid, cessation of the drug, or treatment with neuroleptics.

Dexamethasone has a long half-life and need only be dosed once a day. Typical doses start at 0.1–1.5 mg/kg (maximum 4–10 mg) daily.

Tricyclic antidepressants (TCAs): There are no data that TCAs provide better analgesia than gabapentinoids. The reason that TCAs are often the first adjuvant include once-a-night dosing options (vs. three times per day for gabapentin) and the significant sedative effect at night, often improving insomnia. However, some centers (especially in the setting

TABLE 16.6 Adjuvant analgesia in neuropathic pediatric pain management (Pain Medicine & Palliative Care, Children's Hospitals and Clinics of Minnesota)[a]

Class	Medication	Dose	Route of Administration	Comments/side effects (see text for further details)
Tricyclic antidepressants (TCAs)	Amitriptyline	Starting dose 0.1 mg/kg at bedtime, usually slowly titrated up to 0.5 mg/kg (maximum 1–2 mg/kg)	Oral	Tertiary amine TCA; stronger anticholinergic side effects (including sedation) than nortriptyline
	Nortriptyline	Starting dose 0.1 mg/kg at bedtime, usually titrated up to 0.5 mg/kg (maximum 1 mg/kg)	Oral	Secondary amine TCA; anticholinergic side effects
Gabapentenoids	Gabapentin	Starting dose 2 mg/kg at bedtime, usually slowly titrated up to initial target dose of 6 mg/kg/dose three times daily (maximum 300 mg/dose three times daily). Maximum dose escalation to 24 mg/kg/dose three times daily (maximum 1200 mg/dose three times daily)	Oral	Slow dose increase required; side effects: ataxia, nystagmus, myalgia, hallucination, dizziness, somnolence, aggressive behaviors, hyperactivity, thought disorder, peripheral edema
	Pregabaline	Starting dose 0.3 mg/kg at bedtime, usually slowly titrated up to initial target dose of 1.5 mg/kg/dose twice daily (maximum 75 mg/dose twice daily); maximum dose escalation to 6 mg/kg/dose twice daily (maximum 300 mg/dose twice daily)	Oral	Switch from gabapentin if distressing side effects or inadequate analgesia; side effects: ataxia, nystagmus, myalgia, hallucination, dizziness, somnolence, aggressive behaviors, hyperactivity, thought disorder, peripheral edema; associated with weight gain
Sodium channel blocker/local anesthetic	Lidocaine 5%	Maximum of 4 patches (in patients > 50 kg) 12 h on/12 h off	Transdermal patch	Not for severe hepatic dysfunction
Glucocorticoid	Dexamethasone	0.1–1.5 mg/kg (maximum 10 mg) starting dose, then 0.1–0.25 mg/kg twice/d (for < 14 days) (Malignant spinal cord compression [adult dose]: dexamethason 16–96 mg/d or equivalent)	Oral, IV	Add gastroprotective agent
NMDA receptor antagonist	Ketamine (racemic mixture of S(+)/R(-) enantiomers)	IV: 0.06–0.3 mg/kg/h Oral: 0.2–0.5 mg/kg three or four times daily and as needed	IV, oral, (SC, SL, intranasal, rectal, spinally)	Typical side effects rare at low dose, but would require benzodiazepine administration
α-Agonist	Dexmedetomidine	Infusion: 0.3 μg/kg/h; titrate to maximum 2 μg/kg/h	IV	
	Clonidine	1–3 μg/kg every 4–6 h	Oral	

[a]Used with permission: Stefan Friedrichsdorf, Benioff Children's Hospitals in Oakland and San Francisco, University of California at San Francisco (UCSF).

of QTc prolongation, already significant underlying constipation/urinary retention, etc.) choose gabapentinoids first, possibly followed by a TCA later in the treatment trajectory.

As discussed below, it may take days or weeks for TCAs and/or gabapentinoids to produce an analgesic effect, so in select cases this time period might be bridged by (or combined with) low-dose ketamine.

Adverse effects of all TCAs include arrhythmia and anticholinergic/antihistamine effects, such as dry mouth, constipation, urinary retention, blurred vision, and sedation. Nortriptyline (a secondary amine) may be better tolerated than amitriptyline (a tertiary amine) because it has fewer anticholinergic side effects. The side effect of inducing sleepiness can be particularly helpful for patients with concomitant insomnia when the medication is given at nighttime. Occasionally, the anticholinergic effects of dry mouth, sedation, constipation, and urinary retention limit the usefulness of this medication. However, a slow increase over several days generally reduces the onset of side effects. A rotation from amitriptyline to nortriptyline might decrease the anticholinergic side effects as well.

Both agents, which also come as a liquid, are usually started at 0.1 mg/kg by mouth at bedtime (adult dose 5 mg) and increased to a maximum of 0.4–0.5 mg (maximum 20–25 mg at bedtime). There is anecdotal evidence that increasing beyond that dose (to 1–2 mg/kg [50–100 mg]) does not result in an increased analgesic effect. It may take 1–2 weeks to titrate up to an effective dose and to determine if the analgesic therapy is working, although the induction of sleep will start much sooner. An electrocardiogram to rule out QTc prolongation/Wolff-Parkinson-White syndrome prior to initiation should be considered; however, administered doses for neuropathic pain are usually low compared to "antidepressant" dosing. Of note, despite the name, TCAs do not improve anxiety/depression in children.

Case Part 7

Although Emma had better analgesia since her opioid hydromorphone was titrated to effect, she continued to display significant neuropathic pain in her leg and buttock. An adjuvant analgesic was added. Her weight was 30 kg, and she started with amitriptyline 3 mg once at night, slowly increased every second day by 3 mg to a maximum of 12 mg once at night. She immediately reported improved sleep initiation and felt more rested the next day. Her average pain score in her leg decreased over the next 2 weeks to about 2–3/10. No clear anticholinergic side effects were noted: She already displayed underlying constipation (possibly worsened by the increase in opioid), which did require increases in laxatives, both stool softener "mush" and stimulants "push" plus occasional suppository.* She occasionally might have displayed some urinary retention. However, this was not daily and might have been more attributed to her primary tumor. A rotation to nortriptyline eventually was not necessary.

*No suppositories or rectal medication is administered when a patient is neutropenic and/or thrombocytopenic to reduce risk of bleeding/infection.

Gabapentin (alternative: pregabaline) is commonly used in pediatric pain management. An initial low starting dose is 2 mg/kg/dose (maximum 100 mg/dose) once at night titrated to 6 mg/kg/dose (maximum 300 mg/dose) three times/day. For mild-to-medium neuropathic pain, the titration may take up to 2 weeks to avoid side effects. For severe pain, the titration may be significantly faster (1–3 days). If analgesia is inadequate, the dose may be titrated in steps up to 12 mg/kg/dose (maximum 600 mg/dose) three times daily, then up to 18 mg/kg/dose (maximum 900 mg/dose) three times daily, and finally up to 24 mg/kg/dose (maximum 1200 mg/dose) three times daily. Side effects include lethargy, ataxia, nystagmus, dizziness, thought disorder, hallucinations, headache, peripheral edema, and myalgia; these side effects appear to be mitigated by slow dose escalation. Especially gabapentin and to a lesser degree pregabalin are commonly used in pediatric chronic pain management.[135,136]

Case Part 8

Emma enjoyed a fairly good quality of life and much better sleep and analgesia utilizing her integrated therapies. She especially enjoyed deep breathing and self-hypnosis. The scheduled opioid (hydromorphone) and amitriptyline for the last 4 weeks proved very helpful. Her dexamethasone was successfully weaned 2 weeks ago. Regular assessment of her distressing symptoms with the pediatric Memorial Symptom Assessment Scale (10–18) revealed some constipation, some worry, and increased pain.

Evaluating this further, in the last 2–3 days, she experienced recurrence of significant neuropathic pain in her left leg but did not mention it in order not to worry her parents and her younger brother. In addition to an increase of the hydromorphone by 50%, the decision was made to start her on gabapentin. Due to the acute worsening of her pain, her dose was escalated rapidly over 3 days from 200 mg at bedtime, to 200 mg and then 200 mg. In a less acute situation this titration may take 6–9 days. About a week later, she did not display significant side effects, but she also experienced only somewhat improved analgesia. The dose was escalated slowly to 400 mg and finally 600 mg, which was a dose where she seemed to have much better analgesia.

Lidocaine: A sodium channel blocker, such as intravenous or subcutaneous[137,138] continuous lidocaine infusion, appears to be effective in some children. A case series ($n = 5$) showed it to be effective after anti-GD2 antibody therapy in children with neuroblastoma at a dose of 1 mg/kg/h.[139] The published dose recommendation for lidocaine for neuropathic pain includes 1 mg/kg over 5 minutes or 2 mg/kg over 30 minutes, then 1 mg/h, with a target of 25 μg/mL.[140]

Side effects of intravenous lidocaine include allergic reaction (serious, but rare), and effects are dose related: numbness around mouth, dizziness, slurring of speech, hallucinations, muscle twitches, and seizures.[141]

Lidocaine patches are for localized pain only. The patch can be cut to fit and used for about 12 hours on/12 hours off. A contraindication would be severe hepatic dysfunction. Side effects include skin problems, such as irritation and redness.

Case Part 9

Although Emma's leg pain improved, as the gabapentin was increased, the maximum pain seemed to be localized over her left gluteus maximus muscle. A lidocaine patch (cut to fit) was administered 12 hours on, 12 hours off. Emma described it as "pretty helpful."

Ketamine has been found effective for pediatric neuropathic and acute pain in low (subanesthetic) doses, both alone and in combination with opioids. Ketamine is unique among anesthetic agents in that it does not depress respiratory and cardiovascular systems.

In low analgesic doses, the typical anesthetic dose side effects of ketamine (nystagmus, lacrimation, tachycardia, altered sensorium) are not usually seen, though there are limited pediatric data. Many pediatric centers schedule a low-dose benzodiazepine during the ketamine administration to avoid the rare potential psychomimetic side effects. There is evidence of significant opioid reductions in end-of-life pediatric cancer care after the initiation of low-dose ketamine. The advantage of ketamine in comparison to other frequently used adjuvant analgesia, such as anticonvulsants or antidepressants, is its rather immediate onset of action.

Case Part 10

About 5 weeks later, after good quality of life at home, Emma had a sudden pain crisis, which resulted in a hospitalization. Imagery showed a significant increase of her primary tumor and metastases. Her hydromorphone had been slowly titrated to effect over the weeks to the rather high dose of 7 mg/h intravenously with 7 mg PCA boluses. It was now escalated to 10 mg/h plus 10 mg PCA bolus. In weighing treatment options, her oncology and palliative care teams decided to trial low-dose ketamine prior to a rotation of hydromorphone to methadone.

She was started on 30 µg/min (1.8 mg/h) and slowly titrated over 36 hours up to 150 µg/min (9 mg/h) of intravenous ketamine. She did not display any psychomimetic side effects, so no benzodiazepine (which is ordered on an as-needed basis) was eventually given. Within about 6 hours, Emma reported significant reduction of discomfort.

Over the next 24 hours, her use of the hydromorphone PCA decreased from 55 boluses per day to 12 boluses per day, resulting in an opioid decrease of over 60%. She did not show any signs of opioid oversedation, so the continuous infusion of hydromorphone was not decreased as it would have been if any signs of oversedation had emerged.

Three days later, her hydromorphone was rotated to methadone. Six days later, her intravenous ketamine of 4 mg/h was switched to 25 mg oral ketamine every 4 hours. After discharge to home, 7 days later, Emma decided to change the ketamine to as-needed only, about twice per day, and discontinued the ketamine another week later, stating, "I don't need it anymore."

The **α-2-adrenergic** agonists such as **clonidine** or **dexmedetomidine** can be particularly effective adjuvant analgesics for both nociceptive and neuropathic pain in our experience. Clonidine can be given orally or transdermally or delivered intraspinally (some centers administer it intravenously). Side effects include lethargy, dry mouth, and hypotension.

Dexmedetomidine can also be an effective adjuvant, leading to opioid sparing. It has the advantage of not affecting respirations. However, its use is occasionally limited by side effects of hypotension and bradycardia, leading most institutions to restrict its use to intensive care units.

Case Part 11

During Emma's hospitalization, after initiation of low-dose ketamine, her high-dose hydromorphone was rotated to methadone. She started to display renal dysfunction, with a creatinine rise to 3.4, so the clinical team worried about accumulation of "the bad guy," the metabolite hydromorphone-3-glucoronide, which acts in a nociceptive (e.g., increased pain) fashion and is renally cleared. Some team members expressed worry about opioid-induced hyperalgesia, although Emma did not seem to display this. Additional hydromorphone PCA boluses decreased her pain rather than increased it. However, her constipation had worsened. Since it was unclear how much of this was opioid induced versus caused by her primary tumor, which by this time extended well into her abdomen, rotation methadone (due to its significantly lower dose) with an N-methyl-D-aspartate (NMDA) receptor–blocking mechanism appeared a good choice.

Her very high dose of hydromorphone (10 mg/h) was rotated initially to 30 mg methadone/d orally (conversion range between 30 and 60 mg/d]. On day 1, she received 5 mg methadone every 4 hours by mouth; on day 2, she received 7.5 mg every 6 hours; and on day 3, the dose was 10 mg every 8 hours. The continuous infusion of hydromorphone was discontinued after the second methadone dose, and she continued on a PCA bolus only of 10 mg hydromorphone. On day 5, the methadone dose was increased to 13 mg every 8 hours, which was her final dose for the next 6 weeks. She continued initially with hydromorphone PCA. However, 2 weeks later she requested to be discontinued from all pumps (she had only required about three or four PCA boluses/day), and the as needed dose was switched to 4 mg methadone orally every 4 hours as needed in addition to her scheduled methadone or 13 mg every 8 hours to a maximum of three doses per day. She had daily home visits to ensure the safety of the regimen, and Emma's parents were instructed to hold any methadone administration if she were to show any signs of opioid oversedation. Her constipation and her analgesia improved significantly over the next few days.

Of note: Methadone should not be prescribed by those unfamiliar with its use: Its effects should be closely monitored for several days, particularly when it is first started and after any dose changes.

Marijuana

Cannabis and medical marijuana (including cannabidiol [CBD] and delta-(9)-tetrahydrocannabinol [THC]) lack any evidence to support use for acute or chronic pain.[142,143] The updated American Academy of Pediatrics policy opposes marijuana use,[144] citing lack of research and potential harms, including correlation with mental illness,[145] testicular cancer,[146–148] decline in IQ,[149,150] and increased risk of addiction.[151] In our clinical practice, we do not support the use of marijuana (or medical cannabis) for a child with a primary pain disorder and a normal life expectancy. However, in children with life-limiting conditions, the administration of medical cannabis is often requested by patients and their parents and certainly may be supported on a case-by-case basis, carefully watching for side effects (including pancreatitis, psychosis, etc.).

Regional Anesthesia

The majority of PPC patients with pain due to tissue injury to date unfortunately do not receive one of the most effective analgesic modalities, which would prevent and treat unrelieved pain with the fewest side effects: regional or neuroaxial anesthesia.[152–157] Especially if tissue injury, such as tumor pain, of an extremity or the trunk requires hospitalization, it must now be expected standard of care to ensure assessment of the infant, child, or adolescent by an anesthesiologist for potential regional anesthesia. Blocking pain nociception using a local anesthetic such as bubivacaine, in some cases in conjunction with an opioid and/or α-agonist, can provide complete analgesia without any of the opioid-induced side effects. Pain pathways can be blocked when an anesthesiologist trained in regional anesthesia utilizes central neuraxial infusions, peripheral nerve and plexus blocks or infusions, or neurolytic blocks.[158] Occasionally implanted intrathecal ports and pumps for baclofen, opioids, local anesthetics, and other adjuvants might be considered.

Benefits of regional anesthesia include[159]

- significantly reduced or eliminated need for opioids
- no systemic side effects
- no sedation
- no nausea
- minimal side effects (itching, urinary retention) with epidural
- improved gastrointestinal motility
- fewer postoperative cardiac arrhythmias
- significantly reduced pulmonary complications
- significantly reduced delirium
- improved mobility, which reduces rates of deep vein thrombosis
- extremely high patient satisfaction
- ability to stay awake and remember conversations with clinicians and family
- evidence for reduction of development of chronic pain and phantom pain

Because the nociceptive nerves cannot be numbed independent of all the other nerves that receive local anesthesia, there are side effects such as motor weakness, hypotension, pruritus, or urinary retention.[160] If the patient has breakthrough pain that breaks through a low continuous infusion of the local anesthetic, a PCA bolus allows the patient to give him- or herself additional medication as needed, called patient-controlled regional analgesia (PCRA). Similar to an opioid PCA, the patient can use their PCRA button for breakthrough pain, but without the side effects caused by opioids. Patients can be sent home with a nerve block catheter connected to a disposable pump or one that is returned to the hospital. There are no opioids in the infusion, eliminating misuse potential. That may lead to fewer adverse events, including sedation, delirium, sleep disturbances, and opioid-induced hyperalgesia.

Case Part 12

During Emma's last hospitalization 6 weeks ago she was assessed by a pediatric anesthesiologist, and a tunneled epidural catheter was considered. If the above regimen would not have been successful, she would have been sent home with an epidural catheter. These often last for weeks at home and have been shown to be very effective. However, the team worked hard to keep her care regimen as simple, as least restrictive, and as effective as possible for ease of management at home. Emma continued to receive palliative care visits at home and occasional oncology clinic visits and had a fairly good quality of life. As her condition declined, her parents were able to coach her in using her well-practiced creative visualization skills, which helped her focus on comfort and relax. She celebrated her 13th birthday at home with her family and friends and died peacefully 2 days later, at home.

Physician Assistants in Pain Medicine and Palliative Care

Collaboration with physicians has been a hallmark of PA practice since the profession's inception, and this continues in pediatric pain medicine and palliative care. PAs are formally recognized as part of the interdisciplinary pain and palliative care team and are integral in their role to provide pain and nonpain symptom management. They are also many times the interlocutors with other members of the healthcare team, patients, and their families.

The discipline of pain and palliative care is rooted in a model based on comprehension. The pain and palliative care team seeks to address the patient's physical suffering while simultaneously addressing the individual's psychosocial needs. The discipline's holistic approach encourages the team to address the patient and family as a whole person by treating their mind, body, and spirit in an interdisciplinary fashion.

A multifaceted approach to pain control is typically the optimal approach for the increasingly complex treatment of pain in children and teenagers with potentially life-limiting diseases. The integration of pharmacological and anesthetic interventions can and should be supplemented with holistic approaches that include, but are not limited to, rehabilitation therapy and other integrative (nonpharmacological) therapies that should be applied on an age-appropriate basis. See above for safe and effective age-appropriate modalities, such as massage, distraction, self-hypnosis, biofeedback, acupuncture, acupressure, music and art therapy, and more. Furthermore, evidence-based, pain-minimizing treatments should always accompany elective painful procedures performed on children.

There is a compounding complexity in the field of pediatric pain and palliative care as the assessment of an individual's pain could present itself in a variety of different forms given the child's age and ability to communicate their needs and symptoms. For example, the frequent inability of patients to directly articulate nausea could result in falsely chasing a variety of solutions that will ultimately prove ineffective. Strong associative emotions, such as fear, also cloud the direct path to understanding and subsequently treating root causes of pain.

They are adjacent mechanisms that feed off one another. At times the experience of acute pain from a severely fractured bone in a young child may play a role in the perception of pain that they later experience once the fracture is definitively treated. It is crucial to treat these children's pain appropriately so they realize they no longer need to fear the pain that they previously experienced. This benefits not only the child and family but also the provider in terms of being able to have a more reliable physical examination. Other barriers to solution implementation could range from basic language barriers to effectively level setting expectations versus family's wishes.

The field of pain and palliative care continues to be on an aggressive growth trajectory in its breadth of programs as well as widening the pool of potential caregivers. Not surprisingly, PA-Cs have been a front runner in leading the category's exponential growth. The parallels in teaching methodologies between PA-Cs (physician assistant, certified) and physicians create a natural fit for PAs to benefit from and participate in the palliative care ecosystem. Beyond a conceptual fit, PA-Cs are being formally recognized for their unique qualifications in the field of palliative care. For example, "A recent amendment made to HR 1284—Medicare Patient Access to Hospice Act of 2017—now recognizes PA-Cs as a 'distinct and important part of the hospice interdisciplinary team with the ability to provide care to terminally ill Medicare patients.' This allows PA-Cs to effectively serve as the attending physician for hospice patients, according to the National Hospice and Palliative Care Organization."[160] Not only does this positively impact labor shortages in a high-demand and vital field, but also it inherently expands the role and freedoms of PA-Cs to more directly drive patient care. In addition, recent long-term grants have been funded to incentivize and support educational programs for PAs in the field of pain and palliative care.

The PA's role as a provider is to practice high-quality, patient-centered care. It is imperative and necessary that we value and take into account the physical, psychological, social, spiritual, and emotional toll that therapeutic treatments, procedures, and the overall health-care experience can have on patients and their families. This type of care and understanding is at the forefront in pain and palliative care.

Additional Training in Pediatric Palliative Care
Postgraduate PPC Training

There are different levels of PPC training: primary, advanced, and subspecialty training.[161]

- Examples of *Level 1: Primary PPC* training (i.e., educational content for staff integrating a PPC approach as part of their pediatric clinical services) include the International Children's Palliative Care Network e-learning courses,[162] which are available in 11 languages and free of charge, as well as the End-of-Life Nursing Education Consortium.[163]
- At *Level 2: Advanced Primary PPC/Introductory Subspecialty PPC*, EPEC-Pediatrics (Education in Palliative and End-of-Life Care) has now been developed as the most comprehensive PPC curriculum and dissemination "train-the-trainer" project worldwide. The curriculum originally had not been designed to train PPC specialists, but rather to give clinicians comprehensive tools to teach core PPC to interdisciplinary teams and promote best PPC practices by hematologists/oncologists and other pediatric specialists. However,

since its inception, feedback was received that it is also used for training for PPC specialists, both inside and outside designated fellowship programs.

- *Level 3: Subspecialty PPC* training encompasses postgraduate training for clinicians providing PPC services as a professional career and includes formal physician fellowships, including 47 one-year pediatric (or adult fellowships with a pediatric tract) in hospice and palliative medicine offered in the United States,[164] at least three fellowships in Australia, at least two 2-year fellowships in Canada, plus at least one formal postgraduate training/fellowship in each of New Zealand, United Kingdom, Argentina, Costa Rica, and South Africa. In addition, a very limited number of fellowships exist for social workers and nurse practitioners. University diplomas in PPC are available in Australia,[165] Belgium,[166] Ireland,[167] Portugal,[168] South Africa,[169] Uganda,[170] Italy,[171,172] and the United Kingdom.[173] Advanced leadership courses include Palliative Care Education and Practice, which is offered in the United States by the Harvard Center for Palliative Care in Cambridge, Massachusetts.[174,175]

Conclusion

The effective prevention and treatment of pain in children and teenagers with life-limiting diseases often require intensive "multimodal" pain control. Safe multimodal analgesia[91] may include one, several, or all of the following approaches: pharmacology (e.g., simple analgesia and/or opioids and/or adjuvant analgesia); anesthetic interventions (e.g., neuroaxial analgesia, nerve blocks); rehabilitation (e.g., physical therapy, occupational therapy, sleep hygiene); psychology (e.g., CBT); and age-appropriate positioning and integrative (nonpharmacological) therapies, such as breathing techniques, self-hypnosis, and distraction.

Also, it is inappropriate to perform elective painful procedures (e.g., wound dressing changes, blood draws, intravenous cannulations, injections, lumbar punctures, etc.) in children without evidence-based treatments to avoid or minimize pain.

Acknowledgments

The case scenario of "Emma," and associated parts of this chapter, are based on the Education in Palliative and End-of-Life Care for Pediatrics Curriculum (EPEC-Pediatrics), "Module 12: Neuropathic Pain."[176] For information about the EPEC-Pediatrics train-the-trainer" courses see https://www.bioethics.northwestern.edu/programs/epec/curricula/pediatrics.html or contact EPEC.Pediatrics@childrensMN.org.

References

1. Connor SR, Downing J, Marston J. Estimating the global need for palliative care for children: a cross-sectional analysis. *Journal of Pain and Symptom Management*. 2017;53(2):171–177.
2. World Health Organization. Palliative care. 1998. https://www.who.int/cancer/palliative/definition/en
3. Together for Short Lives. Introductions to children's palliative care.]; http://www.togetherforshortlives.org.uk/professionals/childrens_palliative_care_essentials/definitions. Accessed May 22nd, 2019
4. World Health Organization. *WHO Definition of Palliative Care*. 1998. May 25 2019.

5. American Academy of Pediatrics. Committee on Bioethics and Committee on Hospital Care. *Palliative Care for Children Pediatrics.* 2000 Aug;106(2 Pt 1):351–357. PMID:10920167.

6. Pediatric palliative care and hospice care commitments, guidelines, and recommendations. Section on hospice and palliative medicine and committee on hospital care. *Pediatrics.* 2013;*132*(5):966–972. doi:10.1542/peds.2013-2731

7. Wood F, et al. Disease trajectories and ACT/RCPCH categories in paediatric palliative care. *Palliative Medicine.* 2010;*24*(8):796–806.

8. Feudtner C, Christakis DA, Connell FA. Pediatric deaths attributable to complex chronic conditions: a population-based study of Washington State, 1980–1997. *Pediatrics.* 2000;*106*(1 Pt 2):205–209.

9. Fraser LK, et al. Rising national prevalence of life-limiting conditions in children in England. *Pediatrics.* 2012;*129*(4):e923–e929.

10. Hain R, et al. Paediatric palliative care: development and pilot study of a "directory" of life-limiting conditions. *BMC Palliative Care.* 2013;*12*(1):43.

11. Siden H, et al. Characteristics of a pediatric hospice palliative care program over 15 years. *Pediatrics* 2014;*134*(3):e765.

12. World Health Organization. *Integrating Palliative Care and Symptom Relief Into Paediatrics: A WHO Guide for Health Care Planners, Implementers And Managers.* 2018. https://apps.who.int/iris/bitstream/handle/10665/274561/9789241514453-eng.pdf?ua=1. Accessed May 30th 2019.

13. Wolfe, J., et al. Symptoms and suffering at the end of life in children with cancer. *New England Journal of Medicine.* 2000;*342*(5):326–333.

14. Drake R, Frost J, Collins JJ. The symptoms of dying children. *Journal of Pain and Symptom Management.* 2003;*26*(1):594–603.

15. Heath JA, et al. Symptoms and suffering at the end of life in children with cancer: an Australian perspective. *Medical Journal of Australia.* 2010;*192*(2):71–75.

16. Zimmermann K, et al. When parents face the death of their child: a nationwide cross-sectional survey of parental perspectives on their child's end-of life care. *BMC Palliative Care.* 2016;*15*:30.

17. Contro N, et al. Family perspectives on the quality of pediatric palliative care. *JAMA Pediatrics.* 2002;*156*(1):14–19.

18. Steele AC, et al. Bereaved parents and siblings offer advice to health care providers and researchers. *Journal of Pediatric Hematology/Oncology.* 2013;*35*(4):253–259.

19. Alderfer MA, et al. Psychosocial adjustment of siblings of children with cancer: a systematic review. *Psychooncology.* 2010;*19*(8):789–805.

20. Malcolm C, et al. A relational understanding of sibling experiences of children with rare life-limiting conditions: findings from a qualitative study. *Journal of Child Health Care.* 2014;*18*(3):230–240.

21. Fullerton JM, et al. Siblings of children with life-limiting conditions: psychological adjustment and sibling relationships. *Child: Care, Health and Development.* 2017;*43*(3):393–400.

22. Gaab EM, Owens GR, MacLeod RD. Siblings caring for and about pediatric palliative care patients. *Journal of Palliative Medicine.* 2014;*17*(1):62–67.

23. Jones BL, Contro N, Koch KD. The duty of the physician to care for the family in pediatric palliative care: context, communication, and caring. *Pediatrics.* 2014;*133*(Suppl 1):S8.

24. Himelstein BP, et al. Pediatric palliative care. *New England Journal of Medicine.* 2004;*350*(17):1752–1762.

25. Feudtner C. A commitment to making the emerging field of pediatric palliative care the very best it can be. *Culture of Health Blog.* 2014.]; https://www.rwjf.org/en/blog/2014/06/a_commitment_to_maki.html. Accessed May 30, 2019.

26. Ramsey RJM, M.S. Policy review and recommendations: palliative care for pediatric patients in the United States of America. *Journal of Community and Public Health Nursing.* 2016;*2*:144.

27. Mary J. Labyak Institute for Innovation. *Pediatric Concurrent Care.* 2016. https://www.nhpco.org/sites/default/files/public/ChiPPS/Continuum_Briefing.pdf

28. Goldman A. Symptoms and suffering at the end of life in children with cancer. *New England Journal of Medicine.* 2000;*342*(26):1998.

29. Hongo T., et al. Analysis of the circumstances at the end of life in children with cancer: symptoms, suffering and acceptance. *Pediatrics International.* 2003;*45*(1):60–64.

30. Feudtner C, et al. Pediatric palliative care patients: a prospective multicenter cohort study. *Pediatrics.* 2011;*127*(6):1094–1101.

31. Wolfe J, et al. Symptoms and suffering at the end of life in children with cancer. *New England Journal of Medicine*. 2000;*342*(5):326–333.

32. Wolfe J, et al. Easing of suffering in children with cancer at the end of life: is care changing? *Journal of Clinical Oncology*. 2008;*26*(10):1717–1723.

33. Friedrichsdorf SJ, et al. Improved quality of life at end of life related to home-based palliative care in children with cancer. *Journal of Palliative Medicine*. 2015;*18*(2):143–150.

34. Wolfe J, et al. Symptoms and distress in children with advanced cancer: prospective patient-reported outcomes from the PediQUEST Study. *Journal of Clinical Oncology*. 2015;*33*(17):1928–1935.

35. Friedrichsdorf SJ, et al. Pain reporting and analgesia management in 270 children with a progressive neurologic, metabolic or chromosomally based condition with impairment of the central nervous system: cross-sectional, baseline results from an observational, longitudinal study. *Journal of Pain Research*. 2017;*10*:1841–1852.

36. Friedrichsdorf SJ, Garcia WCG. Assessment, prevention, and treatment of pain in children with serious illness. In J. Downing (Ed.), *Children's Palliative Care: An International Case-Based Manual*. New York: Springer, 2020:65–94.

37. Dame Cicely Saunders [Obituary]. *BMJ*. 2005;*331*(7510):238.

38. Seers T, et al. Professionals underestimate patients' pain: a comprehensive review. *Pain*. 2018;*159*(5):811–818.

39. Krechel SW, Bildner J. CRIES: a new neonatal postoperative pain measurement score. Initial testing of validity and reliability. *Paediatric Anaesthesia*. 1995;*5*(1):53–61.

40. Merkel S, Voepel-Lewis T, Malviya S. Pain assessment in infants and young children: the FLACC scale. *American Journal of Nursing*. 2002;*102*(10):55–58.

41. Willis MH, et al. FLACC Behavioral Pain Assessment Scale: a comparison with the child's self-report. *Pediatric Nursing*. 2003;*29*(3):195–198.

42. van Dijk M, et al. The reliability and validity of the COMFORT scale as a postoperative pain instrument in 0 to 3-year-old infants. *Pain*. 2000;*84*(2–3):367–377.

43. Malviya S, et al. The revised FLACC observational pain tool: improved reliability and validity for pain assessment in children with cognitive impairment. *Paediatric Anaesthesia*, 2006. *16*(3):258–265.

44. Hunt A, et al. Clinical validation of the paediatric pain profile. *Developmental Medicine and Child Neurology*. 2004;*46*(1):9–18.

45. Breau LM, et al. Psychometric properties of the non-communicating children's pain checklist-revised. *Pain*. 2002;*99*(1–2):349–357.

46. Emmott AS, et al. Validity of simplified versus standard self-report measures of pain intensity in preschool-aged children undergoing venipuncture. *Journal of Pain*. 2017;*18*(5):564–573.

47. Hicks CL, et al. The Faces Pain Scale–Revised: toward a common metric in pediatric pain measurement. *Pain*. 2001;*93*(2):173–183.

48. Bailey B, Gravel J, Daoust R. Reliability of the visual analog scale in children with acute pain in the emergency department. *Pain*. 2012;*153*(4):839–842.

49. von Baeyer CL, et al. Three new datasets supporting use of the Numerical Rating Scale (NRS-11) for children's self-reports of pain intensity. *Pain*. 2009;*143*(3):23–27.

50. Taddio A, et al. Inadequate pain management during routine childhood immunizations: the nerve of it. *Clinical Therapeutics*. 2009;*31*(Suppl 2):S152–S167.

51. Taddio A, et al. Reducing the pain of childhood vaccination: an evidence-based clinical practice guideline. *CMAJ*. 2010;*182*(18):E843–855.

52. Friedrichsdorf SJ, et al. A hospital-wide initiative to eliminate or reduce needle pain in children using lean methodology. *Pain Reports*. 2018;*3*(Suppl 1):e671.

53. Taddio A, et al. Impact of parent-directed education on parental use of pain treatments during routine infant vaccinations: a cluster randomized trial. *Pain*. 2015;*156*(1):185–191.

54. Taddio A, et al. Procedural and physical interventions for vaccine injections: systematic review of randomized controlled trials and quasi-randomized controlled trials. *Clinical Journal of Pain*. 2015;*31*(10 Suppl):S20–S37.

55. Postier AC, et al. Pain experience in a US children's hospital: a point prevalence survey undertaken after the implementation of a system-wide protocol to eliminate or decrease pain caused by needles. *Hospital Pediatrics*. 2018;*8*(9):515–523.

56. Goubert L, Friedrichsdorf SJ. Factsheet: Pain in children: management. Global year against pain in the vulnerable. International Association for the Study of Pain. 2019. https://europeanpainfederation.eu/wp-content/uploads/2019/02/8-Pain-in-Children-Management555.pdf

57. Friedrichsdorf SJ, Sidman J, Krane EJ. Prevention and treatment of pain in children: toward a paradigm shift. *Otolaryngology—Head and Neck Surgery.* 2016;*154*(5):804–805.

58. Taddio A, et al. Relative effectiveness of additive pain interventions during vaccination in infants. *CMAJ.* 2016;*189*(5):E227–E234.

59. Koh JL, et al. A randomized, double-blind comparison study of EMLA and ELA-Max for topical anesthesia in children undergoing intravenous insertion. *Paediatric Anaesthesia.* 2004;*14*(12):977–982.

60. Eichenfield LF, et al. A clinical study to evaluate the efficacy of ELA-Max (4% liposomal lidocaine) as compared with eutectic mixture of local anesthetics cream for pain reduction of venipuncture in children. *Pediatrics.* 2002;*109*(6):1093–1099.

61. Lunoe MM, et al. A randomized clinical trial of jet-injected lidocaine to reduce venipuncture pain for young children. *Annals of Emergency Medicine.* 2015;*66*(5):466–474.

62. Lunoe MM, Drendel AL, Brousseau DC. The use of the needle-free jet injection system with buffered lidocaine device does not change intravenous placement success in children in the emergency department. *Academic Emergency Medicine.* 2015;*22*(4):447–451.

63. Schreiber S, et al. Does EMLA cream application interfere with the success of venipuncture or venous cannulation? A prospective multicenter observational study. *European Journal of Pediatrics.* 2013;*172*(2):265–268.

64. Taddio A, et al. Reducing the pain of childhood vaccination: an evidence-based clinical practice guideline (summary). *CMAJ.* 2010;*182*(18):1989–1995.

65. CHEO's Be Sweet to Babies research team and the University of Ottawa's School of Nursing. Be sweet to babies. 2014. https://www.cheo.on.ca/en/clinics-services-programs/be-sweet-to-babies.aspx

66. Shah PS, et al. Breastfeeding or breast milk for procedural pain in neonates. *Cochrane Database of Systematic Reviews.* 2012;*12*:CD004950.

67. Stevens B, et al. Sucrose for analgesia in newborn infants undergoing painful procedures. *Cochrane Database of Systematic Reviews.* 2016;*7*:CD001069.

68. Gao H, et al. Efficacy and safety of repeated oral sucrose for repeated procedural pain in neonates: a systematic review. *International Journal of Nursing Studies.* 2016;*62*:118–125.

69. Stevens B, et al. The minimally effective dose of sucrose for procedural pain relief in neonates: a randomized controlled trial. *BMC Pediatrics.* 2018;*18*(1):85.

70. Gray L, et al. Sucrose and warmth for analgesia in healthy newborns: an RCT. *Pediatrics.* 2015;*135*(3):e607–e614.

71. Gray, L., C.W. Lang, and S.W. Porges, Warmth is analgesic in healthy newborns. *Pain,* 2012;*153*(5):960–966.

72. Campbell-Yeo M, et al. Trial of repeated analgesia with Kangaroo Mother Care (TRAKC Trial). *BMC Pediatrics.* 2013;*13*:182.

73. Campbell-Yeo ML, et al. Co-bedding between preterm twins attenuates stress response after heel lance: results of a randomized trial. *Clinical Journal of Pain.* 2014;*30*(7):598–604.

74. Johnston C, et al. Skin-to-skin care for procedural pain in neonates. *Cochrane Database of Systematic Reviews.* 2014;*1*:CD008435.

75. Campbell-Yeo ML, et al. Understanding kangaroo care and its benefits to preterm infants. *Pediatric Health, Medicine, and Therapeutics.* 2015;*6*:15–32.

76. Benoit B, et al. Staff nurse utilization of kangaroo care as an intervention for procedural pain in preterm infants. *Advances in Neonatal Care.* 2016;*16*(3):229–238.

77. Campbell-Yeo M, et al. Sustained efficacy of kangaroo care for repeated painful procedures over neonatal intensive care unit hospitalization: a single-blind randomized controlled trial. *Pain.* 2019;*160*(11):2580–2588.

78. Karlson K, Darcy L, Enskär K. The use of restraint is never supportive. Poster presented at: Nordic Society of Pediatric Hematology/Oncology (NOPHO) 34th Annual Meeting 2016 and 11th Biannual Meeting of Nordic Society of Pediatric Oncology Nurses (NOBOS); May 2016; Reykjavik, Iceland.

79. Uman LS, et al. Psychological interventions for needle-related procedural pain and distress in children and adolescents. *Cochrane Database of Systematic Reviews.* 2013;(10):CD005179.

80. Schechter NL, Allen DA, Hanson K. Status of pediatric pain control: a comparison of hospital analgesic usage in children and adults. *Pediatrics*. 1986;*77*(1):11–15.

81. Broome ME, et al. Pediatric pain practices: a national survey of health professionals. *Journal of Pain and Symptom Management,* 1996;*11*(5):312–320.

82. Birnie KA, et al. Psychological interventions for needle-related procedural pain and distress in children and adolescents. *Cochrane Database of Systematic Reviews*. 2018;*10*:CD005179.

83. Friedrichsdorf SJ. Nitrous gas analgesia and sedation for lumbar punctures in children: has the time for practice change come? *Pediatric Blood & Cancer*. 2017;*64*(11). doi:10.1002/pbc.26625

84. Hockenberry MJ, et al. Managing painful procedures in children with cancer. *Journal of Pediatric Hematology/Oncology*. 2011;*33*(2):119–127.

85. Pedersen RS, et al. Nitrous oxide provides safe and effective analgesia for minor paediatric procedures—a systematic review. *Danish Medical Journal*. 2013;*60*(6):A4627.

86. Tobias JD. Applications of nitrous oxide for procedural sedation in the pediatric population. *Pediatric Emergency Care*. 2013;*29*(2):245–265.

87. Zier JL, Liu M. Safety of high-concentration nitrous oxide by nasal mask for pediatric procedural sedation: experience with 7802 cases. *Pediatric Emergency Care*. 2011;*27*(12):1107–1112.

88. Livingston M, Lawell M, McAllister N. Successful use of nitrous oxide during lumbar punctures: a call for nitrous oxide in pediatric oncology clinics. *Pediatric Blood & Cancer*. 2017;*64*(11). doi:10.1002/pbc.26610

89. American Society of Anesthesiologists Task Force on Sedation and Anesthesia by Non-Anesthesiologists. Practice guidelines for sedation and analgesia by non-anesthesiologists. *Anesthesiology*. 2002;*96*(4):1004–1017.

90. Friedrichsdorf SJ. Cancer pain management in children. In: Farquhar-Smith P, Wigmore T, eds. *Anaesthesia, Intensive Care, and Pain Management for the Cancer Patient*. Oxford: Oxford University Press; 2011:215–227.

91. Friedrichsdorf SJ. Prevention and treatment of pain in hospitalized infants, children, and teenagers: from myths and morphine to multimodal analgesia. In: Sommer CL, Wallace MS, Cohen SP, Kress M, eds. *Pain 2016: Refresher Courses. 16th World Congress on Pain*. Washington, DC: IASP Press; 2016:309–319.

92. World Health Organization. WHO—principles of acute pain management for children. 2012. http://whqlibdoc.who.int/publications/2012/9789241548120_Guidelines.pdf

93. Moore RA, et al. Faster, higher, stronger? Evidence for formulation and efficacy for ibuprofen in acute pain. *Pain*. 2014;*155*(1):14–21.

94. de Leeuw TG, et al. The use of dipyrone (metamizol) as an analgesic in children: what is the evidence? A review. *Paediatric Anaesthesia,* 2017;*27*(12):1193–1201.

95. Heubi JE, Barbacci MB, Zimmerman HJ. Therapeutic misadventures with acetaminophen: hepatoxicity after multiple doses in children. *Journal of Pediatrics*. 1998;*132*(1):22–27.

96. Drake R, Longworth J, Collins JJ. Opioid rotation in children with cancer. *Journal of Palliative Medicine*. 2004;*7*(3):419–422.

97. Friedrichsdorf SJ. From tramadol to methadone: opioids in the treatment of pain and dyspnea in pediatric palliative care. *Clinical Journal of Pain*. 2019;*35*(6):501–508.

98. Fife A, et al. Methadone conversion in infants and children: retrospective cohort study of 199 pediatric inpatients. *Journal of Opioid Management*. 2016;*12*(2):123–130.

99. Madden K, Bruera E. Very-low-dose methadone to treat refractory neuropathic pain in children with cancer. *Journal of Palliative Medicine,* 2017;*20*(11):1280–1283.

100. Mercadante S Bruera E. Methadone as a first-line opioid in cancer pain management: a systematic review. *Journal of Pain and Symptom Management*. 2018;*55*(3):998–1003.

101. Friedrichsdorf SJ. From tramadol to methadone: opioids in the treatment of pain and dyspnea in pediatric palliative care. *Clinical Journal of Pain,* 2019;*35*(6):501–508.

102. Bussing A, et al. Effects of yoga interventions on pain and pain-associated disability: a meta-analysis. *Journal of Pain*. 2012;*13*(1):1–9.

103. Evans S, et al. Iyengar yoga for young adults with rheumatoid arthritis: results from a mixed-methods pilot study. *Journal of Pain and Symptom Management*. 2010;*39*(5):904–913.

104. Vas J, et al. Acupuncture for fibromyalgia in primary care: a randomised controlled trial. *Acupunct Med*, 2016;*34*(4):257–266.

105. Verkamp EK, et al. A survey of conventional and complementary therapies used by youth with juvenile-onset fibromyalgia. *Pain Management Nursing*. 2013;*14*(4):e244–e250.

106. Friedrichsdorf S, et al. Integrative pediatric palliative care. In: Culbert T, Olness K, eds. *Integrative Pediatrics*. Oxford University Press; 2010:569–593.

107. Kuttner L, Friedrichsdorf SJ. Hypnosis and palliative care. In: *Therapeutic Hypnosis With Children and Adolescents*. Crown House; 2013:491–509.

108. Hunt K, Ernst E. The evidence-base for complementary medicine in children: a critical overview of systematic reviews. *Archives of Disease in Childhood*. 2011;*96*(8):769–776.

109. Evans S, Tsao JC, Zeltzer LK. Complementary and alternative medicine for acute procedural pain in children. *Alternative Therapies in Health and Medicine*. 2008;*14*(5):52–56.

110. Richardson J, et al. Hypnosis for procedure-related pain and distress in pediatric cancer patients: a systematic review of effectiveness and methodology related to hypnosis interventions. *Journal of Pain and Symptom Management*. 2006;*31*(1):70–84.

111. Friedrichsdorf SJ, Kohen DP. Integration of hypnosis into pediatric palliative care. *Annals of Palliative Medicine*. 2018;*7*(1):136–150.

112. Kohen DP, Olness KN. *Hypnosis and Hypnotherapy With Children*. New York, NY: Routledge;2011.

113. National Pediatric Hypnosis Training Institute. Home page. ; http://www.nphti.org. Accessed 2019.

114. Tegethoff M, et al. Comorbidity of mental disorders and chronic pain: chronology of onset in adolescents of a national representative cohort. *Journal of Pain*. 2015;*16*(10):1054–1064.

115. Cohen LL, Vowles KE, Eccleston C. The impact of adolescent chronic pain on functioning: disentangling the complex role of anxiety. *Journal of Pain*. 2010;*11*(11):1039–1046.

116. Palermo TM, et al. Randomized controlled trials of psychological therapies for management of chronic pain in children and adolescents: an updated meta-analytic review. *Pain*. 2010;*148*(3):387–397.

117. Eccleston C, et al. Psychological therapies for the management of chronic and recurrent pain in children and adolescents. *Cochrane Database of Systematic Reviews*. 2014;(5):CD003968.

118. Kashikar-Zuck S, et al. Changes in pain coping, catastrophizing, and coping efficacy after cognitive-behavioral therapy in children and adolescents with juvenile fibromyalgia. *Journal of Pain*. 2013;*14*(5):492–501.

119. Seminowicz DA, et al. Cognitive-behavioral therapy increases prefrontal cortex gray matter in patients with chronic pain. *Journal of Pain*. 2013. *14*(12):1573–1584.

120. Logan DE, et al. A day-hospital approach to treatment of pediatric complex regional pain syndrome: initial functional outcomes. *Clinical Journal of Pain*. 2012;*28*(9):766–774.

121. Eccleston C, et al. Chronic pain in adolescents: evaluation of a programme of interdisciplinary cognitive behaviour therapy. *Archives of Disease in Childhood*. 2003;*88*(10):881–885.

122. Maynard CS, et al. Interdisciplinary behavioral rehabilitation of pediatric pain-associated disability: retrospective review of an inpatient treatment protocol. *Journal of Pediatric Psychology*. 2010;*35*(2):128–137.

123. Palermo TM, Scher MS. Treatment of functional impairment in severe somatoform pain disorder: a case example. *Journal of Pediatric Psychology*. 2001;*26*(7):429–434.

124. Lynch-Jordan AM, et al. Differential changes in functional disability and pain intensity over the course of psychological treatment for children with chronic pain. *Pain*. 2014;*155*(10):1955–1961.

125. Sherry DD, et al. Short- and long-term outcomes of children with complex regional pain syndrome type I treated with exercise therapy. *Clinical Journal of Pain*. 1999;*15*(3):218–223.

126. Odell S, Logan DE. Pediatric pain management: the multidisciplinary approach. *Journal of Pain Research*. 2013;6:785–790.

127. Lee BH, et al. Physical therapy and cognitive-behavioral treatment for complex regional pain syndromes. *Journal of Pediatrics*. 2002;*141*(1):135–140.

128. Wilson AC, Palermo TM. Physical activity and function in adolescents with chronic pain: a controlled study using actigraphy. *Journal of Pain*. 2012;*13*(2):121–130.

129. Jerstad SJ, et al. Prospective reciprocal relations between physical activity and depression in female adolescents. *Journal of Consulting and Clinical Psychology*. 2010;*78*(2):268–272.

130. Ramsey LH, Karlson CW, Collier AB. Mirror therapy for phantom limb pain in a 7-year-old male with osteosarcoma. *Journal of Pain and Symptom Management*. 2017;*53*(6):e5–e7.

131. Hexem KR, et al. How parents of children receiving pediatric palliative care use religion, spirituality, or life philosophy in tough times. *Journal of Palliative Medicine*. 2011;*14*(1):39–44.

132. Borneman T, Ferrell B, Puchalski CM. Evaluation of the FICA Tool for spiritual assessment. *Journal of Pain and Symptom Management*. 2010;*40*(2):163–173.

133. Grossoehme DH, et al. Is adolescents' religious coping with cystic fibrosis associated with the rate of decline in pulmonary function? A preliminary study. *Journal of Health Care Chaplaincy*. 2013;*19*(1):33–42.

134. Reynolds N, Mrug S, and Guion K. Spiritual coping and psychosocial adjustment of adolescents with chronic illness: the role of cognitive attributions, age, and disease group. *Journal of Adolescent Health*. 2013;*52*(5):559–565.

135. Hauer JM, Solodiuk JC. Gabapentin for management of recurrent pain in 22 nonverbal children with severe neurological impairment: a retrospective analysis. *Journal of Palliative Medicine*. 2015;*18*(5):453–456.

136. Edwards L, et al. Gabapentin use in the neonatal intensive care unit. *Journal of Pediatrics*. 2016;*169*:310–312.

137. Peixoto RD, Hawley P. Intravenous lidocaine for cancer pain without electrocardiographic monitoring: a retrospective review. *Journal of Palliative Medicine*. 2015;*18*(4):373–377.

138. Seah DSE, et al. Subcutaneous lidocaine infusion for pain in patients with cancer. *Journal of Palliative Medicine*. 2017;*20*(6):667–671.

139. Wallace MS, et al. Intravenous lidocaine: effects on controlling pain after anti-GD2 antibody therapy in children with neuroblastoma—a report of a series. *Anesthesia and Analgesia*. 1997;*85*(4):794–796.

140. Massey GV, et al. Continuous lidocaine infusion for the relief of refractory malignant pain in a terminally ill pediatric cancer patient. *Journal of Pediatric Hematology/Oncology*. 2002;*24*(7):566–568.

141. Ferrini R, Paice JA. How to initiate and monitor infusional lidocaine for severe and/or neuropathic pain. *Journal of Supportive Oncology*. 2004;*2*(1):90–94.

142. Hill KP. Medical marijuana for treatment of chronic pain and other medical and psychiatric problems: a clinical review. *JAMA*. 2015;*313*(24):2474–2483.

143. Deshpande A, et al. Efficacy and adverse effects of medical marijuana for chronic noncancer pain: systematic review of randomized controlled trials. *Canadian Family Physician*. 2015;*61*(8):e372–e381.

144. Pediatrics, A.A.o. Updated AAP policy opposes marijuana use, citing potential harms, lack of research. 2015. http://aapnews.aappublications.org/content/early/2015/01/26/aapnews

145. Casadio P, et al. Cannabis use in young people: the risk for schizophrenia. *Neuroscience and Biobehavioral Reviews*. 2011;*35*(8):1779–1787.

146. Daling JR, et al. Association of marijuana use and the incidence of testicular germ cell tumors. *Cancer*. 2009;*115*(6):1215–1223.

147. Trabert B, et al. Marijuana use and testicular germ cell tumors. *Cancer*. 2011;*117*(4):848–853.

148. Lacson JC, et al. Population-based case-control study of recreational drug use and testis cancer risk confirms an association between marijuana use and nonseminoma risk. *Cancer*. 2012;*118*(21):5374–5383.

149. Meier MH, et al. Persistent cannabis users show neuropsychological decline from childhood to midlife. *Proceedings of the National Academy of Sciences of the United States of America*. 2012;*109*(40):E2657–664.

150. Moffitt TE, et al. Reply to Rogeberg and Daly: no evidence that socioeconomic status or personality differences confound the association between cannabis use and IQ decline. *Proceedings of the National Academy of Sciences of the United States of America*. 2013;*110*(11):E980–E982.

151. Meier MH, et al. Which adolescents develop persistent substance dependence in adulthood? Using population-representative longitudinal data to inform universal risk assessment. *Psychological Medicine*. 2016;*46*(4):877–889.

152. Sen IM, Sen RK. Regional anesthesia for lower limb burn wound debridements. *Archives of Trauma Research*. 2012;*1*(3):135–136.

153. Cuignet O, Mbuyamba J, Pirson J. The long-term analgesic efficacy of a single-shot fascia iliaca compartment block in burn patients undergoing skin-grafting procedures. *Journal of Burn Care and Rehabilitation*. 2005;*26*(5):409–415.

154. Bussolin L, et al. Tumescent local anesthesia for the surgical treatment of burns and postburn sequelae in pediatric patients. *Anesthesiology.* 2003;99(6):1371–1375.

155. Hernandez JL, et al. Use of continuous local anesthetic infusion in the management of postoperative split-thickness skin graft donor site pain. *Journal of Burn Care Research.* 2013;34(4):e257–e262.

156. Shank ES, et al. Ultrasound-guided regional anesthesia for pediatric burn reconstructive surgery: a prospective study. *Journal of Burn Care Research.* 2016;37(3):e213–e217.

157. Cuignet O, et al. The efficacy of continuous fascia iliaca compartment block for pain management in burn patients undergoing skin grafting procedures. *Anesthesia and Analgesia.* 2004;98(4):1077–1081.

158. Rork JF, Berde CB, Goldstein RD. Regional anesthesia approaches to pain management in pediatric palliative care: a review of current knowledge. *Journal of Pain and Symptom Management.* 2013;46(6):859–873.

159. Burns DA. Using regional anesthesia to manage pediatric acute pain. In: *10th Pediatric Pain Master's Class.* 2017: Minneapolis, MN. https://www.childrensmn.org/events/professional-development-workshop-the-epec-pediatrics-professional-development-workshop-pdw/

160. Morton-Rias D. Certified PA-Cs integral to expansion of palliative medicine. *Provider Long Term & Post Acute Care.* 2018. https://pahpm.org/resources/Authored%20Articles/DMRias_PACs%20ntegral%20Expansion%20Palliative%20Medicine2018.pdf. Accessed August 30, 2019.

161. Friedrichsdorf SJ. From denial to palliactive—practical steps for developing a PPC program: training. Presented at 4th Congress on Paediatric Palliative Care—A Global Gathering; October 24–27, 2018; Rome, Italy.

162. International Children's Palliative Care Network. e-Learning courses. 2018. https://www.icpcn.org/icpcns-elearning-programme/

163. American Association of Colleges of Nursing. Consortium. ELNEC. 2018. https://www.aacnnursing.org/ELNEC164. American Academy of Hospice and Palliative Medicine. Clinical training: hospice and palliative medicine fellowship training. 2018. http://aahpm.org/career/clinical-training#fellowship-directory

165. Students at Flinders University. Master of Palliative Care, College of Nursing and Health Sciences, Flinders University, Australia. 2018. http://www.flinders.edu.au/courses/rules/postgrad/mpc.cfm

166. Université Catholique de Louvain (Brussels, Belgium) and Université Catholique de Lille (France). Multi-university diploma. 2018. mariefriedelcastorini@gmail.com

167. Gaillimh OÉ, NUI Galway. Master/Postgraduate Diploma in Health Sciences. 2018. http://www.icpcn.org/wp-content/uploads/2013/12/Childrens-Palliative-Complex-Care.pdf

168. Portuguese Catholic University. 124-hour course—Portuguese Catholic University School of Public Health and Family Medicine. 2018. http://www.ics.lisboa.ucp.pt

169. University of Cape Town; School of Public Health and Family Medicine. Master of philosophy in palliative medicine. 2018. http://www.publichealth.uct.ac.za/phfm_master-philosophy-palliative-medicine

170. Mildmay Uganda. Diploma in paediatric palliative care. 2018. https://mihs.mildmay.or.ug/programs-courses/academic-programme/higher-diploma-pediatric-palliative-care

171. Bologna Accedemia delle Scienze di Medicina Palliative. Master in PPC. https://www.asmepa.org

172. University of Padova. Medicina del dolore. https://www.unipd.it/corso-perfezionamento-medicina-dolore

173. International Observatory on End of Life Care. Home page. https://www.lancaster.ac.uk/fhm/research/ioelc/

174. Center for Palliative Care, Harvard Medical School. Palliative Care Education and Practice (PCEP). 2018. https://pallcare.hms.harvard.edu/courses/pcep

175. Cardiff University. Palliative medicine for health care professionals. 2018. https://www.cardiff.ac.uk/study/postgraduate/taught/courses/course/palliative-medicine-for-health-care-professionals-msc-part-time

176. Friedrichsdorf SJ, et al. Module 12: neuropathic pain. In: *The Education in Palliative and End-of-Life Care for Pediatrics Curriculum© EPEC-Pediatrics.* 2018. Minneapolis, MN: EPEC-Pediatrics:

17

Older Adult Population

Harry S. Strothers and Dipenkumar Patel

Geriatric Medicine

Geriatric medicine is a specialty of medicine concerned with physical, mental, functional, and social conditions in acute, chronic, rehabilitative, preventive, and end-of-life care in older patients.[1] There is no set age that defines the geriatric population; many use greater than 65 years, although most people don't need geriatric expertise until later.[2]

Geriatric Palliative Care/Medicine

Geriatric palliative care integrates the complementary specialties of geriatrics and palliative care to provide comprehensive care for older patients entering the later stage of their lives and their families.[3]

In aging societies, the last phase of people's lives is changing profoundly, challenging traditional care provision in geriatric medicine and palliative care. In 2017, with a life expectancy at birth of 78.6 years, those who reach 65 have an average life expectancy of 84.4 or 19.4 more years.[4] The increasing life expectancy and the associated changes in end-of-life morbidity forecast major opportunities for healthcare. Increasing life expectancy has led to most older adults accumulating multiple chronic diseases that eventually lead to progressive disability, dependence on others, institutionalization, and frequent hospitalization. Compared to younger adults, older adults are more likely to desire fewer interventions at end of life, likely to have cognitive impairment, likely to have higher functional dependence, and likely to live in institutions.

This chapter provides physician assistants an overview of palliative care in older adults, the differences between palliative care and hospice, understanding and managing geriatrics syndrome, symptom management in older patients and the complexities of end of life, discussion of goals of care, and communicating with geriatric patients and families. Another indispensable component is an overview of physiologic changes in older adults, which leads to differences in the pharmacological and pharmacokinetic effects of medications.

Palliative Care and Hospice

Palliative care is an interdisciplinary approach to improve the quality of life for patients who suffer from severe or chronic terminal illness. Palliative care should be available from the time of diagnosis of a life-altering illness and may be provided concurrently with curative or disease-modifying treatments. Hospice provides comprehensive care to patients and families at the end of life when there is a life expectancy of less than 6 months and when they choose to focus on comfort care, forgoing standard medical therapy.

Physiologic Changes of Aging

Physiological changes occur with aging in all organ systems and influence care during the end of life. These include the following:

- The cardiac output decreases, blood pressure increases, and arteriosclerosis develops.
- The lungs show impaired gas exchange, a decrease in vital capacity, and slower expiratory flow rates.
- The creatinine clearance decreases with age, although the serum creatinine level remains relatively constant due to a proportionate age-related decrease in creatinine production.
- Functional changes, largely related to altered motility patterns, occur in the gastrointestinal (GI) system with senescence, and atrophic gastritis and altered hepatic drug metabolism are common in the elderly.
- Progressive elevation of blood glucose occurs with age on a multifactorial basis.
- Osteoporosis is frequently seen due to a linear decline in bone mass after the fourth decade.
- The epidermis of the skin atrophies with age, and due to changes in collagen and elastin the skin loses its tone and elasticity.
- Lean body mass declines with age, and this is primarily due to loss and atrophy of muscle cells.
- Degenerative changes occur in many joints, and this, combined with the loss of muscle mass, inhibits elderly patients' locomotion.

These changes with age have important practical implications for the clinical management of elderly patients: Metabolism is altered, and changes in response to commonly used drugs make different drug dosages necessary. Understanding these physiologic changes becomes very important in elderly palliative care patients who are terminally ill and have multiple comorbidities. These patients have much higher risks of adverse drug reactions. Proper medication management includes stopping or lowering doses of certain medications and avoiding others to prevent or treat adverse drug reactions in this population.

Dementia

Dementia is a progressive irreversible clinical syndrome characterized by widespread impairment of mental function, which may include memory loss, language impairment, disorientation, personality changes, difficulties with activities of daily living (ADLs), self-neglect, and psychiatric syndromes. It is a life-limiting condition with increasing prevalence and complex needs. Palliative care needs of patients with dementia are often poorly addressed; symptoms such as pain are undertreated.

Dementia usually follows a course characterized by prolonged and progressive disability (Figure 17.1). The level of baseline function is often low as the disease primarily affects older people who may have already accumulated many other comorbidities.[3] This is in contrast to cancer, which usually follows an initial slow overall decline from a high level of function, followed by a relatively rapid decline in function at the end of life, and a fairly predictable terminal phase where there is time to anticipate palliative care needs and plan for end-of-life care.

Palliative care needs of dementia patients are complex and difficult to anticipate. Among major problems in dementia patients are assessment of pain and other needs, such as advance care planning, access to palliative care, prediction of prognosis, multiple other health comorbidities of older patients, and limited research.

Medicare hospice eligibility criteria are as shown in Table 17.1.

Functional Assessment Staging Test

The disease trajectory of dementia makes identification of the terminal phase very difficult, but it is often marked by increasingly frequent infections, disability, and impairment. Palliative care needs of dementia patients start much earlier than the terminal phase. The

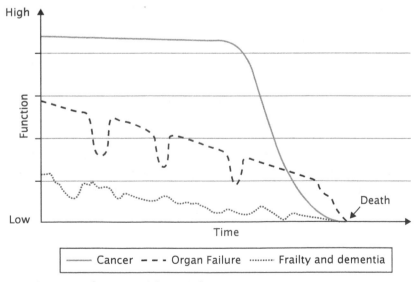

FIGURE 17.1 Trajectory of cancer and dementia.[5]

TABLE 17.1 Medicare Hospice Eligibility[a]

Stage	Characteristics
1	No difficulty either subjectively or objectively
2	Complains of forgetting location of objects. Subjective work difficulties.
3	Decreased job functioning evident to co-workers. Difficulty in traveling to new locations. Decreased organizational capacity.*
4	Decreased ability to perform complex tasks.
5	Occasionally or more frequently over the past week.* A. Improperly putting on clothes without assistance or cueing. B. Unable to bathe properly (not able to choose proper water temp.) C. Inability to handle mechanics of toileting (e.g., forgetting to flush, does not wipe properly or properly dispose of toilet tissue.) D. Urinary incontinence. E. Fecal incontinence.
7	A. Ability to speak limited to approximately = 6 intelligible different words in the course of an average day or in the course of an intensive interview. B. Speech ability is limited to the use of a single intelligible word in an average day or in the course of an intensive interview. C. Ambulatory ability is lost (cannot walk without personal assistance.) D. Cannot sit up without assistance (e.g. the individual will fall over if there are not lateral rests [arms] on the chair). E. Loss of ability to smile. F. Loss of ability to hold up head independently.

[a]From Reference 6. Reprinted with permission.
* Scored primarily on the information obtained from knowledgeable informant.

surprise question, "Would you be surprised if this patient were to die in the next 12 months?" has been suggested as a useful trigger question to help identify patients with nonmalignant disease who are approaching the end of life.

After identifying dementia patients requiring palliative care, the first important steps are to identify goals of care, complete advance care planning, determine the setting for care delivery, and performing a thorough medication review.

Medication review should include stopping unnecessary medication, for example, statin and aspirin for cardiovascular disease prevention or calcium or other vitamin supplements. Use of specific dementia medications in the end-stage dementia patient is questionable, may be harmful, and may be stopped after goals-of-care discussions with family/surrogate decision-makers.

Patients with dementia often lack early access to palliative care in hospice settings and usually do not receive it until the end of life. To maximize quality of life, their needs must be identified and addressed throughout the course of the disease.

Discussion of goals of care and advance care planning with family is very important. Ideally, it should be done when the patient has decision-making capacity, but this does not usually happen. Because of the insidious nature of the disease, families and caregivers may not recognize its onset, so the healthcare provider must work with patient and family to help identify goals of care and plans prior to the inevitable decline of cognition and function.

Discuss with family cardiopulmonary resuscitation, artificial feeding, hospitalization, and appropriate use of antibiotics and intravenous hydration (as well as dialysis if appropriate). Research has shown that aggressive intervention and routine hospital care does not reduce mortality but adds to complications and decreases quality of life. Consideration should therefore be given to relief of pain and other distressing symptoms and minimizing burdensome interventions in this group of patients.

It is very important to identify caregiver burden in family members of dementia patients and provide support and resources for them. Support can be provided as respite care, financial support and benefits, and provision of information and education regarding prognosis and issues such as power of attorney and advance directives.

Frailty

Frailty is a common clinical syndrome in older adults that carries an increased risk for poor health outcomes, including falls, worsening ADL impairment, hospitalization, institutionalization, and death. As frailty progresses, palliative care and hospice, with their focus on quality of life, become more appropriate. The overall prevalence of frailty in community-dwelling older adults aged 65 or older in the United States ranges from 7% to 12%. Prevalence of frailty increased with age from 3.9% in the 65- to 74-year age group to 25% in the 85+ group and was greater in women than men.[7]

Frailty is theoretically defined as a clinically recognizable state of increased vulnerability resulting from aging-associated decline in reserve and function across multiple physiologic systems, such that the ability to cope with everyday or acute stressors is comprised. In the absence of a gold standard, frailty has been operationally defined by Fried et al. as meeting three out of five phenotypic criteria indicating compromised energetics: low grip strength, low energy, slowed walking speed, low physical activity, and/or unintentional weight loss. A prefrail stage, in which one or two criteria are present, identifies a subset at high risk of progressing to frailty.

Older adults who are frail can benefit from comprehensive geriatric assessment, with attention to syndromes such as cognitive impairment, polypharmacy, mobility issues, incontinence, and falls. Medical problems can be optimized, but more importantly, a more global approach to the problem of frailty may be helpful. For example, a patient with severe fatigue can have heart failure, anemia, and hypoxemia optimized, be advised to conserve energy (eat, then rest, then take a bath), and eliminate or reduce the dose of drugs such as β-blockers or tricyclic antidepressants (TCAs). There are some community services for frail older adults, including the Area Agency on Aging, physician home visit programs, visiting nurses, the Program of All-Inclusive Care for the Elderly, and other local and state programs. All of these resources should be provided to frail older adults and their family members.

Palliative care principles should also be woven into the fabric of care for older adults. For healthy patients, ask about goals of care and presence of an advance directive. Dealing with progressive frailty is not hopeless; many interventions ameliorate symptoms. For patients with advanced frailty, screening for occult cancer presents more burdens than benefits. The benefit/burden trade-off is more difficult to assess with early or middle frailty, when the prognosis is less clear. At every stage, readdress the goals of care with open-ended questions, such as: What do you think about balancing quality of life with length of life?

Referral to hospice does not mean that the patient accepts a more accelerated course toward death and needs to forego all treatments. Patients on hospice can continue some or all of their current medications. For example, a patient with low ejection fraction heart failure should continue evidence-based treatment with both medications and devices because these interventions not only prolong life, but also improve the quality of life. Further, a significant minority of patients referred to hospice improve and are discharged, though they may need to reenroll later in the disease trajectory.

Assessment and management of symptoms associated with frailty should be individualized and based on patients' and families' goals of care. For fatigue, patients can modify their environment, such as moving the telephone closer or using a bedside commode, adjusting the room temperature, or reordering tasks to conserve energy. Managing exacerbations of chronic illness at home or in the nursing home often leads to outcomes as good as or better than hospitalization, particularly if the patient wants to avoid hospitalization and aggressive medical interventions at the end of life.[8] Screening older adults who are considering elective surgery for frailty can lead to more nuanced and comprehensive treatment plans and perhaps even reduce perioperative mortality rates. A French randomized trial found that a systematic approach to very old critically ill adults led to twice as many older adults being admitted to the intensive care unit but no reduction in 6-month mortality, suggesting that severity of illness alone should not determine treatment choices.[9]

Polypharmacy

Polypharmacy is defined as the use of more than six medications or the use of more medications than are medically necessary. Polypharmacy is a major risk factor for adverse medication reactions and interactions, particularly in the geriatric population, which can result in excess morbidity and even mortality. Risk factors for polypharmacy are multiple diseases, treating acute problems in patients with multiple comorbidities, misinterpretation and mistreatment of drug interactions and medication adverse reaction, and the involvement of multiple providers in care.

In the palliative care setting, we usually work with patients with very severe and/or life-limiting illness, including advanced dementia or other neurodegenerative diseases (Parkinson disease, amyotrophic lateral sclerosis [ALS], etc.); metastatic cancer; severe end-organ failure (congestive heart failure, cirrhosis/end-stage liver disease, chronic obstructive pulmonary disease, chronic kidney disease [CKD]/end-stage renal disease); and others. At this point, many medications for chronic disease may not confer benefits and may increase symptoms or burden. An important part of this process is de-prescribing, understanding drug interactions, and medication side effects. It is important to discuss with the patient and family about their perception of the need for medication that no longer may be helpful and can even be harmful. Communication with patient and family is very important in this process.

De-prescribing is an effort to taper, reduce dose, or stop medications in an effort to reduce polypharmacy, minimize adverse medication effects, and avoid ineffective or even potentially harmful medications. This can be achieved by coordinating care between treating physicians and palliative care consultants based on goals of care of patients and family. If symptom relief and functional status improvement are the major goals, then many medications, such as antihypertensives, statins, oral hypoglycemics, anticoagulants, vitamins, and supplements, that do not contribute to achieving those goals can often be discontinued.

The most common classes of medications where there is often a great opportunity to "de-prescribe" in the palliative setting with a high likelihood that the benefit (including just reducing the pill "burden" and reducing cost of care) outweighs the harm include

1. Dementia medications—anticholinesterase inhibitors and memantine
2. Statins
3. Anticoagulants and aspirin
4. Antihypertensives
5. Insulin and oral hypoglycemics
6. Vitamins, iron supplements, calcium

The language used in this process is also very important—terms like "optimize, individualize, limit pill burden, maximize benefit and minimize harm" are much better received than terms such as "stopping, quitting, decrease cost, no longer covered, and the like." As with all issues in palliative care, this must be a process of shared decision-making so patients and families do not feel like they are being abandoned or that their treating clinicians are "giving up." Many patients who are taking six, eight, or ten or more separate medications per day and often twice those numbers in terms of pills per day welcome the opportunity for this regimen to be streamlined.[10] Free apps for the iOS and Android operating smartphone systems can be found online (https://deprescribing.org/news/evaluation-of-a-deprescribing-guideline-mobile-application-2/).

Falls and Fractures

Increased risk for falls occurs as part of the aging process, resulting in a major source of morbidity and mortality in elderly patients. Despite the best efforts of the palliative team, fall incidents continue to occur in palliative care patients due to their often complex and debilitating disease processes. Side effects of multiple medications, dementia, delirium, and frailty are major factors associated with and contributors to the falls experienced by palliative patients. Head injuries and hip fractures suffered from a fall further increase health complications, hasten death, and increase distress for the already suffering patients and their families.

Furthermore, inpatient care costs associated with fall-related injuries are devastatingly high, even for the injuries not categorized as life threatening. It is very important to identify risk factors and institute appropriate measures to prevent falls in palliative care patients. These include avoiding polypharmacy, early identification of drug adverse reactions,

TABLE 17.2 One-Year Mortality Risk Among Patients 50 Years or Older Experiencing Hip Fracture

Risk Factor	Points	Score
Male gender	2	
Age ≥ 90 years	2	
Congestive heart failure	2	
Difficulty preparing meals	2	
Not able to drive	1	
Total Score	0–9	

Scoring (points)
0: 1-year mortality 10%; 1: 14%; 2: 20%; 3: 27%; 4: 37%; 5: 45%; 6: 56%; 7–9: 66%.

providing appropriate assistive devices for ambulatory patients, assessment of the home environment, and the need for support at home. The family and palliative care team must be educated on fall prevention.

In patients who sustain injuries, their extent and severity must be considered. Workup and management of injuries after a fall should be based on the goals of care of patients and family. If the goal is symptom management, the focus should be on appropriate pain management. Identifying fractures is very important in palliative care and hospice patients, justifying basic workup with x-rays in such patients and further management based on extent of injury, prognosis, and goals of care. One of the most common fractures in elderly palliative care patients is a hip fracture. It is important to discuss with patient and family risks and benefits of operative versus nonoperative management by coordinating care with orthopedists and palliative care consultants. Again, as always, treatment should be based on a patient's and family's goals of care.

A retrospective cohort study of 857 older adults experiencing fracture led to a mortality index (Table 17.2), which can be used in counseling, probably not to determine whether the patient should have surgery, but rather in assisting decisions after that treatment. Nursing home patients who fracture their hips also have poor outcomes. In a study describing 60,000 nursing home patients who suffered a hip fracture between 2005 and 2009, median survival was 12 months. Outcomes were most dependent on the baseline ability to walk: For those with independent walking at baseline, 33% had died and 27% were still walking at 6 months, while for those who could not walk prior to the fracture, at 6 months 42% were dead and only 3% could walk independently. These poor results do not argue against operating on these patients, because that procedure is palliative, but it does suggest that many of these patients will be hospice eligible after repair, and that many more will become hospice eligible as time passes.[12]

Delirium

Delirium is a neurocognitive syndrome arising from acute global brain dysfunction. Although the global cerebral dysfunction associated with delirium is manifested as multiple symptoms and signs, collectively constituting a neurocognitive or neuropsychiatric disorder, the hallmark of delirium is impaired attention (please refer to the fifth edition of the *Diagnostic and Statistical Manual of Mental Disorders* [*DSM-5*] criteria for delirium). In a palliative setting, prevalence is reported as 13%–42% on admission to inpatient palliative care units, increasing to 88% at the end of life (weeks to hours before death). Delirium is associated with significant patient morbidity and increased mortality in many patient populations, especially palliative care, where refractory delirium is common in the dying phase. Delirium is more common in the geriatrics palliative care group, associated with higher multimorbidity, increasing frailty, and polypharmacy.

Prompt recognition and management of delirium in palliative care is important to improve comfort, quality of life, and decreasing family distress. Depending on its precipitating factors, a delirium episode is often reversible, especially in the earlier stages of a life-threatening illness. Until recently, antipsychotics have played a pivotal role in delirium management, but recent research has failed to demonstrate their efficacy in delirium occurring in palliative care patients. Nonpharmacological strategies for the management of delirium play a fundamental role and should be optimized through the collective efforts of the whole interprofessional team. Refractory agitated delirium in the last days or weeks of life may require the use of pharmacological sedation to ameliorate the distress of patients and usually done in response to increasing distress of family. Constant communication and education of family members about terminal delirium helps to decrease distress of family.

After identifying delirium in palliative patients and whether it is hypoactive, hyperactive, or mixed type, it is important to find its underlying cause and whether it is reversible or terminal delirium. Hyperactive or agitated delirium is usually apparent, but physicians often miss hypoactive delirium because it can be mistaken as sedation due to opioid medication or obtundation near end of life. Delirium is almost always multifactorial, especially in geriatric patients, and causes can be found through medication review, physical examination, and laboratory tests.

Opioids and benzodiazepines used in palliative care may cause substantial alteration in mental status and more subtle, temporary changes in cognition and attention. In the setting of renal failure, opioids, especially morphine, may be less well eliminated, resulting in toxic effects, including delirium. Usually, there is no single medication but a combination of medications causing delirium along with multiple other factors. When medications are identified, most can be switched or their dose can be tapered. Thorough physical examination is also very important to identify causes of delirium such as dyspnea, hypotension, signs of volume depletion, unidentified injuries and related pain, and undertreated pain. A more aggressive search for the cause of delirium depends on the patient's and family's goals of care, which can include some basic blood work like a complete blood count, chemistry, and x-rays to identify fractures. Also, management of delirium should be consistent with the patient's and family's goals of care, for example, giving intravenous fluids for volume depletion and more aggressive measures such as giving blood due to low hemoglobin to help to improve delirium and other symptoms. When death appears imminent, it is appropriate to forgo evaluation beyond history and physical examination and to provide both pharmacological and nonpharmacological interventions to ameliorate symptoms of delirium.

Recent research has shown that antipsychotics do not improve delirium, and benzodiazepines may worsen delirium. Currently, there is no pharmacological intervention that has been shown to improve delirium. It is very important to focus on nonpharmacological measures, which has clearly been shown to reduce delirium in research. HELP (Hospital Elder Life Program) focuses on a combination of nonpharmacological measures that have been shown to improve delirium. Please refer to HELP to learn more about nonpharmacological measures.[13]

Depression

Depression is more prevalent in the geriatric population (1% to 5%) and much more common in geriatric patients with terminal illness.[14] Depression in dying elderly patients who are already frail impairs quality of life by reducing hope, meaning, and a sense of peace. Barriers exist in the recognition and treatment of depression in patients with advanced disease. It is difficult to imagine any patient facing death who would not experience some psychological distress, so clinicians may find it difficult to distinguish normal sadness from clinical depression. Symptoms of coexisting diseases may also overlap with depression.

Risk factors for depression in geriatric palliative care patients are terminal diagnosis, physical disability, frailty, multiple comorbidities, medications, lack of support (social or financial), a previous history of depression, untreated pain, and substance abuse. It is also important to understand that many conditions can mimic depression in terminally ill patients. These include hypercalcemia, brain metastasis, or reaction to medications such as antineoplastics, benzodiazepines, antipsychotics, corticosteroids, or antihypertensives.

The simple question Are you depressed? is a reasonable screen for depression in the palliative setting. If the answer is yes, one strategy might be to use the *DSM*, Geriatric Depression Scale, or Endicott criteria (Table 17.3) to further assess the likelihood of depression.[15] Please

TABLE 17.3 Endicott Substitution Criteria for Depression in the Medically Ill[a]

Physical Symptoms	Psychological or Cognitive Symptoms
Change in appetite or weight	Tearfulness Depressed appearance
Sleep disturbance	Social withdrawal Decreased speech
Fatigue or loss of energy	Brooding Self-pity Pessimism
Psychomotor agitation or retardation	Lack of reactivity

Note: The physical symptoms of depression are replaced by psychological or affective features of depression, enhancing the diagnostic accuracy of depression in the medically ill.
[a] From Reference 11. Reprinted with permission.

refer to *DSM5* criteria for diagnosis of depression in patients with advanced and terminal disease. Teasing out depression in patients with so many physical symptoms can be difficult: The key indicators of depression in dying patients are persistent feelings of hopelessness, worthlessness, and suicidal thoughts. It is important to differentiate grief from depression. Although grief is triggered by loss, it is often experienced in waves, compared with depression, where the patient generally has a persistently flat affect. Grieving patients maintain hope, although the hope may have shifted from cure of disease to comfort. Unlike depression, patients with grief have a preserved self-image, can still experience pleasure, and look forward to special occasions and interactions with friends and family. An active desire for an early death is not part of normal anticipatory grief. If a patient whose symptoms and social needs have largely been met has a persistent and active desire for an early death, this suggests depression.[15]

Suicide rates are higher in patients with advanced disease, and almost half of dying patients have suicidal thoughts. Suicidal patients in hospice and palliative care settings should generally be treated like any other suicidal patient. Even if the patient has clear wishes to avoid heroic and life-sustaining treatments, they should be rescued from suicide attempts such as drug overdoses or trauma.

Nonpharmacological treatment. Various types of psychotherapy, including cognitive behavioral, interpersonal, and problem-solving, may be helpful in both the acute treatment of depression and maintaining remission. Psychotherapy alone, without antidepressants, is reasonable as a first-line therapy for mild depression, but not for severe depression, especially if the patient is either psychotic or bipolar. Combining antidepressants and psychotherapy increases the likelihood of response, reduces relapse, improves quality of life, and increases compliance with medications. For a patient on hospice, social workers, grief and bereavement counselors, or other mental health professionals can often provide or coordinate such services.

Pharmacological treatment. First-line drug treatment of depression in palliative care is usually with an selective serotonin reuptake inhibitors (SSRIs) like sertraline or bupropion or serotonin-norepinephrine reuptake inhibitors (SNRIs) like duloxetine, venlafaxine, or desvenlafaxine, although their efficacy has not been specifically shown in patients with advanced disease. Mirtazapine, an antidepressant that antagonizes noradrenergic, histamine, and serotonin receptors, is a mild antidepressant and associated with sedation and weight gain, but sometimes those side effects are desirable. There is less sedation at higher doses. Duloxetine is an SNRI class antidepressant, which also is useful for chronic pain, especially of neuropathic origin. Avoid TCAs due to the side effects of these medications. It is very important to identify the underlying cause of depression, such as undertreated pain. Psychostimulants may be particularly helpful for treating depression in patients with a limited life span because they work quickly, sometimes with evidence of improvement after the first couple of doses. Psychostimulants are indicated in depressed patients when a prompt response is needed and long-term tolerance is irrelevant. Most commonly used psychostimulants for depression at the end of life are methylphenidate, dextroamphetamine, or modafinil.

Antidepressants Used for Older Adults

It is also important to know about symptoms of serotonin toxicity and serotonin syndrome and management.

- Confusion
- Agitation or restlessness
- Dilated pupils
- Headache
- Changes in blood pressure and/or temperature
- Nausea and/or vomiting
- Diarrhea
- Rapid heart rate

Geriatrics patients are much more susceptible to serotonin toxicity due to polypharmacy, frailty, and multiple comorbidities (Table 17.4).[16]

Syncope

Syncope or presyncope is a frequent symptom in older patients. Its diagnostic and therapeutic management may be complex in older adults, particularly in a palliative care population due to terminal illness, frailty, multiple comorbidities, or cognitive impairment. Morbidity related to syncope is more common in older persons and ranges from loss of confidence, depressive illness, and fear of falling to fractures and consequent institutionalization.

Causes of syncope in a palliative patient usually are the same as for other geriatric patients: orthostatic hypotension, dehydration, cardiac arrhythmia, vasovagal, extreme stress, and neuromediated causes. Dehydration, orthostatic hypotension, or medication adverse drug reactions are much more common in elderly palliative care patients and can be easily managed by improving hydration, intravenous hydration if consistent with the patient's goals of care, or stopping or tapering the medication dose causing hypotension, including antihypertensive medications. It is also important to recognize a cardiac cause of syncope, such as arrhythmia in patients with cardiovascular disease, especially patients with a pacemaker or implantable cardioverter-defibrillator (ICD) in place, which is much more common in the geriatric population. It could be a malfunctioning pacemaker or an ICD firing due to ventricular tachycardia or fibrillation. It is important to remember to deactivate an ICD for patients with a do not resuscitate order if it is not consistent with the patient's goals of care. Contrary to the beliefs of many families, pacemakers in terminally ill patients should not be deactivated. They will not prevent a natural death, but deactivation may precipitate significant symptoms and distress in patients. Aggressive workup, such as an electrocardiogram, cardiac monitor, tilt table test, and management of syncope, of palliative care patients should be based on prognosis of the patient and the patient's and family's goals of care.

TABLE 17.4 Antidepressants for Older Adults[a]

Class, Medication	Initial Dosage	Usual Dosage	Formulations (in mg unless specified)	Comments (Metabolism, Excretion)
SSRIs				Class AEs: EPS, hyponatremia, increased risk of upper GI bleeding, suicide (early in tx), lower BMD and fragility fractures, risk of toxicity if methylene blue or linezolid coadministered. Avoid if hx of falls or fracture; caution if hx of SIADH
Citalopram ▲ (*Celexa*)	10–20 mg every morning	20 mg/d	T: 20, 40, 60; S: 5	20 mg/d is maximum dosage in adults > 60 years old; risk of QTc prolongation
Escitalopram (*Lexapro*)	10 mg/d	10 mg/d	T: 10, 20	10 mg/d is max dosage in adults > 60 years old; risk of QTc prolongation
Fluoxetine ▲ (*Prozac*)	5 mg every morning	5–60 mg/d	T: 10; C: 10, 20, 40 S: 20 mg/5 mL C: SR 90 (weekly 90 mg weekly dose)	Long half-lives of parent and active metabolite may allow for less-frequent dosing: may cause more insomnia than other SSRIs; CYP2D6, -2C9, -3A4 inhibitor (L)
Fluvoxamine ▲ (*Luvox*)	25 mg at bedtime	100–300 mg/d	T: 25, 50, 100	Not approved as an antidepressant in US; greater likelihood of GI AEs; CYP1A2, -3A4 inhibitor (L)
Paroxetine ▲ (*Paxil*)	5 mg	10–40 mg/d	T: 10, 20, 30, 40	Increased risk of withdrawal symptoms (dizziness); anticholinergic AEs: CYP2D6 inhibitor (L)
(*Paxil CR*)	12.5 mg/d	12.5–37.5 mg/d	T: ER 12.5, 25, 37.5 S: 10 mg/5 mL	Increased by 12.5 mg/d no faster than once/week (L)
Sertraline ▲ (*Zoloft*)	25 mg every morning	50–200 mg/d	T: 25, 50, 100 S: 20 mg/mL	Greater likelihood of GI AEs (L)
Additional Medications				
Bupropion ▲ (*Wellbutrin*)	37.5–50 mg every 12 h	75–150 mg every 12 h	T: 75, 100	Consider for SSRI, TCA nonresponders; safe in HF; may be stimulating: can lower seizure threshold. Avoid
(*Wellbutrin SR* ▲)	100 mg every 12 h or every 24 h	100–150 mg every 12 h	T:100, 150, 200	
(*Wellbutrin XL* ▲)	150 mg/d	300 mg/d	T: 150, 300	
Levomilnacipran (*Fetzima*)	20 mg every 24 h × 2 d	40 mg every 24 h; maximum: 120 mg max dose per day	C: ER 20, 40, 8 0	SNRI (L, K 58%)

Drug	Starting dose	Dose range	Formulations (mg)	Comments
Methylphenidate ▲ **BC** (*Ritalin*)	2.5–5 mg at 7 AM and noon	5–10 mg at 7 AM and noon	T: 5, 10, 20	Short-term tx of depression or apathy in physically ill older adults; used as an adjunct. Avoid if insomnia
Mirtazapine ▲ (*Remeron*)	15 mg at bedtime	15–45 mg/d	T: 15, 30, 45	May increase appetite; sedating; ODT (Oral disintegrating tablet) available (L)
Vilazodone (*Viibryd*)	10 mg/d for 7 days, then 20 mg/d	40 mg/d	T: 10, 20, 40	Metabolized by CYP3A4; limited geriatric data: AEs: diarrhea and nausea
Vilazodone (*Brintellix*)	5–10 mg every 24 h; maximum 20 mg per day	5–10 mg every 24 h; maximum 20 mg per day	T: 5, 10, 20	SSRI with 5-HT$_{1A}$ agonist and 5-HT$_3$ antagonist activity (L)
TCAs				Avoid. BC
◆ Desipramine ▲ (*Norpra*)	10–25 mg at bedtime	50–150 mg/d	T: 10, 25, 50, 75, 100,	Therapeutic serum level >115 ng/mL (L)
◆ Nortriptyline ▲ (*Aventyl*)	10–25 mg at bedtime	75–150 mg/d	C: 10, 25, 50, 75 S: 10 mg/5 mL	Therapeutic window (50–150 ng/mL) (L)
SNRs				
◆ Duloxetine (*Cymbalta*)	20 mg/d, then mg	40–60 mg every 24 h or 30 mg every 12 h	C: 20, 30, 60	Most common AEs: nausea, dry mouth, constipation, diarrhea, urinary hesitancy; reduce dosage if CrCl 30–60 mL/min; contraindicated if CrCl < 30 mL/min creatinine clearance (L)
Venlafaxine ▲ (*Effexor*)	25–50 mg every 12 h	75–255 mg/in divided dose	T: 25, 37.5, 50, 75, 100	Low anticholinergic activity; minimal sedation and hypotension; may increase BP and QTc; may be useful when somatic pain present; EPS, withdrawal symptoms, hyponatremia (L)
(*Effexor XR*)	75 mg every morning	75–255 mg/d	C: 37.5, 75, 150	Same as above
Desvenlafaxine (*Pristiq*)	50 mg/d	50 mg; maximum: 400 mg per day	C: 37.5 75, 150	Active metabolite of venlafaxine; adjust dosage when CrCl < 30 mL/min (L, K 45%)

AE, adverse event; BP, blood pressure; ER, extended release; HF, heart failure; hx, history; SR, sustained release; tx, treatment; BMD, bone mineral density; EPS, extrapyramidal side effects.

aFrom Reference 16.

Genitourinary Problems

Genitourinary problems are much more common in the geriatric population. It is important to identify and manage them appropriately in palliative care populations. The most common genitourinary problems in elderly palliative care patients are urinary incontinence (UI), urinary retention, urinary tract infection (UTI), chronic catheter management, and urologic cancers.

Urinary Incontinence

Urinary incontinence can occur at any age but is common in older adults. It is estimated that about 20% of older community-dwelling adults have enough incontinence to limit some part of their lives.[1] It is not normal and may cause significant morbidity and mortality. *Urinary incontinence* is the involuntary loss of urine severe enough to cause social or health problems. Although it is not life threatening, it has a substantial negative impact on quality of life, and it may be overlooked in a patient with multiple comorbidities.

After identifying UI, look for reversible causes, such as infection (UTI, intestinal cystitis, vaginitis); atrophic vaginitis; psychological issues (anxiety, depression); hyperglycemia; restricted mobility; and stool impaction. Once reversible causes are considered, it is important to identify and differentiate types of UI.

There are no guidelines for the evaluation of UI in patients at the end of life. For most patients, the diagnosis is made from history alone. Ask about the pattern of voiding, including onset of UI, frequency, severity, and any precipitating or palliating factors. Ask about urine leakage at night and about any symptoms of outlet obstruction (hesitancy, dribbling, incomplete emptying). Look at the big picture, considering signs and symptoms of delirium, dementia, stroke, parkinsonism, cord or nerve root compression, and peripheral or autonomic neuropathy. Assess for evidence of functional impairment and look at the patient's general medical illnesses and medications. Physical examination rarely adds any information. One might confirm a distended bladder or fecal impaction, detect stress leakage in women, or palpate an enlarged prostate in men. Laboratory testing is also of limited usefulness, but in individual cases, one could order a urinalysis, urine culture, and serum urea nitrogen and creatinine values. All of the workup and treatment should be based on goals of care.

Dialysis in Older Adults

Dialysis or renal replacement therapy (RRT) is a common issue for palliative care patients. Survival after RRT is inversely proportional to age, comorbidities, and poor function. At age 80–84 years, median survival on hemodialysis (HD) is about 16 months; for those over age 85 years, it is less than 12 months. Small inconclusive studies suggested there may be a small survival advantage for those choosing HD, but mainly in those with a higher baseline function.

Renal replacement therapy comes in four varieties: renal transplantation, in-center HD, home HD, and home peritoneal dialysis (PD). Most palliative care/hospice patients are not a candidate for transplant because of comorbidities. If the patient chooses home HD or PD, there are fewer visits to the center, but the family may become overwhelmed. Another option to RRT is active medical management of CKD without RRT.

A cohort study looked at 391 nationally representative adults over age 65 years who initiated HD between 1998 and 2014. All were in fee-for-service Medicare patients. Overall, the 30-day mortality was 23%, 6-month mortality was 44%, and 1-year mortality was 55%. These numbers are higher than other reports, probably because they include all dialysis; the National Registry of Long-Term Dialysis Patients comes from outpatient dialysis centers, not including those who initiate dialysis in the hospital and never make it to an outpatient center. Mortality rose with age: Six-month mortality for age 65–74 years was 35%, for those age 75–84 years was 47%, and for those older than 85 years was 60%. Mortality was higher for those who had substantial comorbidities or baseline dementia, whose first dialysis was as an inpatient, and those whose baseline functional status was dependent. Starting dialysis over age 65 years identifies a group at high risk of death, and comprehensive palliative intervention should be considered to formally assess goals of care, burdens, benefits, and more.[17]

Choice between RRT and medical management should be based on patients' values and goals of care, burdens, and benefits. Patients choosing RRT were four times more likely to die in the hospital. Thus, if a patient chooses in-center HD, they will spend more time away from family. Function will likely decline with either option. In one study of nursing home patients initiating HD, the 1-year mortality rate was 80%, and no patient maintained function. On the other hand, patients on medical management had preserved function until the last month of life. Symptom burden is high with either choice, and there are no studies comparing the effectiveness of symptom management. It is likely that patients would have less dyspnea and pruritus if they choose HD.

Managing Pain in Older Patients

Management of chronic pain does have differences and nuances in older adults, and the American Geriatrics Society (AGS) guideline on this topic is helpful. Older people may be reluctant to complain, may use words other than pain to describe discomfort, are often reluctant to take analgesics, and have comorbidities that make prescribing more difficult. Older patients are undertreated for pain in a wide range of settings. The most important initiative is to ask older adults if they have pain, generally using the 0–10 visual analog scale. Many patients with mild-to-moderate cognitive impairment can also answer questions about pain, and there are specific tools to assess patients with advanced dementia or other causes of severe cognitive impairment. One tool is the Pain Assessment in Advanced Dementia Patient Scale.

Pain Assessment in Advanced Dementia Scale

Instructions: Observe the patient for 5 minutes before scoring his or her behaviors. Score the behaviors according to the following paragraph. Definitions of each item are provided in Table 17.5. The patient can be observed under different conditions (e.g., at rest, during a pleasant activity, during caregiving, after the administration of pain medication).

Scoring: The total score ranges from 0 to 10 points. A possible interpretation of the scores is: 1–3 = mild pain; 4–6 = moderate pain; 7–10 = severe pain. These ranges are based on a standard 0–10 scale of pain but have not been substantiated in the literature for the PAINAD tool.

If cognitively impaired patients have behavioral disturbances or have a condition that should hurt (e.g., a deep pressure sore), an empiric trial of an analgesic is indicated.

Acetaminophen should be considered as the initial analgesic in older adults with chronic pain, with care not to exceed a daily maximum dose of 4 g. GAYF recommends a maximum daily dose of 3 g in frail older adults.[16] Nonsteroidal anti-inflammatory drugs (NSAIDs) at the lowest effective dose are a second choice, despite their GI and renal side effects. Older adults prescribed NSAIDs should take a proton pump inhibitor, H_2 blocker, or misoprostol to reduce the risk of GI bleeding. Avoid cyclooxygenase 2 inhibitors due to increased risk of myocardial infarction and renal impairment. They should also be avoided in severe liver disease.

For older adults with moderate or severe chronic pain, opioids can be considered. Start with around-the-clock medications such as hydrocodone-acetaminophen or immediate-release morphine and convert to long-acting opioids when appropriate using the total daily dose as a guide. Chronic opioids are often safe and effective in frail older adults, although this area needs more research. Please refer to Chapter 14 on pain management.

Older adults with neuropathic pain may be good candidates for adjuvant medications such as gabapentin, pregabalin, other anticonvulsants, and other drugs. Generally, avoid TCAs due to their adverse effects. Start with low doses, titrate up slowly, but keep titrating until analgesia or side effects occur (*Start low, go slow, but get there.*) Many other drugs may be considered in special circumstances, including corticosteroids, topical products containing lidocaine, NSAIDs, menthol, or capsaicin.

Pain management in older adults with cancer is similar to other cancer patients but special consideration should be given to polypharmacy, drug interactions, and drug metabolism, especially in patients with kidney or liver diseases.

Managing Nonpain Symptoms in Older Adults

Evaluation and management of nonpain symptoms such as dyspnea, cough, respiratory secretions, nausea-vomiting, diarrhea, or constipation are very similar to other patients. Special attention should be given to patients with advanced dementia who cannot communicate, patients with multiple comorbidities, and those on multiple medications due to risk of drug interactions and adverse drug reactions.

TABLE 17.5 Pain Assessment in Advanced Dementia Scale[a]

Behavior	0	1	2	Score
Breathing independent of vocalization	• Normal	• Occasional labored breathing • Short period of hyperventilation	• Noisy labored breathing • Long period of hyperventilation • Cheyne-Stokes respirations	
Negative vocalization	• None	• Occasional moan or groan • Low-level speech with a negative or disapproving quality	• Repeated troubled calling out • Loud moaning or groaning • Crying	
Facial expression	• Smiling or inexpressive	• Sad • Frightened • Frown	• Facial grimacing	
Body language	• Relaxed	• Tense • Distressed pacing • Fidgeting	• Rigid • Fists clenched • Knees pulled up • Pulling or pushing away • Striking out	
Consolability	• No need to console	• Distracted or reassured by voice or touch	• Unable to console, distract, or reassure	
			TOTAL SCORE	

[a]From Reference 18. Reprinted with permission.

For dyspnea in patients who cannot self-report, you can use the Respiratory Distress Observation Scale (RDOS) (Table 17.6).

Constipation

Constipation should be actively managed in older adults due to low gastric motility physiologic changes of aging; gastroparesis due to chronic diseases such as diabetes, physical inactivity, or limited activity due to frailty; and medication side effects such as those of opioids commonly used in palliative care. Other medications that cause constipation are aluminum- or calcium-containing antacids, anticholinergics, antihistamines, antidepressants, antipsychotics, calcium channel blockers (especially verapamil), clonidine, corticosteroids, diuretics, iron, levodopa, NSAIDs, ondansetron, and sympathomimetics. Constipation remains a problem even in patients with substantial anorexia, poor oral intake, and weight loss. Stool is still produced in patients without adequate oral intake because feces contain not only the end products of digestion but also GI secretions, shed epithelial cells, and bacteria.

TABLE 17.6 Respiratory Distress Observation Scale

Variable	0 Points	1 Point	2 Point	Total
Heart rate per minute	<90 beats	90–109 beats	≥110 beats	
Respiratory rate per minute	≥18 breaths	19–30 breaths	>30 breaths	
Restlessness; nonpurposeful movements	None	Occasional, slight movements	Frequent movements	
Paradoxical breathing pattern; abdomen moves in during inspiration			Present	
Accessory muscle use; rise in clavicle during inspiration	None	Slight rise	Pronounced rise	
Grunting at end expiration; guttural sound	None		Present	
Nasal flaring: involuntary movement of nares	None		Present	
Look of fear	None		Eyes wide open, facial muscles tense, brow furrowed, mouth open, teeth together	
Total				

Instruction for use:

1. RDOS is not a substitute for patient self report if able.
2. RDOS is an adult assessment tool.
3. RDOS cannot be used when the patient is paralyzed with a neuromuscular blocking agent.
4. RDOS is not valid in bulbar ALS or quadriplegia.
5. Count respiratory and heart rates for one minute, auscultate if necessary.
6. Grunting may be audible with intubated patients on ausculatation.
7. Fearful facial expressions.

From Reference 19. Reprinted with permission.

Diarrhea

By far the most common cause of diarrhea in older adults in palliative care is the overuse of laxatives, often in an attempt to prevent or treat opioid-induced constipation. Perform a rectal examination to ensure that the diarrhea is not passing around a fecal impaction (overflow diarrhea). If diarrhea seems to be caused by laxatives, stop them for a couple of days and then consider restarting them at a lower dose. Before trying to slow the diarrhea with nonspecific treatments, attempt to address the specific causes.

Nausea and Vomiting

Special consideration should be given in geriatric populations with nausea/vomiting who are receiving palliative care via medications such as chemotherapeutics, opioids, other anticholinergic drugs, and others. Gastroparesis, gastric outlet obstruction, constipation, and radiation are common causes often associated with cancer.

Please refer to particular chapters on management of different symptoms in palliative care, such as respiratory secretions, fever, pruritus, anorexia, dysphagia, dyspepsia, and sleep disorders. Keep in mind when managing these symptoms in older adults that these individuals are more prone to adverse drug reactions due to frailty, multimorbidity, and polypharmacy. Always start low and go slow if you are starting medication in older adults.

Discussion of Artificial Nutrition and Hydration

Artificial nutrition and hydration (ANH) is a medical treatment that patients/surrogates may accept or refuse, just as any other medical treatments. ANH is indicated for several conditions but is often used for dubious indications. Short-term (days to weeks) ANH may improve survival in patients with the acute phase of stroke or head injury, in critically ill patients, and in selected patients with advanced cancer who are undergoing intensive radiation therapy or have proximal bowel obstruction. Long-term ANH has a role in patients with persistent vegetative state (not everyone would choose that, but it does work in keeping the patient alive), short bowel syndrome, and ALS. However, evidence suggests that it does not help with cancer patients receiving chemotherapy, patients undergoing major cancer surgery, or in patients with advanced dementia.

Patients with advanced dementia will eventually resist or become indifferent to food, will fail to manage the food bolus properly in the mouth and pharynx, and will aspirate when swallowing. This is inevitable. The median survival of patients with dementia after onset of symptoms is 3–6 years, shorter than previously reported. The Choices, Attitudes, Strategies for Care of Dementia at End of Life (CASCADE) study documented that when demented patients start to have difficulties with feeding, their 6-month survival is close to 50%—this can suggest a need for hospice. These patients are completely dependent in all ADLs and are unable to participate in decision-making. Seventy percent of patients with dementia die in nursing homes. There is wide variation in the use of feeding tubes in demented persons across the country, and caregivers often report no or little conversation around these decisions.[20]

Eating problems are a hallmark of end-stage dementia, and the ability to feed oneself is typically the last ADL to be lost. However, demented patients who cannot feed themselves can sometimes live several years, especially if they have no other competing illnesses and have dedicated caregivers.

There are two main options to address failing nutritional intake at the end of life in patients with dementia: keep trying to feed by mouth or place a percutaneous endoscopic gastrostomy (PEG) tube. Conscientious hand feeding is labor intensive and can take 30–60 minutes per meal, but it does allow the patient the pleasure of tasting food and enhances human interaction. In recent surveys, one-third of severely demented patients nationwide were tube fed.

There are several steps clinicians can take to facilitate informed decision-making. First, clarify the clinical situation. The proxy should understand that dementia is a terminal condition, and that feeding problems indicate the disease has reached the end stage. Other acute and chronic medical conditions may impact decision-making, and potentially modifiable factors should be addressed, such as yeast stomatitis, side effects of medications, or esophageal strictures.

Second, establish the primary goal of care, whether it is life prolongation, maximizing function, promoting comfort, or something else. Only after this is clear can one put the treatment option of PEG feeding into context.

Third, present the treatment options (PEG or comfort feeding), along with the pros and cons of each choice. Ensure there is adequate time for counseling and explain the components of palliative care, which does not necessarily imply stopping other medical treatments. Address common misperceptions of tube feeding (TF; e.g., without it the patient will starve or that the patient will live longer with the tube).

Fourth, weigh the PEG and hand-feeding options against the values and preferences of the patient, as articulated by the proxy. What would the patient want? Follow the principles of substituted judgment, reasonable person, or best interest. Identify and try to follow any advance directives. Promote culturally sensitive discussions.

Finally, regardless of the decision, provide ongoing support. The decision may need to be readdressed as the clinical course evolves. For example, a trial of parenteral hydration may be indicated for a potentially reversible case of dehydration. Engage the interdisciplinary team, including nurses, speech therapists, dieticians, chaplains, and other counselors. Encourage the decision-maker to speak to other trusted advisors, such as family members or clergy. Consider the use of decision aids, such as printed materials, guidelines, and videos.

Explain to families that no evidence suggests that TF leads to improvement in nutrition among demented patients or a reduction in aspiration with TF in patients with dementia. Pressure sores are neither prevented nor treated by TF in patients with end-stage dementia. Instead, placing a feeding tube may increase the risk of pressure sores. Also TF does not provide survival benefit. TF does not reduce infections such as cellulitis, UTI, or pneumonia.[20]

In summary, *there are no clear benefits of TF in patients with dementia*. In addition to lack of benefit, there is a long list of potential complications in patients with either PEG or nasogastric tubes: technical problems such as knotting, tube malfunction, migration, or misplacement; diarrhea, GI bleeding, vomiting, and worsening of gastroesophageal reflux; fluid overload; increased skin moisture; weight loss; metabolic disturbances; lack of the pleasure of eating; anorexia; lack of dignity; loss of the social aspects of feeding; and altered cosmesis. Probably the worst adverse effect of PEG feeding in demented patients is the near-universal need for either physical or chemical restraints.

Both the AGS and the American Association of Hospice and Palliative Medicine have included recommending against TF in patients with advanced dementia as a part of the American Board of Internal Medicine Foundation's Choosing Wisely Campaign.

The AGS has further published a useful position statement on TF in patients with advanced dementia. They have five specific recommendations:

- Feeding tubes are not recommended for older adults with advanced dementia. Careful hand feeding should be offered and is just as good for the outcomes of death, pneumonia, functional status, and comfort. TF increases the risk of agitation, restraints, healthcare use, and pressure sores.
- Enhance oral feeding by altering the environment and creating individual approaches.
- Tube feeding is medical therapy that the surrogate can decline or accept.
- All healthcare professionals should understand and respect previously expressed wishes regarding TF.
- Institutions should promote choice about TF, endorse shared and informed decision-making, and honor individual preferences. There should be no pressure on individuals or providers to institute TF.

Advance Care Planning, Prognosis, and Goals of Care in Older Adults

How and when should clinicians begin to discuss prognosis with older adults, to move from prevention and disease management to looking at the big picture? Clinicians do not routinely discuss overall prognosis and goals of care with older patients, even those with a clearly identifiable terminal illness. However, this undercuts the ability of patients and their caregivers to make informed choices about their futures. Clinicians should routinely offer to discuss prognosis with older adults who have a life expectancy of less than 5 to 10 years or at least by age 85 years. Most older adults welcome this conversation, although a minority are not necessarily as open to the intricacies of the situation.

Older adults with more than 10 years of expected life remaining may benefit from cancer screening and control of blood pressure or blood glucose, while those with life expectancies under 10 years will achieve more benefit from reduction of pill burden and advance care planning. Clinical situations in geriatric practice that present opportunities to discuss overall prognosis and goals of care include cancer screening; modification of standard targets for chronic disease management (e.g., hemoglobin A_{1c}, blood pressure, lipid levels); discussing high-risk surgery, initiation of dialysis, reducing the pill burden, or eligibility for hospice.

Life choices in the very old adults also provide potential opportunities for discussing prognosis, such as financing of long-term care, moving to senior housing, reducing medication copayments, or spending more time with grandchildren. Advanced care planning discussions should be initiated early on with older adults and their family members, especially patients with dementia, patients with limited life expectancy, and those with terminal illness. These include discussions about advance directives, living will, durable power of attorney for healthcare, and Physician Orders for Life-Sustaining Treatment.

Ethnic groups such as Hispanics and African Americans may be less likely to complete advance directives, and some of this is cultural. There is an expectation that the family is supposed to step up and make these decisions, especially for their older members. There is also a fear of being denied medical care, and that this will be facilitated by completing an advance directive. In one study of African Americans, using a faith-based initiative did not increase the use of advance directives, probably because of belief in miracles and a strong conviction that only God can determine when a patient will die. This does not mean that clinicians should give up working with certain groups; clinicians should always talk with patients, realizing that some patients and families may not want any formal written documentation of their preferences.

A large body of research consistently documents that Blacks and Hispanics receive fewer medical services than Whites. For example, Blacks undergo fewer preventive health services and cardiac catheterizations than Whites. More relevant to end-of-life care, compared with White patients, minorities are more likely to have pain underestimated, less likely to receive opioids for pain, and more likely to have pain untreated or undertreated. American pharmacies located in areas with predominantly minority populations are less likely to stock opioids.[21]

However, the underutilization of medical services by minorities is reversed at the end of life. Hanchate studied a random national sample of 160,000 Medicare decedents, oversampled for non-Whites. He tallied all Medicare costs in the last 6 months of life, comparing Whites, Blacks, Hispanics, and other minorities. *Mean Medicare expenses were higher for all three of these minority groups, compared with whites*, and this difference persisted for men and women, across age groups, cause of death, site of death, income, or urban/rural status.

Health Literacy in Older Adults: Additional Challenges

Health literacy is the degree to which individuals have the capacity to obtain, process, and understand basic health information and services needed to make appropriate health decisions. By this definition, nearly half of the US population has some degree of health illiteracy, and limitations in understanding health information are more common among Spanish than English speakers.[22]

The National Assessment of Adult Literacy indicates the following about older adults' health literacy skills:

- 71% of adults older than age 60 had difficulty in using print materials
- 80% had difficulty using documents such as forms or charts
- 68% had difficulty with interpreting numbers and doing calculations

Further, health literacy is related to education, and some older African Americans and Latinos and other minorities may have less education than their offspring. Patients and families with limited health literacy have more difficulty processing both oral and written information about healthcare as well as problems navigating our complex healthcare environment. Low health literacy patients also are less likely to engage in shared decision-making and report that their interactions with clinicians are less helpful. This is magnified by the age factor in general.

Caring for patients and families from other cultures is enhanced through respectful communication, cultural humility, and actively learning their approach to decision-making and medical care; the judicious use of interpreters; and flexibility and understanding of individual variation. These methods can likely bridge many of the disparities and differences documented in the literature.

Summary

Physician assistants take care of older adults in various settings, including clinics, nursing homes, hospitals, and homes. Physician assistants are trained in the medical model and are required to have some geriatric and palliative training by their accreditation agency, but the level and extent of the training varies. Thus, palliative care in the geriatrics population must be part of their expertise.

References

1. Vogel S. Urinary incontinence in the elderly. *Ochsner Journal.* 2001;*3*(4):214–218.

2. Besdine R. Introduction to geriatrics. *Merck Manual.* 2019. https://www.merckmanuals.com/professional/geriatrics/approach-to-the-geriatric-patient/introduction-to-geriatrics

3. Chai E. *Geriatric Palliative Care: A Practical Guide for Clinicians.* Oxford University Press; 2014.

4. Arias E. United States life tables, 2017. *National Vital Statistics Reports.* 2019;*68*(7):207.

5. Teggi D. Unexpected death in ill old age: an analysis of disadvantaged dying in the English old population. *Social Science & Medicine.* 2018;*217*:112–120. doi:10.1016/j.socscimed.2018.09.048. https://www.sciencedirect.com/science/article/pii/S0277953618305446

6. Reisberg B. Functional Assessment Staging (FAST) in Alzheimer's disease: reliability, validity, and ordinality. *International Psychogeriatrics.* 1992;*4*(3):55–69.

7. Collard RM, Boter H, Schoevers RA, Voshaar RCO. Prevalence of frailty in community-dwelling older persons: a systematic review. *Journal of the American Geriatrics Society.* 2012;*60*(8):1487–1492.

8. Ackermann R. Nursing home practice. strategies to manage most acute and chronic illnesses without hospitalization. *Geriatrics.* 2001;*56*(5):37, 40, 43–44.

9. Guidet B, Leblanc G, Simon T, et al. Effect of systematic intensive care unit triage on long-term mortality among critically ill elderly patients in France. *JAMA.* 2017;*318*(15):1450.

10. Farrell B. Evaluation of a deprescribing guideline mobile application. Deprescribing.Org. March 4, 2019. https://deprescribing.org/news/evaluation-of-a-deprescribing-guideline-mobile-application-2/

11. Endicott, J. Measurement of depression in patients with cancer. *Cancer.* 1984;*53*:2243–2248.

12. Palmer A, Taitsman LA, Reid MJ, Nair BG, Bentov I. Utility of geriatric assessment in the projection of early mortality following hip fracture in the elderly patients. *Geriatric Orthopaedic Surgery & Rehabilitation.* 2018;*9*:6–14.

13. Hospital Elder Life Program. Hospital Elder Life Program for prevention of delirium. 2019. https://www.hospitalelderlifeprogram.org/

14. Centers for Disease Control and Prevention. Depression is not a normal part of growing older. 2019. https://www.cdc.gov/aging/depression/index.html

15. Bowers L, Boyle DA. Depression in patients with advanced cancer. *Clinical Journal of Oncology Nursing.* 2003;*7*(3):231–238.

16. Reuben DB, Herr K, Pacala J, et al; American Geriatrics Society, eds. *Geriatrics at your fingertips.* 21st ed. American Geriatrics Society; 2019:260.

17. Wachterman MW, O'Hare AM, Rahman MA, et al. One-year mortality after dialysis initiation among older adults. *JAMA Internal Medicine.* 2019;*179*(7), 987–990.

18. Warden V. Development and psychometric evaluation of the Pain Assessment in Advanced Dementia (PAINAD) Scale. *Journal of the American Medical Directors Association.* 2003;*4*(1):9–15.

19. Campbell M. Tribute to Leslie H. Nicoll, PhD, MBA, RN, BC. *Journal of Hospice & Palliative Nursing.* 2009;*11*(6):303.

20. Goldberg L, Altman K. The role of gastrostomy tube placement in advanced dementia with dysphagia: a critical review. *Clinical Interventions in Aging.* 2014;*9*:1733–1739.

21. Hoffman KM, Trawalter S, Axt JR, Oliver MN. Racial bias in pain assessment and treatment recommendations, and false beliefs about biological differences between blacks and whites. *Proceedings of the National Academy of Sciences of the United States of America.* 2016;*113*(16):4296–4301.

22. Anderson L. Older adults. Centers for Disease Control and Prevention. 2019. https://www.cdc.gov/healthliteracy/developmaterials/audiences/olderadults/index.html

18

LGBTQ Community

Diane Bruessow

Sexual and Gender Minorities: Introduction

The common language used in popular culture, including the terms our patients use to describe themselves and their relationships (e.g., lesbian, gay, bisexual, and transgender [LGBT]), may not correlate with science-based terminology and definitions. In terms of sexual and gender minority (SGM) health,[1] accredited physician assistant (PA) program curriculum was not required until September 2020 to prepare students to provide medical care to patients with consideration for sexual orientation and gender identity.[2]

Sexual orientation is a generic, catch-all term and not a measurable construct. Instead, it is a demographic descriptor of three other constructs: sexual attraction, behavior, and identity. Attraction, behavior, and identity are each a different aspect of sexuality. They are interrelated, with incomplete concordance between them (e.g., a patient's sexual identity and sexual behavior may not completely align).[3]

Sexual attraction is usually established at puberty, before behavior or identity. PAs may inquire about sexual attraction among adolescent patients to normalize sexual development and build rapport. *Sexual identity* is often conflated with orientation in popular culture. This demographic concept is utilized for monitoring disparities in healthcare access, utilization, quality of care, outcomes, and patient satisfaction. People with a sexual minority identity have higher rates of life-threatening diseases like cancer.[4,5] *Sexual behavior* represents any consensual activity or patterns of activity—alone or with one or more people—for sexual arousal. Activities should be defined broadly, beyond genital stimulation. Sex is a self-determined act; if any participant thinks it's sex, it is. Atypical sexual interests are considered *paraphilic disorders* when they meet one of two criteria: (a) involving feelings of distress by the patient about their sexual interests or (b) involving another person's psychological distress, injury or death, or the unwillingness or inability to consent.[6]

Terminology to avoid when speaking with SGM patients includes sexual preference and lifestyle. These terms have been used in arguments to deny civil rights to SGM people and thus have a distinctly negative connotation.

As per the World Professional Association for Transgender Health, "the expression of gender characteristics, including identities, that are not stereotypically associated with one's assigned sex at birth," referred to as *gender diversity*, "is a common and culturally-diverse human phenomenon that should not be judged as inherently pathological or negative," akin to left-handedness.[7] In 2013, the American Psychiatric Association agreed, stating, "Gender non-conformity is not in itself a mental disorder."[6]

In the United States, newborns are *assigned sex at birth* (ASAB), either male (assigned male at birth [AMAB]) or female (assigned female at birth [AFAB]), regardless of genotype or difference of sexual development. *Gender identity* refers to the self-identification of gender. Self-actualization can happen at any age. Sixty percent of transgender adults knew their gender identity before puberty, while 82.6% knew they "felt different" from their ASAB.[8,9] A consistent personal narrative is essential for psychological well-being. In restrictive cultures, including much of the United States, the form taken by sex and gender will present differently from when the culture is permissive.[10] Gender-diverse people may choose to hide their gender identity to avoid stigma, prejudice, discrimination, and violence, ranging from microaggressions (defined as a comment or action that subtly and often unconsciously or unintentionally expresses a prejudiced attitude[11]) to life-threatening while accessing healthcare, housing, public assistance, and other social services.[8,12] In one study, the majority of transgender adults reported psychological pain and suffering as a result of hiding their gender.[9] Emerging data suggest a lack of gender affirmation in crucial developmental areas during childhood has adverse outcomes into adulthood.

Cisgender, reflecting concordance between gender identity and ASAB, and *transgender*, describing discordance between gender identity and ASAB, are descriptors. There are an estimated 1.4 million transgender adults in the United States.[13] While most gender-diverse people are comfortable with the term *transgender* being used to describe them, 14% are uncomfortable. Alternatively, subject matter experts recommend requesting two patient variables during patient intake: ASAB and gender identity. With this approach, the Centers for Disease Control and Prevention identified gender diversity 64% more often than when using a one-question approach.[3] Approximately two-thirds of transgender adults in the United States reported identifying only as male or female. The remaining one-third of transgender adults identified as *nonbinary*, that is, a gender that is neither entirely male nor entirely female.[8] Some countries offer an alternative to male/female (M/F) gender markers (e.g., X, T, I, E, O, or a blank) on official identity documents, including passports. Within the United States, a growing number of states recognize nonbinary gender identities on state-issued identification documents. A smaller number of states allow amendments to birth certificates, though a smaller portion allows a nonbinary gender designation.

By employing gender identity and ASAB in medical records, other documentation, and even case presentations, healthcare professionals can respect the wishes of patients who are uncomfortable with the transgender descriptor being used to describe them. For example, Jax Doe is a 60-year-old nonbinary, AFAB, or Jane Doe is a 60-year-old female, AMAB. This approach respects patients who experience discomfort with the term *transgender*, while the patient's gender identity and ASAB are communicated.

As per Healthy People, an initiative of the US Department of Health and Human Services intended to develop measurable objectives related to improving human health, "In order to effectively address LGBT health issues, we need to securely and consistently collect Sexual Orientation Gender Identity (SOGI) information in national surveys and health records."[14] Healthcare providers' reluctance to inquire about sexual behaviors and sexual health is a significant barrier to improving the care of SGM patients receiving palliative and end-of-life care. The result is a lack of data that limits our understanding of SGM health disparities, maintaining the status quo of inadequate care.[15] Additionally, disclosure of sexual identity, sexual behavior, and gender identity has been linked to improved psychological well-being.[16]

The term *SOGI* has been part of the electronic health record (EHR) meaningful use criteria since 2015. Yet research suggests that PAs are unaware that this information may have been collected during patient intake by nonclinical staff or on a patient intake form, or they are uncertain where to find it documented within the EHR.[17] This may in part be the result of poor EHR design. Documentation of patient SOGI is visible on an administrative page of the EHR along with other demographics, such as race and ethnicity, rather than within the clinical pages that are part of most PAs' workflow.

There are four opportunities within the delivery of healthcare services when knowing SOGI matters most: patient intake and registration, clinical encounters, patient satisfaction, and outcomes.

- Patient intake—which may be done by a nonclinician—provides an opportunity for SGM patients to ensure their legal rights in visitation, advanced directives, billing, preferred name, and so forth. Guardianship, whether foster, incarcerated, or associated with other facilities, and military service, presents unique challenges for SGM patients as well as SGM parents with dependent minors.
- Clinical interactions should reflect an awareness of SGM health, and PAs should approach each patient with cultural humility.[18] Transitions in care between palliative, hospice, bereavement, and aftercare raise particular challenges for SGM patients and their support network. These range from lack of provider knowledge and experience in SGM health, resulting in suboptimal communication; difficulty in assessment; lack of respect for patients' definitions of family, intimacy, and spirituality; and patient concerns for safety and acceptance at the point of care.[19]
- Patient satisfaction evaluations and health outcomes should track the experiences of SGM patients.[18]
    o In 2019, Press Ganey, the leading provider of patient satisfaction scores, introduced variables relevant to SOGI and ASAB, while simultaneously expanding their services beyond emergency rooms and hospitals.
    o The Patient Protection and Affordable Care Act of 2010 allowed Medicare to reduce reimbursement fees for clinicians with less-than-stellar patient satisfaction scores, enhancing clinician motivation for improved patient satisfaction.
    o Meaningful use inclusion of SOGI demographic data collection during patient intake will contribute, in part, to tracking of health outcomes.

SGM Caregivers

Sexual and gender minority individuals are overrepresented among caregivers.[20] SGM caregivers experience several disproportionate burdens, among them physical, emotional, spiritual, and financial stress compared to the non-LGBT caregiver population. This may also result in disenfranchised grief because SGM adults without family acceptance experience more isolation as caregivers.[21] This is compounded by the support groups for caregivers that operate from a cisgender-heterosexual-normative culture, deterring SGM caregivers from accessing them.[21]

Resilience

High levels of resilience have been identified among SGM people in response to often severe challenges.[22] Quality of life among SGM people is negatively associated with hostile cultures, being presumed to be heterosexual and cisgender, victimization, homophobia, transphobia, the anxiety associated with coming out, adverse reactions to disclosure of SOGI, in addition to the stress of SOGI self-concealment and discriminatory laws causing minority stress.[22,23] At end of life in particular, SGM concerns involve institutionalization, staying out of the closet, and recognizing the need for different social support networks.[24] Resilience, in the form of lower reported experiences with discrimination, results from social support and a larger social network.[22] In other words, a network of support is needed to counteract systemic, institutional, and interpersonal bias, especially as it pertains to advocating against discriminatory practices and behaviors. Isolation from social network and social support and hidden SOGI diminishes these positive factors—whether intentionally; due to the invisibility of sexual attraction, behavior, and identity; or by passing privilege (defined as being assumed to be cisgender).[21,23] SGM patients whose SOGI is hidden or unaccepted have a higher occurrence of isolation and loneliness.[15]

Cisgender-heterosexual family members who are legally recognized may be ill-equipped to respond to any bias and discrimination toward the patient they may observe, as well as the anticipation of discrimination.[21] There is a high risk of alienation where legally recognized family members command power while the patient's family of choice has no legal standing.[21] Connection with the family of choice is essential throughout the continuum of care for serious illness, including palliative care, hospice, and end-of-life care. All PAs, including those who practice palliative care medicine, should have an awareness of the documentation, specific to the jurisdiction in which you are practicing, necessary to ensure access for visitation by SGM patients' de facto family members and possibly restricting access by legally recognized family if that is the patient's wish.

Another obstacle of concern is when seriously ill SGM patients anticipate bias, marginalization, and discrimination.[25] This distrust leads to self-protective practices like nondisclosure of SOGI to healthcare professionals and delaying or avoiding access to medical care and other health and social services.[26,27] If the anticipation of bias inhibits access to care, a more substantial burden falls to their caregivers.[22] The growth and acceptance of hospice in the United States has been attributed to the organization of LGBT grassroots social networks that joined together to provide end-of-life care to partners, friends, chosen family, and neighbors during the AIDS crisis.[28]

Recommendations

Studies have concluded that SOGI and sexual health are essential but rarely discussed.

One approach might be to ask, on a scale of 1 to 10, a patient's comfort level in talking about sex and modifying the conversation accordingly, emphasizing plain language rather than euphemisms. The comfort level of the provider also plays a role. In palliative care medicine, compassionate discussions on the quality of life—including sex and sexuality, identity issues, and patients' support systems—are essential.[29]

It is the responsibility of everyone on the palliative medicine team to be proactive in creating a warm and welcoming patient-centered environment. For SGM patients and caregivers, this involves the need to

- reinforce confidentiality,
- provide an appropriately timed referral to palliative care and meet quality standards for pain and symptom management[30];
- practice inclusive communication skills such as asking patients how they would like to be addressed and starting with gender-neutral language in discussions about identity and relationships, which signals to the patient that the provider is not making assumptions;
- create an opportunity for patients to disclose SOGI and respond to SGM disclosure in a positive, matter-of-fact manner;
- celebrate affectional bonds and interpersonal connections by acknowledging spouses, partners, chosen family and friends and their roles as sources of support;
- explore the relationship with the family of origin with the recognition that familial reconciliation may not be needed or welcomed[30];
- respect patient wishes for care plans, surrogate decision-maker, medical proxy, custody of dependent children, hospital visitation, and burial rights;
- seek continuing medical education from SGM community organizations such as the LBGT PA Caucus to be informed on insights that inform optimal care.[19,21]

Recognition of intersectionality, co-occurring domains of social identities such as race, ethnicity, socioeconomic status, faith communities, and kinship networks, is crucial. With each added dimension, provider-patient rapport increases in complexity, as does the risk of bias and discrimination.[31]

Affirmation of a patient's identities at end of life helps to facilitate self-acceptance. The hospice and palliative care provider has a vital responsibility to affirm patient identity and to facilitate and reinforce self-acceptance, so that the patient may successfully come to terms with their identity and life experience.[32] This has been referred to as social cure, though "the real remedy that is needed is the antidote to intolerance."[33]

Affirmation has also been shown to have a remarkable impact on transgender children. While transgender children who are not supported in their gender journey experience higher rates of internalizing psychopathology such as depression and anxiety, transgender children whose gender identity is affirmed in all domains do not differ in levels of anxiety and depression from cisgender controls.[34] In other words, with affirmation they are psychologically indistinguishable. This illustrates the value of SOGI affirmation for our patients regardless of where they are across the life span.

References

1. Morgan RE, Dragon C, Daus G, et al. *Updates on Terminology of Sexual Orientation and Gender Identity Survey Measures.* Federal Committee on Statistical Methodology; August 2020. FCSM 20-03.
2. Accreditation Review Commission on Education for the Physician Assistant. *Accreditation Standards for Physician Assistant Education.* 5th ed. Johns Creek, GA: ARC-PA; 2019. http://www.arc-pa.org/wp-content/uploads/2019/11/Standards-5th-Ed-Nov-2019.pdf. Accessed May 20, 2020.
3. Institute of Medicine. *Collecting Sexual Orientation and Gender Identity Data in Electronic Health Records: Workshop Summary.* Washington, DC: National Academies Press; 2013.
4. Burkhalter JE, Margolies LS, Igurdsson HO, et al. The national LGBT cancer action plan: a white paper of the 2014 National Summit on Cancer in LGBT Communities. *LGBT Health.* 2016;3:19–31.
5. Maingi S, O'Mahony S, Bare M, et al. National guidelines for the best practices in palliative and end-of-life care for lesbian, gay, bisexual, and transgender cancer patients and their families. *Journal of Clinical Oncology.* 2015;33:126.
6. American Psychiatric Association. *Diagnostic and Statistical Manual of Mental Disorders.* 5th ed. Arlington, VA: American Psychiatric Association; 2013.
7. Coleman E, Bockting W, Botzer M, et al. Standards of care for the health of transsexual, transgender, and gender-nonconforming people, version 7. *International Journal of Transgenderism.* 2012;13(4):165–232.
8. James SE, Herman JL, Rankin S, Kesiling M, Mottel L, Anafi M. *The Report of the 2015 U.S. Transgender Survey.* Washington, DC: National Center for Transgender Equality; 2016.
9. Beemyn G, Rankin S. Introduction to the special issue on "LGBTQ campus experiences." *Journal of Homosexuality.* 2011;58(9):1159–1164.
10. Nichols M. *21st Century LGBT: Clinical Work With Gender Diversity, Kink, and Consensual Non-monogamy.* New York, NY: Greater New York Association of Imago Relationship Therapists; December 9, 2016.
11. Casey LS, Reisner SL, Findling MG, et al. Discrimination in the United States: experiences of lesbian, gay, bisexual, transgender, and queer Americans. *Health Services Research.* 2019;54(Suppl 2):1454–1466.
12. Grant J, Mottet L, Tanis J, et al. *Injustice at Every Turn: A Report of the National Transgender Discrimination Survey.* Washington, DC: National Center for Transgender Equality and National Gay and Lesbian Task Force; 2011.
13. Flores A, Herman J, Gates G, Brown T. *How Many Adults Identify as Transgender in the United States?* Los Angeles, CA: Williams Institute; June 2016.
14. US Department of Health and Human Services, Healthy People 2020. Lesbian, gay, bisexual, and transgender health. https://www.healthypeople.gov/2020/topics-objectives/topic/lesbian-gay-bisexual-and-transgender-health. Accessed August 1, 2020.
15. Cathcart-Rake EJ, Breitkopf CR, Kaur J, O'Connor J, Ridgeway JL, Jatoi A. Teaching health-care providers to query patients with cancer about sexual and gender minority (SGM) status and sexual health. *American Journal of Hospice and Palliative Care.* 2019;36(6):533–537.
16. Morris JF, Waldo CR, Rothblum E. A model of predictors and outcomes of outness among lesbian and bisexual women *American Journal of Orthopsychiatry.* 2001;71:61–71.
17. Department of Health and Human Services, Office of the Secretary. *2015 Edition Health Information Technology (Health IT) Certification Criteria, 2015 Edition Base Electronic Health Record (EHR) Definition, and ONC Health IT Certification Program Modifications.* Office of the National Coordinator for Health Information Technology (ONC), Department of Health and Human Services (HHS),

eds. *Federal Register. 45 CFR Part 170, RIN 0991-AB93*. Vol. 80 FR 62601. National Archives; 2015:62601–62759.

18. Bruessow D. Keeping up with LGBT health: why it matters to your patients. *Journal of the American Academy of Physician Assistants*. 2011;*24*(3):14.

19. Cloyes KG, Hull W, Davis A. Palliative and end-of-life care for lesbian, gay, bisexual, and transgender (LGBT) cancer patients and their caregivers. *Seminars in Oncology Nursing*. 2018;*34*(1):60–71.

20. Boehmer U, Clark MA, Heeren TC, Showalter EA, Fredman L. Differences in caregiving outcomes and experiences by sexual orientation and gender identity. *LGBT Health*. 2018;*5*(2):112–120.

21. Brotman S, Ryan B, Collins S, et al. Coming out to care: caregivers of gay and lesbian seniors in Canada. *Gerontologist*. 2007;*47*(4):490–503.

22. Fredrikson-Goldsen K, Kim H, Emlet C, et al. *The Aging and Health Report: Disparities and Resilience Among Lesbian, Gay, Bisexual, and Transgender Older Adults*. Seattle: Institute for Multigenerational Health; 2011.

23. Hanl J, Koeck S. *Hospice Care: Health Services, Quality and Clinical Management*. New York: Nova Science; 2013.

24. Wilson K, Kortes-Miller K, Stinchcombe A. Staying out of the closet: LGBT older adults' hopes and fears in considering end-of-life. *Canadian Journal on Aging*. 2018;*37*(1):22–31.

25. Walker RV, Powers SM, Witten TM. Impact of anticipated bias from healthcare professionals on perceived successful aging among transgender and gender nonconforming older adults. *LGBT Health*. 2017;*4*(6):427–433.

26. Institute of Medicine (US), Committee on Lesbian G, Bisexual, and Transgender Health Issues and Research Gaps and Opportunities. *The Health of Lesbian, Gay, Bisexual and Transgender (LGBT) People: Building a Foundation for Better Understanding*. Washington DC: Institute of Medicine; 2011.

27. Lambda Legal. When health care isn't caring: Lambda Legal's survey of discrimination against LGBT people and people with HIV. 2010. https://www.lambdalegal.org/health-care-report. Accessed August 1, 2020.

28. Boyle DA. The caregiving quandary. *Clinical Journal of Oncology Nursing*. 2017;*21*(2):139.

29. Cathcart-Rake E, O'Connor J, Ridgeway JL, et al. Patients' perspectives and advice on how to discuss sexual orientation, gender identity, and sexual health in oncology clinics. *American Journal of Hospice and Palliative Care*. 2020;*37*(12):1053–1061.

30. Stevens EE, Abrahm JL. Adding silver to the rainbow: palliative and end-of-life care for the geriatric LGBTQ patient. *Journal of Palliative Medicine*. 2019;*22*(5):602–606.

31. Duma N, Maingi S, Tap WD, Weekes CD, Thomas CR Jr. Establishing a mutually respectful environment in the workplace: a toolbox for performance excellence. *American Society of Clinical Oncology Educational Book*. 2019;*39*:e219–e226.

32. O'Mahony S, Maingi S, Scott BH, Raghuwanshi JS. Perspectives on creating an inclusive clinical environment for sexual and gender minority patients and providers. *Journal of Pain and Symptom Management*. 2020;*59*(3):e9–e11.

33. Suppes A, Napier JL, van der Toorn J. The palliative effects of system justification on the health and happiness of lesbian, gay, bisexual, and transgender individuals. *Personality & Social Psychology Bulletin*. 2019;*45*(3):372–388.

34. Olson KR, Durwood L, DeMeules M, McLaughlin KA. Mental health of transgender children who are supported in their identities. *Pediatrics*. 2016;*137*(3):e20153223.

19

Patients With Substance Use Disorder

Hunter Woodall

Introduction

Over 20 million adults in the United States have substance abuse disorder[1] (SUD) involving alcohol, opioids, amphetamines, cocaine, or other drugs. Many families feel the effects of a loved one with SUD. Thus, palliative care providers, including physician assistants, frequently encounter SUD in patients or their families.

Many patients with SUD remain undiagnosed at the time of palliative care referral, with most patients with these issues having preexisting conditions. Alcohol use disorder (AUD) is the most common problem affecting management, with issues of intoxication, nonadherence, increased suicide risk, and medical complications.[2] Opioid use disorder (OUD) remains quite common and requires specific strategies with pain management.[3]

Palliative care teams must be able to

- Detect SUD and differentiate addiction behaviors from incompletely managed symptoms
- Diagnose and manage associated psychosocial issues
- Communicate clear expectations regarding treatment
- Safely prescribe controlled medications
- Manage intoxication or withdrawal
- Develop plans to deal with drug diversion

SUD Definition and Screening

SUD Definition

Substance abuse disorder involves continued use of a substance despite negative consequences to one's mental, physical, and social health. The *Diagnostic and Statistical Manual of Mental Disorders* requires two or more of 11 criteria be present for 12 months for the diagnosis (see Box 19.1).[4] The manual rates the severity of SUD higher as the number of criteria present increases.

BOX 19.1 *DSM-5* Criteria for SUD

Two or more manifested over a 12-month period for diagnosis:

1. Alcohol is often taken in larger amounts or over longer period than was intended.
2. There is a persistent desire or unsuccessful efforts to cut down or control alcohol use.
3. A great deal of time is spent in activities necessary to obtain alcohol, use alcohol, or recover from its effects.
4. Craving, or a strong desire or urge to use alcohol.
5. Recurrent alcohol use resulting in a failure to fulfill major role obligations at work, school, or home.
6. Continued alcohol use despite having persistent or recurrent social or interpersonal problems caused or exacerbated by the effects of alcohol.
7. Important social, occupational, or recreational activities are given up or reduced because of alcohol use.
8. Recurrent alcohol use in situations in which it is physically hazardous.
9. Alcohol use is continued despite knowledge of having a persistent or recurrent physical or psychological problem that is likely to have been caused or exacerbated by alcohol.
10. Tolerance, as defined by either of the following:
    a. A need for markedly increased amounts of alcohol to achieve intoxication or desired effect.
    b. A markedly diminished effect with continued use of the same amount of alcohol.
11. Withdrawal, as manifested by either of the following:
    a. The characteristic withdrawal syndrome for alcohol.
    b. Alcohol (or a closely related substance, such as benzodiazepine) is taken to relieve or avoid withdrawal symptoms.

From Reference 4.

SUD Screening

Substance abuse disorder is often hidden, requiring practitioners to actively screen for it. The best validated screens evaluate for AUD, which is by far the most common SUD seriously affecting palliative care.[2] The simplest screen to use for AUD is the NIDA (National Institute on Drug Abuse) Quick Screen (Box 19.2).[5] It has a sensitivity of 81.3% and a specificity of 79.3%.[6]

When the NIDA quick test is positive, one can gain more information with the Alcohol Use Disorders Identification Test (AUDIT).[7] Developed by the World Health Organization, this 10-question test may be self-administered by patients and has a sensitivity of 92% and a specificity of 94%. Copies and directions for the AUDIT are available from the National Institute for Drug Abuse.[8] The higher the AUDIT score, the more likely that a patient will display intoxication, withdrawal, or aberrant behaviors that increase morbidity and complicate management.[2]

The NIDA quick test has been modified for drug abuse. Instead of asking about standard drinks, the screen asks one question: "How many times in the last year have you used an illegal drug or used a prescription drug for nonmedical reasons?"[9] Any positive response is considered problematic. Reported sensitivity is 93%–97%, and specificity is 79%–93%.[5]

Managing Life-Limiting Illness and SUD
General Concepts

Communicating with patients and families about the diagnosis of SUD should be done gently, emphasizing it is a brain disease and not a choice or moral failing (Box 19.3).[2] Sometimes a frank supportive discussion with the patient and/or their caregiver is all that is required. Forthright communication builds trust, and identifying potential complications enhances treatment. Teams must set clear expectations for pain reduction and handling of controlled substances.[3] Patients and caregivers should realize that eradicating all pain is unrealistic, and the goal of daily pain management is maintaining function without undue side effects. Patients with SUD may use pain medications to modify mood. They may often signal undermanaged emotional or existential suffering with increased pain complaints,[2,3] signaling a need for further spiritual assessment. Large numbers of SUD patients also have psychiatric comorbidities, particularly anxiety and depression.[2,3] Evaluating and handling the patient's

---

BOX 19.2 NIDA Quick Screen

How many times in the past year have you had 5 or more drinks in a day? (men)
How many times in the past year have you had 4 or more drinks in a day? (women)
Any answer of 1 or more is considered positive and requires further screening.

From Reference 6.

BOX 19.3 Resources for Families of Patients With SUD

Al-Anon Family Groups
Nar-Anon Family Groups
Ala-Teen Groups
Co-Dependents Anonymous
Adult Children of Alcoholics
Individual or family counseling with addiction-savvy counselors

From https://www.projectknow.com/support-groups/families-of-addicts-alcoholics/. Accessed September 14, 2019.

---

affect well is critical to successful management. Teams must learn as much as possible about the patient's social and religious support. The team can also provide the extra support that caregivers require.

Since patients with SUD and those with undermanaged psychiatric issues have higher rates of both unintentional and intentional overdose,[3,10] extra care is needed in handling opioids and benzodiazepines (Box 19.4). The team must ensure that coexisting psychiatric issues are properly managed, being especially alert for major affective disorder, post-traumatic stress disorder, and anxiety. The team can address these complex illnesses using risk-reduction strategies[11] and cognitive therapies like motivational interviewing or the BATHE technique.[12]

BOX 19.4 SUD Issues Affecting Palliative Care Patients

Decreased adherence to medical advice
Emotional or existential suffering reported as pain
Chemical coping—treating anxiety and/or sadness with opioids or alcohol
Family member and caregiver frustration and mistrust
Intoxication or withdrawal
Legal issues
Dangerous or inadequate living situation
Diversion by patients or family members
Continued compulsive use with medical and psychiatric complications
Inadequate closure of relationships
Delayed planning of legacy

From Reference 3.

Safety With Opioids

In 2016, the Centers for Disease Control and Prevention (CDC) issued 12 guidelines[10] for handling opioids in patients with chronic pain (Box 19.5). Although these guidelines were not intended to apply to hospice patients, they still inform present regulations and palliative care practice. Following the guidelines should reduce the risk of unintentional overdose in patients with chronic nonmalignant pain, and the principles expressed by the guidelines can be helpful even in patients with limited life expectancy.

Safety Tools

When one starts opioid therapy, CDC guidelines recommend assessing the potential for dependence in the patient using a risk stratification tool such as the Opioid Risk Tool (ORT).[13] However, in 2019, a systematic review by Kilmas et al.[14] found none of the risk stratification tools, including the ORT, had high-quality evidence for efficacy, and none of them produced clinically useful predictions about opioid risk (see Box 19.6).

States now require prescribers to consult their prescription-monitoring program before the first controlled substance prescription and periodically thereafter; hospice patients are often excused from this scrutiny. The CDC guidelines[10] encourage urine drug testing similarly. Pill counts can be useful to monitor adherence as well as diversion, often revealing that patients do not fully understand their regimen. Controlled substance agreements ensure communication of the risk and benefits of opioid therapy. These also include expectations for patient behavior, including handling and storing medications properly, avoiding increased dosing without permission, refusing to sell or give the medication to others, and cooperating with ongoing monitoring.

Pain Management in Patients on Medication-Assisted Treatment

Clinicians will encounter patients on methadone or buprenorphine for opioid maintenance who require adjustments for optimal pain management. Utilization of palliative care medication in this population is complex, and this knowledge or skill set will enhance their ability to counsel the patient and improve adherence and health literacy in complicated pain management situations. Patients on methadone can be continued on the drug, but instead of a once-daily dose, to avoid withdrawal they should split the baseline dose for use three or four times daily for smoother analgesic effect.[15] There is no limit to a patient's methadone dose, but higher doses (over 100 mg) often prolong the QTc interval and are likely to increase drug interactions. Acute exacerbations of pain can be treated with additional methadone or with other short-acting opioid analgesics.

Palliative care patients on buprenorphine who have stable needs can stay on it, and spreading the total dose through the day provides smoother symptom relief.[16,17] Acute pain exacerbations can be handled according to their severity. Mild exacerbations respond well to continuing or perhaps increasing the buprenorphine and adding oral nonsteroidal anti-inflammatory drugs (NSAIDS) and acetaminophen. Parenteral ketorolac (NSAID) and acetaminophen can be useful in some cases. More severe episodes may require adding other short-acting opioids or temporarily changing from buprenorphine to another opioid

BOX 19.5 CDC Guidelines for Opioid Prescribing in Chronic Pain

Nonpharmacological therapy and nonopioid pharmacological therapy are preferred for chronic pain. Clinicians should consider opioid therapy only if expected benefits for both pain and function are anticipated to outweigh risks to the patient. If opioids are used, they should be combined with nonpharmacological therapy and nonopioid pharmacological therapy, as appropriate.

Before starting opioid therapy for chronic pain, clinicians should establish treatment goals with all patients, including realistic goals for pain and function, and should consider how opioid therapy will be discontinued if benefits do not outweigh risks. Clinicians should continue opioid therapy only if there is clinically meaningful improvement in pain and function that outweighs risks to patient safety.

Before starting and periodically during opioid therapy, clinicians should discuss with patients known risks and realistic benefits of opioid therapy and patient and clinician responsibilities for managing therapy.

When starting opioid therapy for chronic pain, clinicians should prescribe immediate-release opioids instead of extended-release/long-acting (ER/LA) opioids.

When opioids are started, clinicians should prescribe the lowest effective dosage. Clinicians should use caution when prescribing opioids at any dosage, should carefully reassess evidence of individual benefits and risks when considering increasing dosage to ≥50 morphine milligram equivalents (MME)/day, and should avoid increasing dosage to ≥90 MME/day or carefully justify a decision to titrate dosage to ≥90 MME/day.

Long-term opioid use often begins with treatment of acute pain. When opioids are used for acute pain, clinicians should prescribe the lowest effective dose of immediate-release opioids and should prescribe no greater quantity than needed for the expected duration of pain severe enough to require opioids. Three days or less will often be sufficient; more than seven days will rarely be needed.

Clinicians should evaluate benefits and harms with patients within 1 to 4 weeks of starting opioid therapy for chronic pain or of dose escalation. Clinicians should evaluate benefits and harms of continued therapy with patients every 3 months or more frequently. If benefits do not outweigh harms of continued opioid therapy, clinicians should optimize other therapies and work with patients to taper opioids to lower dosages or to taper and discontinue opioids.

Before starting and periodically during continuation of opioid therapy, clinicians should evaluate risk factors for opioid-related harms. Clinicians should incorporate into the management plan strategies to mitigate risk, including considering offering naloxone when factors that increase risk for opioid overdose, such as history of overdose, history of substance use disorder, higher opioid dosages (≥50 MME/day), or concurrent benzodiazepine use, are present.

Clinicians should review the patient's history of controlled substance prescriptions using state prescription drug monitoring program (PDMP) data to determine whether the patient is receiving opioid dosages or dangerous combinations that put him or her at high risk for overdose. Clinicians should review PDMP data when starting opioid therapy for chronic pain and periodically during opioid therapy for chronic pain, ranging from every prescription to every 3 months.

When prescribing opioids for chronic pain, clinicians should use urine drug testing before starting opioid therapy and consider urine drug testing at least annually to assess for prescribed medications as well as other controlled prescription drugs and illicit drugs.

Clinicians should avoid prescribing opioid pain medication and benzodiazepines concurrently whenever possible.

Clinicians should offer or arrange evidence-based treatment (usually medication-assisted treatment with buprenorphine or methadone in combination with behavioral therapies) for patients with opioid use disorder.

From Reference 11.

---

agonist.[16] Patients with progressive pain syndromes such as metastatic cancer should consider converting from buprenorphine to methadone,[17] which provides greater dosing flexibility. Eight milligrams of buprenorphine is approximately an equianalgesic equivalent to 30 mg of methadone (10 mg three times daily), but wide patient-to-patient variation exists, and clinicians should start low, frequently reassess, and slowly increase the dose. Ideally, methadone should be reserved for use by clinicians experienced with its risks and benefits.

BOX 19.6 Klimas et al. Strategies to Identify Patient Risks of Prescription Opioid Addiction When Initiating Opioids for Pain: A Systematic Review

The 2019 systemic review found that none of the risk stratification tools, including the ORT, had high quality evidence for efficacy and none of them produced clinically useful predictions about opioid risk. The review did find that a history of SUD, chronic pain disorder, personality disorder, somatoform disorder, or psychotic disorder indicated higher risk for prescription drug abuse. In addition concomitant use of atypical antipsychotics or anxiolytics, duration of opioid prescriptions more than 30 days, and daily doses more than 120 morphine milligram equivalents are associated with greater risk of developing OUD.

From Reference 15.

Dealing With Aberrant Behaviors

Substance use disorder is a chronic relapsing disease, so clinicians must be prepared to manage behaviors such as intoxication, higher than customary opioid doses, family chaos, and even diversion. SUD patients often use opioids for chemical coping with anxiety, sadness, and loneliness, not just for pain. SUD patients often require higher than usual doses of opioid medications, and they often present with complaints of insufficiently controlled pain. The term *pseudoaddiction* refers to behaviors that seem driven by SUD but when investigated are due to undermanaged suffering. Pseudoaddiction responds to properly focused palliative interventions such as increasing pain medication or addressing emotional or existential problems (Box 19.7).[18] True SUD behaviors require interventions focused on the substance abuse problem. The differential diagnosis of unrelenting pain includes physical causes, such as new fractures or previously unrecognized neuropathic pain. It includes unrecognized amplifiers of pain, such as depression, anxiety, or existential distress. The differential in SUD patients must also include using pain medicines for emotional coping, seeking purposeful intoxication or sedation, and intentional misuse for secondary gain. Diversion should be suspected when medication counts are expectantly short, particularly if any family members manifest symptoms of SUD.[19]

BOX 19.7 Strategies for Management of Opioids in SUD patients

Obtain a substance use history, including past and present use

Discuss expectations for pain management

Maximize nondrug approaches to symptom control

Discuss medication safety, risks, and benefits

Mandate a controlled substances agreement

Dispense just a few days of opioid at a time with close monitoring and close follow-up

Consider pill counts and urine drug screening

Consider addiction medicine consultation and comanagement

Encourage ongoing SUD treatment, including Medication Assisted Treatment (MAT) and support groups

Be sure comorbid psychiatric disease is properly diagnosed and treated

Take a differential diagnosis approach to escalating requests for pain medication

Recognize chemical coping and recruit team members to address emotional and spiritual issues

Develop policies for handling possible diversion using a case-by-case team-based approach

Develop policies and procedures for orderly patient dismissal

From References 22–24.

Reducing Risk of Aberrant Behaviors

Teams can reduce the risk of aberrant behaviors in patients with SUD by careful prescribing habits. Clinicians should limit prescriptions for short-acting pain medications to just a few days at a time and monitor carefully with short visit intervals.[20] Tamper-proof medications may be considered but are generally much more expensive. Preferential use of transdermal patches or buprenorphine for long-acting medicine may reduce risk. Controlled substance agreements and pill counts are often recommended but have no proven efficacy. Urine drug testing can be beneficial but may be considered intrusive in patients with limited life expectancy.[21] It may also be cost prohibitive for SUD patients, and results can be difficult to interpret. Perhaps its best use is to aid in detection of possible diversion, where a negative urine may indicate that the patient is not ingesting the prescribed drug. Additionally, prescribers must exercise extra care in prescribing benzodiazepines for patients receiving chronic concurrent opioid therapy.[22]

Possible diversion is the most serious of SUD behaviors, with ethical and legal ramifications. Diversion can be as innocent as sharing a few pills with family or can involve selling medications. Diversion can be voluntary or the patient can be a victim of theft.[23] Clinicians are under no obligation to continue to prescribe medications in the face of diversion, even if withdrawal is possible. Teams should be ready to treat withdrawal. Each case is different, but written policies regarding missing medications provide accountability to patients, caregivers, and the palliative care team.

Dissolving the Therapeutic Relationship

At times aberrant behavior cannot be successfully managed by the team, and the therapeutic relationship must be severed. Sometimes this happens voluntarily when team members unite to make it clear to patients and families that their demands exceed what the team can safely deliver. Other times the team must insist. Patients should be notified verbally and in writing. The team should follow their institution's policy and procedures for patient dismissal. The team should arrange for a smooth transition to other providers whenever possible and should remain available to patients for at least 30 days after dismissal for emergencies.[24]

Managing Intoxication

Alcohol Intoxication

Acute alcohol intoxication becomes more dangerous when alcohol is mixed with other drugs with sedative effects, such as benzodiazepines and opioids. Prescribers must exercise extra caution when writing for these drugs for persons who still actively abuse alcohol. The risk for both intentional and unintentional overdose is higher[3,10] in such persons. Severe intoxication is managed with supportive care, and sometimes even requires emergency hospitalization and ventilation.

Opioid Overdose

Palliative care patients are often on high doses of opioids. The higher a patient's morphine milligram equivalent (MME) dose, the higher their risk of unintentional overdose and death.[10] Naloxone, which can be injected or taken nasally,[25] has current guidelines that recommend prescribing nasal naloxone for patients and for caregivers to keep it on hand when the daily opioid dose rises above 50 MME.[10]

Opioid overdose manifests as stupor progressing to loss of consciousness with bradypnea and constricted pupils. Death can result from prolonged apnea.[25] Patients with liver disease and renal disease can build up toxic metabolites more rapidly than others and are at higher risk. Apnea is also the final manifestation of approaching death in hospice patients, and naloxone can precipitate a withdrawal syndrome. So, teams must be very clear about goals of care and code status, differentiating disease progression from opioid overdose and symptoms with supportive care in patients who desire no further resuscitation attempts.

Managing Withdrawal

Alcohol Withdrawal

Alcohol withdrawal syndrome (AWS) may begin 24–48 hours after a precipitous reduction in alcohol use. It is manifested by autonomic dysregulation, anxiety, and tremor, which can advance to hallucinations and psychosis. Generalized seizures can happen at any stage of the process. Benzodiazepine therapy is the cornerstone of AWS prevention and treatment.[26] The severity of AWS can be measured with the clinical institute withdrawal assessment for alcohol scale,[27] and it can be used to direct benzodiazepine dosing. With proper safeguards, patients with AWS can be detoxified as outpatients.[26]

Opioid Withdrawal

Opioid withdrawal manifests as tremor, rhinorrhea, inability to sit still, anxiety, dilated pupils, tachycardia, yawning, and increased pain. Withdrawal starts in hours after cessation of short-acting drugs like heroin or fentanyl and up to 3 days after cessation of long-acting drugs such as methadone or buprenorphine. Clinicians may use the clinical opioid withdrawal scale[28] to confirm the syndrome and monitor its severity. α-Adrenergic blockers[29] with acetaminophen or NSAIDS can block symptoms, but replacing the missing opioid with a long-acting drug such as methadone or buprenorphine provides more rapid and dependable relief.[30] Once withdrawal has been successfully managed, a reassessment of the patient's medication regimen should follow.

Benzodiazepine Withdrawal and Tapering

Benzodiazepine withdrawal is more subtle than other sedative withdrawal syndromes but can be uncomfortable. Rebound anxiety is the hallmark symptom. Seizures can occur with abrupt cessation of short-acting benzodiazepines such as alprazolam. Restarting a benzodiazepine will rapidly ameliorate symptoms, but reassessing the drug regimen is crucial. Sometimes patients may need to be tapered off chronic benzodiazepine therapy to reduce risk of falls, motor vehicle accidents, and unintentional overdose. This arduous task takes commitment from the prescriber and patient together and may take weeks to months.[31]

Nicotine Withdrawal

Nicotine withdrawal manifests as craving, irritability, anxiety, restlessness, and difficulty concentrating. Palliative care patients residing in their own homes have little onus to stop tobacco use or vaping, but these patients may be required to stop on entering smoke-free facilities. Nicotine replacement in the form of patches, gum, lozenges, or nasal spray enhances patient comfort.[32,33] Daily patches are the most convenient replacement, but some patients will do better with other forms or with combinations.

Summary

Palliative care patients are often profoundly affected by SUD in themselves or close family members. Management of these patients requires proper screening and diagnosis. Teams must establish clear expectations about pain management and handling controlled substances. Teams must differentiate between aberrant behaviors and uncontrolled pain or anxiety. Teams should be ready to handle intoxication and withdrawal. Ongoing timely multidisciplinary communication is paramount in managing these challenging illnesses.

Recommendations

1. Institute routine screening for SUD in palliative care populations.
2. Develop policies for managing opioid medication in SUD patients.
3. Consult addiction medicine colleagues to assist with difficult cases.
4. Evaluate all patients on an MME greater than 50 for emergency naloxone provision.
5. Develop policies and procedures to deal with controlled substance diversion.
6. Develop an integrated approach with a multidisciplinary team for patients with SUD.

References

1. Substance Abuse and Mental Health Services Administration. *Results From the 2014 National Survey on Drug Use and Health: Mental Health Findings*. Rockville, MD: SAMHSA; 2015. NSDUH Series H-50, HHS Publication No. (SMA) 15–4927.
2. MacCormac A. Alcohol dependence in palliative care: a review of the current literature. *Journal of Palliative Care*. 2017;*32*(3–4):108–112.
3. Gabbard J, Jordon A, Mitchell A, et al. Dying on hospice in the midst of an opioid crisis: what should we do now? *American Journal of Hospice & Palliative Medicine*. 2019;*36*(4):273–281.
4. American Psychiatric Association. *Diagnostic and Statistical Manual of Mental Disorders*. 5th ed. Washington, DC: American Psychiatric Association; 2013:490–491.
5. National Institute on Drug Abuse. Resource guide: screening for drug use in general medical settings. http://www.drugabuse.gov/publications/resource-guide. Accessed May 31, 2021.
6. Smith P, Schmidt S, Allensworth-Davies D, Saitz, R. Primary care validation of a single-question alcohol screening test. *Journal of General Internal Medicine*. 2009;*24*:783–788, 881–883.
7. Babor T, Higgins-Biddle J, Saunders J, Monterio M. *The alcohol use disorders identification test, guidelines for use in primary care*. 2nd ed. Department of Mental Health and Substance Dependence, World Health Organization; 2001.

8. Saunders OB, Aasland OG, Babor TF, et al. Development of the Alcohol Use Disorders Identification Test (AUDIT): WHO Collaborative Project on Early Detection of Persons with Harmful Alcohol Consumption—II. *Addiction*. 1992 June; *88*(6):791–804. https://www.drugabuse.gov/sites/default/files/files/AUDIT.pdf. Accessed May 16, 2019.

9. Smith PC, Schmidt SM, Allensworth-Davies D, et al. A single question screening test for drug use in primary care. *Archives of Internal Medicine*. 2010;*170*:1155–1160.

10. Dowell D, Haegerich TM, Chou R. CDC guideline for prescribing opioids for chronic pain. *JAMA*. 2016;*315*(15):1624–1645.

11. Walsh A, Brogllio K. Pain management in the individual with serious illness and comorbid substance use disorder. *Nursing Clinics of North America*. 2016;*51*:433–447.

12. Searight H. Counseling patients in primary care: evidence-based strategies. *American Family Physician*. 2018;*98*(12): 719–728.

13. Witkin LR, Diskina D, Fernandes S, Farrar JT, Ashburn MA. Usefulness of the opioid risk tool to predict aberrant drug-related behavior in patients receiving opioids for the treatment of chronic pain. *Journal of Opioid Management*. 2013;*9*(3):177–187.

14. Klimas J, Gorfinkel G, Fairburn N, et al. Strategies to identify patient risks of prescription opioid addiction when initiating opioids for pain: a systematic review. *JAMA Network Open*. 2019;*2*(5):e193365. doi:10.1001/jamanetworkopen.2019.3365

15. Taveros M, Chuang E. Pain management strategies for patients on methadone maintenance therapy: a systematic review of the literature. *BMJ Supportive & Palliative Care*. 2017;*7*:383–389.

16. Jonan A, Kaye A, Urman D. Buprenorphine formulations: clinical best practice strategies recommendations for perioperative management of patients undergoing surgical or interventional pain procedures. *Pain Physician*. 2018;*21*:E1–E12.

17. Childers JW, Arnold RM. Treatment of pain in patients taking buprenorphine for opioid addiction. Palliative Care Fast Facts and Concepts #221. Palliative Care Network of Wisconsin. https://www.mypcnow.org/blank-zi1e3. Accessed May 25, 2019.

18. Weissman DE. Pseudoaddiction. Palliative Care Fast Facts and Concepts #69. Palliative Care Network of Wisconsin. https://www.mypcnow.org/blank-bua5r. Accessed June 3, 2019.

19. Weissman DE. Is it pain or addiction? Palliative Care Fast Facts and Concepts #68. Palliative Care Network of Wisconsin. https://www.mypcnow.org/blank-xn3i1. Accessed June 3, 2019.

20. Reisfield GM, Paulian GD, Wilson GR. Substance use disorders in the palliative care patient. Palliative Care Fast Facts and Concepts #127. Palliative Care Network of Wisconsin. https://www.mypcnow.org/blank-iicww. Accessed June 3, 2019.

21. Kennedy AJ, Arnold RM, Childers JW. Opioids for pain in patients with history of substance abuse disorders part 1: assessment and initiation. Palliative Care Fast Fasts and Concepts #311. Palliative Care Network of Wisconsin. https://www.mypcnow.org/blank-bhvai. Accessed June 3, 2019.

22. Lembke A, Humphreys K, Nemark J. Weighing the risks and benefits of chronic opioid therapy. *American Family Physician*. 2016;*95*(12):982–990.

23. Kennedy AJ, Arnold RM, Childers JW. Opioids for pain in patients with history of substance abuse disorders part 2: management and monitoring. Palliative Care Fast Fasts and Concepts #312. Palliative Care Network of Wisconsin. https://www.mypcnow.org/blank-hro12. Accessed June 3, 2019.

24. Willis DR, Zerr A. Terminating a patient: is it time to part ways? *Family Practice Management*. 2005;*12*(8):34–38.

25. Chou R, Korthus P, McCarty D, et al. Management of suspected opioid overdose with naloxone in out-of-hospital settings: a systematic review. *Annals of Internal Medicine*. 2017:*167*(12):867–875.

26. Muncie H, Yasinian Y, Oge L. Outpatient management of alcohol withdrawal syndrome. *American Family Physician*. 2013;*88*(9):589–595.

27. Sullivan JT, Sykora K, Schneiderman J, Naranjo CA, Sellers EM. Assessment of alcohol withdrawal: the revised Clinical Institute Withdrawal Assessment for Alcohol Scale (CIWA-Ar). *British Journal of Addiction*. 1989;*84*(11):1353–1357.

28. Wesson R, Lang W. Clinical opioid withdrawal scale. 2003. https://www.drugabuse.gov/sites/default/files/files/ClinicalOpiateWithdrawalScale.pdf. Accessed June 5, 2019.

29. Royall M, Garner K, Hill S, Barnes M. Alpha-andrenergic agonists for the management of opioid withdrawal. *American Family Physician*. 2017;93(1):98.

30. Gordon D, Dahl J. Opioid withdrawal. Palliative Care Fast Facts and Concepts #95. Palliative Care Network of Wisconsin. https://www.mypcnow.org/blank-nonh6. Accessed June 4, 2019.

31. Jennifer Pruskowski J, Rosielle D, Pontiff L, Reitschuler-Cross E. Deprescribing and tapering benzodiazepines. Palliative Care Fast Facts # 355. Palliative Care Network of Wisconsin. https://www.mypcnow.org/fast-fact-355. Accessed June 4, 2019.

32. Shuckit M. *Drug and Alcohol Abuse: A Clinical Guide to Diagnosis and Treatment*. 6th ed. Springer; 2006.

33. Drugs for tobacco dependence. *Medical Letter*. 2016;59:27–30.

20

Veteran Population

Holly Pilewski

Introduction to Veterans Affairs

The Department of Veterans Affairs (VA) is a large, multilayered administration of the federal government. Federal assistance for veterans can be traced back to the year 1636, when the Pilgrims instituted a law for the colony to provide support for disabled soldiers. After World War I, the Veterans Bureau was established. In 1930, President Herbert Hoover signed an executive order that made the Veterans Bureau an official federal administration and renamed it the Veterans Administration. In 1989, the Department of Veterans Affairs became what it is today, a cabinet-level position with a dedicated secretary of the Department of Veterans Affairs.[1]

Structure of the VA

Many think the Department of Veteran Affairs is just the "VA" or the veteran's healthcare system; however, the Veterans Health Administration (VHA) is only one piece of this department. All providers should be aware of the major branches of the current VA (Table 20.1): the VHA, the Veterans Benefits Administration (VBA), and the National Cemetery Administration (NCA).

Veterans Health Administration

The VHA is one of the largest integrated healthcare systems in the world and provides training for many of America's healthcare professionals. The VHA comprises 1600 healthcare facilities, including 144 VA Medical Centers and over 1200 outpatient facilities.[1,2] More than 9 million veterans are enrolled in the VA, and in 2018, the VA provided care to 6.34 million unique patients.[2] There are a projected 19.6 million living veterans,[2] suggesting that a majority of veterans receive their care outside the VHA.

TABLE 20.1 Major Branches of the Department of Veterans Affairs[3]

Veterans Health Administration	Veterans Benefits Administration	National Cemetery Administration
• Medical benefits ○ Primary care/home-based primary care ○ Specialty care, including hospice and palliative care ○ Mental health ○ Community care programs ○ Long-term care ○ Pharmacy	• Service connection • Compensation and pension • Aide and attendance • Survivors' benefits • Life insurance • Education • Home loans • Vocational rehabilitation	• Burial services • Cemeteries • Headstone and markers • Memorial services • Presidential memorial certificates

Healthcare providers outside the VHA must understand the basics of the system and the unique qualities of veterans' health. Eligibility for healthcare from the VHA is based on active military service in the Army, Navy, Air Force, Marines, Coast Guard, or reservists or National Guard members who were called to active duty by a federal executive order. Eligibility is not restricted to veterans in combat or with a medically or service-connected disability, but all veterans must be honorably discharged in order to be eligible for care. A veteran who was dishonorably discharged cannot receive care or any veteran benefits. Once a veteran applies for care, the length of active military service and Veteran's Character of Discharge from active military service is reviewed.[3]

Once enrolled in the VHA, veterans may receive healthcare at any VHA facility nationwide. The medical benefits package from VHA includes preventive care services; outpatient diagnostic and treatment services, including primary care, emergency department care, outpatient specialist care, home care services, and telehealth services; acute care hospitalization for treatment and evaluation or surgery; medications and supplies; hospice and palliative care; and long-term care services (there are restrictions on the long-term care benefit).[3]

For the rest of this chapter, veterans' healthcare services will be referred to the more commonly used term, VA.

Veterans Benefit Administration

The VBA is the second major branch under the VA. The VBA provides financial and other forms of assistance to not only veterans, but also their dependents and survivors. The major benefit programs under the VBA are disability compensation, compensation and pension, and aid and attendance. Other benefits include survivors' benefits, life insurance, education, home loans, and vocational rehabilitation.

If a veteran was injured or acquired an illness related to or aggravated by military service, the veteran may be eligible for a service-connected disability benefit. A service-connected disability is a compensation for the injury or illness and is not subject to federal or state income tax. This disability can range from 0%–100% based on severity of the medical problem.[3] Service-connected disability may qualify veterans for additional benefits, including a survivors' compensation benefit at death. For a veteran's survivors or dependents to apply for the Compensation for Surviving Spouse and Dependents, the veteran's service-connected disability should be written on the death certificate as long as it caused or contributed to the death.[4] Application for disability and determination of severity is done by a Veterans Service Representative or Officer (VSO) through the VBA.[3,4] It is recommended that all veterans establish with a VSO to help determine eligibility for all benefits.[5]

National Cemetery Administration

The third major branch of the Department of Veterans Affairs is the NCA. The NCA oversees 136 national cemeteries in the United States and territories as well as soldier's lots, confederate cemeteries, and monument sites.[3,6] The NCA provides burial services, state grant programs, headstones and markers to private cemeteries, maintenance of cemeteries as national shrines, presidential memorial certificates, and memorial services.[3] The mission of the National Cemetery Association is to "honor Veterans and their eligible family members with final resting places in national shrines and with lasting tributes that commemorate their service and sacrifice to our Nation."[6] Veterans are eligible for reimbursement of burial expenses and other benefits upon death.[7] Veterans and family members should be referred to the Decedent Affairs Department at their local VA medical facility for more information on services and eligibility.

Hospice and Palliative Care in the VA

Of the 19 million living veterans, almost half (47.1%) are over than 65 years old.[2] Each year, approximately one-quarter of Americans (680,000)[2,8] who die are veterans. Of these deaths, 21,000 die in VA inpatient care.[8] It is projected that these numbers will continue to increase, which supports the need for VA-provided hospice and palliative care services.

VA End-of-Life Directive

In 1996, the Veterans' Health Care Eligibility Reform Act mandated that VA offer hospice and palliative care services to enrolled veterans.[3,8,9] Specifically, the VA must provide palliative care consultation teams and hospice care either at the VA or purchased through community providers.[10] The VA defines hospice and palliative care as "a continuum of comfort-oriented and supportive services provided across settings, including hospital, extended care facility, outpatient clinic, and private residence."[2] The VA has shown continued commitment to high-quality end-of-life care through ongoing funding of these programs, development of new programs focusing on discussion of life-sustaining treatments earlier in the disease trajectory, and expanded quality metrics.

Palliative Care Consult Teams

In 2003, the Comprehensive End of Life Care Initiative provided funding to VA facilities to establish palliative care consult teams, regional palliative care program managers for these teams, and quality metrics for palliative care. Facility palliative care teams must include at least a 0.3 full-time equivalent of a physician, nurse, social worker, psychologist (or other mental health provider), administrative support, and chaplain. Teams may also consist of pharmacy support, advance practice practitioners (certified nurse specialist, physician assistant [PA], or nurse practitioner [NP]), physical therapist, occupational therapist, recreation therapist, and/or dieticians.[8] All palliative care teams also have a coordinator who serves as a leader for the program, liaison for community hospice agencies, and educational resource for VA staff, patients, and families.[9]

Palliative care consult teams perform consultations in the hospital, VA nursing homes (community living centers), and/or outpatient clinics. While the VA does not provide in-home palliative care, VA home-based primary care teams provide primary palliative care services in the home.[3] Like civilian teams, VA palliative care teams assist with symptom management, prognostication, goals of medical treatment, advance care planning, psychosocial and spiritual support, and referrals to hospice care.[8] However, VA palliative care teams are often managing veterans who have numerous chronic illnesses with longer trajectories than civilians and more complex psychosocial issues.[9]

Research shows that veterans with palliative care support are more likely to set goals of care, less likely to be admitted to the intensive care unit, undergo fewer diagnostic tests, and have increased satisfaction with the healthcare experience.[9,11] Palliative care has numerous benefits due to its focus on communication, aggressive symptom control, and addressing the many pillars of quality of life.

Levels of Hospice Care

Hospice care in the VA is provided in a variety of settings and follows similar eligibility criteria as the Medicare Hospice Benefit. In order to receive hospice care from the VA, veterans must be enrolled in the VA system, diagnosed with a life-limiting illness with expected prognosis of 6 months or less if the disease runs its natural course, choose comfort-focused care, and be accepting of hospice care.[10] However, hospice care paid for by the VA is not confined by Medicare guidelines. Veterans can receive aggressive interventions such as palliative cancer treatments (chemotherapy, immunotherapy, or radiation) or blood transfusions and hospice care as long as the goals remain comfort, quality, and palliation of symptoms.[9] If a veteran is identified in the community setting who is not enrolled in the VA and may benefit from VA resources, community hospice agencies can coordinate with VA staff to determine veteran eligibility for care and complete enrollment.

Home hospice care for veterans is provided by community hospice agencies who have contracted with the VA. The veteran has the option of utilizing another insurance, such as Medicare, or can request VA payment for the home hospice care. In order to get approval for VA paid home care, a VA physician must certify the veteran for hospice services in addition to the agency hospice medical director.[3] VA-purchased hospice care includes home visits by interdisciplinary hospice team members, medications, supplies, biologicals, durable medical equipment, and bereavement services for families.[10]

Inpatient hospice care within the VA is provided in several locations: VA inpatient hospice units, skilled nursing facilities, and acute care hospital settings. Inpatient hospice care is recommended when pain or other symptoms cannot be managed at home or the veteran is no longer able to be cared for at home due to either lack of caregiver support or caregiver fatigue.

The VA inpatient hospice units are often located within the VA community living centers. These units are frequently staffed by dedicated hospice nurses; hospice-trained physicians, NPs, or PAs; and supportive, interdisciplinary team members. Each unit is managed differently from VA to VA; nonetheless, many units can provide care for weeks to months at a time as long as there is evidence of decline.[3,9] The VA recognizes the complex psychosocial issues and chronic, terminal illness of veterans, permitting them to remain as an inpatient longer than in a community inpatient hospice unit, which is typically 2 weeks or less. Veterans may also choose to utilize another insurance to cover inpatient hospice care in a community hospice facility or request VA payment for inpatient hospice.[3]

The VA facilities that do not have an inpatient hospice unit utilize the acute care setting or community nursing homes for hospice care. The Hospice in Acute Care treating specialty exempts veterans from copays they may normally have for acute care.[3] This treating specialty can also be used for veterans who are too ill to transfer to a hospice unit.

For hospice care in a community nursing home, the veteran can utilize another insurance benefit to pay for residential care at the nursing home of veteran's choice, and the VA will pay for the home hospice care. The veteran can also elect to go to a VA-contracted nursing facility. The VA will pay for room and board in a contracted facility in addition to the hospice services, or the veteran may utilize Medicare or another insurance to pay for hospice in this setting. All this care is coordinated by VA palliative care consult teams and community health nurse coordinators.[3,10]

Finally, for all veterans who die in a VA facility, the caregiver or next of kin will receive an end-of-life survey assessing the family's perception of communication, emotional and spiritual support, personal care, and pain management in the last months of life. This is one of many quality metrics the VA uses to ensure ongoing high-quality care.

National Hospice and Palliative Care Organization and VA Partnership

As noted previously, approximately a quarter of American deaths annually are veterans. Most of these veterans are not dying in the VA or receiving their care from the VA.[2,12] It is important to ensure these veterans' unique needs are being met and they have access to excellent end-of-life care. The VA Hospice and Palliative Care Initiative created Hospice-Veteran Partnerships (HVPs) to improve veterans' access to hospice and palliative care and enhance VA and community agency relationships. Members of the HVPs are state hospice organizations, community hospices, VA facilities, military hospitals, state veterans homes, and other organizations. The goals of these HVPs are to

- Improve veterans' access to quality hospice and palliative care
- Enhance communication among VA and non-VA providers and healthcare organizations
- Ensure that every veteran receives hospice care when needed
- Strengthen relationships between VA and community hospice agencies
- Ensure community agency understanding of VA benefits and resources
- Initiate end-of-life community engagement plans for veterans, for example, conducting community education programs for Veterans' groups about advance care planning and

available hospice resources or educating community hospice agencies about veterans' needs[3,9,13]

The We Honor Veterans program is an HVP between the National Hospice and Palliative Care Organization (NHPCO) and VA.[13,14] This partnership provides hospice organizations locally and statewide with tools and resources for caring for veterans, quality and outcome measures, navigating the VA, and the ability to collaborate with hospice providers across the country.[15] NHPCO has created several toolkits, podcasts, and webinars to set standards of end-of-life care for veterans and augment relationships with the VA.[13]

Defining a Veteran

Thus far, the services available through the multilayered system of the VA have been reviewed, but the question "Who is a veteran?" has yet to be answered. Speaking with veterans will provide a variety of answers to this question. Some veterans may not consider themselves such if they did not serve in combat; some veterans simply view being a veteran as a required duty (and for those who were drafted, it was); and many are prideful about being a veteran, viewing their service as a meaningful period of life making a difference for their country.

The federal government defines a veteran as someone who has "served in the active military, naval, or air service and was discharged or released under conditions other than dishonorable."[16] A veteran may be someone who served only several months in the service but was injured during training and medically discharged; someone who made a career of the military and has retired; or someone who served the 2–4 years of their contract and has been honorably discharged.[3,16]

Culture Experiences of Veterans and End of Life
Military Culture and Feelings About Service

The United States was born out of a military culture with the American Revolution giving the United States its independence over 200 years ago. The military culture continues to exert its importance in multiple generations. Veterans share a distinctive, common bond through their military experience. This experience may be positive or negative and impacts how a veteran feels about their health and, ultimately, affects their end-of-life care. There are four specific questions that should be asked of every hospice and palliative care veteran to best understand the veteran's military experience (Box 20.1).[3,13]

Most veterans were very young when they enrolled or were drafted into the military. In basic training, veterans were transformed from individuals to common units or squads working together with a sense of duty and privilege. They were taught to be warriors and develop stoicism and courage in order to cope with battle or other tribulations during service. Even though many veterans were not in combat situations, all were prepared for this possibility in training.[17] The stoicism developed in basic training never goes away and may lead to psychological, emotional, social, physical (from underreported symptoms), and spiritual suffering while living with chronic illness, especially at the end of life.

BOX 20.1 Questions to Define Veterans' Military Experience

Where did you serve?

When did you serve?

What did you do in the service?

Tell me about your time in the service.

Most veterans take great pride in their service and the unity they created with their squads. This pride may be exhibited at end of life with sharing stories about their service and is expressed by the desire to have veteran-specific ceremonies before and after death. But, for others, their service resulted in anger, guilt, or negative feelings toward the military and government. Some of these veterans were never able to fully reintegrate into civilian society after their service. They may have developed post-traumatic stress disorder (PTSD) or other psychological issues and avoided healthcare settings, especially in the VA.[17]

Veterans who served during a specific war, conflict, or era each has personal unique experiences and feelings toward their service as well. Combat veterans carry at least some emotional, spiritual, or social burden from their service that can be escalated during a terminal illness. This is especially true in the veterans whom acquired a disability or injury in the service or those whom were exposed to certain toxins, extreme weather conditions, and other trauma that resulted in their terminal disease.[17] There are some veterans who did not see combat and have guilt about not participating in a conflict during their service, especially if they had a friend or relative who did go to war. This may have a negative impact on their view of their military experience, and some will not even consider themselves a veteran.

Experience of Veterans in Different War Eras

World War II

There are less than half a million World War II veterans still living, and it is estimated that 348 die per day.[2] The World War II veterans had a mission that enhanced unity and were enthusiastically supported by Americans during and after the war. These veterans won the war and usually are very proud of their service to the country. PTSD was not a diagnosis during their service, and many remained stoic about their duties, never talking about direct combat experiences. Delirium or nightmares directly related to military service or unresolved grief from service are common at end of life.[17] Some of these veterans will begin to share their stories with friends and families for the first time in the final months of life, providing the veteran closure to this period of their life but sometimes resulting in guilt for families who may not have known the burdens the veteran carried. At the end of the war, these vets were exposed to radiation and mustard gas, which may have resulted in injuries such as neuropathy, sensitivity to temperatures, and again, increased risk of delirium, which is more pronounced at end of life.[17,18]

Cold War

The Cold War was defined as an "arms race" that started at the end of World War II but did not end until the mid-1990s. During this time, there was a great deal of above-ground testing of nuclear weapons due to the United States' fear of a nuclear war. These veterans are referred to as the "atomic veterans" because of their exposure to significant amounts of radiation. The Ionizing Radiation Registry recognizes these exposures. Veterans can have an examination to determine if any of their medical conditions are related to this exposure. Some of the illnesses associated with radiation exposure include leukemia, various other cancers, and cataracts. These veterans may have mistrust and anger toward the government and therefore receive most of their care outside the VA.[17,19]

Korean War Era

The Korean War was never officially declared a war, but more than half a million Americans served in Korea and nearly 40,000 died in this conflict. Soldiers in Korea were exposed to extreme heat and cold and often did not have the equipment needed for these temperatures, resulting in trench foot and other disorders. Because the Korean War is often referred to as the "forgotten war" and there was no clear victory, many veterans feel their service was unappreciated and minimize their war experience. This often causes them to relive this experience at end of life, which can trigger delirium and agitation. Additionally, the cold exposure may have caused neuropathy, skin cancers in frostbite scars, Reynaud phenomenon, and changes in skin, muscle, ligaments, and bone. These injuries can result in a sensitivity to touch, underreported pain, and discomfort with moving/repositioning.[17,18] Caregivers and hospice staff should be sensitive to these needs, especially during personal care.

Vietnam War

Perhaps the most controversial war in history, the Vietnam War resulted in a distrust of political leadership in the United States. Over 7 million veterans served in Vietnam in lengthy deployments with frequent rotation of troops.[17,20] Vietnam was the first televised war exposing civilians to its trauma. Vietnam was also the first guerilla war, meaning it was hard to distinguish between civilians and enemy, so US soldiers were never able to let their guard down. On return home, US soldiers were often shamed and dishonored because the mission of the Vietnam War was poorly understood, and the previous glorification of war was gone due to its television exposure.

Vietnam veterans were more likely to survive severe wounds than in past war settings due to the improvement in medical and surgical therapies. Many of these veterans returned with significant physical and psychological injuries, which escalated with the shame and dishonor perceived by or projected by the civilians of the country. Consequently, they had difficulty reintegrating into society and developed high rates of substance use disorder, mental health issues, hepatitis C, social isolation, and unemployment.[17]

Perhaps one of the biggest consequences of the Vietnam War was exposure to the chemical Agent Orange, a herbicide that was used to clear trees and plants in Vietnam. Agent Orange exposure has been connected to several cancers and other diseases (Box 20.2). These

BOX 20.2 Diseases Related to Agent Orange[21]

Amyloidosis

Chronic B-cell leukemia

Chloracne or similar acneform disease

Diabetes mellitus type 2

Hodgkin lymphoma

Ischemic heart disease

Multiple myeloma

Non-Hodgkin lymphoma

Parkinson disease

Peripheral neuropathy

Porphyria cutanea tarda

Prostate cancer

Respiratory cancers including lung, larynx, trachea, and bronchus

Soft tissue sarcomas (not including osteosarcoma, chondrosarcoma, Kaposi
    sarcoma, or mesothelioma)

illnesses can result in veterans' deaths and complicate terminal illness by impacting symptom burden and the way these veterans cope with their disease.[21] Veterans can undergo examinations to be on the Agent Orange Registry and receive service-connected disability, including financial compensation for these injuries.[17]

Additionally, Vietnam veterans more often have poor social supports and complex physical and psychosocial needs in the last months of life. It is estimated that 30% of Vietnam veterans experience PTSD symptoms.[9] PTSD and other mental illnesses are associated with higher rates of delirium as well as war flashbacks. Even those veterans who fully reintegrated into society without PTSD symptoms can have flashbacks and PTSD symptoms at end of life.[9,17] These veterans may also have anger toward their service, especially if it resulted in their terminal illness, and never utilized the VA or sought medical treatment altogether. Nevertheless, anecdotally numerous Vietnam veterans state they would serve again. Interdisciplinary teams are essential for management of the multiple complex issues within the Vietnam era of veterans.

Gulf War

The Persian Gulf War was a short conflict (from early 1990 to June 1991). These veterans were exposed to many environmental toxins, including depleted uranium used in weapons, large burning oil fields, and multiple vaccinations for endemic diseases in the regions served. On return home, these veterans complained of many similar symptoms, and the Gulf War syndrome was identified. The Gulf War syndrome is defined by memory loss, fibromyalgia symptoms, and other nonspecific symptoms. Amyotrophic lateral sclerosis (ALS) and respiratory problems are also correlated with the Gulf War. Veterans in general have higher rates of ALS than nonveterans, but Gulf War vets are twice as likely than other veterans to develop ALS.[17,22] In turn, the VA provides 100% service-connected disability and significant amounts of home services to all veterans with ALS.[21] More associated health problems could be identified as these veterans age.

Operation Enduring Freedom/Operation Iraqi Freedom

Operation Enduring Freedom (OEF) and Operation Iraqi Freedom (OIF) began after the September 11, 2001, terrorist attacks on the United States. Over 1.7 million soldiers deployed as part of this conflict, and many experienced multiple, long deployments.[17] Much more research will be needed to fully define the physical and psychological impacts on these veterans, but we do know these veterans have increased rates of traumatic brain injuries, traumatic amputations and other blast injuries, PTSD, depression, and suicide in part due to the type of combat and prolonged, multiple deployments.[17,23] Other health problems not yet fully identified may occur from environmental exposures, infectious diseases, occupational hazards, and side effects of mefloquine, a drug given to veterans to protect against malaria (Box 20.3).[24,25]

Military Checklist

The We Honor Veterans program, a partnership between NHPCO and VA, established the Military Checklist to ensure veterans are identified and their unique needs are met.[3,13] The Military Checklist is a free resource, available to anyone, that acts as a guideline and standardization for evaluating military experience. The checklist identifies a veteran, determines the branch and time of service, determines if a veteran was in combat, determines the impact of the military experience on the veteran, and identifies if there are benefits for which the veteran and caregiver may be eligible. There are many resources available to learn more about this tool.[26,27]

Psychological Issues of Veterans

Veterans have complex psychological problems, such as PTSD, moral injury, substance abuse, and homelessness, that add to distress and difficulty coping with advanced illness and at end of life. The treatment and diagnosis of these issues is beyond the scope of this chapter. Consultation with a mental health professional as well as involvement of social work and chaplain services is recommended. However, in order to reduce suffering providers should have a good understanding of the psychological problems that plague many veterans.

Post-Traumatic Stress Disorder

During the Civil War, PTSD was known as "soldier's heart." It evolved into "shell shock" during WWI and "battle fatigue" in WWII. It was not until after the Vietnam War that PTSD earned its current name. In 1980, PTSD became more fully defined in the Diagnostic and Statistical Manual of Mental Disorders (*DSM*). Simply, PTSD is an anxiety disorder that can occur in someone who has experienced a traumatic event.[27-29] The fifth edition, *DSM-5*,

BOX 20.3 OEF/OIF Health Issues[17,24,25]

Environmental exposures

    Sand, dust, particulates

    Sulfur fire

    Burn pits

    Depleted uranium (used in military armor and some bullets)

    Heat and cold exposures

    Chromium

Toxic-embedded fragments (shrapnel, other metals)

Noise from guns, explosives, rockets, aircraft, etc.

Infectious diseases

    Malaria

    Brucellosis

    Campylobacter jejuni

    Coxiella burnetii (Q fever)

    Mycobacterium tuberculosis

    Nontyphoid salmonella

    Shigella

    Visceral leishmaniasis

    West Nile virus

Rabies

Occupation-related hazards/exposures

    Chemicals

    Paints

    Machinery

    Radiation

Mefloquine side effects

Traumatic brain injury

has eight categories of criteria for diagnosis: The person must be exposed to death, threatened death, actual or threatened serious injury, or actual or threatened sexual violence in one of several ways; traumatic event is persistently reexperienced; avoidance of trauma-related stimuli after the trauma; negative thoughts or feelings that began or worsened after the trauma; trauma-related arousal and reactivity that began or worsened after the trauma; symptoms last for more than 1 month; symptoms create distress or functional impairment; and symptoms are not due to medication, substance use, or other illness.[30]

There are many screening tools for PTSD for both veterans and civilians. Even so, key symptoms that clinicians should be aware of are reliving the event, avoiding situations that remind the veteran of the event, and hyperarousal.[28] Specifically, veterans may experience recurring memories and flashbacks of the traumatic event; these flashbacks occur at any time or are triggered by sights, sounds, smells, emotions, dates or anniversaries, and other sensory feelings.[30] For example, fireworks may trigger PTSD by reminding a veteran of gunfire; cold weather can bring back memories of combat for Korean War veterans, who experienced extreme cold temperatures; and shortness of breath may trigger PTSD if shortness of breath was felt during the event. During flashbacks, veterans may not be able to differentiate the flashback from current reality. At end of life, this may be misinterpreted as delirium.[28] The avoidance of situations that remind veterans of the traumatic event may not be verbalized by veterans but can still be recognized by the complications of this symptom. Avoidance may lead to depression, social isolation, strained relationships, substance abuse to cope with the situations, significant anxiety and depression, suicidal ideation, and inability to experience emotions.[28,31] The persistent feelings of hyperarousal may present as anger, irritability, increased awareness, being "keyed up," insomnia, difficulty concentrating, fear, being on guard, and being easily startled.[28]

Most often, PTSD symptoms occur soon after the provoking event; however, PTSD symptoms can arise for the first time when diagnosed with a terminal illness in any veteran, but especially those who have never received treatment. In fact, 17% of veterans have PTSD-related symptoms during the last month of life.[32] For combat veterans, terminal illness and facing death in and of itself can be a trigger as it may remind them of death on the battlefield and the vulnerability of being in combat.[28,31]

The PTSD symptoms have many implications for not only the veteran, but also the friends and families of veterans. PTSD can result in marital problems, difficulty parenting, substance abuse, depression, fear, criminal activities, and unemployment, all causing strain on the veteran's relationships and often leaving them with limited social supports.[28] There is also increased suicide risk in veterans with PTSD compared to veterans without PTSD.[30] The social isolation may lead to veterans relying on the medical team as their "family" and support in the last months of life. Veterans may exhibit regret of loss of relationships and seek to reach out to lost friends and family members for reconciliation.

Finally, PTSD may produce spiritual distress for veterans who have lost their faith; total pain resulting in difficulty managing symptoms; substance abuse leading to increased pain tolerance or misuse of medications to cope with symptoms; anger toward authority figures, especially the VA or government; and difficulty with the loss of independence and feeling confined, resulting in increased agitation and anxiety. Research has also shown that PTSD is associated with increased morbidity and mortality for veterans, increased pain, and overall increased medical problems.[28]

It is imperative to recognize the symptoms of PTSD, provide adequate mental health support, and utilize medications for associated symptoms of PTSD.[28,31] Life review with the veteran and family may also help, but providers should recognize that an escalation of symptoms can take place through reliving the event. A mental health provider such as a psychologist or licensed social worker should be available to support veterans and families.

Military Sexual Trauma

Military sexual trauma (MST) is not a recognized diagnosis by the *DSM*, but it is a recognized disability by the VA. Military sexual trauma is defined by Title 38 U.S. Code 120D. It states that MST is "psychological trauma resulting from a physical assault of a sexual nature, battery of a sexual nature, or sexual harassment which occurred while a veteran was serving on active duty, active duty for training, or inactive duty training."[33]

Military sexual trauma affects both male and female veterans and results in increased rates of PTSD, anxiety, panic disorder, depression, insomnia, nightmares, suicide, substance use disorders, eating disorders, and other physical symptoms.[28,34] MST is often underreported by veterans due to fear, perpetrator being a superior, or military failing to act on their complaint. Many veterans do not want to talk about MST, so it is important for providers to be empathetic, ensure privacy and safety, and provide support when having these discussions.[28]

Like PTSD, MST can cause physical and psychological symptoms at the end of life. Certain personal care, such as that involving touch, bathing, or toileting, can trigger the traumatic experience. All care should be explained in detail, and special observation should occur among caregivers for physical reactions to personal care or other triggers. Asking permission for all care is also important to lessen the suffering associated with MST at end of life.[28,34] The VA will provide free counseling and treatment of mental and physical symptoms associated with MST.[34] These resources should be explored for all veterans.

Moral Injury

Unlike PTSD and MST, moral injury is not a diagnosis or eligible for service-connected disability. Yet moral injury is a very real syndrome in veterans that is still being researched and needs to be better understood.

Moral injury was first defined by Dr. Jonathon Shay as a betrayal of what's right either by a person in legitimate authority or by one's self and in a high-stakes situation.[35] Per the VA "Moral Injury in Context of War," "the key precondition for moral injury is an act of transgression, which shatters moral and ethical expectations that are rooted in religious or spiritual beliefs, or culture-based, organizational, and group-based rules about fairness, the value of life, and so forth."[36] For veterans, moral injury often results from combat, especially if it involves killing or harming others, but also may result from betrayal of expectations by leaders or unintentional mistakes.

Like PSTD and MST, moral injury can result in anger, shame, guilt, isolation, despair, and self-destructive behaviors like substance abuse or suicide. However, moral injury is not a diagnosed mental disorder, but rather a dimensional problem, which means that at any given time a veteran may have no moral injury or it may be extreme. It is important to recognize this syndrome as it can result in increased psychological distress in the setting of a serious or advanced illness and end of life. Treatment for moral injury is still not well understood, but cognitive behavioral therapy programs are being trialed.[36]

Substance Abuse and Homelessness

Substance abuse, including of nicotine, and homelessness are more prevalent among veterans than nonveterans. Exposure to combat increases the likelihood of substance use, which in turn increases the risk for homelessness. In fact, 23% of the homeless population are veterans, and 47% of these veterans served in the Vietnam era.[28] Substance abuse and homelessness are also correlated with increased morbidity and mortality and lack of family and social support networks. Untreated substance issues can result in difficulty managing symptoms such as pain at the end of life because of higher tolerance for pain medications, lower pain thresholds, and poor adherence to treatment plans.[28,37] The VA has many programs in place to support these veterans, but it is critical for non-VA providers to know how to access and gain support from the VA. Resources for homeless veterans can be found on the US Department of Veterans Affairs Homeless Veterans webpage[38] and through HVP programs.

Veterans Caregivers

In the United States, there are over 65 million individuals who provide care to a chronically ill or disabled family member or friend.[39] Caregivers experience emotional burdens, mental health issues, physical health issues, and financial burdens from loss of time at work and assistance with cost of medical care.[40] Similar to the unique needs of veterans, research has indicated that veterans' caregivers also have unique and more complex needs than caregivers for nonveterans.[39,41]

A RAND corporation report in 2013 revealed that veterans' caregivers are often younger with dependent children, often live with the person they are caring for, provide care for up to a decade longer than nonveteran caregivers, and must navigate within the large, complex healthcare, financial, and legal system of the VA.[41] In addition, over half of veterans requiring caregivers have cognitive impairment, 60% have PTSD, and 70% have some other mental illness, such as depression and anxiety disorder.[39]

Caregivers of veterans have extra financial hardship due to longevity of required care, 10 or more years, and many have stopped working.[41] There is a higher emotional stress among veterans' caregivers, often due to the multiple, complex health problems of veterans, the higher degree of mental illness and cognitive impairment, and the navigation of the VA. Veterans' caregivers are also more likely to live with the veteran, and more than 80% of veterans' caregivers report having to be an advocate for the veteran.[39]

It is crucial for all caregivers, but especially those of veterans, to receive support from the medical team. The VA has an extensive caregiver program that is continuing to grow and adapt to meet the needs of the aging veteran population.[41,42] Caregivers should receive frequent and truthful communication from the medical team, education about advance care planning and medical decision-making, information about medical home care support, and mental health support, including empathy, resources for caregiver support groups, and grief support at end of life.[40]

Summary: Warrior at End of Life

Veterans maintain their warrior mentality throughout their entire life, and often many of the physical, mental, psychosocial, and spiritual issues related to their service arise during advanced illness and end of life. All providers must be aware of this complex population and how best to care for them.

It is important to have a basic knowledge of the VA and know how to access this extra layer of support for veterans. Resources such as the Military Checklist and the We Honor Veterans program can help with VA access, initial assessment, perceptions of military service, and better understanding of veterans overall. It is also essential to understand how veterans' caregivers need significant support for increased emotional, financial, and physical stressors, but also extended time caring for veterans.

The warrior mentality may make veterans stoic about their physical and psychological symptoms at end of life, but ultimately their final mission should be about comfort, quality of life, and reconciliation.

References

1. United States Department of Veterans Affairs. VA History Office. Updated August 6, 2018. https://www.va.gov/about_va/vahistory.asp. Accessed August 1, 2019.
2. United States Department of Veterans Affairs. VA benefits and health care utilization. Updated July 31, 2019. https://www.va.gov/vetdata/docs/pocketcards/fy2019q4.PDF. Accessed August 1, 2019.
3. Emanuel LL, Hauser JM, Bailey FA, Ferris FD, von Gunten CF, Von Roenn J. Plenary 3: caring for veterans in VA setting and beyond. In: *EPEC for Veterans: Education in Palliative and End-of-Life Care for Veterans*. Chicago, IL; 2011:P3-1–P3-29.
4. VA Benefits and Health Care. Compensation for surviving spouse and dependents. U.S. Department of Veterans Affairs. https://www.va.gov/burials-memorials/dependency-indemnity-compensation/. Accessed September 7, 2019.
5. US Department of Veterans Affairs. Veterans Benefits Administration. https://benefits.va.gov. Accessed September 7, 2019.
6. US Department of Veterans Affairs, National Cemetery Administration. About NCA. Updated August 26, 2019. https://www.cem.va.gov/about/index.asp. Accessed September 2, 2019.
7. US Department of Veterans Affairs, Veterans Benefits Administration. Burial and plot interment allowance. Updated October 2018. https://www.benefits.va.gov/benefits/factsheets/burials/Burial.pdf. Accessed August 23, 2019.
8. US Department of Veterans Affairs, Veterans Health Administration. Palliative care consult teams (PCCT) and VISN leads. June 14, 2017. VHA Directive 1139. https://www.va.gov/vhapublications/ViewPublication.asp?pub_ID=5424. Accessed August 1, 2019.
9. Antoni C, Silverman MA, Nasr SZ, Mandi D, Golden AG. Providing support through life's final chapter for those who made it home. *Military Medicine*. 2012;177(12):1498–1501. doi:10.7205/milmed-d-12-00315
10. US Department of Veterans Affairs, Veterans Health Administration. Community hospice care: referral and purchase procedures. March 1, 2005. VHA Handbook 1140.5. https://www.va.gov/vhapublications/ViewPublication.asp?pub_ID=1229. Accessed August 1, 2019.
11. Penrod JD, Deb P, Luhrs C, et al. Cost and utilization outcomes of patients receiving hospital-based palliative care consultation. *Journal of Palliative Medicine*. 2006;9(4):855–860. doi:10.1089/jpm.2006.9.855
12. US Department of Veterans Affairs. Fact sheet. North Carolina and the U.S. Department of Veterans Affairs. November 2017. https://www.va.gov/opa/publications/factsheets/State_Summaries/docs/North_Carolina.docx. Accessed August 1, 2019.
13. We Honor Veterans. Hospice-veteran partnerships. https://www.wehonorveterans.org/va-veteran-organizations/hospice-veteran-partnerships. Accessed August 2, 2019.
14. We Honor Veterans. Partners: hospice and VA working together. Updated June 6, 2015. https://www.wehonorveterans.org/sites/default/files/public/WHV_Hospice-VA_Partnering.pdf. Accessed August 2, 2019.

15. National Hospice and Palliative Care Organization. We Honor Veterans campaign fact sheet. https://www.wehonorveterans.org/sites/default/files/public/WHVeteransFactSheet.pdf. Accessed August 2, 2019.

16. US Department of Veterans Affairs, Veterans Benefits Administration. Chapter 6. Determining veteran status and eligibility for benefits. M21-2, Part III, Subpart ii. January 28, 2016. https://www.benefits.va.gov/WARMS/docs/admin21/m21_1/mr/part3/subptii/ch06/M21-1III_ii_6.docx. Accessed August 2, 2019.

17. Emanuel LL, Hauser JM, Bailey FA, Ferris FD, von Gunten CF, Von Roenn J. Module 9: the experiences of veterans from different war eras. In: *EPEC for Veterans: Education in Palliative and End-of-Life Care for Veterans.* Chicago, IL; 2011:M9-1–M-16.

18. We Honor Veterans. WWII Health Risks. https://www.wehonorveterans.org/veterans-their-needs/needs-war-or-trauma/wwii/wii-health-risks. Accessed September 1, 2019.

19. We Honor Veterans. Peacekeeping (Cold War) health risks. https://www.wehonorveterans.org/veterans-their-needs/needs-war-or-trauma/peacekeeping-cold-war/peacekeeping-cold-war-health-risks. Accessed September 1, 2019.

20. We Honor Veterans. Vietnam. https://www.wehonorveterans.org/veterans-their-needs/needs-war-or-trauma/vietnam/vietnam. Accessed September 1, 2019.

21. US Department of Veterans Affairs. Public Health. Veterans' diseases associated with Agent Orange. Updated June 3, 2015. https://www.publichealth.va.gov/exposures/agentorange/conditions/index.asp. Accessed September 1, 2019.

22. We Honor Veterans. Gulf War. https://www.wehonorveterans.org/veterans-their-needs/needs-war-or-trauma/gulf-war/gulf-war-health-risks. Accessed September 1, 2019.

23. We Honor Veterans. OEF/OIF Health Risks. https://www.wehonorveterans.org/veterans-their-needs/needs-war-or-trauma/afghanistan-and-iraq-oef-oif/oefoif-health-risks. Accessed September 1, 2019.

24. US Department of Veterans Affairs. Operation Enduring Freedom veterans health issues. Updated June 14, 2019. https://www.va.gov/health-care/health-needs-conditions/health-issues-related-to-service-era/operation-enduring-freedom/. Accessed October 25, 2019.

25. US Department of Veterans Affairs. Public Health. Iraq War exposures. Updated March 19, 2015. https://www.publichealth.va.gov/exposures/wars-operations/iraq-war.asp. Accessed October 25, 2019.

26. We Honor Veterans. Intake/admission. https://www.wehonorveterans.org/get-practical-resources/resources-topic/intakeadmission. Accessed September 1, 2019.

27. US Department of Veterans Affairs. Office of Academic Affiliations. Military health history pocket card for health professions trainees and clinicians. Updated June 4, 2019. https://www.va.gov/OAA/pocketcard/. Accessed August 26, 2019.

28. Emanuel LL, Hauser JM, Bailey FA, Ferris FD, von Gunten CF, Von Roenn J. Module 8: psychosocial issues in veterans. In: *EPEC for Veterans: Education in Palliative and End-of-Life Care for Veterans.* Chicago, IL; 2011:M8-1–M.29.

29. US Department of Veterans Affairs. Mental health. PTSD. https://www.mentalhealth.va.gov/ptsd/index.asp. Accessed August 26, 2019.

30. US Department of Veterans Affairs. PTSD: National Center for PTSD. PTSD and DSM-5. Updated September 26, 2018. https://www.ptsd.va.gov/professional/treat/essentials/dsm5_ptsd.asp. Accessed September 9, 2019.

31. We Honor Veterans. Post-traumatic stress disorder (PTSD). https://www.wehonorveterans.org/veterans-their-needs/specific-populations/post-traumatic-stress-disorder-ptsd. Accessed September 7, 2019.

32. Alici Y, Smith D, Lu HL, et al. Families' perceptions of veterans' distress due to post-traumatic stress disorder-related symptoms at the end of life. *Journal of Pain and Symptom Management.* 2010;39(3):507–514. doi:10.1016/j.jpainsymman.2009.07.011

33. US Department of Veterans Affairs, Veterans Benefits Administration. Disability compensation for conditions related to military sexual trauma (MST). Updated August 2018. https://www.benefits.va.gov/BENEFITS/factsheets/serviceconnected/MST.pdf. Accessed August 26, 2019.

34. We Honor Veterans. Sexual trauma. https://www.wehonorveterans.org/veterans-their-needs/specific-populations/sexual-trauma. Accessed September 7, 2019.

35. Shay J. Moral injury. *Psychoanalytic Psychology.* 2014;*31*(2):182–191.
36. Maguen S, Litz B. Moral injury. PSTD: National Center for PTSD. Updated June 6, 2019. https://www.ptsd.va.gov/professional/treat/cooccurring/moral_injury.asp Accessed September 7, 2019.
37. We Honor Veterans. Substance use disorder. https://www.wehonorveterans.org/veterans-their-needs/specific-populations/substance-use-disorder. Accessed September 7, 2019.
38. US Department of Veterans Affairs. Veterans experiencing homelessness. https://www.va.gov/homeless. Accessed September 10, 2019.
39. Dupke N, Plant K, Kosteas J. Supporting caregivers of veterans online: a partnership of the national council on aging and VA. *Federal Practitioner.* 2016;*33*(1):41–46.
40. Rabow M, Hauser J, Adams J. Supporting family caregivers at the end of life: "they don't know what they don't know." *JAMA.* 2004;*291*(4):483–491. doi:10.1001/jama.291.4.483
41. Ramchand R, Tanielian T, Fisher MP, et al. Hidden heroes. America's military caregivers. *Rand Health Quartly.* 2014;*4*(2):14.
42. US Department of Veterans Affairs. VA Caregiver Support. Caregiver Support Program (CAP) events page. https://www.caregiver.va.gov/index.asp. Accessed August 26, 2019.

21

Prisoners' and Ex-Offenders' Community

Catherine R. Judd and Marguerite R. Poreda

From 1999 to 2016 the number of inmates in federal and state prisons over the age of 55 increased 280%,[1,2] while the population of younger adults grew by only 3%.[3]

Consequently, the percentage of older inmates increased from 3% of the total inmate population to 11%. Inmates in correctional facilities have higher rates of chronic disease and significantly higher rates of mental illness. The cost of medical care for older inmates is significantly higher than for younger inmates.[3]

All inmates have basic rights that are protected by the Eighth Amendment of the Bill of Rights of the US Constitution. The rights of inmates include the rights to humane facilities, to adequate medical care to treat both acute and chronic diseases, to appropriate mental health care, and to be free from "cruel and unusual punishment," a basic concept of human dignity.

Establishing standards for end-of-life care for incarcerated individuals will ensure inmates who are terminally ill do not die alone and die in comfort with dignity.

Adequate healthcare as a right protected under the Eighth Amendment to the US Constitution was further defined by the courts arising from case law.

In the mid-1970s, the courts established that adequate healthcare was a right that must be extended to all inmates and is not a privilege that could be offered as a reward or denied as a punishment. The courts ruled that healthcare includes basic medical, dental, and mental health needs of all inmates and must be provided by jails and prisons. The Supreme Court has interpreted this responsibility for adequate healthcare as the duty to avoid "deliberate indifference" to serious medical needs of inmates and established standards of care (*Estelle v. Gamble*).[4]

Federal and state courts specifically included psychiatric needs within the standard (*Bowring v. Godwin*).[5-7]

Initially healthcare standards were defined and described by the American Public Health Association (1976) and the American Medical Association (1977, 1979). The minimum standards are now set forth by the National Commission on Correctional Health Care Standards addressing medical and mental healthcare in jails and prisons.[8–10]

Compassionate release offers a humane and economical alternative for cost containment in caring for inmates who are terminally ill; however, it is rarely granted. Providing palliative care and hospice care in correctional facilities challenges prevailing attitudes of correctional staff and the criminal justice system toward punishment and suffering at the end of life.

Introduction

In order to develop and implement strategies and standards of care for addressing the end-of-life care needs of the prison population, it is important to understand the criminal justice system, theories of punishment, how inmates and correctional facilities are classified, and the multiple entry and exit points of imprisonment.

Theories of Punishment

Corrections refers to the local, state, and federal agencies and programs under whose jurisdiction individuals who have been arrested and accused of a crime or convicted of a crime interface. The correctional system is integrally related to police, prosecutors and defenders, judges, and the courts.

There are four components to punishment: (1) retribution, derived from the Latin word *retribo,* which means "pay back"; (2) deterrence: if individuals are held accountable for their illegal behavior, others will be deterred from the same behavior; (3) rehabilitation: if individuals are incarcerated, they have the opportunity to learn from their mistakes and be reformed through education, training, and counseling; and (4) incapacitation: incarceration will prevent the individual from repeating a criminal act.[11]

The prison population continues to age because of rising crime rates in the 1980s and the "tough-on-crime" public sentiment that drove longer sentences for even nonviolent crimes and the belief that all offenders should receive the same sentence for the same crime regardless of individual differences and potential risks of reoffending.

Correctional Facilities

The US correctional system is multilayered with a diverse organizational structure. It includes a federal system; 50 separate state correctional systems; District of Columbia and an infinite number of county and local systems. Differences do exist from state to state in organization and in how crimes are defined, sentenced, and adjudicated. Facilities at the state level consist of lockups, jails, and prisons. Lockups are local and temporary, operated by local police departments, separate from jail, with length of stays usually less than 48 hours.[11]

Jails are for confinement of individuals who have been arrested, awaiting trial or awaiting release on bond, or charged with lessor misdemeanor crimes and for temporary housing of individuals who will be transferred to other state or federal authorities, held in protective custody, or held by courts as witnesses. Jails may also serve to detain and house noncitizens in custody of United States.

Citizenship and Immigration Services. Of the total number of incarcerated individuals in the United States, approximately one-third are held in local jails.[12]

Few young offenders are incarcerated in adult facilities; in 2015, state prisons held an estimated 1000 prisoners 17 years or younger; federal prisons held 21 persons under 18 years old and 2204 inmates 18 to 21 years old; fewer than 4000 juveniles were in local jails.[13]

Prisons are operated under state and federal correctional systems, and as a rule, house individuals convicted of felonies, considered more serious than misdemeanors. Prisons house a larger number of inmates than jails. Prisons as a rule are housing inmates who have been convicted of a crime and who are serving sentences of longer than a year. The fundamental difference between jail and prison is the expected length of stay of inmates. Jails by definition hold individuals awaiting trial or who are serving a short sentence, usually less than a year. Prisons are designed to hold inmates convicted of more serious crimes, usually a felony, and serving sentences on average from a year to life.[14]

In 1930, the Federal Bureau of Prisons (BOP) established a nationwide system of federally run prisons and detention facilities. There are 109 federal prisons and 1000 state prisons. In addition to those facilities under the oversight of the Federal BOP, there are 3163 local jails and 80 Indian Country jails, as well as military prisons, immigration detention facilities, civil commitment centers, and state and federal psychiatric hospitals.[15]

Civil Commitment

A civil commitment is a court-ordered involuntary confinement of a person suffering from mental illness or alcohol and/or drug addiction and usually with a finding that the person is dangerous to him-/herself or others. This generally applies to sexually dangerous persons but has been used for persons who pose a high threat to themselves or others and may include those individuals with mental illness, developmental disabilities, or chemical dependencies. Instead of punishment for past crimes, this involuntary confinement is based on the risk that an individual may commit offenses in the future. The US Supreme Court upheld civil commitment (*Kansas v. Hendricks*),[16] finding that such laws do not violate the US Constitution's double jeopardy. Civil commitment laws are constitutionally permissive and exist at the federal and state levels; detainees are held in state and federal facilities.[17,18]

In 2019, the majority of criminal offenses were drug related (45.3%), an increase from 16% in 1970. The remaining offenses were for weapons charges, explosives, arson (18.8%); and robbery (3.5%); homicide, aggravated assault, kidnapping (3.2%); and sex offenses (10.1%).[19] There has been an increase in the privatization and contracting of privately operated facilities to alleviate overcrowding in state and federal systems.[20] The federal system and 27 states contract for beds in private facilities. According to the US Department of Justice, as of 2013 there were 133,000 state and federal prisoners housed in privately owned prisons in the United States, constituting 8.5% of the overall US prison population. The war on drugs and harsher sentencing, including mandatory minimum sentences, have fueled a rapidly expanding prison population that began in the 1980s, resulting in a rise in the number of for-profit privately owned and operated prisons.[21]

Comparative outcome studies between state-run prisons and private for-profit prisons are not available, but there are anecdotal reports of poor quality care at many private prisons, with an increase in inmate mortality, deficiencies in care, and allegations of increased risk of serious harm and preventable injury due to the conditions at those facilities. As a result, there have been multiple court cases and judgments by the Department of Justice against those facilities.[22-25]

Typically, the housing of inmates is based on a classification determined by level of security required, level of supervision required, and services required by the inmate. Services may include accommodations for disabilities, medical illnesses and medical care required, as well as accommodations for developmental disabilities and mental illness.

Changing Demographics

The demographics of incarcerated individuals in the United States are changing with implications for the economic burden of caring for an aging prison population. There are increasing numbers of inmates serving life sentences today, more than the entire prison population in the early 1970s. The number of inmates serving life sentences is at an all-time high and includes those inmates serving life without the possibility of parole (53,290), life with the possibility of parole (108,667), and "virtual" life sentences of 50 years or more (44,311). Over 6000 women are serving life or "virtual" life sentences, with the number of women rising faster than that of men in recent years. Older individuals have a higher incidence of chronic illnesses, such as HIV/AIDS, cancer, chronic obstructive pulmonary disease, heart disease, hypertension, diabetes, hepatitis, and hepatic failure and other ailments that require significant increases in healthcare budgets.[26]

The Centers for Disease Control and Prevention published a survey of prison healthcare. Among the most frequently screened for health issues of inmates were hepatitis A, B, and C; tuberculosis; mental health issues; traumatic brain injury; cardiovascular conditions; elevated lipids; and hypertension.[27]

The National Research Council reported half of the 222% growth in the state prison population between 1980 and 2010 was due to an increase in the time served in prison for all offenses.[28]

From 1999 to 2019, the number of people 55 or older in state and federal prisons increased nearly three-fold. The Federal BOP reports 11.2% of the prison population is over the age of 55 (Table 21.1). As of 2016, of prisoners sentenced to more than 1 year in state or federal prison 11% were age 55 or older. Sixteen percent of White male prisoners were age 55 or older, compared to 10% of Black male and 8% of Hispanic male prisoners. Eight percent each of White and Black female prisoners were age 55 or older, compared to 5% of Hispanic female prisoners.[29-31]

TABLE 21.1 Percentage of Inmates Over Age 55[29,30,31]

White males	16
Black males	10
Hispanic males	8.0
White females	8.0
Black females	8.0
Hispanic females	5.0

Like senior citizens outside prison walls, older individuals in prison are more likely to experience cognitive decline, including dementia, impaired mobility, and loss of hearing and vision. In prisons, these ailments present special challenges and can necessitate increased medical and correctional staffing levels and enhanced officer training to accommodate those who have difficulty understanding and complying with orders from correctional officers. This senior population requires structural access adaptations in housing and accommodations.

Additionally, as the Bureau of Justice Statistics found, older inmates are more susceptible to costly chronic medical conditions. Older inmates typically experience the effects of aging earlier than people outside prison because of substance abuse, inadequate preventive and primary care prior to incarceration, the stressors linked to isolation, and the prison environment.

For these reasons, those inmates older than 55 have a negative impact on prison budgets. Estimates of the increased cost vary. The National Institute of Corrections calculates the annual cost on average of incarcerating those 55 or older who have chronic or terminal illnesses at two to three times that for all others in the prison population. More recently, other researchers have found that the cost differential may be even greater, approaching $34,000.00 per year to keep a healthy younger inmate locked up and twice that amount for elders.[3,32]

For prisoners over the age of 50, the United States currently spends about $16 billion on incarceration.[33]

Palliative Care and Hospice Care in Prisons

Prison Legal News reported on a California medical facility, one of only two licensed hospices in correctional facilities in the state, where inmates were trained and volunteered to work in a hospice program begun in the early 1990s during the height of the AIDS crisis. It now houses more elderly prisoners dying from other causes. To meet eligibility for one of the 17 hospice beds, an inmate must receive a diagnosis with a life expectancy of no more than 6 months and sign a do not resuscitate (DNR) order. The goal of hospice is "to help prisoners find peace while dying." The inmate hospice volunteers undergo a series of interviews, submit to random urine drug screens, and have their disciplinary record reviewed before accepting one of the lowest paying job details in the California prison system. Training of the volunteer caregivers is by the prison chaplain and includes 70 hours of training on hospice care and comfort, psychological and end-of-life issues, appropriate bedside care, stages of grief, and compassion fatigue. In the final stages of dying, pastoral care staff maintains the 24-hour bedside vigil.[34]

Prisoners are used as hospice caregivers in approximately 80 prisons nationwide. The program in California is modeled after a program begun in 1988 by the Louisiana-Mississippi Hospice and Palliative Care Organization at the Louisiana State Penitentiary in Angola, where over 80 percent of the 6500 prisoners are serving life sentences and will die behind bars. Selected younger prisoners serve as volunteer caregivers to join a terminally ill inmate's four-person rotation team.

The inmate hospice volunteers received 40 hours of training in the principles of hospice care.

Prison management noted more compassion and less violence among inmates as the program grew within the institution.[34-36]

Pennsylvania implemented its first inmate hospice volunteer program in 2004. A group of inmate hospice volunteers at Graterford State Correctional Institution (SCI) became a source of comfort for those destined to die behind bars. Although families are limited to visits of 1 hour a day, the inmate hospice volunteers assist with feeding, grooming, and personal hygiene. In 2016, all Pennsylvania prisons were ordered to implement a hospice program; however, not all facilities have opted to use inmates as hospice volunteer caregivers.[3]

Standards of Palliative Care and Hospice

Hospice care is similar to palliative care; however, there are some important differences, especially as these two models are applied to the care of incarcerated inmates. The objective of both hospice and palliative care is pain and symptom management, but the prognosis and goals are different. The definition of hospice care is compassionate comfort care. Based on the healthcare provider's estimate, if the disease runs its course, the patient has a prognosis of 6 months or less, and the patient no longer has curative treatment options or has chosen not to pursue further treatment.[37] Palliative care is compassionate comfort care that provides relief from the physical and mental symptoms of a serious or life-limiting illness. Palliative care takes a preventive and holistic approach to healthcare, and does not pursue all possible treatments to prolong life unnecessarily, such as feeding tubes, tracheostomy, and ventilators. Palliative care can be pursued at the time of diagnosis, during the course of curative treatment, or at the end of life.[37,38]

Patients seeking palliative care do not have to meet the same requirements as for Medicare or Medicaid. The expense of palliative care, medication, and other costs vary by healthcare provider and insurance. Hospice requires that two physicians or healthcare providers document that the patient has less than 6 months to live if the disease follows its expected course.

Palliative care is begun at the discretion of the physician or healthcare provider and the patient and can be initiated at any time and at any stage of illness, regardless of whether or not the diagnosis is terminal.

The interdisciplinary palliative and hospice care team focuses on supporting those with serious illness from diagnosis to the very end of illness and death, addressing the needs of the patient and the patient's significant others. The focus is to improve care, mitigate suffering, and improve quality of life. The ultimate goal is a "good death," free from preventable distress and suffering for patients/inmates, family members if involved, and the healthcare team. End-of-life issues addressed by the interdisciplinary healthcare team are related to medical/physical symptoms, psychological symptoms, and existential distress and include pain, confusion, delirium, depression, anxiety, fatigue, breathlessness, insomnia, nausea, constipation, diarrhea, anorexia, fear of dying, and emotional suffering, which may be exacerbated by mental illness and religious, spiritual, and existential concerns. The compassionate care rendered to the incarcerated person will result in decreased pain, decreased loneliness, decreased hopelessness, and improved emotional well-being while actively dying.[39]

Advance care planning for terminally ill and dying inmates can provide compassionate, dignified, palliative, and end-of-life care for the terminally ill and those who are destined to die in prison. It can provide for a good death and a good grief experience for those caring for the inmates, including the prison and institutional healthcare staff and the prisoner hospice volunteer caregivers who are inmates who have been trained to provide palliative and end-of-life care. These volunteer caregivers provide support and companionship to these incarcerated patients at the end of life. For the prisoner hospice volunteers, it is not about them, but for the dying inmate, who gives them purpose and an increased opportunity to express compassion and empathy and to realize a sense of their own humanness in the prison setting.[40]

Delivery of palliative care and hospice care behind bars is not the same as on the "outside" of prison walls. The following are barriers to palliative and hospice care in the correctional setting:

a. informational barriers exist related to medical care/treatment decisions within the inmate population; barriers may be related to illiteracy or general unfamiliarity with healthcare/advance care planning, such as cardiopulmonary resuscitation, DNR orders, feeding tubes, and other medical interventions;

b. lack of autonomy, or lack of decision-making capacity since prisoners are accustomed to having no power or decision-making ability for the years they have been housed in a correctional facility; or they may be cognitively impaired and have advanced disease, such as dementia;

c. custody versus compassionate care; the goals of corrections is punishment, incapacitation, and custody and are in conflict with goals of compassionate care;

d. mistrust between staff and inmates; it is easier to care for people you know and trust;

e. safety concerns, especially in high-security prisons regarding such prisoners or in the event an inmate attempts escape or is released back into society;

f. concern over the potential for inmates to misuse, abuse, or traffic medications, especially pain medications, or cause intentional self-injury in order to receive medical care or medication that may or may not be indicated;

g. ethical and moral dilemmas resulting in stress and burnout among medical and correctional staff dealing with caring for aging and dying population following prison regulations;

h. institutional and medical staff attitudes, lack of compassion or apathy toward terminally ill patients;

i. public and (estranged) family isolation from inmate population.

Compassionate Release/Reduction in Sentence

Freedom from torture and "cruel and unusual punishment" is a fundamental right afforded inmates; this should include an inmate's right to an appropriate level of care. These rights are guaranteed, regardless of the nature of the crime or prior prison placement(s). Compassionate release describes a range of policies and procedures offering early release or parole to incarcerated inmates with serious or debilitating illnesses. However, in many states that have compassionate release policies, few inmates are actually granted release. When palliative care is unavailable, the ongoing incarceration of inmates with debilitating or terminal illness may represent a violation of human dignity and human rights.[41]

Compassionate release is a process by which inmates in the criminal justice system may be eligible for immediate early release on grounds of "extraordinary" or compelling circumstances that could not reasonably have been foreseen by the court at the time of sentencing. If inmates with terminal illness are granted a compassionate release, which is rare, they may not have health insurance coverage in place at the time of release. However, by virtue of their terminal illness, they may meet criteria for Medicare and Medicaid coverage. Reasons for release denial range from concerns regarding risk to public safety, inmate's original crime or criminal history is too serious to justify early release, inmate not felt to be a model prisoner, or inmate does not meet medical criteria such as life expectancy estimates or is not felt to be "sick enough."[40]

According to the Marshall Project Report (2018), compassionate release dates back to the early 1980s when federal sentencing laws were revised. Congress created a mechanism for compassionate release as a means by which inmates such as those terminally ill could be released, providing judges the authority to retroactively reduce sentences in "extraordinary and compelling circumstances" that could not have reasonably been predicted by the court at the time of sentencing. However, a court could only do so if, and only if, the BOP filed a motion with the court on behalf of the inmate.

The BOP received approximately 5400 applications for compassionate release between 2013 and 2017. Of those, 312 were approved; during the same period, 266 inmates who filed applications died in custody.[42]

The US Department of Justice Statistics reported in 2016 that as of the year ending in 2014, there were approximately 1,433,800 prisoners in state and federal facilities. A total of 3483 inmates died in state prisons and 444 in federal prisons, the highest number of deaths recorded since the bureau started compiling data in 2001. Between 2001 and 2014, there were a total of 50,785 deaths in state and federal facilities.[43]

In view of the increasing population of aging prisoners, the number of deaths will continue to rise. For many years, the BOP only approved those inmates who were near death for compassionate release. Although the reality is the federal inmate population is getting older and the cost of their care is escalating, a report by the inspector general in 2013 found not a single application for compassionate release was approved over the previous 6-year period. The inmates who would meet criteria for compassionate release are among the oldest, frailest, and terminally ill. The BOP budget for healthcare was $1.3 billion for fiscal year 2016. In 2019, inmates over 55 made up 11.2%, and many of those will end their lives behind bars, and some will die in shackles.[32,42]

The application process for the compassionate release of an inmate from prison is as follows:

a. The warden approves physician/medical officer recommendation and documentation of compelling and extraordinary circumstances.
b. The director of the BOP may file a motion with an inmate's sentencing court for reduction in sentence (RIS) for an inmate presenting extraordinary and compelling circumstances.
c. The BOP may consider both medical and nonmedical circumstances (see 18 U.S.C. § 3582 and Program Statement on Compassionate Release/Reduction in Sentence).
d. The BOP consults with the US Attorney's Office that prosecuted the inmate and will notify any victims of the inmate's current offense.
e. If the RIS is granted, the judge will issue an order for the inmate's release; he or she will then usually begin serving the previously imposed term of supervised release.
f. If an inmate's RIS request is denied, the inmate will be provided a statement of reasons for the denial; the inmate may appeal a denial through the Administrative Remedy Procedure.
g. Denials by the general counsel or the director are final agency decisions and cannot be appealed.
h. Inmates who feel their request is of an emergency nature (i.e., a terminal medical condition) may state as such in accordance with the regulation (see 28 CFR part 542, subpart B).

State prison systems have similar provisions for compassionate release, sometimes referred to as medical parole, emergency parole, or medical release. Physician assistants (PAs) working in correctional care and as a member of the healthcare team are in a position to provide care within their scope of practice as delineated by the institution.

Dozens of states have passed sentencing and prison reforms in an effort to safely reduce prison populations and save healthcare costs.

Forty-nine states and the District of Columbia have a mechanism for early release of disabled or seriously ill inmates; however, it is rarely used. There are multiple barriers for compassionate release, including confusing rules, unrealistic time frames, poor communication, and public safety concerns. Patient advocacy groups, including Families Against Mandatory Minimums, put forth best compassionate release practices that would include involving families, clarity of processes, simplifying rules and regulations, and reasonable time frames for processing requests.[44,45]

Caring for Ex-Prisoners on Probation, Parole, or Compassionate Release

As of December 31, 2016, there were more than 4.5 million adults on community supervision (parole or probation) in the United States, representing one out of 55 adults in the US population. Ex-prisoners released on probation or parole, and among them those terminally ill who, in the rare instance, have been granted compassionate release, are more likely than the general population to have severe and persistent mental illness, have prior criminal offenses, a higher incidence of antisocial personality disorder, and a history of violence/aggression and substance abuse.[46]

Many inmates do not have health insurance while they are incarcerated since Medicaid benefits are terminated while inmates are incarcerated and must be reapplied for on release. This has implications for their eligibility to receive hospice and palliative care benefits as well as for receiving mental health services if and when they are released. In addition, these inmates are more likely to be homeless, unemployed, and lack health insurance than the general population never incarcerated. Often, psychiatric treatment is a condition of release, and those who do not engage in treatment face reincarceration.[46]

For inmates who are terminally ill and granted the rare conditional or compassionate release, it is likely predicated on family involvement with a documented family caregiver and a place to live. Nonetheless, for those who are at the end of life, actively dying, palliative and hospice care services will afford them a more compassionate death than they would have had behind bars. Please see the sidebar for supplemental information related to the pandemic.

Pandemic Covid-19—Implications and Consequences for Prisons and Jails

The first cases of Covid-19 began to appear in the United States in early 2020. The first reported case in the prison population, which includes over 2 million men and women, was diagnosed at the main jail complex in New York City at Riker's Island. The number of cases soared to 200 in 2 weeks.[47]

Until mid-April 2020, the case rate in prisons was lower than in the general population. As the disease spread across the United States, it also did in jails and prisons. Between March 31 and June 6, 2020, the number of cases in federal and state prisons was 5.5 times higher than in the general population. Data from the Covid-19 Behind Bars Project looked at multiple sources and databases. By summer 2020, it was estimated 42,107 of 1,295,285 prisoners had been infected at a case rate of 3.25% versus 0.59% in the general population. In some prisons, outbreaks involved 65% of inmates. As the death rate in the United States was approaching 100,000, the death rate among the incarcerated population was three times higher than the general population. According to data collected by researchers from Johns Hopkins University and the University of California Los Angeles, the Covid-19 Behind Bars Data Project estimated the true prevalence may be even higher.[48]

Infectious diseases that are highly and rapidly transmissible are difficult to manage in overcrowded prisons and jails, where inmates are unable to adhere to the measures needed to contain and mitigate spread of the virus. They are housed in close confinement, cannot practice social distancing, do not have access to personal protective equipment, and, in addition, suffer higher rates of underlying medical conditions, such as congestive heart failure, hypertension, and respiratory disease, which are known to increase morbidity/mortality. In addition, correctional officers and other jail staff entering facilities from the outside are all too often the carriers of the virus into an otherwise-isolated environment where social distancing is physically impossible.

The lack of testing and adequate infection control creates a potentially lethal environment. Few facilities are prepared for the surge and numbers of patients reporting for sick call. Some facilities require copayments for sick call, which poses severe challenges and prevents inmates from seeking care.

Prisons have attempted to slow transmission and decrease the number of infections through early release of nonviolent offenders. However, the aged population at greatest risk for complications and more life-threatening illness are frequently the same inmates who are serving longer sentences for more serious crimes. Thus, they are not considered eligible for compassionate release, and this presents a similar obstacle for the terminally ill. Depending on the policies set by the locale and the warden, the terminally ill are also unable to be visited by their loved ones and/or whomever they have designated as family.

In April 2020, US Attorney General William Barr ordered release of as many such inmates as possible with high-risk and underlying medical conditions. There is limited information available regarding the extent to which his directive has been implemented.[49]

Infection with Covid-19 is considered an acute illness, not unlike influenza, mumps, or other contagious diseases. These patients, unfortunately, would not be considered eligible for hospice care or palliative care, despite the fact that those who are terminally ill are among the most vulnerable and at high risk.

Summary

Providing humane and compassionate end-of-life care in correctional facilities presents multiple challenges and obstacles for the criminal justice system, correctional staff, healthcare providers, and hospice and palliative care providers. It is infinitely more challenging than providing hospice care and palliative care in hospitals, nursing homes, and private homes in the "free world" (a term used in correctional care by inmates and staff to describe life outside of prison walls). Adapting hospice care in prisons frequently runs counter to prevailing, long-held attitudes and behaviors toward the punishment and suffering of inmates. Punishment at the end of life is in direct conflict with the philosophy of hospice, which is to provide dying inmates a dignified and peaceful death regardless of criminal offense or original sentencing.

References

1. Human Rights Watch. Old behind bars: The aging prison population in the United States. 2012. https://www.hrw.org/sites/default/files/reports/usprisons0112_brochure_web.pdf. Accessed October 25, 2019.

2. Glaze LE, Kaeble D. Correctional population in the United States, 2013. Bureau of Justice Statistics. 2014. http://www.bjs.gov/index.cfm?ty=pbdetail&lid=5177. Accessed October 25, 2019.

3. McKillop M, Boucher A. Aging prison populations drive up costs. February 20, 2018. https://www.pewtrusts.org/en/research-and-analysis/articles/2018/02/20/aging-prison-populations-drive-up-costs. Accessed May 1, 2019.

4. *Kansas v. Hendricks*, 521 U.S. 346 (1997). https://caselaw.findlaw.com/us-supreme-court/521/346.html. Accessed October 25, 2019.

5. https://caselaw.findlaw/us-supreme-court/521/346.html. Accessed October 25, 2019.

6. https://www.prisonpolicy.org/reports/pie2020.html. Accessed September 1, 2019.

7. National Commission on Correctional Health Care. Standards: a framework for quality. 2018. https://www.ncchc.org/standards. Accessed October 27, 2019.

8. https://www.ncchc.org/standards. This is a consensus statement, and specific areas mentioned. Accessed April 28, 2019.

9. American Bar Association Standards for criminal justice treatment of prisoners is outlined in ABA Criminal Justice section on health care standards. 23-6.1–23-6.5. https://www.americanbar.org/content/dam/aba/publications/criminal_justice_standards/treatment_of_prisoners.pdf

10. Scott CL, Gerbasi JB. *Handbook of Correctional Mental Health*. Washington, DC: American Psychiatric Press; 2005.

11. Harrison PM, Karberg JC. *Prison and Jail Inmates at Midyear 2003 (BJS Bulletin, NCJ 203947)*. Washington, DC: Office of Justice Programs, Bureau of Justice Statistics, US Department of Justice; May 2004.

12. Caroline Cournoyer. States Seek Shortened Probation and Parole for Many. https://www.governing.com/topics/public-justice-safety. Accessed April 27, 2017. https://www.governing.com/archive/sl-states-probation.html

13. HG.org. https://www.hg.org/legal-articles/what-is-the-difference-between-jail-and-prison-31513. Accessed April 25, 2019.

14. https://www.prisonpolicy.org/reports/pie2020.html. Accessed September 1, 2019.

15. FindLaw. https://caselaw.findlaw.com/us-supreme-court/521/346.html

16. *Estelle v. Gamble* 429 U.S. 97 (1976).

17. *Bowring v. Godwin* 551 F.2d 44 (4th Cir.1977).

18. *Kansas v. Hendricks* 521 U.S. 346 (1977). https://caselaw.findlaw.com/us-supreme-court/521/346.html

19. Bureau of Prisons. Inmate Offenses. https://www.bop.gov/about/statistics/statistics_inmate_offenses.jsp. Accessed September 1, 2019.

20. https://www.bop.gov/resources/research_projects/published_reports/cond_envir/oreprscott1.pdf

21. Gotsch K, Basti V. Capitalizing on mass incarceration: U.S. Growth in private prisons. The Sentencing Project. August 2, 2018. https://www.sentencingproject.org/publications/capitalizing-on-mass-incarceration-u-s-growth-in-private-prisons/

22. Stern MF. Report on ICSI medical and mental health. Case 1:81-cv-01165-BLW. 2012. Position paper from AAFP: https://www.aafp.org/about/policies/all/incarceration.html

23. Clark M. Court's expert says medical care at Idaho prison is unconstitutional in *Prison Legal News*. *Prison Legal News*. 2016.

24. Clark M. Arizona prison conditions unconstitutional alleges ACLU class-action federal lawsuit in *Prison Legal News*. *Prison Legal News*. 2016.

25. American Civil Liberties Union. *Gamez v Ryan* final complaint. 2012. https://www.aclu.org/other/gamez-v-ryan-final-complaint

26. McKillop M, Boucher A. Topics: fiscal & economic policy & U.S. state policy projects: state fiscal health. February 20, 2018. https://www.pewtrusts.org/en/research-and-analysis/articles/2018/02/20/aging-prison-populations-drive-up-costs

27. Chari KA, Simon A, DeFrances CJ, Manuschak L. National Survey of Prison Health Care: selected findings. *National Health Statistics Reports*. 2016;(96):1–23.

28. https://www.sentencingproject.org/publications/capitalizing-on-mass-incarceration-u-s-growth-in-private-prisons/. Accessed September 2, 2019.

29. U.S. Department of Justice Office of Justice Programs Bureau of Justice Statistics. Prisoners in 2016. NCJ 251149. January 2018. Updated August 7, 2018. https://bjs.ojp.gov/content/pub/pdf/p16_sum.pdf

30. https://www.bjs.gov/content/pub/pdf/p16.pdf. Accessed May 1, 2019.

31. https://www.bop.gov/about/statistics/statistics_inmate_age.jsp. Accessed September 1, 2019.

32. http://www.npr.org/2018/08/9/630515551.

33. Neumann A. What hospice care looks like for dying patients in America's prisons. *The Atlantic*. Health Section. https://www.theatlantic.com/health/archive/2016/02/hospice-care-in-prison/462660/. Accessed April 20, 2019.

34. Bliss KW. Humane treatment for terminally ill prisoners. *Prison Legal News*. May 2, 2019, p. 18.

35. Maull F. Issues in prison hospice: toward a model for the delivery of hospice care in correctional setting. *Hospice Journal*. 1998;13(4):68–70.

36. Evans C, Herzog R, Tillman T. The Louisiana State Penitentiary: Angola prison hospice. *Journal of Palliative Medicine*. 2002;5(4):553–558.

37. National Hospice Organization. Standards of hospice program of care. *Hospice Journal*. 1994;9(4):39–74.

38. *Oxford Textbook of Palliative Medicine*. 4th ed. New York, NY: Oxford University Press.; 2010: 513–572.

39. National Hospice Organization. Standards of hospice program of care. *Hospice Journal*. 1996;9(4):65–73. https://www.tandfonline.com/doi/abs/10.1080/0742-969X.1994.11882777

40. https://www.nytimes.com/2018/03/07/us/prisons-compassionate-release-.html

41. Mitchell A, Williams, B. Compassionate release policy reform: physicians as advocates for human dignity. *AMA Journal of Ethics*. 2017;19(9):854–861. https://journalofethics.ama-assn.org/article/compassionate-release-policy-reform-physicians-advocates-human-dignity/2017-09.   Accessed September 3, 2019.

42. Thompson C. Old sick and dying in shackles. Marshall Project. March 3, 2018. https://www.themarshallproject.org/2018/03/07/old-sick-and-dying-in-shackles

43. Clarke M. Department of Justice releases reports on prison and jail deaths. *Legal News*. January 2018, p. 28.

44. Price M. Everywhere and nowhere: Compassionate release in the states. Families Against Mandatory Minimums (FAMM). June 27, 2018. https://stoprecidivism.org/the- history-behind-mandatory-minimums/?   gclid=Cj0KCQjwh_eFBhDZARIsALHj   IKcks9vKKnEMyocv16GNIMZ3mRD9 HRfKstRnIo0lGqAgw21 NtOaePCcaAjsHEALw_wcB

45. https://famm.org.wp-content/uploads/Exec-Summary-Report.pdf. Accessed September 3, 2018.

46. Holoyda B, Landess J. Caring for patients on probation or parole. *Current Psychiatry*. 2019;18(6):27–32.

47. Hawks L, Woolhandler S, McCormick D. COVID-19 in prisons and jails in the United States. *JAMA Internal Medicine*. 2020;180(8):1041–1042. doi:10.1001/jamainternmed.2020.1856

48. Van Beusekom M. US prison inmates among those hit hard with COVID-19. CIDRAP News. July 9, 2020. https://www.cidrap.umn.edu/news-perspective/2020/07/us-prison-inmates-among-those-hit-hard-covid-19

49. Pavlo W. Barr's memo to release federal inmates fails to address BOP policies to release them. *Forbes*. April 4, 2020. Accessed April 4, 2020. https://www.forbes.com/sites/walterpavlo/2020/04/04/barrs-memo-to-release-federal-inmates-fails-to-address-bop-policies-to-release-them/#3d71de014ff3

Care Transitions Including End of Life

22

Withdrawal of Life Support

Richard Ackermann

Withdrawal of potentially life-sustaining treatments should occur when the burdens outweigh the benefits, consistent with the patient's values, preferences, and goals of care. This situation is imprecise but reflects clinical reality.[1]

Over 2.5 million Americans die every year. Median life expectancy in the United States is 80 years, and most of these older adults die from chronic diseases that occur over several years, with a final event in an impersonal environment, such as an intensive care unit (ICU). At this point, fewer than 10% can directly participate in medical decision-making, except through advance directives. Family members are faced with difficult decisions to forgo cardiopulmonary resuscitation (CPR) or other potentially life-sustaining treatments.[2]

In a 2013 survey of 458 hospitalized adults, 75% wanted to die at home, with another 10% wanting to die in an institution such as a hospital, nursing home, or inpatient hospice. However, of the 123 patients who died during follow-up, 80% died in institutions, with only 37% dying in their preferred site.[3] In 2017, patient's homes replaced the hospital as the most common site of death for Americans.[4]

Helping patients and their families make difficult decisions about life-sustaining treatments is a core competency of physician assistants (PAs). The PA needs to understand the legal and ethical framework as well as practicalities of medical decision-making. All states have laws and regulations regarding informed consent and withholding or withdrawing treatments. Although the American default position is to provide all available therapies unless there are specific orders to the contrary, most hospital deaths occur following a decision to withdraw life support. Box 22.1 provides a summary of guidance for PAs managing end-of-life care and withdrawal of life support.[5,6]

Why would a PA withhold or withdraw a potentially life-sustaining treatment? First and most important, this is done to comply with the goals and preferences of a competent adult or their surrogate. Second, stopping treatment is indicated if the proposed therapy cannot meet the overall goals of treatment. Finally, stop a treatment if it has failed or is

---

BOX 22.1 End-of-Life Policies From the American Academy of Physician Assistants

Among the ethical principles that are fundamental to providing compassionate care at the end of life, the most essential is recognizing that dying is a personal experience and part of the life cycle.

Physician assistants should provide patients with the opportunity to plan for end-of-life care. Advance directives, living wills, durable power of attorney, and organ donation should be discussed during routine patient visits.

Physician assistants should assure terminally ill patients that their dignity is a priority and that relief of physical and mental suffering is paramount. PAs should exhibit nonjudgmental attitudes and should assure their terminally ill patients that they will not be abandoned.

To the extent possible, patient or surrogate preferences should be honored, using the most appropriate measures consistent with their choices, including alternative and nontraditional measures.

Physician assistants should explain palliative and hospice care and facilitate patient access to those services.

End-of-life care should include assessment and management of psychological, social, and spiritual or religious needs.

While respecting patients' wishes for particular treatments when possible, PAs also must weigh their ethical responsibility, in consultation with supervising physicians, to withhold futile treatments and to help patients understand such medical decisions.

Physician assistants should involve the physician in all near-death planning. The PA should only withdraw life support with the supervising physician's agreement and in accordance with the policies of the healthcare institution.

Adapted from the AAPA Policy Manual as amended in 2018.

---

prolonging the dying process. For example, consider stopping hemodialysis in a previously vigorous patient who becomes comatose after an intracranial hemorrhage, leaving him in a state he would regard as very low quality. Ideally, the PA will have a long-term relationship with the patient, managing chronic diseases from diagnosis all the way to final illness. However, in many cases, withholding and withdrawing decisions are managed by clinicians who have not previously met the patient and family.[1,7,8]

The Legal Framework

US laws and court decisions have established a right to withhold or withdraw potentially life-sustaining treatments. In 1914, Justice Cardozo wrote that *every human being of adult years and sound mind has a right to determine what shall be done with his own body.*

In 1976, the parents of Karen Ann Quinlan, a 22-year-old woman in a chronic vegetative state, petitioned the New Jersey Supreme Court to remove her ventilator. The court held that the parents had the right to remove life support. In 1990, the parents of Nancy Cruzan, another young woman in a persistent vegetative state, petitioned to remove her from artificial hydration and nutrition. The US Supreme Court affirmed that, through her parents, she had this right, but the court also ruled that states could set their own levels of evidence to make these decisions. Some states have *clear and convincing* statutes, where a strict, usually written, level of evidence is required before withdrawal of artificial nutrition and hydration can occur. Other states do not require that high level of evidence, and physicians and PAs can utilize, withhold, or withdraw any life-sustaining intervention based on conversation with patients or their surrogates.

Following the Cruzan case, in 1990 the federal Patient Self-Determination Act was passed, which requires healthcare facilities to ask about the presence of advance directives and counsel patients about them if requested. Most recently, the Terry Schiavo case in Florida pitted her parents against her husband; they were arguing about continuing percutaneous endoscopic gastrostomy feedings in a woman in a persistent vegetative state. All the courts upheld the right of a legal surrogate to direct medical care.[9,10]

Competence is a legal term that refers to an adult who has *decision-making capacity* (DMC). Adults are competent unless deemed incompetent by a court. On the other hand, DMC generally has four requirements: The patient must be able to

(1) understand relevant information,
(2) communicate this information,
(3) appreciate the situation and its consequences, and
(4) reason about the choices.

Details of DMC vary by state. In many states, DMC can be determined by any physician. There is generally no requirement for consultation with a psychiatrist or other medical specialist, although such consultation may be useful in some cases. For patients living in nursing homes, before an order to restrict life support is valid in some states, it must be signed by two physicians.[9]

Invoking futility is rarely useful in clinical practice. *Physiologic* futility indicates that the intervention is unlikely or cannot maintain or restore function; for example, physicians may stop efforts at resuscitation when further efforts cannot restore function. *Quantitative* futility uses a low probability of success to argue against the intervention; for example, third-line chemotherapy for small cell lung cancer has a less than 2% chance of leading to a sustained remission. *Qualitative* futility assesses that the benefits of the proposed intervention are not worth its risks. For example, an older man with metastatic lung cancer who experiences severe weakness and dyspnea may opt against mechanical ventilation and CPR because these interventions cannot restore him to a level of health that would permit him to live outside the hospital setting. Probably a better term than *futile* is *potentially nonbeneficial*.[11]

Ethical Decision-Making

The primary ethical basis behind withholding or withdrawing medical treatments is patient autonomy. Competent adults may decide which medical interventions they want, including the right to refuse treatment, even if that decision could lead to an earlier death. If the patient does not have DMC, then in every state a surrogate has full authority to act. All medical treatments are included, including artificial hydration and nutrition. Patients who die because life support is withdrawn die from the underlying disease process, not from assisted suicide (physician-assisted death) or euthanasia.[8]

Distinguishing *ordinary* from *extraordinary* treatments is not useful because those terms are relative and can only be defined by the individual. However, the Roman Catholic Church and other religions may provide specific guidance. Review the benefits and burdens of each proposed intervention. For example, the ordinary treatment of hydration for a vigorous patient with pneumonia might be considered extraordinary in a patient with advanced malignancy. The use of vasopressors and hemodialysis might be fully justified in a patient with cancer who experiences a complication of chemotherapy. Ask this question: *What are the benefits and burdens of the proposed treatment in this patient, at this time in the illness?*

Ideally, patient preferences will have been clearly established in advance directives and operationalized in all clinical settings by a Physician Order for Life-Sustaining Treatment (POLST) or some other method. However, advance directives may not be present, and if they are, they are often violated or ignored.[5]

A PA may have a long-term relationship with the patient in a community setting, which facilitates end-of-life communication. In such a setting, discussions may occur naturally and in small pieces over several months or years. However, in most circumstances in modern American medicine, the clinician who needs to urgently address resuscitation status is a stranger without a long-term relationship. Consultation with the primary care provider or a palliative care team may improve decision-making and reduce the use of nonbeneficial treatments. The PA should support the patient's and family's preferences throughout this time of biomedical and psychosocial complexity.

Patients with advanced diseases have many potentially life-sustaining treatments to consider, including CPR, artificial hydration and nutrition, cancer therapies, mechanical ventilation, dialysis, blood transfusion, imaging and laboratory tests, antibiotics, and even whether to be admitted to the hospital or to an ICU. The complexity and pace of treatment choices often accelerates as the patient becomes overwhelmed by disease and treatment complications. For example, cancer patients may initially want to cure the cancer, with no treatment restrictions. If the malignancy does not respond to treatment, they may opt first for a do not resuscitate (DNR) status, with progressively more treatment restrictions as the disease progresses. As a cancer patient approaches the end of life, patients and clinicians tend to withdraw/withhold treatments, starting perhaps with restricting blood products and then progressing through restrictions on dialysis, vasopressors, ventilation, parenteral nutrition, even on tube feeding, intravenous fluids, or antibiotics.[12]

Helpful communication strategies include frequent, timely, and consistent communication about prognosis; being available to answer questions to enhance health literacy;

encouraging family discussions to facilitate their goals of care; and excellent symptom management. On the other hand, avoid burdensome strategies such as delaying discussions of life support withdrawal, physically avoiding the family as death approaches, or relegating end-of-life discussions to junior clinicians. PAs should provide frankly directive advice to patients about these matters, following state laws and institutional regulations. This advice is based on science, experience, and the goals and preferences of the patient.[13,14] For example, it may be appropriate to say:

> Your cancer is very advanced. We can't alter that, but there is a lot we can still do. We could insert a feeding tube into your stomach to increase the number of days you will live, but the quality of the days you have left would be worse. I wouldn't advise that.

Patients and families make serious decisions in different ways. In a study of women with breast cancer, 9% wanted to make decisions herself, 14% wanted to make the decision herself after getting advice from the physician, 44% wanted a decision jointly made by the patient and physician, 17% wanted the physician to make the decision after hearing her input, and 18% preferred a completely paternalistic model, where the physician makes decisions.[15] You won't know what the preferred style is unless you ask.

Find out what the patient/family already know about the medical situation. Often, there are misunderstandings, or someone may blame a physician or family member for the current predicament. Listen calmly and accept this, even if you disagree. Use vocabulary appropriate for the audience, who may have differing degrees of medical knowledge. Provide your honest opinion and don't be afraid to express doubt if that is appropriate, especially if physicians disagree about the appropriate next step. Ask the family if they have enough information or would like another opinion. The PA might summarize:

> This is what I hear you saying.

If the patient no longer has DMC, ask the surrogate to express the patient's own values and preferences, if those are known. This is the legal principle of *substituted judgment*, in which the family member transmits to the physician what the patient would say. This may reduce guilt or decisional paralysis because the family member doesn't want to make the decision to end life support. If the family disagrees on the appropriate approach, spend more time on clarifying the goal of care before proceeding to specifics such as dialysis or intubation. For example, if the family can't agree on a full code or DNR, go back to the goal:

> Given that your primary goal for your mother is comfort, how do you think an attempt at CPR fits with that?

Some patients want the clinicians to *do everything*. This is broad, easy to misunderstand, and implies that the decision is between doing everything and nothing, which is never true. It also assumes that medicine has power over disease, and you simply decide to use that power or not. If the patient is dying, establish context:

> Your mother is dying, despite the current treatment. Sadly, she will likely die in the next few days.

Don't use the phrase *do everything* in counseling. Instead of saying,

> You want us to do everything?

or

> Do you want us to hook mom up to the breathing machine and restart her heart?

Rather, reframe the question:

> If her heart or breathing stops, do you want us to use "heroic" measures?

or

> Do you want us to compress her chest and put a tube in her lungs to try and restart her heart and lungs?

Once the goal is clear, move to specific treatment options, providing this information in small pieces. For example, if at this session you just told your patient she has cancer, she may not hear anything else you said that day.

> I'm afraid I have bad news. The biopsy work came back positive for cancer of your pancreas, and it looks like the cancer has already spread.

Then sit quietly, waiting. Patients are often very distressed at key points in an illness, such as diagnosis, failure of therapy, or a life-threatening complication. You may call on counselors, chaplains, or palliative care specialists to help. Despite the emotional trauma, patients are usually grateful for the presence and continued advice of physicians and PAs, even if the advice is to stop aggressively treating the disease.

Patients need a clear understanding of what is wrong with them and the reasonable treatments. Don't sugarcoat the prognosis, hiding behind euphemisms or medical jargon, or use false reassurance such as *everything will be all right*. As the disease advances, routinely include a discussion of palliative options. Most patients will move to a comfort-based goal at some point.

After this discussion, establish a plan and implement it. Sometimes this isn't possible because the situation is overwhelming, the family needs time, there are religious objections, and so on.[16] In that case, summarize how the meeting has been helpful and arrange for follow-up:

> I think this meeting helped to clarify what you know about your dad's illness. It looks like you need time to reflect on what's happening before we make any changes. Let's meet again in a couple days while you talk about this among yourselves. I know you want to do what's right for your father.

The FICA Tool

The FICA (Faith, Importance, Community, Address) Tool may help clarify spiritual issues. Patients often feel they are being forced into choosing between fighting the disease and giving in to death. But hoping for a cure and preparing for eventual death are not mutually exclusive. These conversations should occur early and often during the disease, not just when the patient is in the last few days of life. Support both hope and preparation as you continue to develop a trusting, continuing relationship with the patient. Patients with aggressive diseases expect active curative care, but they also want a sense of control, dignity, and symptom relief.[17]

> At this point, I think we should continue to hope for a cure, but let's also be realistic and face whatever happens together.

Cardiopulmonary Resuscitation

Cardiopulmonary resuscitation was first utilized in the operating room in 1960, and it wasn't until 1974 that the American Medical Association recommended that code status be documented for hospitalized patients. An attempt at CPR occurs in 1% of hospital admissions, but most hospitalized patients who die have a DNR status at the time of their death. Half of patients who undergo in-hospital CPR regain circulation, but only 13%–19% survive to hospital discharge. Of these, 11% have no neurologic disability, 5% have a moderate disability, and 3% are left with severe disability, either a vegetative state or conscious but totally dependent on others. Patients value these outcomes differently; for some patients, immediate death is better than a prolonged death in the hospital, and that is better than being alive in a vegetative state.[18]

A DNR order withholds all components of resuscitation in an unresponsive, pulseless patient, including chest compressions, cardiac medications, defibrillation, and intubation and mechanical ventilation. However, having a DNR order does not imply that other medical procedures should be withheld. For example, if a woman with a DNR order is hospitalized for atrial fibrillation with a rapid ventricular rate, the DNR does not prevent cardioversion to relieve her symptoms. A DNR order is usually chosen along with do not intubate (DNI), although some patients may authorize temporary mechanical ventilation for a potentially reversible condition, while still prohibiting CPR.

An interesting question is whether a DNR order remains valid in the operating room. Many of the interventions in CPR (intubation, vasoactive drugs) are also routinely used in the operating room, cardiac arrest can be induced by anesthesia or surgery, and the results of resuscitation in this setting are better than other settings. In all cases, the discussion and decisions regarding DNR in the operating room should be part of the surgical consent process. If a patient decides to maintain the DNR after counseling, that wish should be respected. The order and length of resuscitation should be part of this discussion in order to honor the patient's wishes since the patient may lack capacity following the procedure. For example, a patient requiring palliative surgery (e.g., a venting gastrostomy) should not have the procedure withheld because of a DNR order.

The decision not to use CPR (DNR) can also be articulated in a more natural, positive way: allow natural death or do not attempt resuscitation.

If a DNR order is chosen, reassure the family that this restriction does not apply to other aspects of care, such as transfusion, surgery, or medications.

> I am writing the DNR order, but please know that we will always provide comfort care and use maximal, aggressive medical therapy to try to meet your goals.

Patients and families sometimes advocate for CPR (full code) when the treating clinicians disagree. This conflict may arise from several concerns. While most people believe that CPR is usually successful, survival to hospital discharge of those who receive in-hospital CPR is less than 20%, and it is much lower (1%–5%) for those who also have metastatic cancer, renal failure, or AIDS. Guilt can drive decision-making. For example, a daughter who lives thousands of miles away may not have visited her dying mother for months or years. For some family members, the DNR order is equivalent to choosing to die. If following skillful counseling, the family continues to desire CPR, accept their wishes, but return to the discussion later.[13]

Families from minority or disenfranchised populations may not trust the medical system, especially if they have received poor quality care in the past. Address this possibility directly:

> Your decisions for your dad make me wonder if you trust those who are treating him here at the hospital. I could be wrong, but do you have any concerns like that?

If the PA believes that CPR cannot work, and the family insists on its use, there are several options. Mostly commonly, you accede to the CPR request and continue to gently counsel against its use and offer an alternative treatment option. However, clinicians are not required to act in a way they find unethical. Options include transferring care to another provider or to another hospital, but this is often impractical. However, disagreements between patients/families and the medical team are best handled through continued respectful negotiation and meetings and not through avoidance of responsibility. Obtain a spiritual consultation from a chaplain or local pastor known to the patient and family. It is important to allow some time to pass for the patient to process the information. Finally, this is a definite indication for a palliative team consultation.

If the patient endorses DNR or other restrictions such as DNI in the hospital, that order may need review and reassessment in other settings, such as the patient's home or a skilled nursing facility for acute or long-term care. Most states now have a POLST or similar document, which delineates specific orders related to the patient's wishes to be legally transmitted to other settings.[19]

Mechanical Ventilation

Mechanical ventilation is one of the few interventions in which withdrawal can cause pain and suffering. It is the only intervention where weaning is often appropriate; one can simply turn off vasopressors, a balloon pump, or a defibrillator. Ventilator withdrawal usually occurs in the hospital intensive care setting, but it can also sometimes be accomplished at home, in the nursing home, or in inpatient hospice.[20]

Consent for ventilator withdrawal or terminal extubation requires a discussion of the process. Agreement about the goals of care and the decision to withdraw is fundamental to this decision. Other forms of life support, such as enteral feeding, intravenous fluids, vasopressors, and dialysis, are withdrawn before the ventilator to avoid volume overload symptoms and thereby complicate the terminal extubation. Contingency plans for transfer out of the ICU may be necessary if death is delayed after ventilator withdrawal.[21]

Ventilator withdrawal involves two options: immediate extubation or weaning. With immediate extubation, suction the patient, remove the endotracheal tube, and provide humidified oxygen to keep the airway moist. This method is preferred if the patient is awake, secretions are minimal, and the airway will be intact after extubation.

The second method is weaning, in which the tidal volume, oxygen fraction, positive end-expiratory pressure, and respiratory rate are progressively decreased, leaving the endotracheal tube in place. This can be done over 30–60 minutes or more slowly. If the patient survives weaning, the clinician sometimes leaves the endotracheal tube in place and disconnects the ventilator, with oxygen provided through a T piece. Use this method of ventilator withdrawal when the patient requires high levels of ventilator support or cannot protect his airway. This includes patients with severe facial or airway swelling, facial trauma, or profound neurologic impairment. If the endotracheal tube is left in when the ventilator is withdrawn, it can be removed later.

The PA should counsel the patient/family about the possible outcomes of withdrawal. Discuss any prognostic uncertainty. Some patients die within minutes, and most patients die within hours to days, depending on their medical condition and the use of other support. Occasionally, a patient survives compassionate ventilator withdrawal, even surviving to hospital discharge.

Explain the procedure in simple terms. Decide whether the endotracheal tube will be removed. Review how you will use oxygen and medications to manage anxiety or breathlessness. Tell the family that the patient will likely require some sedation to manage symptoms. The procedure of ventilator withdrawal should be supervised by a clinician at least for several minutes after withdrawal. An order for "terminal wean" that leaves the details to the other team members and the respiratory therapist is not appropriate.

Encourage the family to gather around the bedside and participate in any special music, religious observation, or ritual. Inquire if a chaplain would be helpful. Document the clinical conditions leading to withdrawal, a summary of the discussion with the patient or surrogate, and the plan. Deactivate and remove monitors and alarms, particularly the oxygen saturation monitor. Deactivate an implanted cardiac defibrillator but leave any pacing function intact. This often requires consultation with cardiology or electrophysiology. In an emergency, deactivate the defibrillator component by placing a magnet over the device.

Always withdraw a paralytic agent before the ventilator is withdrawn, wait for spontaneous movement and attempt at respirations to return. Paralysis eliminates your ability to assess discomfort, and maintaining paralysis may hasten death because the patient has no chance to resume breathing.

Remove restraints and medical equipment such as a nasogastric tube, telemetry, and leg compression devices. Ensure an intravenous line is functioning solely to provide comfort medications. Before turning off the ventilator, discontinue inotropic agents, antibiotics, dialysis, vasopressors, prophylaxis for thromboembolism and gastrointestinal bleeding, and any other nonbeneficial treatments. Usually discontinue hydration or enteral feeding several hours before in order to reduce the burden of respiratory secretions, but this can be negotiated with the family.

Create space for the family. Allow them to be present for the withdrawal, although not all family members and loved ones will want to do that. Offer chairs and tissues. Get permission to allow more visitors than usual around the bed, even outside visiting hours.

Ensure that symptoms such as pain, dyspnea, and agitation are well managed before you begin the extubation. An opioid and benzodiazepine should be readily available. There may be a reflexive "gasp" from the patient during the actual removal of the endotracheal tube, which can be distressing to family members.

If you decide to remove the endotracheal tube, ask a respiratory therapist to do that while you stand at the foot of the bed, and the nurse can give medications. The therapist should have suction and a washcloth ready, deflate the endotracheal tube and remove it into a towel. If the patient remains awake, ask them if they need to be suctioned. Silence the ventilator and move it out of the way. Stay with the patient for a few minutes to support the family and manage any symptoms. After the death, allow the family to spend as much time as they need at the bedside.

Common symptoms following ventilator withdrawal are anxiety and dyspnea; you should both prevent and treat these problems. An opioid for dyspnea and a benzodiazepine such as midazolam or lorazepam for anxiety are typical, often at doses that cause mild sedation. When treating dyspnea associated with ventilator withdrawal, start with an opioid, adding a benzodiazepine if needed. Do not withhold sedation out of fear that death will be hastened. On the other hand, there is also no justification for using doses beyond what is needed to secure sedation. Evidence documents that titrated doses of these drugs do not hasten death. They relax the patient and allow death to occur at its own pace. Provide sedation, usually with an opioid and benzodiazepine, to all patients undergoing compassionate ventilator withdrawal, even if the patient is deeply comatose.[22]

For an opioid-naïve patient, prescribe 2–5 mg morphine IV, followed by a morphine infusion at 50% of the bolus dose per hour. Another option is fentanyl 50–200 µg intravenously every 3–5 minutes. Also give lorazepam or midazolam 1–2 mg IV, followed by a 0.5–1 mg/h intravenous drip. Titrate these medications to achieve good control of dyspnea and anxiety prior to extubation.

After extubation, if respiratory distress or anxiety appear, an extra bolus of both the opioid and benzodiazepine, every 5–10 minutes, may be necessary until symptoms are better managed. Reasonable goals are to keep the respiratory rate less than 30 breaths per minute and heart rate less than 100 beats per minute and to reduce grimacing and agitation.

Comprehensive prevention and management of symptoms of dying patients helps both the patient and his family. A clinician's calm competence helps to normalize the dying process.[23]

References

1. Prendergast TJ. Withdrawal of life support. Intensive caring at the end of life. *JAMA*. 2002;*288*:2732–2740.

2. Loertscher L, Reed DA, Bannon MP, Mueller PS. Cardiopulmonary resuscitation and do-not-resuscitate orders: a guide for clinicians. *American Journal of Medicine*. 2010:*123*:4–9.

3. Fischer S, Min S-J, Cervantes L, Kutner J. Where do you want to spend your last days? Low concordance between preferred and actual site of death among hospitalized adults. *Journal of Hospital Medicine* 2013; *8*:178–183.

4. Cross SH, Warraich HJ. Changes in the place of death in the United States. *New England Journal of Medicine*. 2019;*381*:2369–2370.

5. The SUPPORT Principal Investigators. A controlled trial to improve care for seriously hospitalized patients. The Study to Understand Prognoses and Preferences for Outcomes and Risks of Treatments (SUPPORT). *JAMA*. 1995;*273*:1591–1598 (published erratum appears in *JAMA*. 1996;*275*:1232).

6. Guideline for ethical conduct for the PA profession, and end of life decision making. In: *American Academy of Physician Assistants Policy Manual*. https://www.aapa.org/downloads/51507. Accessed August 22, 2019.

7. Ackermann RJ. Withholding and withdrawing life-sustaining treatment. *American Family Physician*. 2001;*62*:1555–1560.

8. Ackermann RJ. Withholding and withdrawing potentially life-sustaining treatment. In: Berger AM, Shuster JL, Van Rosen JH, eds. *Principles and Practice of Palliative Care and Supportive Oncology*. Lippincott, Williams, and Wilkins; 2007:697–705.

9. Applebaum PS. Assessment of patients' competence to consent to treatment. *New England Journal of Medicine*. 2007;*357*:1834–1840.

10. Goston LO. Ethics, the constitution and the dying process. The case of Theresa Marie Schiavo. *JAMA*. 2005;*293*:2403–2407.

11. Swetz KM, Burkle CM, Berge KH, Lanier WL. Ten common questions (and their answers) on medical futility. *Mayo Clinic Proceedings*. 2014;*89*:943–959.

12. Lynn J. Serving patients who may die soon and their families. The role of hospice and other services. *JAMA* 2001;*285*:925–932.

13. Ngo-Metzger Q, August KJ, Srinivasan M, Liao S, Meyskens FL. End-of-life care: guidelines for patient-centered communication. *American Family Physician*. 2008;*77*:167–174.

14. Wiegard DL, Cheon J, Netzer G. Seeing the patient and family through: nurses and physicians experiences with withdrawal of life-sustaining therapy in the ICU. *American Journal of Hospice and Palliative Care*. 2019;*36*:13–23.

15. Lee SJ, Back AL, Block SD, Steward SK. Enhancing physician-patient communication. *Hematology. American Society of Hematology. Education Program*. 2002;*464*–483.

16. Murray SA, Boyd K, Sheikh A. Palliative care in chronic illness. We need to move from prognostic paralysis to active total care. *BMJ*. 2005;*330*:611–612.

17. Back Al, Arnold RM, Quill TE. Hope for the best, and prepare for the worst. *Annals of Internal Medicine*. 2003;*138*:439–443.

18. Bosch FH, Fleming DA. Moving to high-value care: more thoughtful use of cardiopulmonary resuscitation. *Annals of Internal Medicine*. 2015;*162*:790–791.

19. Lee SJ, Back AL, Block SD, Steward SK. Enhancing physician-patient communication. *Hematology. American Society of Hematology. Education Program*. 2002;*464*–483.

20. O'Mahony S, McHugh M, Zallman L, et al. Ventilator withdrawal: procedure and outcomes. Report of a collaboration between a critical care division and a palliative care service. *Journal of Pain and Symptom Management*. 2003;*26*:954–961.

21. Asch DA, Faber-Langendoen K, Shea JA, et al. The sequence of withdrawing life-sustaining treatments from patients. *American Journal of Medicine.* 1999;*107*:153–156.
22. Chan JD, Treece PD, Engelberg R, et al. Narcotic and benzodiazepine use after withdrawal of life support. Association with time to death? *Chest.* 2004;*126*:286–293.
23. White DB, Angus DC, Shields AM, et al. A randomized trial of a family-support intervention in intensive care units. *New England Journal of Medicine.* 2018;*378*:2365–2375.

23

Last Days and Hours of Life

Richard Ackermann

The terminal phase of an illness is the period of inexorable decline in functional status prior to death. Other terms include *actively dying* or *imminent death*, defined as the last few hours or days of life. The two primary goals during this period are to provide the best possible quality of life for the patient and to help the patient and family navigate the best treatment *option* among a list of choices.[1] The skills required for management of patients at the end of life are an integral part of the core practice competencies of physician assistants (PAs).

Physiology of Dying

As many as 85% of patients take the usual, peaceful, and physiologic road to death, in which the patient moves from being sleepy, to lethargic, obtunded, and comatose, to death. Others take a more difficult road, manifested by progressive restlessness, confusion, tremors, myoclonus, *and* sometimes even seizures.

The patient will reduce oral intake of both foods and fluids, eventually to nothing. This can be explained as "the body cannot properly use the food that it takes in." The patient will become weaker and may not be able to raise their head or clear secretions.

Most dying patients develop hypotension, tachycardia, a slight elevation of temperature, and hypoxemia. However, on the day prior to death, half have normal vital signs, and no combination of vital signs accurately predicts imminent death. Other signs commonly seen in the last 2–3 days of life are nonreactive pupils, decreased response to stimuli, inability to close the eyes, drooping of the nasolabial fold, neck hyperextension, and grunting.[2,3]

There may be noisy respiratory secretions, mottling and cooling of the extremities, and fever. Many patients experience periods of apnea interspersed with crescendo/decrescendo pattern tachypnea; these are Cheyne-Stokes respirations, with respiratory pauses as long as a minute. This pattern reflects normal dying, not dyspnea. Tachypnea in dying patients often signifies respiratory compensation for metabolic acidosis, so irregular breathing or tachypnea should not be treated unless there are other signs of respiratory distress.[1,4,5]

Managing Symptoms and Medications

Because of a decline in neuromuscular control, the patient will be unable able to take oral medications. Review the medication list, discontinue many, and consider nonoral routes. Stop lipid-lowering drugs, taper off antihypertensives, and individualize medications for heart failure, coronary artery disease, and diabetes (see Table 23.1). If used for seizures, maintain anticonvulsants and consider switching to subcutaneous or intravenous lorazepam. Many palliative medications can be given rectally, including acetaminophen, anticonvulsants, benzodiazepines, corticosteroids, and most opioids and nausea medicines. Avoid the rectal route in the presence of severe thrombocytopenia, neutropenia, or coagulopathy. Nearly all palliative medications (opioids, lorazepam, haloperidol, phenobarbital, dexamethasone, furosemide, and octreotide) can also be given subcutaneously, although the evidence for this route is weak.[6,7]

Discontinue monitoring such as telemetry, oxygen saturation, and fingerstick sampling for glucose. It is often reasonable even to stop recording vital signs. However, some families find peace and security from the knowledge of vital signs or measurements like blood glucose or oxygen saturation.

Aggressively prevent and treat the symptoms of dying, such as pain, dyspnea, dry mouth, dry eyes, agitation, and noisy respiratory secretions. For each symptom, consider physical, social, spiritual, and psychological contributors. If the patient has a central line or percutaneous endoscopic gastrostomy in the last days of life, maintain them. They may provide useful routes for medicines even if you are not utilizing them for hydration or nutrition.

Change long-acting opioids to immediate-release oral forms or to intravenous or subcutaneous boluses or continuous infusions. Convert from the patient's prior use of an opioid and provide both basal and bolus drug, rather than starting everyone on an intravenous

TABLE 23.1 The OncPal Describing Guideline: Drugs That May Be Suitable for Discontinuation in Palliative Care Populations[a]

Drug/Drug Class	Comments
Aspirin for primary prevention	Time to benefit exceeds life expectancy
Lipid-lowering agents	Few short or intermediate risks of stopping drug
Medications for mild or moderate hypertension	
Osteoporosis medications	Time to benefit exceeds life expectancy
Proton pump inhibitors or H_2 blockers, unless there is a history of Gastrointestinal bleeding, peptic ulcer, gastritis, reflux, or use of nonsteroidal anti-inflammatory drugs	Time to benefit exceeds life expectancy, except for the treatment of bony metastasis
	Unnecessary
Oral hypoglycemic	Short-term complications outweigh potential benefits in most patients
Vitamins or minerals for general use	Ineffective

[a]Adapted from Reference 6.

morphine drip at 1 mg/h. One choice is concentrated morphine solution (20 mg/mL) placed in the buccal space or under the tongue. It is vital to communicate with caregivers, providers, patients, and families about the potency of this formulation to avoid accidental overdose. Half of dying patients need an increase in their opioid dose during the last few days of life. Many patients become anuric near death, which could cause accumulation of opioid, and some experts recommend reduction of opioid doses. This is not advised because it poses the double risk of precipitating opioid withdrawal as well as worsening pain or dyspnea. A better approach is cautious dosing as death approaches.[8]

For patients on a fentanyl patch who are actively dying, there are several choices, depending on the setting and clinical circumstances: (1) remove the patch and replace it with another oral or intravenous opioid; (2) leave the patch on and add another short-acting opioid for use as needed; or (3) switch to a fentanyl infusion at the same or slightly lower dose.

Try to avoid radiation therapy or interventional procedures close to death. For example, if a patient with advanced lung cancer in inpatient hospice progresses to stupor while receiving a course of radiation therapy, consider canceling the remaining treatments. Avoid complex interventions in dying patients, but consider on a case-by-case basis antibiotics, red cell transfusion, dexamethasone for superior vena cava syndrome, or thoracentesis for a large pleural effusion.

For dyspnea, consider possible contributing factors. Elevate the head of the bed and direct a fan at the face. For hypoxemic patients, titrate oxygen to the dyspnea, not to the oxygen saturation or the respiratory rate. Oxygen is not helpful in treating dyspnea in dying patients without hypoxemia. Oxygen can sometimes *prolong* dying *without* making the patient more comfortable. In selected patients, consider withdrawing the oxygen for several minutes, observing if this enhances distress or seems to have no effect. Some families request that the oxygen be discontinued. Titrated opioids are usually the best medication for dyspnea in the last few days of life. Add a benzodiazepine if dyspnea and anxiety remain troublesome.[9]

For delirium in the last days of life, diagnostic workup with laboratory testing or imaging is not recommended, except for checking something simple, such as a fingerstick for glucose. Try nonpharmacological treatments such as a quiet dark room, the constant presence of family, and other familiar routines, such as wearing personal clothes, glasses, and hearing aids. No pharmacological agent is clearly effective, but severe agitation is usually treated with an antipsychotic or short-acting benzodiazepine. Some patients with severe terminal delirium may require palliative sedation with drugs such as chlorpromazine, phenobarbital, or propofol. Opioids, while useful for pain and dyspnea, are not effective for delirium.[10]

Treating noisy respiratory secretions in a comatose patient does not make the patient feel better, but it may relieve the distress of family and visitors. The best way to prevent noisy respiratory secretions is to stop hydration, especially in patients who are volume overloaded; have dyspnea, edema, or diarrhea; and have a low serum albumin. Another useful technique is positioning; patients may have less-audible secretions on one side or the other, and it is not necessary to turn patients every 2 hours when they are dying.[11] At the end of life, comfort for the patient and family is the primary goal, and prevention of pressure sores is not a priority.

For patients with noisy respiratory secretions who are still awake, treat with the anticholinergic drug glycopyrrolate (Robinul), which, because it does not cross the blood-brain barrier, poses less risk of delirium. Once the patient becomes comatose, a recent randomized trial has documented that early treatment with an anticholinergic drug substantially reduces noisy respiratory secretions in the last hours and days of life. Although a scopolamine patch is not approved by the Food and Drug Administration (FDA) for noisy respiratory secretions, it is widely used in palliative medicine, and experts recommend using up to three patches at a time. An inexpensive alternative commonly used by hospice nurses is atropine eye drops, which can be placed onto the tongue. All these drugs appear to be equally effective. Avoid suctioning, particularly deep into the trachea, as this is uncomfortable, even in comatose patients.[12,13]

Dry eyes and mouth are nearly universal in the dying patient. Dry eyes can be caused by the dehydration of natural dying, as well as medications such as anticholinergic drugs, beta-blockers, or selective serotonin reuptake inhibitors. In dying patients, the eyelids may not close completely. Prescribe a lubricating gel. For dry mouth in patients who are still alert, consider having the patient suck on frozen or semifrozen liquids, taking frequent sips of cold water or a water spray, humidifying the ambient air, and rubbing petroleum jelly on the lips. Avoid glycerin swabs, which further dry the mucosa, as well as lemon juice, which exhausts salivary secretions. For the actively dying, coat the lips and nares with a small amount of petroleum jelly and keep the oral cavity clean. There are two drugs FDA approved to stimulate salivation (pilocarpine and cevimeline), but these are not recommended in dying patients.[14–16]

Teach the Family What to Expect

Most family members have little experience with dying and will be unprepared for the reality of death. It is within the PA role to educate the patient's family, caregivers, and other members of the hospice and/or palliative care team about the process. Teach the family what to expect: decreasing level of consciousness, decreasing interaction with family and environment, minimal-to-no oral intake, decreasing urine output, an increase in pulse and decrease in blood pressure, cool extremities, mottling, tachypnea, accessory muscle use, shallow breathing, Cheyne-Stokes respirations, and then eventually lack of respiration, followed by cardiac arrest. The patient may lose control of sphincters, the ability to swallow, or even to shut the eyes.

Family members often ask how long the patient has; unfortunately, there is no way to be precise. Offer a range, such as by saying, "Although I can't be sure, I expect her to die in the next few hours to days."

As the patient loses the ability to communicate, make the environment familiar. The patient can wear her own clothes, have her favorite pillow, be surrounded by family pictures and beloved objects, and listen to music. The family can give her permission to let go, touch her hands and face, or lie next to her. Ira Byock recommends phrases that patients and families can consider saying while they still can: *I forgive you; forgive me; thank you; I love you; goodbye.* Even if the patient cannot express herself or understand speech, it is likely that familiar voices may reach her. Encourage the family to use phrases such as *it's OK to go; I love you; we'll be fine;* or whatever feels comfortable.[17]

If the family will not be with professionals at the time of death, teach them the actual signs of death—The heart stops beating, breathing stops, the pupils become fixed and dilated, body color becomes pale and waxen, body temperature drops, muscles and sphincters relax, urine and stool may be released, the eyes may remain open, and the jaw can fall open. Internal trickling of fluids may still be heard.[4]

Declaring Death

The PA should follow a routine in declaring death, consistent with state law and institutional guidelines. If the patient is unknown to you, take a few minutes with the chart and staff to inquire into the circumstances of illness and death. Consider asking a chaplain or counselor to accompany you.

Ask if family is present and how they are doing. Steady yourself, enter the room, and introduce yourself. Explain what you are doing and do *not* ask those present to leave. Identify the patient by her hospital ID tag. Ascertain if she responds to tactile stimulus, but do not provide a painful stimulus. Verify the absence of heart sounds and carotid pulse. Look and listen for the absence of respirations. If there is any doubt, for example, in a very obese patient not on telemetry or a patient who had periodic breathing, pause for several minutes during the examination while looking and listening for respirations. Communicate that the patient has died, using the word *died*, not a euphemism such as "passed away" or "gone." Offer your condolences (e.g., "I'm so sorry for your loss").

Pause for an anticipated grief reaction and don't speak too much. Console as you feel appropriate. Allow the family to spend time with the body prior to an autopsy, notification of others, or calling the funeral home. Write a brief note in the chart documenting your examination and the time of death, following state law and institutional guidelines. Call the attending physician. Sometimes the PA may need to notify family of death via telephone. Inquire where the person is and whether they are alone. If they are driving, ask them to pull over. Identify yourself and your relationship, give a warning shot (e.g., "I'm sorry I have some bad news") and then give the news in a brief sentence. Listen before you speak again, allowing a few seconds of silence. If questions arise, answer them briefly. Suggest that they do not have to come in right away. Rather, give permission to let feelings settle, suggesting they come in with a family member or friend. Give clear instructions where to go and whom they should contact when they arrive at your facility. End with an expression of empathy, such as, "This must be very hard for you. Let me know if there is anything else I can do to help."[1]

Early Grief and Bereavement

Bereavement is the experience of losing a loved one to death, *grief* is the response to loss, and *mourning* is the process of adapting to the loss. Common early symptoms of acute grief include somatic distress, numbness, preoccupation with the deceased, anger, and guilt. Distress often occurs in waves and may include uncontrolled crying, loss of concentration, and hearing the deceased's voice. Sometimes, a family member experiences *derealization*, a perception that the external world is unreal. Some cultures are quiet at the time of death, while others may wail, chant, or "fall out." Resist the urge to fix this with an anxiolytic. Pharmacotherapy is not a routine part of the treatment of grief, and you should not prescribe to family members for whom you do not have a patient-clinician relationship and a chart. Your physical presence for a few minutes can provide a calming and supportive effect.

Allow the family time with the deceased. Warn that the next few days will be difficult, that they should support one another and cancel everything else. Facilitate religious rituals and ceremonies. Hospice chaplains are skillful in assisting families of different faiths, even those who aren't religious. Normal grief typically lasts 6 to 12 months but has no set duration. Grief therapy can be managed by grief and bereavement counselors, psychologists, social workers, chaplains, and volunteers. Hospice provides grief and bereavement services for at least a year following death.[18,19]

Near-Death Awareness

There is anecdotal evidence of *near-death awareness*, where patients near death describe what dying is like and what they need for a peaceful death. Patients sometimes report talking with someone who has died, preparing for travel, describing a place in a new realm, or knowing when they are going to die. These visions are part of normal dying and do not represent psychosis; do not prescribe medications. Occasionally, this is difficult to distinguish from delirium, but the appropriate response is to listen, gather more information, and help the patient achieve a peaceful death. Accept what the patient is telling you, even if you don't understand it or if your personal belief system differs from theirs.[20]

References

1. Ferris FD, von Gunten CF, Emanuel LL. Competency in end-of-life care: last hours of life. *Journal of Palliative Medicine.* 2003;6:605–613.
2. Hui D, Dos Santos R, Chisholm G, et al. Bedside clinical signs associated with impending death in patients with advanced cancer: preliminary findings of a prospective, longitudinal cohort study. *Cancer.* 2015;121:960–967.
3. Bruera S, Chisholm G, Dos Santos R, et al. Variations in vital signs in the last days of life in patients with advanced cancer. *Journal of Pain and Symptom Management.* 2014;48:510–517.
4. Hallenbeck J. Palliative care in the final days of life. "They were expecting it any time." *JAMA.* 2005;293:2265–2271.
5. Plonk WM, Arnold RM. Terminal care: the last weeks of life. *Journal of Palliative Medicine* 2005;8:1042–1054.
6. Lindsay J, Dooley M, Martin J, et al. The development and evaluation of an oncological palliative care deprescribing guideline: "OncPal deprescribing guideline." *Supportive Care in Cancer.* 2015;23:71–78.
7. Masman AD, van Dijk M, Tibbrel D, Baar FPM, Mathôt RAA. Medication use during end-of-life care in a palliative care centre. *International Journal of Clinical Pharmacy.* 2015;37:767–775.
8. Anderson SL, Shreve ST. Continuous subcutaneous infusion of opiates at end-of-life. *Annals of Pharmacotherapy.* 2004;38:1015–1023.
9. Kamal AH, Magure JM, Wheeler JL, Currow DC, Abernathy AP. Dyspnea review for the palliative care professional: assessment, burdens, and etiologies. *Journal of Palliative Medicine.* 2011;14(10):1167–1172. doi:10.1089/jpm.2011.0109

10. Kamal AH, Maguire JM, Wheeler JL, Currow DC, Abernethy AP. Dyspnea review for the palliative care professional: treatment goals and therapeutic options. *Journal of Palliative Medicine.* 2012;*15*:106–114.

11. Breitbart W, Alici Y. Agitation and delirium at the end of life. "We couldn't manage him." *JAMA.* 2008;*300*:2898–2910.

12. Ellershaw JE, Sutcliffe JM, Saunders CM. Dehydration and the dying patient. *Journal of Pain and Symptom Management.* 1995;*10*:192–197.

13. Prommer E. Anticholinergics in palliative medicine: an update. *American Journal of Hospice and Palliative Medicine.* 2012;*30*:490–498.

14. Mercadente S, Marinangeli F, Masedu F, et al. Hyoscine butylbromide for the management of death rattle: sooner rather than later. *Journal of Pain and Symptom Management.* 2018;*56*:902–907.

15. Drugs and Therapeutic Bulletin: The management of dry eye. *BMJ.* 2008;*47*:1270–1276.

16. Wiseman M. Palliative care dentistry: focusing on quality of life. *Compendium of Continuing Education in Dentistry.* 2017;*38*:529–534.

17. Regnard C, Allport S, Stephenson S. ABC of palliative care: mouth care, skin care, and lymphoedema. *BMJ.* 1997;*315*:1002.

18. Byock I. *Dying Well: Peace and Possibilities at the End of Life.* New York, NY: Riverhead Books, 1997.

19. Widera EW, Block SD. Managing grief and depression at the end of life. *American Family Physician.* 2012;*86*:259–264.

20. Marks A, Marchand L. Fast Facts and Concepts #118. Near death awareness. October 2015. https://www.mypcnow.org/fast-facts/

24

Transitions in Palliative and End-of-Life Care

Karl Steinberg and Michael Fratkin

Transition is defined as the process or period of changing from one state or condition to another. Change is inevitable in life, and many people, as they near the end of their lives, experience a number of transitions—in their functional status, their physical location, their cognitive abilities, and their goals of care. In the hospice field, the word *transitioning* also has a specific meaning, sometimes referred to as the preactive phase of dying that may begin weeks to days before the "active dying process." This chapter focuses on care transitions in location and in medical treatment preferences and discusses some of the potential pitfalls of transitions, along with telemedicine as a palliative care tool to reduce the burden of transitions.

During the twentieth century, the most common paradigm for medical care was for patients to have a community-based primary physician, usually a family physician, internist, or general practitioner, who essentially followed them across all care settings—in the outpatient primary care setting, the acute care hospital, the nursing facility, and perhaps even with home visits for patients too debilitated to access the clinician's office or facility. Obviously, the benefit of such a system is that wherever the patient goes, the clinician or provider who knows them and their family will be managing care, often as part of an interdisciplinary team. With the advent of hospital medicine as a specialty in the 1990s, though, this paradigm began to fade as medical groups favored the efficiency of having their outpatient clinicians concentrate on productivity and maximizing billing. Since 2000, more and more outpatient practices have also moved away from following their own patients in nursing homes, relying on "SNFists" or postacute and long-term care specialists who are similar to hospitalists, but do skilled nursing facility (SNF) care. So today, in many markets, primary care physicians care for their patients only in the clinic and never set foot in a hospital or nursing facility. This may be good for efficiency, but is not so good for continuity of care because patients who transition across care settings are likely to see different clinicians (physicians, physician assistants [PAs], advanced practice nurses) in each setting—often a new provider whom they have never seen before.

The hospital medicine movement had been around for at least a decade before substantial attention was given to the lack of continuity of care under this model and the risks of poorly engineered transitions from hospital to home. Eric Coleman, MD, MPH, was a pioneer in identifying and devising strategies to address unsafe care transitions in the early 2010s. Coleman's care transition intervention, which included a new member of the care team, the "transitions coach," was among the first of many programs designed to improve the quality of care transitions, mostly between the acute care hospital back to the community.[1] In 2012, the Centers for Medicare and Medicaid Services (CMS) rolled out the Hospital Readmissions Reduction Program (HRRP) as part of their Value-Based Purchasing initiative, and this scheme—still operational today—essentially penalized hospitals with excessive readmission rates in the 30 days after patients were discharged with specific diagnoses.[2] Programs such as Project BOOST,[3] Project RED,[4] and many others sprang up as hospitals suddenly had an acute financial interest in ensuring that their patients were discharged with a safe, appropriate discharge plan and follow-up. Prior to that, if a patient was sent home with a diagnosis of congestive heart failure exacerbation but failed to pick up their prescription for the new diuretic and if they landed back in the hospital a few days later, the hospital actually stood to gain because they would be paid for a whole new hospitalization. The HRRP marked the first time meaningful dialogue between acute hospitals and post–acute care settings and institutions, especially SNFs and home health agencies, occurred to any appreciable degree, and it was a catalyst for the interest in ensuring safe care transitions.

Since 2017, SNFs have had a similar program through the CMS, called the Skilled Nursing Facility Value-Based Purchasing (SNF VBP) program.[5] This program authorizes 2% withholding of Medicare funds to all US nursing facilities and redistributes much of this withholding to facilities based on their performance on quality measures, including rehospitalizations. Such programs have created a further incentive for nursing homes to plan carefully for safe discharges and to provide excellent, proactive care in the facility to avoid unnecessary trips to the hospital and other burdensome transitions.

Among the most important factors associated with safe transitions are

- ensuring the patient (and a caregiver) understand the diagnosis(es), the plan of care, the specific medical follow-up needed, how to contact primary care and/or specialty offices, and clinical signs and symptoms that would require sooner follow-up or emergency evaluation;
- ensuring access to all needed prescription and over-the-counter medication, durable medical equipment, supplies, and transportation if applicable;
- considering basic needs, including shelter, temperature control, food security, and absence of abuse or neglect (including physical, sexual, fiduciary, emotional abuse; and self-neglect);
- in palliative care, ensuring that advance care planning documents and corresponding orders (e.g., medical power of attorney, do-not-resuscitate, POLST [Physician Orders for Life-Sustaining Treatment] paradigm orders) are complete and accessible to first responders—such as posting on a refrigerator or other customary location; and

- with patients who are taking medications that may be prone to theft, diversion, or misuse (e.g., opioids, benzodiazepines and others), ensuring that there is a plan to prevent others from depriving the patient of needed comfort medication.

Medication reconciliation deserves special mention. A pharmacist may be a valuable member of the team, especially a geriatric pharmacist if dealing with older patients, but if no pharmacist is available, another clinician should take the time to fully review the medication list and determine for each medication whether it is truly necessary. Many medications that are commonly used in younger patients may have significant adverse effects in older patients, including drugs with anticholinergic effects often used for overactive bladder or insomnia; overly vigorous diabetic or hypertensive control can result in life-threatening hypoglycemia, syncope, falls, and other serious adverse outcomes. Efforts to discontinue unnecessary medications (sometimes referred to as de-prescribing) should be undertaken at every transition of care. In palliative care, it is often not appropriate to continue medications prescribed to reduce future adverse events (e.g., statin drugs in hypercholesterolemia) if a patient's life expectancy is too brief to derive any appreciable benefit. Similarly, preventive medicine screening tests (e.g., mammography, colorectal cancer screening) should not be performed if there is little or no benefit to be derived from the information they may provide. Of course, each patient and each situation should be assessed individually, and documentation in the medical record of the reasoning (and ideally shared decision-making) behind de-prescribing and forgoing screening tests is advisable.

Transitions in care location can be difficult and harmful to patients and in general should be undertaken only when the expected benefits of a move clearly outweigh the burdens. "Transfer trauma" or relocation stress syndrome has been a recognized phenomenon since the 1970s, most commonly identified in patients with preexisting cognitive impairment, where there is a sudden deterioration in cognition, attention, behavior, or functional status associated with a change in physical location.[6-9] The etiology of transfer trauma is thought to be multifactorial, but certainly includes loss of familiar surroundings and cues, changes in caregivers, and variations in daily routine. To the extent routines can be kept consistent between two locations, this should be the goal. Sometimes, patients will return to baseline after transfer trauma, but it is not unusual for them to suffer an enduring decline in one or more parameters, and family members should be made aware of this possibility before any transfer is planned. If resources are available to allow a patient to remain in a stable, long-standing stable and enduring care setting (e.g., the ability to retain a paid caregiver to assist with care in a private home), that should be encouraged before proceeding to relocate the patient.

The most common general care settings encountered in day-to-day clinical practice are as follows, from most medicalized/institutional to least:

- General acute care hospital—In this setting, the patient is usually seen by at least one physician on a daily basis, and generally the condition requires close monitoring by nursing or access to specialty services (e.g., operating room, interventional radiology, cardiac catheterization laboratory, etc.). In the Intensive Care Unit, access to intravenous pressors, ventilators, continuous cardiac monitoring, and other high-level medical technology is also available. (*Note*: Even the transitions between units or floors in the hospital can be fraught, and errors can be made in these transitions.) A great majority of US hospitals today have access to some level of palliative care practitioner consultation and associated services (e.g., spiritual care/chaplain, social work), but many communities do not have full-service palliative care available short of actual hospice enrollment.

- Long-term acute care hospital (LTAC or LTCH)—The LTACs are for patients who have chronic complex needs, including ventilator dependence, extensive wounds, or the requirement to see multiple specialists on a frequent basis. Usually a daily physician or practitioner visit is made. Palliative care consultation services are sometimes available in LTACs, but in general it is a setting that is focused on prolonging life as a primary goal of care. Usually, LTAC stays are covered by Medicare for Medicare beneficiaries, and Medicaid generally covers LTAC for those who do not have Medicare.

- Skilled nursing facility—Both postacute (skilled) and long-term (custodial) care are provided in the SNF setting, and some of these facilities (e.g., subacute units) are able to manage chronically ventilator-dependent patients. Residents of SNFs vary from highly medically complex patients to those with mild cognitive and/or functional deficits. SNFs are highly regulated by the federal government via the CMS. Usually a physician, PA, or advanced practice nurse visit is required no less frequently than once every 30 days in a nursing facility for the first 90 days, then every 60 days for stable long-term care residents. For skilled/postacute residents, it is usually recommended (but requirements are variable in different states) that the initial visit take place within a few days of admission, then roughly weekly depending on medical complexity and stability throughout the skilled stay. During the Covid-19 pandemic, the ability for advanced practice practitioners to perform initial comprehensive visits in nursing facilities has been allowed under a federal 1130 waiver. These waivers also have allowed initial visits and subsequent visits to be done via telehealth technologies during the pandemic. Rehabilitation services (physical therapy, occupational therapy, speech and language pathology); social services; dietary/nutrition; and some on-site specialty and ancillary services (e.g., podiatry, dentistry, optometry, psychology, psychiatry) are usually available. The availability of palliative care is highly variable in SNFs depending on community resources, but often are scant beyond primary palliative care from the regular attending practitioners and formal hospice enrollment. Some communities have hospice agencies or affiliated organizations that provide at least partial palliative care services in the nursing home (and assisted living, independent living, and regular community residences) as a charitable service and/or as a loss leader with the expectation that when the patient becomes philosophically and prognostically appropriate for hospice, they will sign on with that hospice. Most skilled/postacute nursing home residents are primarily covered short term (up to 100 days) by Medicare or other medical insurance, and skilled care is expensive, often over $500 per diem. Most custodial/long-term nursing home residents are covered by Medicaid, at a significantly lower rate. For those who do not meet the economic criteria for Medicaid, other long-term residents pay privately until they "spend down" and qualify for Medicaid, while a few are covered by other long-term care insurance, structured settlements or third-party payers, and other sources. Certain criteria must generally be met for long-term care insurance to be covered, including a minimum duration of disability and a minimum number of activities of daily living (ADLs) with which the person needs assistance. Hospice agencies may help provide care, but in general do not provide room and board except when patients meet criteria for inpatient care or short-term respite (usually limited to 5 days at a time). Physicians or other advanced practice practitioners usually must affirm the documentation regarding a patient's clinical and functional status to demonstrate that they meet such criteria.

• Assisted living communities (also called assisted living facilities), including other "nonmedical," residential care settings like small group homes (sometimes called personal care homes, board-and-care facilities, residential care facilities for the elderly, dedicated dementia or "memory care" units, and other designations) are for generally non–medically complex persons who require some assistance with their ADLs and instrumental activities of daily living or need supervision because of cognitive deficits. Usually, assisted living communities will provide food, activities, laundry services, transportation, medication administration, incontinent care, assistance with ambulation/locomotion/transfers, and limited supervision, such as checking vital signs in some facilities. There is no requirement for a nurse on site, but some larger facilities will employ a "wellness nurse" or other nursing professional to help monitor residents' medical status. There are no federal regulations governing the licensure or operating requirements for assisted living communities, so each state has its own regulations, which vary significantly. Most states do not have a specific requirement for how often an assisted living resident must be seen by a physician or other advanced practice practitioner, and often these residents will still go to their community outpatient clinics or specialty offices. However, there has been increasing availability in many areas for these residents to be seen on site—which is desirable especially for those for whom being transported to a clinic may represent a significant burden, whether because of functional dependence, dementia-related behavioral issues, or other considerations. As with SNFs, the availability of palliative care services is highly variable and often lacking in these settings, other than formal hospice admission. These facilities and the assisted living industry have clung to the notion of nonmedical care for decades, but since the turn of the century, it has become increasingly clear that there are in fact significant numbers of medically complex patients residing in assisted living. Often, home health agencies and their professionals (nursing, physical therapy, occupational therapy, speech and language pathology, social work, home health aides) provide services of a medical and rehabilitative nature in assisted living communities.

• Independent living communities—these are often not licensed or regulated, but merely provide limited services such as communal dining, laundry and housekeeping services, shopping, transportation, and other assistance to elders who choose to live in this type of congregate setting. Many of these communities have some communal activities like music, crafts, and lectures. There is no requirement for physician or other practitioner supervision in this residential setting, and palliative care services are usually limited to hospice agencies, except in geographic areas with robust community-based palliative care providers available. These are covered by private payments.

• Another care paradigm provides wraparound services for "aging in place," often referred to as continuing care retirement communities. Most of these require a significant buy-in for a contract to reside there, and residents typically start out in the independent setting, then if their needs increase, they can transition to the assisted living wing or floor, then if they actually meet the criteria for requiring skilled nursing care, they can move into the nursing facility wing. These are generally covered by private payment, especially initially, but sometimes with help from private long-term care insurance if the resident meets criteria for the need for long-term care assistance.

- Programs of All-Inclusive Care for the Elderly[10] are another care paradigm that provides extensive care services, both medical and nonmedical, and including adult day care services, with the goal of allowing enrollees to remain in their own community/home setting for as long as possible. It is usually considered an alternative to SNF placement. These are capitated programs through CMS, and there is generally no cost to the recipient.
- Community/home living—This is usually the preferred care setting for people who have the resources to continue residing in their own or a family member's or friend's home. Sometimes if there are medical or nonmedical needs, assistance such as that provided by a private (often unlicensed/uncertified) caregiver, or from a certified home health agency, can be provided in the home along with help from other family or household members.

Many patients may transition back and forth from these (and other) care settings many times during the course of a chronic illness. Again, to the extent transitions can be minimized, that is a worthy goal. Clearly, financial and psychosocial concerns may drive the ability to remain in place versus having to move to a different care setting, and these must be explored. Social workers may be invaluable in helping determine optimal current and future care settings, and their assistance should be sought in situations where there is not a clearly outlined direction.

Most patients have a strong preference to remain in their comfortable, familiar "home" setting—however the patient defines that—as long as possible, which is understandable. At times, remaining in a private home situation without sufficient resources to meet care needs represents an unsafe situation. Patient autonomy is extremely important, and it should always be a goal to respect people's right to make their own decisions with respect to their care. A person has a right to make ill-advised decisions and exercise poor judgment, even when it places them at risk. This occurs throughout the life cycle and in a variety of contexts. When patients and their families make potentially risky decisions as far as location of care and amount of services they will receive, it is important to document discussions of risks, benefits, and alternatives. In situations where significant safety concerns are present, including the possibility of neglect (on the part of others or self-neglect) or abuse, notifying adult protective services is advisable in addition to documenting the clinician's recommendations for a different care setting or situation. Also, if the patient's capacity to understand and appreciate the ramifications of such a decision is in question because of dementia, delirium, or other cognitive or psychiatric disorder, mental health evaluation, adult protective services referral, and involvement of family members and other close contacts (to the extent permissible by the Health Insurance Portability and Accountability Act [HIPAA]) should be sought.

Patients who have stabilized medically during an acute care hospitalization often want to go home, but it may not be appropriate for a return directly to the community. Clinicians can help hospital discharge planners, social workers, and often family members to encourage patients to consider a safe transition to an SNF or other care setting with adequate support and/or medical resources. The physician, PA, or advanced practice nurse can give medical reasons why the recommendation is being made for a nonhome discharge and what the negative consequences may be if the patient goes home. Similarly, when a patient has completed a postacute skilled admission in a nursing home (when the rehabilitation process is completed or the need for skilled medical treatment such as intravenous antibiotics), there may still be concerns about the safety of returning home, and a move, possibly temporary, into an assisted living community may be appropriate. In any of these situations, it may be reasonable for the clinician to say—without making any promises—that "our hope is that you will go home after you have recovered enough, and that will be plan A. But for now, you are not at that point, and I think it would be best for everyone, and safest, for you to go to [type of facility]." It is surprising how often, in the author's experience, a patient who has resided in the same home for four or five decades and who is dead set against moving into assisted living—once they have agreed to try it, even on a trial basis—will come back and say, "I wish I had done that 10 years ago." Social isolation in a private home can be difficult and challenging, and managing a home alone or even as a couple may be difficult and compromised when they are frail. The social intercourse, prepared food, laundry services, housekeeping, and other services can turn out to be a wonderful bonus to what was expected to be a miserable transition and a step toward the grave.

No chapter on transitions in medical care would be complete without a discussion of transitions in a patient's goals of care. Some patients have clarity about what medical interventions they do or do not want at a given phase in the trajectory of their illness, while for many others there is a process that often includes bargaining and weighing of burdens versus benefits. It is common for relatively healthy people to say, for example, "If I were ever diagnosed with metastatic cancer, I would not take chemo, and I would seek out medical aid in dying" (or take an overdose, etc.). Yet, when they actually receive such a diagnosis, they often reassess their options in light of current reality and may elect one or more courses of toxic chemotherapy because they have decided they do not want to die—or want to survive at least for some important event (e.g., wedding, birth, graduation). Similarly, patients with severe illness who have completed advance healthcare directives and have received POLST[11] orders from their attending practitioners for do not resuscitate/do not attempt resuscitation and do not intubate, yet when they arrive in the emergency room in acute respiratory distress, they may change their mind and request intubation when they are failing noninvasive attempts at ventilation.

On the other side of the coin, patients commonly change their treatment preferences as a serious chronic illness progresses. As front-line clinicians, it is important for us to elicit discussion about treatment preferences and goals of care multiple times over time, as our patients' conditions evolve. It is assumed (although not entirely accurate) that most people without significant medical morbidities want, at least initially, aggressive and invasive attempts at prolonging life—and our medical system defaults to all-out efforts, including cardiopulmonary resuscitation, defibrillation, intubation, and the like. Our emergency medical system, first responders, emergency departments, and hospitals all act on the presumption that all patients, even chronically and even terminally ill ones, want to live for as long as possible—unless there is substantial evidence to the contrary, like POLST orders or an advance directive. Indeed, most reasonably healthy people do not object to aggressive attempts to prolong their life and restore them to a satisfactory functional and cognitive status if there is a reasonable expectation that even burdensome interventions may have that result. But as a person with a serious chronic illness experiences progressive functional decline and troubling symptoms during the trajectory of their illness, they usually will come to the point where they do not want burdensome measures to prolong their lives—or even to a point where only comfort-focused treatments are desired (e.g., no antibiotics for an infection). In other words, some patients get to the point where they do not want any interventions that may prolong their life—even antibiotics or hand feeding in some instances. POLST paradigm orders can help translate patients' treatment preferences into actionable orders, memorializing a conversation between the physician or advanced practice practitioner and the patient and/or family. These orders should be reviewed and updated/revised on a regular basis as appropriate.

Clinicians must remain vigilant to transitions in patients' treatment preferences along the course of their illness. In palliative care, an empathetic listening ear is one of the best tools for assessing and monitoring these transitions in order to help patients make informed decisions and get through these changes. It is important to ensure that the patient, and whenever possible their family or other close circle of humanity, understands the risks and benefits of different courses of action—just as we want them to understand the ramifications of their choice of physical location.

Telemedicine

Telemedicine Applications

Telemedicine has provided a rapidly advancing paradigm for improving the safety and efficiency of care transitions and also can help prevent unnecessary and burdensome transitions in care location. Technology use has advanced communications between people with illness and their healthcare providers, as well as communications between members of the healthcare delivery structure and each other. *Synchronous* communications link sender and receiver in real time without a requirement they be in the same place, whereas *asynchronous* communications are transmission of data between two or more parties without the requirement that all recipients respond immediately. Beginning at the turn of the twentieth century, telephones began to provide unprecedented synchronous means of engaging healthcare providers and coordinating medical interventions in real time. By the mid-1980s, fax-based communication provided dramatic improvements in speed and fidelity of asynchronous data transmission. The development of the Internet and its rapid adoption, availability, and bandwidth have allowed for a vast array of both synchronous and asynchronous innovations with revolutionary impact on developing models of healthcare delivery in all settings.

Definitions and Competencies

There is some variability in the terminology used to describe these technologies; telehealth is defined by the Health Resources and Services Administration as "the use of electronic information and telecommunications technologies to support and promote long-distance clinical health care, patient and professional health-related education, public health and health administration. Technologies include videoconferencing, the internet, store-and-forward imaging, streaming media, and terrestrial and wireless communications."[12] In common use, the term *telemedicine* tends to be reserved for synchronous videoconferencing that links a patient and a provider with a real-time audiovisual link and for asynchronous "store-and-forward" video and still image communications. In a recently published document, telehealth is further defined to include patient portals, eConsults, video visits, and remote patient monitoring (Association of American Medical Colleges [AAMC] Telehealth Competencies.[13]

As noted above, effective care transitions from one care setting to another require impeccable communication among all members of the care team, including patient and family. This is defined as caregivers or whomever the patient designates as "family"; for example, there may be an individual who has technological capabilities, such as a smartphone, who assists for the purpose of the televisit. Over the last 5 years, telehealth broadly and telemedicine technology more specifically have been successfully applied to palliative care delivery by interdisciplinary teams to people with serious illness at home, in assisted living facilities, SNFs, other rehabilitation and LTACs, and in acute hospital settings. The use of videoconferencing for the direct care of seriously ill people at home has been dramatically accelerated during the Covid-19 pandemic through relaxation of federal restrictions on billing and limitations related to HIPAA enforcement during the Public Health Emergency Declaration. The provisions have allowed reimbursement for videoconferencing for clinical encounters in parity to outpatient clinic visits. This reimbursement and the services have dramatically impacted the delivery of healthcare in the community setting as a whole and will evolve over time to persist in some form or another. Early indications are that they demonstrate efficacy, cost reductions, increased coordination of care, and prevention of hospitalization, which results in greater overall satisfaction of patients and caregivers. Incorporation of best practices in this arena will ensure the continued success of this initiative since communication skills are at the core of the competencies detailed for all providers and students in the healing arts.

Best Practices in Telehealth

Best practices for the use of telehealth technology in palliative care are defined as their effectiveness to deliver improved quality of life to people with serious illness, the experience of support for those that care for them, and an adequate channel of communication for healthcare professionals to assess and intervene at the right time and in the right setting. Six general domains were identified in the AAMC Telehealth Competencies[13] that apply well to the technology-enabled practice of palliative care.

1. Patient Safety and Appropriate Use of Telehealth: Clinicians will understand when and why to use telehealth, as well as assess patient readiness, patient safety, practice readiness, and end-user readiness.
2. Data Collection and Assessment via Telehealth: Clinicians will obtain and manage clinical information via telehealth to ensure appropriate high-quality care.
3. Communication Via Telehealth: Specific to telehealth, clinicians will effectively communicate with patients, families, caregivers, and healthcare team members using telehealth

modalities. They will also integrate both the transmission and receipt of information with the goal of effective knowledge transfer, professionalism, and understanding within a therapeutic relationship.

4. Ethical Practices and Legal Requirements for Telehealth: Clinicians will understand the federal, state, and local facility practice requirements to meet the minimal standards to deliver healthcare via telehealth. Clinicians will maintain patient privacy while minimizing risk to the clinician and patient during telehealth encounters while putting the patient's interest first and preserving or enhancing the doctor-patient relationship.

5. Technology for Telehealth: Clinicians will have basic knowledge of technology needed for the delivery of high-quality telehealth services.

6. Access and Equity in Telehealth: Clinicians will have an understanding of telehealth delivery that addresses and mitigates cultural biases as well as physician bias for or against telehealth, accounts for physical and mental disabilities, and non–health-related individual and community needs and limitations to promote equitable access to care

Choosing the proper and safe channel for communication depends on recognition of strengths and weaknesses of each channel. For example, in the assessment of symptoms that are a manifestation of a chronic progressive illness, like a cancer patient with worsening pain, videoconferencing-based evaluation and intervention may be satisfactory or even superior to burdening a patient to be seen in a clinic setting. However, if evidence of acute decompensation in cardiovascular function is revealed, as with an exacerbation of heart failure or chronic lung disease with moderate or severe dyspnea during a videoconferencing visit, rapid escalation that allows physical assessment can be critically needed when aligned with a patient's preferences. Remote patient monitoring data (e.g., serial weights, oximetry, blood pressure, pulse rate) may guide the intensity and pace of intervention. Recognition of the limitations of an audiovisual assessment is an essential best practice. For example, remote monitoring, synchronous versus asynchronous monitoring, and the availability of technology such as a remote stethoscope head for the patient with a critical need can be problematic. The education in the use of a device is an equally important part of the physical assessment of the patient.

Ease and facility in the practice of medicine via telehealth depend on the mastery of verbal and nonverbal communication skills that are at the core of all medical specialties but are absolutely essential during detailed conversations about goals of care in the serious illness patient population. A human connection of trust must be established to gain access to information that illuminates the lived experience of patients with serious illness, their caregivers, and families. Palliative care values the best possible management of physical symptoms. This fundamentally depends on the ability of the provider to understand the complex multidimensional dilemmas faced by patients, their caregivers, and families. The practice competencies of the PA profession align with these best practices in conceptual and actual terms (Core Competencies for New PA Graduates).

Pragmatic advantages of telemedicine/telehealth include reduction in patient symptom burden; reduction in family and caregiver stress by locating more care in the home; reduction in travel requirements in the context of serious and advanced illness; and realization of cost and time savings in the holistic care of the patient. In addition to convenience, the home visit provider(s) are further able to perform an immediate evaluation of safety issues in the home environment. They can collaborate with the patient, caregivers, and other interdisciplinary team members to target and address important needs and preventive care, for example, fall prevention and medication reconciliation. These are not issues that can be replicated easily in the office setting.

Telemedicine can be used to assess goals of care, complete advance care plans and documents such as POLST/MOLST (Medical Orders for Life-Sustaining Treatments) orders, and integrate primary care and specialty care, including therapists of physical, occupational, speech and language, and nutritional expertise. Much of the care coordination between site-specific providers, such as hospitalists and SNFists, relies on flawed asynchronous communications of faxed electronic health records and encounter reports. On the other hand, videoconferencing provides opportunities for efficient multispecialty and interprofessional and family meetings that anticipate problems. This will result in development and facilitation of treatment programs to realign unrealistic treatment goals of care. Additionally, such communication can assess and promote medication adherence, safe use of scheduled and as-needed medications, and home safety. This is seen, for example, in the provision of durable medical equipment to enhance function and autonomy of the patient and to avoid caregiver injury.

The facilitation of comprehensive family meetings, including members and caregivers who are dispersed and important, can reliably prevent some of the common difficulties that disparate information and fragmented communication cause. Urgent, and even emergent, videoconferencing-based assessment can be initiated instantaneously. This provides an unprecedented opportunity to triage and/or treat a developing issue promptly or avoids an emergency ambulance call. This also preempts the default choice of waiting for a scheduled appointment or an often unnecessary, undesired, and potentially dangerous visit to the emergency department. This is particularly true in times of pandemic. A brief and timely audio and/or visual connection with a trusted healthcare provider can reassure patients, family, and healthcare staff more effectively. At the same time, this type of connection provides the healthcare provider team a plethora of contextual, objective, and actionable information for assessment that is required to make a safe and sensible plan of care. Coupled with the availability of an increasing number of remote devices that can augment or substitute for a physical examination, this can prevent an unwanted hospitalization and transition of care.

Some types of visits may lend themselves to telemedicine better than others: diagnostic dermatology and psychiatry are certainly among the more established areas to date. But other types of encounters—for example, orthopedic problems amenable to video and self-examination techniques—are also expanding into this arena. Body language, eye contact, and other typical nonverbal cues are essential in the history-taking process and may be difficult to pick up when on a smartphone screen or monitor. However, they are present and more essential to recognize in the course of a telemedicine encounter. PAs are compassionate listeners who recognize the value of and practice a comprehensive history to formulate a diagnosis, create a management plan, and establish a trusting and open relationship with the patient and their caregivers.

While there are some areas where telemedicine cannot substitute for in-person care—including provision of actual, hands-on care and the comfort provided in an actual human touch or hug—it is an excellent solution to logistical problems. This is not unusual in palliative care practice. As in the general medical practice, this is especially true in remote and rural areas. With the increasing availability of telemedicine applications and wearable technology, it is expected that in the near future this will allow for unprecedented and exciting opportunities for clinicians and teams and patients. It has great potential to avoid unnecessary transitions; enable smooth transitions to occur; and provide prompt and effective assessment of changes in medical, psychosocial, or existential conditions in the patient care scenario. This will enhance patient and family/caregiver education and optimize symptom management. It opens up unlimited possibilities for home and community-based hospice, in real time, and has the additional advantage of adding support that was not previously available. End-of-life care and home hospice are an important aspect of palliative care that avoids the emergency room, enhances patient dignity, and preserves the patient-centered care paradigm.

Legal and Ethical Considerations

The legal and ethical context of technology-enabled palliative care delivery demands on-going attention to rapidly changing guidelines, while demonstrating the highest possible standard of respect for the patient and family's interest and preserving the provider-patient relationship. In entering the home of people we serve, we must recognize the importance of explaining our role and obtaining informed consent to evaluate the environment of their home. There is an important reason for this: to assess the safety of the home environment. This can determine whether or not the patient needs to transition to a different setting or facility. We must have adequate capacity to troubleshoot the technology we are using or have ready access to "teammates" in the form of another individual or institutional support that can keep the management of the technology from interfering with the clinical work itself. As we use these technologies to "leave" the constraints of the controlled context of the hospital or clinic, disparities in access to technology and comfort with its use must be addressed along with programmatic investments that ensure equity, language translation, and cultural sensitivity in the communities we serve. The success in the implementation of best practices is dependent on these variables being addressed and thus the success of the individual provider or clinician who invests time and effort to successfully treat their patients.

Summary

Transitions are inevitable in life, and they may range from extremely positive experiences to dismal, miserable ones. As palliative care clinicians, our duty is to walk the path with our patients and their families, ideally as part of an interdisciplinary team—and wherever the path takes them. To the extent we are able to smooth transitions in care location and in goals of care for the patients we serve—by educating, listening, respecting, and advocating—palliative care clinicians should always provide compassionate, holistic counsel.

References

1. The Care Transitions Program. Home page. https://caretransitions.org/
2. Centers for Medicare & Medicaid Services. Hospital Readmissions Reduction Program (HRRP). Last modified August 24, 2020. https://www.cms.gov/Medicare/Medicare-Fee-for-Service-Payment/AcuteInpatientPPS/Readmissions-Reduction-Program
3. SHM Project BOOST. The 8P Screening Tool. Identifying your patient's risk for adverse events after discharge. https://www.hospitalmedicine.org/globalassets/clinical-topics/clinical-pdf/8ps_riskassess-1.pdf
4. Agency for Healthcare Research and Quality. Re-engineered Discharge (RED) toolkit. Last reviewed February 2020. https://www.ahrq.gov/patient-safety/settings/hospital/red/toolkit/index.html
5. Centers for Medicare & Medicaid Services. The Skilled Nursing Facility Value-Based Purchasing (SNV VBP) program. Last modified March 8, 2021. https://www.cms.gov/Medicare/Quality-Initiatives-Patient-Assessment-Instruments/Value-Based-Programs/SNF-VBP/SNF-VBP-Page
6. Hitov SA. Transfer trauma: its impact on the elderly. *Clearinghouse Review*. 1974–1975;8:846. https://heinonline.org/HOL/LandingPage?handle=hein.journals/clear8&div=179&id=&page=
7. Ryman VM, Erisman JC, Darvey LM, Osborne J, Swartsenburg E, Syurina EV. Health effects of the relocation of patients with dementia: a scoping review to inform medical and policy decision-making. *Gerontologist*. 2018. Advance access publication April 28, 2018. doi:10.1093/geront/gny031. https://www.researchgate.net/publication/324920089_Health_Effects_of_the_Relocation_of_Patients_With_Dementia_A_Scoping_Review_to_Inform_Medical_and_Policy_Decision-Making
8. Coleman EA, Barbaccia JC, Croghan-Minhane MS. Hospitalization rates in nursing home residents with dementia: a pilot study of the impact of a special care unit. *Journal of the American Geriatrics Society*. 1990;38(2):108–112. https://onlinelibrary.wiley.com/doi/abs/10.1111/j.1532-5415.1990.tb03470.x
9. Weaver RH, Roberto KA, Brossoie N. A scoping review: characteristics and outcomes of residents who experience involuntary relocation. *Gerontologist*. 2020;60(1):e20–e37. https://academic.oup.com/gerontologist/article-abstract/60/1/e20/5494575
10. Note: The term *elderly* has fallen out of favor in recent years as somewhat pejorative, with "elder" or "older" preferred. However, it is explicitly in the title of PACE as designated by CMS. For more information about PACE programs, see https://www.medicaid.gov/medicaid/long-term-services-supports/pace/programs-all-inclusive-care-elderly-benefits/index.html
11. POLST originally was an acronym for Physician Orders for Life-Sustaining Treatment, but now is used as a word designating portable patient orders that are valid across care settings. Different states have different names and acronyms for POLST paradigm orders. More information can be found at https://polst.org/.
12. US Department of Health and Human Services, Health Resources and Services Administration (HRSA). 2019.
13. https://www.aamc.org/system/files/2020-09/hca-telehealthcollection-telehealth-competencies.pdf

Social, Cultural, and Legal Aspects of Care

25

Family Stress
Including Cultural Context

Denis Snow and Mary Ellen Lasala

Social, Financial, and Legal Needs of Individuals and Families With Serious Illnesses

Social Determinants of Health and Health Outcomes

Social determinants of health refer to a broad set of social factors (income, education, race and ethnicity, transportation, housing, insurance, food access) that influence health outcomes.[1] It has been postulated that these determinants are responsible for more than a third of all deaths annually in the United States.[2] The recognition of the effect of social determinants on health outcomes has generated initiatives within the Centers for Medicare and Medicaid Services to establish models that look at the nonmedical factors that affect health outcomes. An example of such a program is the Delivery System Reform Incentive Payment. This initiative links Medicaid funding for providers to process performance metrics, which include social needs targets such as supportive housing.

"Health care outcomes are driven by an array of factors, including underlying genetics, health behaviors, social and environmental factors and health care. Studies suggest that health behaviors, such as smoking, diet and exercise and social and economic factors are the primary drivers of health outcomes, and social and economic factors can shape individuals' health experience."[2] Healthy People (https://wwwhealthypeople.gov/2020) identifies five key determinant areas affecting health outcomes: health and healthcare, social and community context, education, neighborhood and built environments, and economic stability. Palliative care, in treating the whole person, is intertwined with all the key areas, especially health and healthcare. Of the key determinants, social and community context and economic stability create some of the greatest challenges for the palliative care patient. For many individuals, access to healthcare, including primary care, may be limited geographically or by economic status. Health literacy deficits further interfere with care and outcomes. Thus, it is not surprising that availability of a palliative care consult is not universal. For communities and healthcare systems that are palliative care barren, the clinician must become familiar with treatment goals of palliative care and be adept at identifying the sociofinancial/legal issues and be skilled in communicating with the palliative care patients and their families.

Being poor can make you sick; being sick can make you poor. This is particularly true within the context of palliative care. The clinician working in the sphere of palliative care quickly becomes aware of the relationship of serious illness to the financial and legal needs of individuals and families. As stated by the Center to Advance Palliative Care, "Palliative care sees the person beyond the disease" with a goal to ease emotional suffering and improve quality of life.[3] The emotional suffering encountered when providing care to palliative care patients encompasses the socioeconomic, financial, and legal aspects has been appropriately coined "medical-legal suffering"[4,5] since the medical issues have created or exacerbated the nonmedical problems an individual or family experiences. Because relieving the stress of illness is a primary goal of palliative care, it is critical the clinician has a deep understanding of the nonmedical factors affecting both the palliative care patient and the family. Patients face many social and legal issues during the course of an illness. It is important that physician assistants become aware of these issues; otherwise, the care may be less effective. This chapter explores some of the common but critical issues faced by the palliative care patient during the course of treatment.

Economic Stability: Employment, Income, Medical Debt Support

Chronic serious illness jeopardizes the stability in almost all aspects of a family's financial situation. The effects of health status on social and financial status can be loss of employment, loss of housing, bankruptcy, and food insecurity, which in turn create healthcare disparity. In terms of healthcare outcomes, this aspect of disparity is identified as a potentially modifiable or avoidable difference in health that is not justifiable by the underlying health condition or treatment preferences of the patients.

Serious illness is never someone's single story. The impact of nonmedical determinants of health of a multiyear serious illness can have long-lasting legal and financial burdens for the individual and the family unit (Box 15.1). One should consider that chronically ill individuals may lose their source of income, and they may experience extended periods without work. Spouses may also need to stop working to take care of the ill spouse. The cultural impact of the current pandemic further exacerbated this situation, with children who are at home and unable to socialize or attend school. This forces the parent(s) to include yet another unexpected stress into the picture of care for their spouse or loved one. This is especially taxing on nonprofessional workers, whose paycheck depends on hours worked, and they may also lack healthcare benefits. As employment income diminishes, household bills continue to mount, which adds stress on coping mechanisms for the individual coping with a serious illness. Loss of income will result in further food insecurity, housing instability (eviction or foreclosure), utility shutoffs, and loss of health insurance. This creates, in effect,

BOX 25.1 The Nonmedical Needs Checklist

Medical-Legal Checklist

Health Insurance

Problems obtaining health insurance

Concerns with insurance through employment

Copay concerns

Claims being denied or not paid to medical providers

Medicare coverage

Medicaid: application, spend downs, or denial

Housing Problems

Fear of eviction

Fear of foreclosure

Utilities shutoff concerns

Need for emergency housing, homelessness

Financial Concerns

Income reduced

Employment-related concerns

Social Security Disability denial

Medical debt

Consumer or other debt

Planning if you become too sick

Concerns of who will make medical decisions

Concerns of who will make financial decisions

Need for a will

Need for a guardian for minor or adult disabled child

---

an economic class of the "sick poor." This may be particularly difficult for those who lack knowledge about resources and who have no previous interface with government-based social programs (i.e., Medicaid, food stamps, and disability payments).

Advocacy begins with recognizing the patient's unmet nonmedical needs[4,5] (Figure 25.1). Hence, communication skills and recognition of "red flags" are critical skills for the physician assistant. Here are common red flags that are seen in the palliative care patient:

- **Finances:** Uninsured, sole wage earner, pursuing benefits/statuses, employment status, discrimination
- **Dependents:** Single parent, minor children, domestic partnership where survivor has no guardianship, disabled children of any age
- **Family:** Unmarried couples, food and energy insecurity, poor environmental or housing conditions, domestic violence
- **Legal Status:** Immigrant status, in divorce proceedings, other legal problems

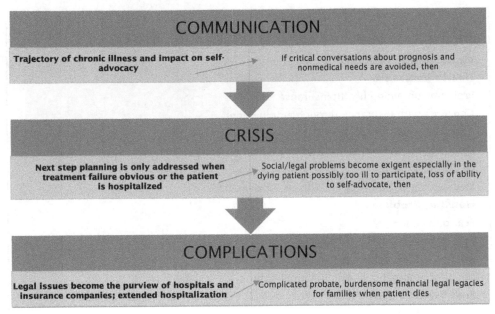

FIGURE 25.1 Trajectory of chronic illness and impact on self-advocacy.

Nonmedical Needs Evaluation

Commonly, clinicians ask, "Why is the patient non-compliant?" The following case study illustrates the many nonmedical needs affecting care.

Case Study

You are meeting a patient in the emergency room 1 month after her initial admission; she is now being evaluated for worsening back pain. You read her history, which is that she is a 46-year-old woman with a history of breast cancer diagnosed 7 years ago who was admitted 1 month ago with severe low back pain and leg weakness. She was subsequently found to have metastatic disease, including spinal involvement with impending cord compression. Emergency spinal surgery was done and follow-up chemotherapy was recommended. After being sent to a "subacute rehab" for 2 weeks for recovery from back surgery, she did not show up for her oncology appointment.

The physician assistant speaks with her and learns that the patient is a single mother of two minor children and a sole wage earner who is estranged from the children's father. She works as a hairdresser and is not paid when she is not at work. Through her job, she has basic healthcare coverage with a large copay. She relies on the public bus for transportation and has only intermittent help from her mother to babysit her young school-aged children. Since being discharged from the rehab facility, she has had ongoing pain in her back and is unable to walk more than a few feet. She currently relies on a credit card and a small amount of savings to pay for food and rent since she is still not able to return to work. She cannot afford the pain medication she was prescribed in rehab. She attempted to take a taxi to her follow-up visit, but they showed up 45 minutes late, and she missed the appointment. What steps can the clinician take to assist this patient to promote quality care?

The following are some of the critical issues to be evaluated by the clinician.

Access to Care

Is the patient insured? Is it adequate? Most Americans have private insurance through employment; however, many palliative care patients will lose that coverage during the course of an illness. They may choose to purchase private health insurance, but the cost may be prohibitive to the palliative care patient. Monthly premiums cost hundreds of dollars, and the insurance plan may have high copayments (fixed payment for services) for treatments and prescriptions, further burdening the patient. Patients need to be aware that they can be billed by specialists who are not in network with their insurance plan. Called "balance billing," the specialist bills the patient for the amount billed but not paid by the patient's insurance company. Therefore, any referrals made by the clinician should include confirmation that the patient will not incur any out-of-pocket charges.

Additionally, insurance companies will often deny authorization for medication, diagnostic tests, or treatment that a clinician has prescribed. Insurers can deny authorization for one of three reasons: (1) The treatment/service is not covered under the plan. (2) The treatment or service is not medically necessary. (3) The service or treatment is investigational or experimental.

The most common denial is for "not medically necessary." To successfully appeal this denial, the clinician must state why the prescribed treatment is appropriate care for this particular patient, not patients in general. For example, if the clinician orders a computed tomographic (CT) scan and the insurer denies the service based on the diagnosis, the explanation should detail the reasons why a CT scan is medically necessary in this case. If a treatment is denied because it is deemed "investigational or experimental," the appeal must show some type of peer-reviewed support for the use of the procedure, diagnostic test, or medication, and the appeal should discuss the medical justification and reason(s) that standard treatment is not appropriate for this patient. This is also done by a case manager, social worker, or designated office personnel, depending on the facility and state.

For the patient without private insurance, the designated office/hospital/clinic personnel or social worker may assist the individual in obtaining public insurance. There are two types of public, government-based health insurance plans: Medicare and Medicaid. Medicare is the federal public insurance program for those aged 65 or older or the blind or disabled. In certain medical conditions, Medicare can also be automatically granted, such as renal dialysis for end-stage renal disease. Medicare has monthly premiums that are taken out of the individual's Social Security monthly payment. The Medicare recipient is responsible for a coinsurance for most visits, prescriptions, diagnostics, and procedures. Medicaid is the state- and county-managed public insurance program that provides health insurance to low-income and disabled individuals. Eligibility is based on assets and income. However, if the disabled person is otherwise asset eligible, but over the income limit, they are able to "spend down" that excess income in several ways. The clinician should learn about the best ways to spend down that excess income in their state. There are special income and asset rules for the disabled. The clinician should have a basic knowledge of what the income and asset thresholds are for their state.

The federal program that provides health insurance coverage for children is the Children's Health Insurance Program (CHIP). Each state program has its own rules about who qualifies for CHIP and how much of a monthly premium is charged, but no state can charge more than 5% of a family's income. CHIP provides comprehensive coverage. There is no copayment on well visits and dental visits.

Medicaid is also the insurance that covers nursing home care and home care. Low-income disabled individuals may have both Medicare and Medicaid. These are called "dual eligibles." The provider's role (MD, DO, physician assistant, nurse practitioner) is to understand the eligibility requirements for Medicaid and to provide any documentation requested from the local social service department regarding the patient's medical condition. If the patient will need long-term care or home care, the provider should know the community resources that can help them apply for those services. The seriously ill patient may need extensive assistance in the home. Documentation from the provider will make the difference between a patient getting that assistance or struggling without it. Administrative forms may seem repetitive and time consuming, but completing them on time is essential for the patient with a serious illness.

Planning Documents

Does the patient have a healthcare/medical power of attorney? The healthcare/medical power of attorney should be an individual who knows the patient's wishes for medical decisions. When obtaining a medical power of attorney form (also called a healthcare proxy form), the patient should be instructed to speak to their agent and let their wishes be known. Involve the medical agent: Does the agent know what the patient wants?

Healthcare proxy/medical power of attorney documents should be readily available, such as keeping a picture of the document in the patient's medical record. The agent's contact information should be readily available in the medical record as well.

If the patient does not have anyone to act as their healthcare/medical power of attorney, do they have a living will? A living will is a document signed by a person with decisional capacity that contains his or her instructions about treatment to be followed if he or she becomes incapable of making treatment decisions directly. A living will is an advance directive. The living will provides guidance and may limit an agent or surrogate's decision-making authority. Healthcare agents are required to make decisions consistent with the patient's wishes and instructions as set forth in the living will. A healthcare agent or surrogate cannot make a decision contrary to the instructions given in the living will unless the agent or surrogate has a valid reason for disregarding the living will, such as the patient revoked the living will or the patient gave more recent, superseding instructions. A healthcare agent and surrogate has no legal authority to override a patient's living will in order to replace the patient's wishes with the agent's beliefs.

Healthcare providers are obligated to disseminate information about a patient's right to execute advance directives to take effect when the patient no longer has capacity. When an advance directive has been presented to a physician or healthcare provider, a copy of the directive must be placed in the patient's medical record. In multiple states, a document that substantiates the medical orders (Physician Orders for Life-Sustaining Treatment, Medical Orders for Life-Sustaining Treatments, Physician Orders for Scope of Treatment, or Medical Orders for Scope of Treatment) will substitute for advance directives. The PA should be aware of these documents and whether or not they can sign them. This is a vital skill in the discussion of advance care planning.

Does a patient have a power of attorney document or someone to act on their behalf if they become incapacitated? A power of attorney is an important document for the patient to have in place, especially if prolonged hospitalization is anticipated. This allows a trusted person to act as an agent for the patient in the event they become physically or mentally unable to manage their financial matters, such as banking, insurance, benefits, and many other needs. In the event the patient becomes incapacitated, the agent can manage the patient's financial affairs. However, if the patient becomes incapacitated and has not named an agent, then it becomes complicated to obtain benefits, work with insurance companies, pay bills, perform bank transactions, manage real estate property, and many other matters that need to be done on the patient's behalf.

Does the patient want or need a will? Patients may express concerns about not having made estate plans. This is an appropriate time to ask if they have updated beneficiary status on all investments, life insurance, bank accounts, annuities, or retirement accounts. Taking care of these matters will reduce time, cost, and possible conflict for the survivors. It is critical to talk to the patient about these issues while the client has capacity. On occasion, it becomes too late to execute these important documents.

Income Maintenance

Individuals who are not able to work for 12 months or more should be encouraged to apply for permanent disability through the Social Security Administration (SSA). If the individual has a work history (i.e., has contributed to their Social Security through their employment), they will be eligible for Social Security Disability Insurance benefits. The patient or representative can apply online for disability benefits. The provider can assist with all necessary medical documents requested by SSA to expedite the process. If the patient's condition is severe (e.g., metastatic cancer), the applicant can ask that the application be expedited. There is a 6-month waiting period from the onset of the disability to when benefits will be issued. The amount of monthly benefit will be based on the work history. Therefore, the patient should be encouraged to apply for short-term disability (26 weeks) through their employer. Twenty-four months after SSA finds the person disabled, the individual will receive Medicare health insurance.

But if there is no work history and the individual has not contributed to Social Security through employment, the disabled person may receive Supplemental Security Income (SSI). This is a set amount of money that all SSI recipients receive in the United States. All SSI recipients are eligible for Medicaid health insurance.

For the patient whose income has been greatly reduced, the clinician may recommend that the patient apply for food, utility, and housing assistance. The Supplemental Nutritional Assistance Program (SNAP) is a federal program under the US Department of Agriculture and administered by the states. Previously known as food stamps, SNAP provides nutrition benefits to supplement the food budget of needy families so they can purchase healthy food. Utility shutoffs can be prevented by the clinician's intervention with the utility company, such as providing a letter of medical necessity. Thus, the clinician's documentation is critical to the patient receiving benefits. However, many clinicians feel unsure of how to fill out forms or do not recognize the importance of doing so. However, the patient may not obtain desperately needed benefits with these forms, such as monthly income or health insurance. The clinician should assess the timing: When does the form need to be returned? To complete the form, review the medical record. In general, the more inclusive the medical diagnoses, the more likely approval will be granted. It is not the clinician's role to make a disability determination; the agency will do that. The clinician's role is to provide objective, descriptive, medical evidence regarding the patient's condition and to link the diagnosis to the limitation in the comment section of the form. For example,

> *Diagnosis* → Asthma
> *Limitation* → Walks less than 3 blocks
> *Comment* → Patient suffers from shortness of breath due to asthma and as a result cannot walk more than 2 blocks

Family Maintenance

Child Care Benefits . Parents of minor children who become disabled due to illness may need assistance with child care. Parents may rely on other family members for support, but if the social history reveals a lack of such support systems, then a recommendation for child care benefits provided through local social services programs may be made. This benefit may pay for some or all of the child care costs, such as afterschool programs or day care.

Guardianships of Children. If the history of a seriously ill patient shows the patient is a single parent of a minor child, this must be explored further. Specifically, are there plans in place for the minor child in the event the parent becomes incapacitated or dies. The parent needs to identify a person who can become the guardian of the child. This is necessary for school-related interface, travel, benefits, and many other basic issues. Otherwise, the minor child could be placed into the foster care program. The most important task for the clinician is to identify the issue. Once identified, the clinician can begin to discuss this with the patient so the patient can begin to consider who to name as a proposed guardian of the child(ren). The next step is to then put that plan into a legal document. There are two ways to ensure that the patient's wishes are realized. The first and simplest is to document a "standby guardian." The patient can name a person to act as standby guardian in the event he or she is incapacitated. The signature of the patient is witnessed by two people. It comes into effect when the patient becomes incapacitated or dies. However, this is not a binding legal document and can be challenged. The other avenue to take is a petition to the court asking for a standby guardian to be named. This will be more complicated, and the patient will most likely need legal assistance, but once ordered, it is binding, and guardianship will reside with the person the patient has chosen to take care of the child(ren).

Adult Disabled Individuals. If the social history reveals that the patient is a parent of an adult disabled child, the clinician should address this immediately. Often, parents will take care of their developmentally child individually. However, once the parent is no longer able to take care of the adult child, plans need to be made for the disabled adult child's care. There may be resources in the patient's community specific to the child's need and child needs to begin to interface with these services. The child may no longer be able to remain in the family home once the parent is hospitalized or dies, so housing should be a primary consideration for the adult disabled child.

Spousal and Child Support. Complicating matters for the seriously ill patient is lack of financial support from a spouse or the parent of a child. Legal issues involving family matters are difficult because they often involve the family court system. Although family courts are designed to allow a person seeking support to act "pro se," meaning without an attorney, the process can be exhausting, frustrating, prolonged, and adversarial. The clinician should be aware of this. The other way the clinician can assist the patient is to provide documentation of treatment "interfering with a court date" when necessary.

Community Resources for Nonmedical Needs

The clinician should explore the community. There can be many resources that will assist the patient with nonmedical needs. The following is a brief list of community resources:

- Home care/hospice agency manager and staff members who visit the patients at home
- Director of a local family or elder services agency or the Area Agency on Aging
- Public interest law firms, law school clinics
- Legislative aides for the patient's elected officials, such as national and state congress persons
- An office for disabilities
- Others to consider: local library staff, post office staff, local bank staff, local food establishments or food banks

An important aspect of practice is to establish relationships with others in the community that provide the above services. Develop a list of community resources and make the connections *before* your patient has an urgent need for their services.

Communication: Advocacy Begins With Communication Skills

Physician assistants know that their patient's social problems are as important as their physical health problems but may not be confident in their ability to help patients with social challenges and barriers (see Box 25.1). Specifically, the clinician can ask, "Are there any financial or legal concerns you have that are affecting your ability to cope with your illness or affecting you or your family?" There is greater recognition that unmet social needs directly lead to worse health outcomes for all Americans—particularly in the current pandemic. Clinicians may not have adequate skills and practice competence to address social/financial/legal issues that impact the individual, the family, and the caregivers of a seriously ill patient.

Cultural Context of Serious Illness: Support Systems

Family Dynamics

Family members of patients receiving palliative care may be overwhelmed by the patient's illness. However, family involvement and support are both critical for optimal care for the patient. Failure to involve the family of the patient and respond to their perceptions and experience of the situation results in disjointed care.[6] The composition of families can vary from patient to patient. Physician assistants understand that the concept of family extends far beyond blood relatives. Family is defined by the patient and can include anyone the patient identifies as having involvement in their care.

Cultural Issues

Another important aspect of palliative care is ensuring that the patient is provided culturally appropriate care. Culture is a broad concept that includes factors such as ethnicity, age, gender, abilities/disabilities, sexual orientation, religion and spirituality, and socioeconomic status.[7] Understanding of one's own cultural identity and biases and being cognizant of the impact on how our biases shape the care we provide is extremely important. The physician assistant must first explore their own personal and professional biases. Once this is accomplished, then one can begin to become acquainted with common attitudes, norms, and beliefs of a given culture or group.[8] This process is not a finite task, and in order for the provider to provide quality, culturally appropriate care, continuous self-evaluation and education about different cultural groups and individuals must occur.

Faith-Based Support

The importance of spirituality and religion in the lives of our patients cannot be overstated. Balboni et al.[9] found that 68% of participants identified that religion and spiritual support were of great importance. In this study, religion and spirituality were found to be key factors for the participants, which assisted in guiding decision-making during illness and at the end of life.

Additionally, the 2018 National Consensus Project for Quality Palliative Care, *Clinical Practice Guidelines for Quality Palliative Care*, identified spiritual, religious, and existential aspects of care as an important domain. The guidelines recommended the regular assessment, reassessment, and documentation of spiritual concerns, as well as interventions to address issues that have been identified. All health-care providers are charged with being advocates for patients' religious and spiritual rituals, especially at the end of life.[10]

Furthermore, supportive relationships with the clergy are important to include in the spiritual assessment and provision of care for the patient. For example, the Joint Commission for the Accreditation of Healthcare Organizations' 2008 *Comprehensive Accreditation Manual for Hospitals* made specific references to the importance of religion and spirituality, stating that patients are entitled to care and services that protect their spiritual values.[11]

Spiritual care and physical well-being are connected.[9] The clergy is able to bridge the gap between the patient, family, and healthcare provider. The provider should be acquainted with the clergy in the healthcare setting to ensure that the patient is receiving a holistic approach to their care both in the hospital and on discharge into the community. In the hospice and hospital setting, chaplains are members of the core interdisciplinary palliative care team, consult on patients with spiritual concerns, and serve as liaison with the clergy in the community. Ideally, the palliative care team will involve the chaplain or other clergy in daily patient care rounds. Specific training for clergy in palliative care is not the topic of this chapter, but palliative care is rapidly evolving as a specialty for the faith-based community. When this occurs, and a patient is transitioned to any other setting, including home, better patient outcomes are noted, including increased longevity and quality of life.[12]

References

1. US Department of Health and Human Services, Office of Disease Prevention and Health Promotion, Healthy People 2020. Social determinants of health. 2019. https://www.healthypeople.gov/2020/topics-objectives/topic/social-determinants-of-health

2. Kaiser Family Foundation. The U.S. government and non-communicable disease. January 29, 2019. https://www.kff.org/global-health-policy/fact-sheet/the-u-s-government-and-global-non-communicable-diseases/

3. Center to Advance Palliative Care. About palliative care. https://www.capc.org/about/palliative-care/. Accessed November 17, 2019.

4. Hallarman L, Snow D. The medical-legal partnership: an alliance between doctors and lawyers in the care of patient-clients with advanced life-limiting illness. *New York State Bar Association Health Law Journal.* 2012;*17*(1):44–47.

5. Hallarman L, Snow D. The medical-legal partnership. *Journal of Palliative Care Medicine.* 2012;*15*(1):123–124.

6. Sudore RL, Casarett D, Smith D, Richardson DM, Ersek M. Family involvement at the end-of-life and receipt of quality care. *Journal of Pain and Symptom Management.* 2014;*48*(6):1108–1116.

7. Cain CL, Surbone A, Elk R, Kagawa-Singer M. Culture and palliative care: preferences, communication, meaning, and mutual decision making. *Journal of Pain and Symptom Management.* 2018;*55*(5):1408–1419. doi:10.1016/j.jpainsymman.2018.01.007

8. Patel B. Providing culturally appropriate palliative care. *Pharmacy Practice and Research.* 2014;*44*(3):78–79.

9. Balboni TA, Vanderwerker LC, Block SD, et al. Religiousness and spiritual support among advanced cancer patients and associations with end-of-life treatment preferences and quality of life. *Journal of Clinical Oncology.* 2007;*25*:555–560.

10. National Consensus Project for Quality Palliative Care. *Clinical Practice Guidelines for Quality Palliative Care.* 4th ed. Richmond, VA: National Coalition for Hospice and Palliative Care; 2018. https://www.nationalcoalitionhpc.org/ncp

11. Penn Medicine. *Comprehensive Accreditation Manual for Hospitals. The Official Handbook.* 2008. http://www.uphs.upenn.edu/pastoral/resed/jcahorefs.html

12. Puchalski CM, Vitillo R, Hull SK, Reller N. Improving the spiritual dimension of whole person care: reaching national and international consensus. *Journal of Palliative Medicine.* 2014;*17*(6):642–656.

26

Ethical and Legal Issues
Evaluation and Management

Bonnie K. Cole-Gifford and Kathlyn F. Wohlrabe

As stated in the "Guidelines for Ethical Conduct for the PA Profession,"[1] physician assistants (PAs) are expected to behave both legally and morally, knowing and understanding the laws and understanding the ethical responsibilities of their profession—understanding that "the law describes minimum standards of acceptable behavior, and ethical principles delineate the highest moral standards of behavior."[1] These two issues can overall and often be confusing. This chapter examines the case of Mr. S., an 80-year-old male who presents to the office complaining of back pain. His straightforward complaint and its treatment can have various legal and ethical implications that must be considered. The sections of this chapter discuss both evaluation and management of legal and ethical aspects of the profession, taking into consideration that the PA practice flows out of a relationship between the PA, the physician, and the patient.

Law and Ethics
What Is "the Law"?

"The law" is a system of rules that a society or government develops to deal with crime, business agreements, and social relationships. Laws are "laid down, ordained, or established." A law is a rule that orders or permits or forbids.[2] These rules are divided into criminal law and civil law, with civil law being further divided into contract law and tort law. There are consequences for breaking the law, and in the criminal case, the consequences are the loss of liberty and/or fines or restitution. The consequences for violating contract law and tort law lie in liability, which means a monetary compensation. Laws can also be divided into categories identifying their origins: common law, with its authority stemming from tradition and usage (the fundamental law of the United States, is derived from English common law);

constitutional law; statutory law (laws passed by a legislative body); administrative or regulatory law; and case law, which comes from court decisions. Legal issues are decided by juries or judges. In many instances, laws contain the word, or are governed by the words, *shall* or *must* or the opposite (*shall not, must not*).

Ethics

As opposed to laws, ethics are often governed by the words *ought, should, right, good,* and their opposites. Many times, in making a medical ethical decision, one must look at the specific problem and use values to decide the best course of action. This determination can be quite complex as well as confusing. Professional standards can be of some help; however, they cannot address every issue. This is apparent when trying to reconcile two conflicting values.

There are four basic values or principles that PAs can use to help decide ethical issues:

- Autonomy
- Justice
- Beneficence
- Nonmalfeasance

Autonomy asserts patients basically have the right to determine their own healthcare. Justice requires that benefits and burdens of care should be distributed across society. Beneficence requires that all medical providers do good for the patient. This is closely associated with the fourth, nonmalfeasance, which requires that one not harm the patient. In addition to these four principles, it is important to consider the values of truth, transparency, respect, people skills in presenting your decisions, and good listening skills.

The PA should be aware that ethics is traditionally seen as outlining the PA's responsibilities to clients and to society. Ethics also provides a standard of practice. Last, ethics protects the public and the profession. A PA should use these guideposts to direct their decisions and actions, especially if there is an ethical dilemma.

In the case of Mr. S., these four core ethical principles may come into play. Honoring Mr. S.'s autonomy would allow him to decide what diagnostic test or treatment approach he would or would not want to participate in. Justice would ensure he had access to appropriate treatment while working around any barriers to his care, such as ability to pay or transportation to an office. Beneficence and nonmalfeasance would be appropriate when determining the overall benefit of a diagnostic x-ray weighed against potential radiation exposure. Although basic, these values are woven into the treatment of Mr. S.'s presenting complaint.

Who Decides?

In a legal matter, the judge or jury is the decision-maker. In an ethical dilemma, there is no similar decision-maker. There may be an ethical committee in place in a hospital; however, these committees are not final authorities. They are educators and advisors. The ultimate arbiter of clinical medical ethics is the caregiver, the person who gives care to an individual who needs help taking care of himself or herself, working hand in hand with the patient.

The types of tasks that caregivers do may include[3]

- Help with daily tasks like bathing, eating, or taking medicine
- Doing housework and cooking
- Running errands such as shopping for food and clothes
- Driving the patient to appointments
- Providing company and emotional support
- Arranging activities and medical care
- Assistance with making health and financial decisions

Thus, the integrity of the caregiver is of vital importance. (Note: eligibility and standards of conduct of caregivers are governed by federal and state laws, which vary by state.) In Mr. S.'s case, perhaps he is accompanied to his visit by a caregiver. This brings out additional legal and ethical considerations, such as the appropriateness of the caregiver being in the room for the visit. Does the caregiver have decision-making authority? What should the caregiver know to best facilitate medical treatment?

Confidentiality

"Confidentiality is one of the core duties of medical practice."[4] Confidentiality usually refers to protection of information shared with attorneys, therapists, physicians, and other medical providers, including PAs, from being revealed to third parties without the consent of the patient/client. Privacy refers to the legal protection of personal medical information from being shared on a public platform. Privacy provides a legal protection of such information. The Health Insurance Portability and Accountability Act is a federal privacy rule of law that restricts personal health information from being disclosed as a public record.

Physician assistants, like other medical providers, should maintain confidentiality regarding their patients' identity, their medical complaints, and all treatment. This "code of confidentiality" should be relayed to the patient so that the patient will feel freer to divulge all information, including sensitive disclosures, to the PA. A patient, therefore, can trust the PA not to share personal information about his or her address, lifestyle, health, medical treatment, or any other "identifying" personal information. If this patient information were not protected by confidentiality, the relationship between the PA and the patient would be compromised.

The PA needs to understand that for possible "stigmatizing" conditions, such as reproductive, sexual, public health, and psychiatric health concerns, confidentiality assures the patient that such private information will not be disclosed to family or employers or any other entity or individual without the consent of the patient. The PA should take care that only authorized access of information occurs.

There are several cases where authorized access of information does occur:

- Concern for patient safety
- Legal requirement to report
- Suspected abuse or neglect
- Suspicion of criminal action

The first includes concern for the safety of other specified persons. The PA must weigh the mandate of confidentiality with the duty to protect identifiable individuals from serious, credible threat of harm. "The determining factor is whether there is good reason to believe specific individuals (or groups) are placed in serious danger depending on the medical information at hand."[4] The second exception is where legal requirements exist to report certain conditions or circumstances. With this exception, the state's interest in protecting public health outweighs the individual's interest in confidentiality. In the pandemic situation or in the context of any disaster, this is even more imperative to preserve the relationship of the PA, patient, and caregiver(s). The PA must look to the laws of the state in which he or she is practicing for a list of these conditions. Also, there are circumstances in which PAs (and other individuals) have a duty to report information they have obtained from their patients/clients. Those circumstances include cases of suspected child abuse and elderly abuse. In addition, medical providers in hospitals must report situations that could be a crime, such as gunshot or knife wounds. Local municipal code and institutional policies can vary regarding what is reportable. PAs, as well as other medical providers, should stay informed about individual state laws and local policies governing exceptions to patient confidentiality.[4]

In many states, adolescents can seek treatment for certain conditions without the permission of their parents. Some of these conditions are pregnancy, sexually transmitted disease, mental health issues, and substance abuse. PAs should be familiar with the laws of the state and locality in which they practice regarding these conditions.

In Mr. S.'s case, he may have previously authorized his caregiver to have access to his medical records, and the caregiver can be briefed on his condition while maintaining confidentiality. If he has not given access, you will need to protect his confidentiality by asking the caregiver to leave the room, if appropriate. Confidentiality is of utmost importance and is not always straightforward.

The Patient and the Medical Record

According to the "Guidelines for Ethical Conduct for the PA Profession," PAs have an obligation to keep information in the patient's medical record confidential.[1] In order for any information from this record to be released, the PA must have written consent of the patient or the patient's legal representative. Specific exceptions to this general rule may exist in the laws and regulations of the PA's individual jurisdiction. Some of these exceptions are workers' compensation, communicable disease, HIV, knife/gunshot wounds, abuse, neglect, and substance abuse. In addition, some issues fall under elevated requirements for confidentiality. This includes genetic testing results and mental health records. The PA should know how to access this information and be thoroughly familiar with these exceptions.

Perhaps in treating Mr. S.'s back pain you discover he has cancer, and he does not wish to inform his family. This information is part of his medical record and cannot be divulged without a release of information and consent to break confidentiality.

However, as of March 9, 2020, the federal government (the US Department of Health and Human Services [HHS]) finalized two rules that transformed this area in giving patients unprecedented access to their health information and data. "Putting patients in charge of their health records is a key piece of giving patients more control in healthcare, and patient control is at the center of the Trump administration's work toward a value-based healthcare system."[5] These rules require both public and private entities to share health information between patients and other parties while keeping the information private and secure. These rules are intended to put patients at the center of their own healthcare.

The guidelines also provide that both legally and ethically, the patient has certain rights to his or her own medical record. Although the chart is legally the property of the institution or agency, the information in the chart is the patient's property.[1] Again, the state law provides guidance in this arena, and the PA should know the laws relevant to this issue in his or her own jurisdiction. An area of concern is the increasing computerization of medical records. With this new technology and the consolidation of the healthcare system, patients have a valid heightened concern that their records remain confidential. Additionally, this new computerization of their medical records may make their access to their own records easier. The PA should be ready to help the patient navigate this access.

Mandatory Reporting

In most states, professionals that regularly deal with children and the elderly are listed as mandated reporters, which means they are under mandate of law to report abuse if they suspect such is taking place. To ascertain whether their profession is on the mandatory reporting list in the state in which they practice, PAs should consult the statutory laws of that state. In most states, such reports can be made anonymously. The laws also do not punish people for making such reports as long as the reports are made in good faith and not out of malice.

In some states there are no mandated reporter lists. Anyone who knows or suspects child or elder abuse is required by law to make a report. The federal HHS maintains a list of mandatory reporters by state, and PAs should check this list to determine whether they are on the list of mandatory reporters. It should be noted, however, that everyone is permitted to report child and elder abuse.

If the x-ray reveals Mr. S.'s back pain shows signs consistent with elder abuse, then a breach of confidentiality would be required in order to report the case to adult protective services. In this case, there is an additional responsibility for the provider—who may not want to reveal this to the caregiver if they are under suspicion of the abuse. Although the breach of confidentiality is warranted, it becomes a larger discussion: what to share, whom to share it with, and when to share it.

Informed Consent

Informed consent is the basis on which the ethical principle of autonomy in medical treatment is upheld. Informed consent is both an ethical and a legal obligation of the provider. This process allows patients to have choices in their evaluation and care plan. For medical procedures and treatment, informed consent has four components.[6] The first is ensuring the patient has the capacity or ability to make decisions for themselves. Refer to the section on capacity for more information regarding determining the capacity of a patient. The second is the disclosure of information, by the medical professional, regarding the risks and benefits of treatment, withholding treatment, and alternative options. A patient's decision-making must be informed by the provision of as much information as possible. The third component is the patient's comprehension of all information presented. The last component is the ability of the patient to consent to treatment without coercion or duress. This coercion can be from multiple sources, including family, friends, and medical professionals. Informed consent for treatment should be documented in the patient's medical record at the time of service.

Consent and Assent

Although related, consent and assent to medical treatment are different. Both are based on the ethical principle of autonomy and respect for people. Both are agreements, or objections, to undergoing certain medical treatment or procedures. However, consent can only be given by a person who has reached the legal age of consent, typically 18 years old in the United States, although this may differ based on individual state laws. Assent is the agreement of someone not able to give legal consent to participate.[7] Assent from a minor is an important consideration in their treatment. However, it is only a consideration. Ultimately, the legally binding consent from their parent/guardian is what informs and dictates medical decisions. Care should be taken when treating a child of divorced parents. It is necessary to ascertain which parent/parents have legal custody, which then grants the right to medical decision-making. Consult local family law in your area of practice to determine how to proceed in cases of dispute between parents with joint custody.

Conflict can occur when the legally binding consent conflicts with the assent, or lack thereof, from the child. In some cases, it may be a matter of a conversation with the child to help them understand the benefits and risks of a specific treatment. It may involve a conversation with the parent(s) to help them acknowledge their adolescent child, enhancing their sense of independence and autonomy. This may require a family meeting with child life specialists and other caregivers. In most cases, tension between parent and child can be resolved. However, there are cases where this may not be true, and consent from the parent may not be necessary to render treatment. In this case, the ethics committee and the legal system are involved with the conflict and become the final arbiters.

In Mr. S.'s case, there is an added feature that complicates the decision-making process: His daughter is his healthcare proxy. He may be capable of making decisions and can give both legal consent to treatment and assent to treatment procedures. However, he may *not* be able to consent to treatment. His daughter is his healthcare proxy and can consent, but he does not assent to it. Although the provider is protected on a legal basis, this case may warrant a family meeting with the ethics hospital committee. The goal is to honor the autonomy of the patient and arrive at the next best steps in his treatment.

Additional Exceptions

In most scenarios, parents are required to give consent for treatment of children and adolescents. However, in all 50 states, there is legislation that permits minors to seek treatment without parent's permission for health concerns such as sexually transmitted infections, substance use/abuse, and pregnancy or birth control.[8] Additionally, laws exist that cover areas of dispute in cases such as suspected child abuse when the parent may not have the child's best interest in giving or withholding consent for treatment. These laws vary from state to state, and it is important to be aware of the legislation in your practice area.

In general, consent must be given in every situation. However, much like any rule, there are exceptions. The first is when consent is understood. For example, taking a patient's blood pressure during a physical examination often does not require an explicit informed consent process explaining the benefits and risks of the test. This procedure can fall under the general informed consent of the office visit. Other procedures, especially ones that are invasive or exploratory, require a more explicit, often written, informed consent. Additionally, there are special cases and populations that require additional exceptions to the typical informed consent process.

There are situations that allow for an exception to the informed consent process for individuals who would otherwise be able to consent to treatment, for example, in an emergency situation where medical care is immediately necessary and waiting for informed consent could cause serious or irreversible harm.[8] Additionally, if a patient is incapacitated at the time of needing treatment, informed consent is not necessary to obtain. However, effort should be made to contact a designated decision-maker for this patient. If there is no specified decision-maker, states have unique laws to determine who is next in the hierarchy of decision-makers. If no one is able to be reached, the court can assign a legal guardian to make decisions on behalf of the patient.

Capacity

A person's capacity describes his or her ability to make a decision, specifically concerning choices in treatment options. This differs from competency, a legal term requiring a global assessment and legal determination made by a judge in court. In general, adults are considered to possess the capacity to make their own decisions unless determined otherwise.

Components of Capacity

There are four components to be considered when determining the capacity of a patient[9]:

- Communication
- Understanding
- Appreciation
- Reasoning

The patient must have the ability to communicate his or her decision regarding medical treatment. Additionally, the patient's communication must be stable enough over time in order to provide a course of treatment. This does not preclude a patient from modifying the decision. However, the patient should be able to communicate an explanation for the change. In regard to understanding, the patient not only must be able to understand the information presented to him or her, but also must be able to process the information in such a way as to be able to determine causal relationships between treatment and outcomes. Difficulties with memory, attention, and language comprehension can affect understanding and should be considered. Health literacy in general is culturally determined and is a responsibility of the healthcare provider(s) to address in the continuum of the patient's care. Appreciation of information involves the ability to discern how the information presented applies to them personally. Denial of an illness, either from lack of understanding or an emotional response, can influence a patient's appreciation of their illness and treatment. The patient's deep sense of spirituality and meaning can fundamentally shape their decision-making process. A patient must be able to reason or rationalize the information in order to weigh risks and benefits of whether to undergo or refuse a specific treatment.

During the appointment with Mr. S., it becomes apparent that he has an altered mental status, and this brings into question his capacity for medical decision-making. A first step would be to consult his medical record, if available, for any history of similar episodes and if an alternative decision-maker has been identified. However, it may also be possible that his mental status and therefore his capacity are not clearly impaired, and this would require further observation. In this case, capacity is a situational variable and can change over time. This is exemplified by cases of delirium where the patient's mental capacity is temporarily challenged until the causes of the condition are treated.[10] In the care of the palliative serious illness patient population, this can arise in multiple settings. The potential risk/benefit of the proposed treatment—even when it is a palliative modality—can also create greater distress and suffering.

Formally Measuring Capacity

The primary tool for measuring patient capacity is a clinical interview. This is assessed during the patient encounter and is often readily apparent. However, there are situations should prompt further, more formal, investigation.[11] The first is when a patient displays an abrupt change in mental status. Regardless of the underlying reason, capacity should be called into question, and it should be reestablished. The second scenario when capacity should be given further testing is when a patient refuses a recommended treatment and is unwilling or unable to discuss their rationale for that decision. It is important to note that a patient does not necessarily lack the capacity to make a decision when they make a choice against medical advice. Although these decisions can be frustrating for the provider, a person who has the capacity to make healthcare decisions has the right to refuse treatment. The third situation in which capacity should be carefully examined is when a patient consents to a risky or invasive treatment seemingly without careful consideration. The last scenario in which capacity should be questioned is when a patient has a known risk factor and/or history of impaired decision-making. This occurs with patients who have chronic intellectual and developmental disorders, neurological/psychological conditions, a significant cultural and/or language barrier, or a genuine concern about their health literacy, which is their educational level specifically regarding processing medical information. Further investigation is necessary in each of these instances.

If following the clinical interview the provider feels there is still inconclusive information gathered from direct questioning, there are more formal assessment tools available.

Common tools are the Aid to Capacity Evaluation and the Hopkins Competency Assessment Test.[9] Each test has its own use and limitations, and care should be taken when choosing a formal assessment tool. Whichever method is chosen, responses and findings should be documented in the patient's medical record. If uncertainty remains after using informal and formal assessment tools, it can be helpful to consult with another professional, such as a psychiatrist.

Conflicts of Interest

The *Journal of the American Medical Association* defines a conflict of interest as "a situation in which a person is or appears to be at risk of acting in a biased way because of personal interests."[12] This definition is not inherently negative and does not assume wrongdoing. It is important to note that being *at risk* of acting in a biased way is sufficient to be considered a conflict of interest. Additionally, merely the appearance of a conflict, even where there is none, can be problematic.

Often, financial conflicts of interest are most readily recalled; however, they are not the sole type of conflict. Conflicts may arise between professional duty and personal beliefs, managed care and patient care, research interests, professional reputation, teaching/education duties, organizational demands, professional affiliations or memberships, leadership or volunteer positions, even ties of the PA's immediate family. Each of these areas brings conflicts that must be managed in a way that upholds the PA's ethical and legal obligations.

One area that is providing increased opportunity for conflicts of interest is in managed care. PAs have reported managed care interfering with the ability to provide quality care for their patients,[13] specifically, perceiving influence to mislead insurers to aid patients in receiving care, including pressure to exaggerate the patient's condition. This conflict places the PA between providing appropriate and necessary care and being factual in reporting and not knowingly creating a financial burden for their patient. Each of these obligations is important, and this situation creates both a moral and legal quandary for the provider. Unfortunately, there is often not one right path forward in these instances, and legal and ethical principles must be used to make sound decisions while managing these conflicting interests.

It is important to note the existence of a conflict does not inherently signify a legal or ethical misstep. In fact, conflicts of interest can occur in a variety of situations without being considered illegal or unethical. For example, a PA has a duty to treat his or her patients and provide appropriate care. However, this PA also has an obligation to their personal life outside the clinic or practice. These two obligations may sometimes be concurrent with appointments scheduled outside clinic hours and thus appear to create a conflict of interest. In order to handle these situations appropriately, the conflicts need to be managed by the provider, which is the PA in this case. This conflict can be managed without compromising patient care or the PA's obligations.

The best tool to mitigate conflicts of interest is disclosure. An important detail to remember concerning conflicts of interest is even the appearance of a conflict can undermine trust in the practitioner and suggest impropriety when there is none. As a result, disclosure of areas where a potential conflict of interest may exist can help prevent future issues. Additionally, the American Academy of Physician Assistants (AAPA) Code of Ethics suggests declining gifts, trips, hospitality, or other items as a manner of preventing actual or perceived conflicts of interest.[1] Consultation with a peer or other professional can also be a helpful tool to determine best practice in decision-making to avoid conflicts of interest.

While the above is true in all general contexts of PA ethical practice, there are distinctions that require a more nuanced approach in the world of palliative care and hospice. For example, in the course of treatment of a dying patient, especially in the home-based setting, there is a deep and long-standing relationship that often involves a network of caregivers and others related to the patient. The PA is part of the palliative and hospice processes as well as one of those grieving when the patient has died. This is distinct from a typical conflict of interest situation and can include gifts, attendance at funerals, and other legacy events. By the same token, the PA needs to be aware of the context in which these events occur.

Competency-Impairment

In the Physician Assistant Code of Conduct developed by the AAPA, PAs are called to provide competent and empathetic healthcare in every patient encounter.[1] In addition, they are called to maintain and increase their knowledge and subsequent quality of the care provided. This is accomplished through hands-on experience, formal study and education, and lifelong learning. Continuing education requirements in the practice arena should be considered the minimum standard necessary to maintain competency. Additional education and specialty training are often essential as different situations present themselves throughout a career.

Physician assistant practice competencies were outlined by four national PA organizations between 2003 and 2004 and were updated in 2012.[14] Competent care has been measured as having five core dimensions:

- Application of medical knowledge
- Interpersonal and communication skills
- Patient care with professionalism
- Practice-based learning and improvement
- Systems-based practice

The AAPA has a sample competency assessment tool that can be used to evaluate the competency of a PA across each of these domains. It should be noted these competencies are not static or measured at only one point during the PA's career. The PA should continually learn and grow in competency throughout his or her practice. In a recent document (PAEA, 2019), the task force that reviewed these categories and aligned them with other groups such as American College of Critical Care Medicine (ACCM), said the Core Competencies for New Physician Assistant Graduates has a "distinct focus on health rather than on disease—a focus in which the needs of patients are considered above those of educators, students, or providers in determining the knowledge, skills, attitudes, and behaviors that new PA graduates need to demonstrate."

Competencies are a guideline from which to determine both competent and incompetent or inadequate care. There are clear situations when a PA should not practice due to impairment, such as being under the influence of drugs or alcohol. However, other situations may not be as apparent, for example, engaging in clinical practice after the death of a family member or another emotionally taxing event. Care should be taken to assess personal level of impairment, and it may be beneficial to consult a colleague to ensure quality of care does not suffer. In the case of the apparent impairment of another professional, PAs have a duty, according to their code of ethics, to protect patients by identifying those that are impaired. It is important not only to be able to recognize impairment in others but also to know the appropriate actions to take and procedures to follow to ensure proper care within the organization the PA is practicing.

In palliative and end-of-life care, PAs are particularly vulnerable not only to issues related to the specialty but also to the additional burden of maintaining their competency on the interdisciplinary team in which they are collaborating with multiple other professionals and caregivers. Burnout should be named and responded to in order to maintain and develop resilience and prevent situations in which the PA's competency is degraded or compromised. See Chapter 9, Caring for the Palliative Clinician.

Disclosure

Although potentially avoidable, medical errors are an unfortunate consequence of practicing medicine as a fallible human. Discovery of a medical error and its disclosure is layered for the PA. The Guidelines for Ethical Conduct for the PA Professions outlined by the AAPA state PAs should disclose discovered errors to their supervising physician.[1] Afterward, when it "is significant to the patient's interests and wellbeing," these errors should also be disclosed to the patient. However, when the discussion of goals of care takes into account the potential for disclosure of medical error, the PA needs to thoroughly review the situation with the team. This is essential to avoid additional distress and suffering on the part of the patient. This can potentially jeopardize not only the efficacy of the goals of care but also the trust inherent to the relationship between the patient, caregivers, and the palliative care team.

It should be noted that an advance directive alone may not be sufficient to halt all life-saving treatment. Do not resuscitate orders may be required. Do not forget that a patient, as long as possessing the capacity to do so, has the right to override decisions of a representative, change the terms in the living will or power of attorney, or revoke an advance directive.

Rationing of Care in Futile Treatments

Hippocrates counseled physicians not to treat patients who were "overmastered by their disease." Hence, the issue of medical treatment in futile situations is an ancient one for clinicians, and the issue of rationing medical care raises many fears and strong feelings about a number of issues. These issues include fears about unfair treatment, lack of patient autonomy, and costs. In the twenty-first century healthcare arena, natural disasters and pandemics spotlight the fundamental issues of ethnic, geographic, and cultural disparities, and this requires constant medical and public health evidence-based literature review as it relates to the care of all populations.

Most definitions of rationing medical treatment focus on the denial of a potentially beneficial treatment to a patient on the grounds of scarcity. Treatment setting may further determine decision-making such as clinical practice in a resource-poor area or within a specific demographic category. Denial of treatment can also focus on the age, condition, and evaluation of potential recovery of the patient. In other words, whether the "medicine offers certain benefit for an individual patient and . . . whether the potential benefit is large enough or likely enough to offer in order to justify the expense."

The individual PA, especially when working in end-of-life environments, will likely encounter these very issues in his or her practice. It is wise to know the thoughts and feelings of the team, the hospital, and the locality, as well as confronting individual biases and prejudices regarding this issue(s). It is ideal for the palliative care team to align with the patient and caregivers in all respects, and this is a primary purpose of the interdisciplinary team meeting, as well as family meetings with the team members.

References

1. American Academy of Physician Assistants. Guidelines for ethical conduct for the PA profession. 2013. https://www.aapa.org/wp-content/uploads/2017/02/16-EthicalConduct.pdf
2. Black HC, Garner BA. *Black's Law Dictionary*. 11th ed. St. Paul, MN: West Group; 2019.
3. Caregivers. MedlinePlus. Updated May 28, 2020. https://medlineplus.gov/caregivers.html. Accessed June 8, 2020.
4. De Bord J, Burke W, Dudzinski DM. Confidentiality. UW Medicine Department of Bioethics and Humanities. 2013. https://depts.washington.edu/bhdept/ethics-medicine/bioethics-topics/detail/58
5. Centers for Medicare and Medicaid Services. HHS finalizes historic rules to provide patients more control of their health data [Press release]. Centers for Medicare and Medicaid Services. March 9, 2020. https://www.cms.gov/newsroom/press-releases/hhs-finalizes-historic-rules-provide-patients-more-control-their-health-data. Accessed June 8, 2020.
6. Van Staden CW, Krüger C. Incapacity to give informed consent owing to mental disorder. (2003). Consent and Assent. https://jme.bmj.com/content/medethics/29/1/41.full.pdf. Accessed July 31, 2019.
7. University of Alaska Fairbanks: Institutional Review Board. Consent and assent. https://www.uaf.edu/irb/faqs/consent-and-assent/. Accessed 2019.
8. Gossman W, Thornton I, Hipskind JE. Informed consent. Updated July 10, 2019. StatPearls. Treasure Island, FL: StatPearls; January 2019. https://www.ncbi.nlm.nih.gov/books/NBK430827/
9. Barstow C, Shahan B, Roberts M. Evaluating medical decision-making capacity in practice. *American Family Physician*. 2018;98(1):40–46.
10. Lim T, Marin DB. The assessment of decisional capacity. *Neurology Clinics*. 2011;29:115–126. https://www.neurologic.theclinics.com/article/S0733-8619(10)00128-3/pdf
11. Tunzi M. Can the patient decide? Evaluating patient capacity in practice. *American Family Physician*. 2001;64(2):299–308.
12. Muth C. Conflict of interest in medicine. *JAMA*. 2017;317(17):1812. doi:10.1001/jama.2017.4044
13. Ulrich C, Danis M, Ratcliffe S, et al. Ethical conflict in nurse practitioners and physician assistants in managed care. *Nursing Research*. 2006;55(6):391–401.
14. American Academy of Physician Assistants. Competencies for the physician assistant profession. 2012. https://www.aapa.org/wp-content/uploads/2017/02/PA-Competencies-updated.pdf

Index

For the benefit of digital users, indexed terms that span two pages (e.g., 52–53) may, on occasion, appear on only one of those pages.

Tables, figures, and boxes are indicated by an italic *t*, *f*, and *b* following the page number.